DONALDSONS' ESSENTIAL PUBLIC HEALTH
Third Edition

LIAM J DONALDSON

and

GABRIEL SCALLY

Radcliffe Publishing
Oxford • New York

Radcliffe Publishing Ltd
18 Marcham Road
Abingdon
Oxon OX14 1AA
United Kingdom

www.radcliffe-oxford.com
Electronic catalogue and worldwide online ordering facility.

First Edition 1993 (published by Kluwer Academic Publishers)
Second Edition 2000 (published by LibraPharm Ltd)
Second Edition revised 2003

British Library Cataloguing in Publication Data

A catalogue record for this book is available from the British Library.

ISBN-13: 978 184619 209 8

Typeset by Pindar NZ, Auckland, New Zealand
Printed and bound by TJ International, Padstow, Cornwall, UK

DONALDSONS' ESSENTIAL PUBLIC HEALTH

Third Edition

Contents

Preface

This is the first new publication of the book without its co-author Raymond 'Paddy' Donaldson, a towering figure in post-war British public health, who died recently in his mid-eighties. He is greatly missed.

The book has been in continuous print for 25 years, first as *Essential Community Medicine*, then as *Essential Public Health Medicine*, latterly as *Essential Public Health*. Its longevity is an indication of just how important public health is to our society.

For this third edition, my co-author is Dr Gabriel Scally. Gabriel knew my father well. From this vantage point, and bringing his depth of knowledge and experience of public health, he was ideally placed to respect the origins and traditions of the book as well as helping with a new edition.

As always, the text aims to bring together, in one volume, the principles and applications of epidemiology, the main health problems experienced by populations and by the main groups within them, the strategies for intervention to promote health and prevent disease, the main themes underlying health policy formulation and a description of the provision of health services.

The fact that *Essential Public Health* has become a standard text in so many institutions of learning and training, as well as the large and very positive response we have had from students and practitioners in a variety of disciplines, emboldens me to claim that we largely fulfil these aims. Students, both undergraduate and postgraduate, in a number of disciplines, have even written that they were successful in examinations through reading the book and receiving no other teaching. As an experienced teacher, I would neither encourage nor condone such an approach. Nevertheless, I am pleased that the book provided the breadth and depth of knowledge required.

For this third edition, each chapter has been revised. Many new themes have been introduced. Many new subjects dealt with in the previous edition have been brought up-to-date. We have also introduced new material of direct practical relevance.

Chapter 1 of *Essential Public Health* describes the ways in which an assessment can be made of the health and health needs of a population. The main sources of information on health and health services are reviewed, with examples of their uses. The common measures of morbidity and mortality are described together with illustrations about how they are used to describe health problems in populations. Throughout this first chapter, we have placed special emphasis on providing simple descriptions and definitions of the concepts involved and on explaining the origins of the common types of routinely available and specially collected data.

Chapter 2 draws together the main approaches of public health investigation, starting with the ways in which descriptive epidemiological data can be used to examine the frequency of diseases within and between populations and over time. The main study methods of epidemiology – cross-sectional or prevalence studies, cohort studies, case-control studies and randomised controlled trials – are described. Emphasis is placed not just on the conceptual bases of these important methods of investigation but also on their strengths and weaknesses and their applicability in particular situations. The final section of Chapter 2 gives examples of practical investigations in public health, most from my own public health practice. I draw attention to the reality of carrying out such investigations, as well as how to interpret and act upon the findings which emerge from them. The field of study is sometimes referred to as 'quick and dirty' investigation. I do not subscribe to this philosophy, and my emphasis is on the need for rigour even when a pragmatic approach is necessary in deciding the scope and urgency of a study.

Chapter 3 discusses the concept of health. The main strategies in health promotion are described in this chapter, along with the main health problems amenable to intervention. There are strengthened sections on drug and alcohol abuse, obesity, and public health policy. The previous sections on coronary heart disease, stroke, accidents and pre-symptomatic screening have been expanded and brought up-to-date.

Special emphasis is given in Chapter 3 to the promotion of health in the younger age groups, where the foundations of healthy living can be laid. Many young people become involved in different types of risk-taking behaviour during their teenage years. In the case of smoking, drinking and drug or solvent misuse, such behaviour

has considerable impact on both current and future health. Unhealthy patterns of behaviour can be developed in younger years that are carried through into maturity and adulthood. Not only must young people be informed and educated, they must be encouraged and helped to adopt an approach to life that will safeguard their health in the years ahead. Chapter 3 discusses these issues and the challenges of, and strategies for, achieving behaviour change in all age groups, particularly young people. Chapter 3 also discusses inequalities in health and the powerful underlying influence of social and economic determinants on health.

In the first three chapters, many of the scientific foundations of public health are laid down. Throughout, the reader is made aware of: the strengths and limitations of data, how data are turned into information, the challenges of changing human behaviour and the need to design programmes to promote health and prevent disease.

The modern welfare state is a large and complex structure with diverse origins and traditions. In each decade it has undergone major reform. The period since the last edition of the book has been no exception. Chapter 4 brings together in one place a description of the present structure, organisational framework and method of functioning of the National Health Service (NHS). Individual sections deal with quality in health care, including a description of clinical governance and the structure and processes that support it. The emerging discipline of patient safety is also discussed. The sections on the management and design of the health care system have also been expanded substantially to include topics such as commissioning, regulation of health care providers and professions, and the rules and incentives that drive the internal market in the NHS. The implications of the NHS Next Stage Review are also part of this chapter.

Early life is the time when the foundations of health are laid and when some of the risks are greatest. Chapter 6 deals with the health of mothers and children. The main epidemiological features of health and disease in infancy and childhood are described, as are the risks to foetal and maternal health. The main measures of fertility in a population are described, along with the main trends in fertility over time and the factors that can influence it in a population. The causes of death at different periods of infancy are discussed, and the various mortality rates in early life are defined. The range of approaches to promote health in pregnancy and childhood are described, as are the maternity and child health services themselves.

Increasingly, more and more people in many countries of the world are living into late old age. They will have needs that must be met not just by those services that diagnose and treat illness but also by those that enhance capacity for independent living and provide appropriate support where this is not possible. There are other groups within the population with special needs: adults and children with physical disability, people with mental health problems and those with learning disability. All these groups need services that are broad-based and delivered by a wide range of agencies within the community working towards a common purpose. They also need services that are based upon a clear assessment of their needs. This means being familiar with all relevant sources of data and the ways in which they can be used to describe the needs of a group within the population. Chapter 5 (Physical Disability), Chapter 7 (Mental Health and Learning Disability) and Chapter 8 (Health in Later Life) are concerned with these groups. In these chapters, greater emphasis has been placed on defining needs, as well as on describing the framework of health and social care provision required. The development of care in the community and the need for coordination of the work of different care agencies and the professional staff working within them is particularly emphasised. The importance of taking account of, and meeting, the needs of family members and other informal carers is also stressed.

Chapter 9 deals with infectious diseases. We have retained the approach used in the previous edition, that of describing individual diseases, but we have also introduced a new classification of these important health problems. Particular emphasis is given to the so-called 'new and emerging diseases' like SARS, vCJD, resurgent tuberculosis and antimicrobial resistance. A completely new section on the threat of pandemic influenza is also included. There is also a new section on health care-associated infection, particularly MRSA and *Clostridium difficile*. The practical approaches to the surveillance of infectious diseases are also covered, especially the handling of outbreaks and untoward incidents. Since the last edition, a number of important organisations have come into being, notably the Health Protection Agency and the Food

Standards Agency. The role and functions of each is described, as is a new European agency for communicable disease control. The International Health Regulations came into force in 2008 and were incorporated into new public health legislation in this country. These developments are covered in this chapter.

The importance of the relationship between the quality of the environment and people's health has long been recognised. Moreover, there have been a number of major incidents around the world that have all too dramatically highlighted some of the contemporary threats and hazards, both to the well-being of individuals and to the planet itself. There is still an enormous amount to be learned about the influence of the environment on health. The growth in interest and rapidly rising concerns about wider climate change highlights many clear and direct links with health. In Chapter 10, we describe the impact of the environment on health, as well as strategies for promoting health through the adoption of the principles of sustainable development, and we discuss risk and its communication.

In introducing the third edition of *Essential Public Health* to readers both old and new, we believe we have built upon the successful formula of its predecessor. However, looking at it afresh, revising and introducing much new material, we have been able to encompass the entire scope of modern public health, as well as describing and discussing the range of services required to provide a comprehensive system of care. We look forward to continuing to receive the views of readers in providing the kinds of constructive comments so valuable in the past.

We would like to acknowledge our special thanks to a large number of colleagues who have so generously provided their specialist expertise in commenting on the book. We have not named them all here, but our gratitude to them is deep nonetheless. We would like to thank in particular: Louis Appleby, Richard Caves, Sandy Clarke, Kevin Cleary, Gerald Dziekan, Emma Gordon, Muir Gray, Sheila Hollins, Rachel Jenkins, Richard Lilford, Graham MacGregor, Jon Moore, Ian Philp, June Raine, Chris Shaw, Julie Storr, Sian Thomas, Andrew Wadge and Kent Woods. In addition, Liam Donaldson would like to thank his colleagues in the Department of Health for the accuracy checks and suggestions they made to the final drafts of the chapters, in particular Scott Binyon, Sarah Connelly, Brian Duerden, Felix Greaves, Rowena Jecock, Linda Johnson-Laird, Bill Kirkup, Dorian Kennedy, Mary Mulvey, Douglas Noble, Karen Noakes, Mark Noterman, Kay Orton, Gerry Robb, Meredith Vivian, Ailsa Wight and Patience Wilson. Fiona Mackichan assisted with the figures and tables on several chapters. We owe a deep debt of gratitude to Lee Morris. Any omissions or errors of fact and interpretation are our own. Any opinions expressed are our own and not those of any body we represent or may have represented in the past.

Liam J Donaldson
January 2009

About the Authors

Sir Liam Donaldson has been the Chief Medical Officer for England and the United Kingdom's Chief Medical Adviser since 1998. He is only the fifteenth person to hold this important and historic post since it was established in 1855.

Since coming into the post, Sir Liam has authored a series of groundbreaking reports aimed at transforming a wide range of areas of health, health care and medical science, for example: producing the country's first comprehensive health protection strategy; proposing new legislation to allow carefully regulated stem cell research; addressing poor clinical performance; introducing a comprehensive programme for patient safety; and empowering patient self-management of chronic disease.

Sir Liam is probably best known for three of his achievements. The first is his trailblazing annual reports, which have brought major health concerns to public attention, in particular the need for smoke-free public places, the obesity 'time bomb' and the problems of binge drinking. The second is his creation of the concept of clinical governance – a clinically led way to assure high standards of care – which is now an internationally recognised approach in health care. The third is his leadership of patient safety as a priority for health care systems around the world. His report *An Organisation with a Memory* shaped policy on patient safety in the United Kingdom, and his chairmanship of the World Health Organization's World Alliance for Patient Safety has moved action to a global scale.

He has worked in all sectors of health care, having held posts in hospitals, general practice, universities, health service management and government. He currently holds honorary chairs in the universities of Leicester and Newcastle upon Tyne.

Sir Liam has received honours and awards from many public bodies. His published writing and research on health and health care subjects is very extensive. He has given many keynote addresses at conferences. He is an experienced broadcaster and public communicator.

Gabriel Scally has been a Regional Director of Public Health in England since 1993 and works for both the Department of Health in England and the South West Strategic Health Authority. The South West is the largest region in England and has a population of more than five million people.

Gabriel studied medicine in Belfast, and prior to moving to England he was Chief Administrative Medical Officer and Director of Public Health of the Eastern Health and Social Services Board in Northern Ireland.

The range of professional activities that he has undertaken covers the full span of public health practice, from championing the provision of sexual health services for young people to campaigning for sustainable development and dealing with serious clinical failures in hospitals.

In addition to his Department of Health and NHS posts, Gabriel is a visiting professor in the University of the West of England in both the School of Health and Social Care and the School of the Built and Natural Environment.

For the enhancement of personal psychological well-being, Gabriel also takes every opportunity to enthusiastically support the London Irish Rugby Football team.

List of Tables and Figures

TABLES

FIGURES

Acknowledgements

We are grateful to individual publishers, institutions, editors, authors and organisations for permission to reproduce material in figures or tables. In most cases we have been able to cite the source as a footnote to the presentation. We take the opportunity here to give the fuller acknowledgement requested by some copyright holders.

We have tried very hard to be thorough in this process, but in the flurry of activity associated with bringing a major text to publication we may have made oversights. If so, we would be very pleased to acknowledge any missing attributions in future printings.

We acknowledge and are grateful to a number of agencies that provide population health statistics for the use of official data in tables or graphs. Specifically, we wish to thank the Office for National Statistics in the United Kingdom, the World Health Organization and the United Nations.

The Office for National Statistics prepared some special analyses for which we are particularly grateful. Two other agencies in the United Kingdom provided key statistics: the Health Protection Agency and the Food Standards Agency. Our gratitude also goes to them.

We acknowledge further with **kind permission** the following, in relation to individual presentations:

American Journal of Epidemiology: Figure 9.3.

British Journal of Cancer: Figure 9.14.

British Medical Journal: Figures 1.3, 2.3, 4.11, 4.12; Tables 2.15, 2.16, 2.17, 4.3, 4.8, 8.9.

Canadian Journal of Ophthalmology: Figure 2.2.

Canadian Medical Association Journal: Table 4.10.

Carnegie United Kingdom Trust: Table 8.1.

Crown Copyright (ONS): Figures 7.5, 7.6, 7.7, 7.8 reproduced under the terms of the Click-Use Licence.

Diabetes Research and Clinical Practice: Figure 2.5.

Epidemiologic Reviews: Table 7.6.

Hayward Medical Communications: Figure 1.8.

Healthcare Computing & Communications Canada Inc.: Figure 1.9.

Health Trends: Table 1.6.

Hospital Medicine: Tables 2.1 and 2.11.

Joseph Rowntree Foundation 8.12 (from *Monitoring poverty and social exclusion 2007*. Guy Palmer, Peter Kenway and Tom MacInnes. Joseph Rowntree Foundation.

Journal of Epidemiology and Community Health (BMJ Publishing Group Ltd): Figures 2.12, 2.13, 2.17; Tables 2.20 and 2.21.

King's Fund Publishing: Tables 3.6 and 10.5.

Lancet: Figures 2.4, 7.1, 9.10, 9.18.

McMillan Press Ltd and Professor Klim McPherson: Table 2.4.

Organisation for Economic Co-operation and Development (OECD): Figure 4.15.

Oxford University Press: Figures 2.1, 3.23; Tables 2.27, 7.7.

Parliamentary Office of Science and Technology: Table 1.1.

Professor Adrian Davis: Figure 5.5.

Professor James Reason: Figure 4.14.

Professor David Sackett: Table 4.7.

Royal Society of Medicine: Figure 8.10.

Royal College of Psychiatrists: Tables 2.25, 2.26, 2.27.

Sainsbury Centre for Mental Health: Figures 7.2, 7.9, 7.13; Table 7.11.

UNAIDS: Figure 9.7.

Wellcome Institute Library for supplying historical pictures in Chapters 3, 7 and for the cover.

CHAPTER 1
Assessing the Health of the Population

INTRODUCTION

One of the great strengths of the National Health Service (NHS) in the United Kingdom, and one which has endured since its inception in 1948, is the concept of responsibility for the health of geographically defined populations, not just the patients who actively seek help from the service.

This is in contrast to the health care systems of some other countries, where the population for which health care is provided is not so readily defined or where it comprises, for example, those subscribing to a health insurance plan. In Britain a framework of service provision helps to ensure that a comprehensive range of care, based in primary care, in hospital and in the community, is made available to local populations on the basis of their health needs.

The assessment of a population's health needs is not, however, a straightforward process. Health is not easily defined, other than in broad terms such as the definition used in the preamble to the constitution of the World Health Organization (Box 1.1), and it certainly cannot be measured with precision. Instead, wide-ranging data sources are available, some used as proxies, to illustrate, with appropriate analysis, different aspects of the health of a population living in a particular place: its size and composition; the people's lifestyles; the illnesses and diseases that are experienced; and those of its number who are born or who die. By piecing together information from different sources, of different types and to which different levels of importance are attached, it is possible to begin to develop an understanding of the health of a population.

This first chapter describes the main ways of obtaining data that can contribute to the assessment of a population's health. In looking at all of the sources of data relevant to population health and health care, it is useful to consider three distinct groups. Firstly, there are data which describe populations. Without knowledge of the numbers and characteristics of people at risk of ill health or death, it is impossible to make sense of morbidity or mortality data. Secondly, there are what may be termed health event data, triggered by occurrences related to an individual's health that are then recorded. The starkest of these is death certification, which provides relatively accurate and complete information on the last illness of all individuals but says little about previous health. This category also includes the recording of contact with the hospital services and with primary care. The third group comprises a variety of population-based health information, including lifestyle factors and other aspects of health status. In theory, this is often what is desirable in order

---

BOX 1.1

'Health is a state of complete physical, mental and social well-being and not merely the absence of disease or infirmity.'

— Preamble to the Constitution of the World Health Organization, as adopted by the International Health Conference, New York, 19 June to 22 July 1946; signed on 22 July 1946 by the representatives of 61 states and entered into force on 7 April 1948.

to study population health, but in practice the data tend to be patchy, incomplete and irregularly available.

All sources of health data, to a varying degree, are subject to quantitative and qualitative deficiencies that limit the conclusions which can be drawn from them. These drawbacks are best appreciated by being familiar with the way in which the data are gathered.

POPULATION DESCRIPTION

Fundamental to any examination of population is a periodic count of all the people and households in a given area. This is known as a population census.

THE CENSUS

A census has been carried out every 10 years in Great Britain since 1801, except in 1941 during World War II. The first census asked five questions and counted 10 million people living in two million households. The 2001 census asked 40 questions and counted 60 million people living in approximately 24 million households. Authority for the census is enshrined in an act of parliament, the 1920 Census Act. Before each census there is extensive public consultation on conduct and content and a programme of field testing.

The law requires that all people alive on the night of the census are enumerated, traditionally in the household or establishment where they spent that night. A household is defined as one person living alone or a group of people, not necessarily related, living at the same address, with common housekeeping – sharing at least one meal a day or a living room, temporary residents being included.

Up to and including 2001, England and Wales were divided into some 117 000 enumeration districts for the purpose of administering the census. These were the smallest areas for which results could be provided. Enumeration districts are now used solely for administration of the census and have been superseded by Output Areas (OA) for the purpose of analysing and presenting census data. Output Areas were introduced at the 1981 census in Scotland and the 2001 census in England, Wales and Northern Ireland. There are 175 000 of them in England and Wales, and on average each comprises 125 households and approximately 300 residents. In order to preserve confidentiality, all Output Areas are above a threshold of 100 residents and 40 households. Their boundaries were set to create areas as compact and homogeneous as possible. Due to their smaller average size, they can provide finer-grained data output.

Until the 2001 census, electoral wards were used as the main analytical building block. The problem with wards was that they varied substantially in size across the country and were subject to change as electoral boundaries were reviewed. Super Output Areas (SOA) have now been introduced to provide more consistency of size and over time. In England and Wales, up to three different layers of Super Output Areas have been created to provide different scales of aggregation. In Scotland, Output Areas have been combined to create 6505 Data Zones, which can then be further aggregated to a higher level.

In the 2001 census, data were collected using three separate forms. A census form was provided to each household in England and Wales (with a bilingual form used in Wales). In addition, individual forms were available to people who were not in a traditional household but resided in some form of communal establishment such as a nursing home. A third form was used to collect information about the communal establishment itself. The household form had 10 questions relating to the household, and it collected information including postcode, type of building, number of rooms, tenure, the presence of certain amenities (bath, shower, toilet, central heating) and the number of cars or vans. The person completing the household form then had to list the names of people in the household and their relationship to other members of the household (for example, wife, daughter). Up to 35 questions were then asked about each individual member of the household. The information gathered included: sex; date of birth; marital status; address one year previously; country of birth; ethnic group; the presence of long-term illness, health problem or handicap which limits daily activities; whether working and details of occupation and employment; higher education; the address of students and school children; and usual means of travel to work. In Scotland, Wales and Northern Ireland, questions were asked about people's ability to speak, read or write Scottish Gaelic, Welsh and Irish.

The census in England and Wales is planned and carried out by the Office for National Statistics (ONS). It collates and processes all of the census data under conditions of strict confidentiality. The General Register Office for Scotland and the Northern Ireland Statistics and Research Agency carry out similar functions for their respective countries. Names are not entered into computers for processing but used only for internal checking of completeness and accuracy of forms. In analysis, great care is taken not to differentiate very small communities in which an individual person might be identified.

Completeness of a census is important if the data are to be reliable. The response rate is an important component of this. In 2001 the response rate was 94%, compared with 96% for the 1991 census. The response rate varied with age and sex, with the lowest response rates in 2001 being amongst men and women aged 20 to 24 years (Figure 1.1). The rate also varied geographically. For example, it was 78% in Inner London, 10 percentage points lower than in 1991. In contrast, 17 local authority areas had response rates of over 99%.

A number of methods are used to improve the completeness. In 2001 a new approach was taken using a sample re-enumeration. For the first time this enabled the publication of results that represented 100% of the population.

Publication of census results takes a number of forms and includes output in print, CD, DVD, and on the web. The results are usually made available in tabular form, and there are three main standard sets produced: Key Statistics, Standard Tables and Census Area Statistics. Non-standard customised statistics can be specially commissioned from the ONS. A fee may be charged for this service.

Ethnic Minority Populations

The provision of appropriate and effective access to health services for those from ethnic minorities is an important public health concern (Table 1.1). According to the former Commission for Racial Equality (now replaced by the Commission for Equality and Human Rights), anyone who would tick a box other than 'White British' in response to an ethnicity question on a census form can be said to belong to an ethnic minority. On this basis, 12.5% of the population were from ethnic minorities in the 2001 census, but on a more limited definition used in analysis of census data, 4.6 million people (or 7.9% of the population) belong to ethnic minorities. The largest minority group was Indians, followed by Pakistanis, those of mixed ethnic backgrounds, Black Caribbeans, Black Africans and Bangladeshis. In Britain the ethnic minority population

had grown by 53% between the 1991 and 2001 censuses. This analysis did not include other recognised ethnic minority groups such as the Irish, who counted for 0.7 million people in 2001.

The ethnic minority population is very unevenly distributed within Britain, with a high concentration in London, where, according to the 2001 census, the 'White' population made up 71% of the population. In contrast, the 'White' component of the population of the South West region was 98%.

Generally, the age structure of ethnic minority populations is younger than the indigenous population due to a mixture of immigration patterns and fertility. Among the distinct ethnic groups, the Bangladeshi community has the highest proportion of people under the age of 16 years (38%). This is double the proportion of under-

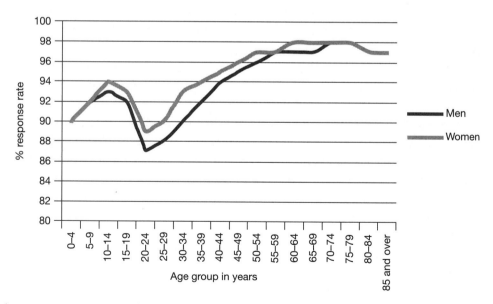

Figure 1.1 Response rate by age group in 2001 census
Source: Office for National Statistics.

Table 1.1 Issues relating to health and the provision of services for ethnic groups

- Physical barriers such as area deprivation
- Socio-economic status
- Discrimination
- Poor delivery of health care
- Cultural/lifestyle differences
- Biological susceptibility

Source: Parliamentary Office of Science and Technology. Postnote no. 276. July 2007. Parliamentary copyright.

16s in the 'White' community (19%). As the population ages amongst some of the longest-standing ethnic minority groups in Britain, the special problems of their elder members will pose challenges for services in the future.

BIRTH AND DEATH REGISTRATION

Populations do not remain constant. Over time, individuals die and new ones are born, and it is important to track both processes to understand how populations are changing. This is primarily done through the registration of births and deaths and through the periodic censuses.

In Britain and most developed countries, the registration of births and deaths is a legal requirement placed on an individual known as the qualified informant – usually the nearest available relative. In England and Wales the process is organised by the General Register Office, which is part of the ONS, through a network of local registration districts and sub-districts throughout the country, administered by superintendent registrars and registrars of births and deaths.

Traditionally, the certificate of cause of death, issued by a doctor or coroner, is used by the registrar to register the death along with information from the informant. He or she then gives the informant a certified copy of the death register entry ('death certificate'), which is used for a variety of legal and administrative purposes. This system came under scrutiny in the course of the Public Inquiry into the activities of Harold Shipman, the general practitioner who murdered large numbers of his patients. Weaknesses were identified in the third report of the Inquiry, published in 2003, which dealt with death certification. These criticisms dealt with the absence of independent medical scrutiny in the process in general and the need for a system for routine analysis of the information on death certificates.

POPULATION ESTIMATES AND PROJECTIONS

While the population census takes place every 10 years, it is necessary to produce statements of population size and characteristics for periods between census points.

Such statements are produced annually and are called population estimates. Population estimates are derived by taking the census as a baseline, adding births, subtracting deaths and making an allowance for migration. Since registration of births and deaths is required by law, these components of estimation are reasonably sound. The weakness is the allowance made for migration. Information on external migration (that is, in and out of Britain) is reasonably accurate, but an understanding of internal migration has to be based on an accumulation of local knowledge, including factors such as new housing development, clearance of old housing estates and the mass movement of population to other areas.

Population estimates become less reliable as proximity to a census year recedes but for most uses are adequate.

While population estimates assess populations between census points, population projections attempt to predict the characteristics and size of populations in the future. They make assumptions about fertility, mortality and migration. Population projections can be accurate in the short term. For example, a projection of the number of people aged 65–74 years in 20 years' time will be quite accurate, as the number of people now aged 45–54 years is known, as is the expected mortality of this age group. On the other hand, a projection of the number of school children in 30 years' time will be less accurate because current fertility experience may not be maintained for the next 15 to 25 years. Fresh population projections are produced by the Government Actuary's Department every two years. As well as a 'principal' projection, a series of six 'variants'

are published using alternative assumptions of low or high levels of mortality and fertility.

POPULATION LOCATION

Classification of the population by place of residence is important in health care for both epidemiological and health service planning purposes. For example, mapping people with a particular disease permits exploration of that disease's relationship with specific geographical features, or it can allow calculation of disease rates for specific communities. The precision of geographical location needed will depend on the particular analysis being performed. It makes sense, therefore, to use a building block from which appropriately sized 'patches' can be assembled. An ideal measure would be the map-grid reference for each person's home, but this is not collected routinely.

Postcodes

One of the most common tools for examining data is the postcode. The first experiment with postcodes took place in Norwich in 1959. The current postcode is based on an eight-character designation that always includes one or two central 'blanks' – for example, NE30 4ET. In this example, 'NE' denotes the postcode area, of which there are 124 in the country. The '30' represents a postcode district (of which there are just over 2900) and the '4' represents the postcode sector within a district. Finally, the 'ET' identifies a small geographical area (commonly about 15 postal delivery points in residential areas) within a sector, which is known as the unit postcode. There were a total of 1 764 875 separate postcodes in the United Kingdom in 2007.

There are problems with the use of post-codes. For example, not all people know or remember them accurately, and, inevitably, there are delays in the issuing of new postcodes to cover housing development. In a partnership between the Royal Mail, the ONS and the Department of Health, postcodes are made available to the NHS, updated regularly, and are becoming increasingly reliable in their translation to other area-based classifications.

All birth and death data and most patient-based service data are now postcoded. This fact and the availability of computer programs to assign postcoded data to local authorities or areas covered by health bodies (through direct links provided by postcode look-up files or through a postcode's grid reference and the use of digital boundaries) means that postcodes are a very powerful tool for geographical analysis of health data, although the data is often presented in relation to Super Output Areas (Figure 1.2).

Deprivation Measures

Exploration of health differences between population groups whose social and economic circumstances differ may be based on classifications derived from occupation, such as social class or other socio-economic groupings (see Chapter 2). However, these classifications have come under increasing criticism from social scientists as reflecting too rigidly a particular hierarchical view of society that has become outmoded in other contexts. Increasingly, inequalities in health (see Chapter 3) are examined through analyses based on measures of material and social deprivation that are unrelated to occupation. A variety of indicators of the deprivation status of populations have been proposed, generally based on variables recorded in population censuses. They differ according to the nature of the concept of deprivation that underlies them (for example, encompassing wealth, income, social isolation, environment) and according to which factors are selected to differentiate groups on this basis (such as employment status, overcrowding or car ownership). Because these factors are generally restricted to census variables and because the underlying concepts of deprivation are often quite complex (and sometimes not made explicit), it must be remembered that all of the various indices and scores are more or less indirect indicators rather than direct measures.

Two deprivation indicators have come to be used frequently in Britain in public health research and in the surveillance of local population health. These are the Townsend Material Deprivation Score and the Jarman Underprivileged Area Score (both named after the researchers who first put them forward). The Townsend Material Deprivation Score is based on four census variables – the percentage of private households with more than one person per room; the percentage of private households with no car; the percentage of private households that are not owner-occupied and the percentage of residents eligible for employment who are unemployed. These four factors were explicitly selected to reflect different aspects of material deprivation and are combined

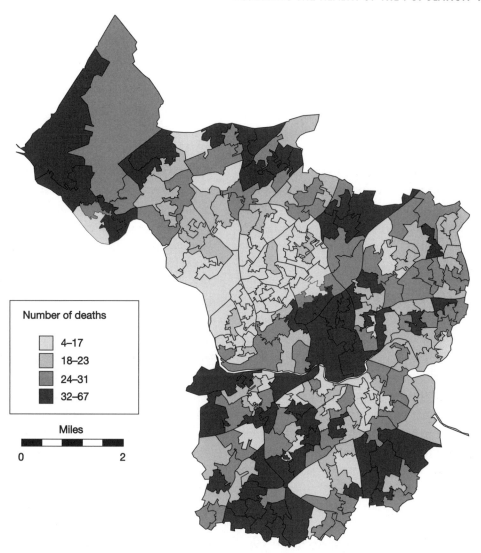

Figure 1.2 Number of deaths under-75 years of age, Lower Super Output Areas, Bristol, 2002–06
Source: Office for National Statistics.

into a single overall deprivation index. The Jarman Underprivileged Area Score was not actually constructed as a measure of deprivation but as a measure of general practice workload. The variant of the Jarman Underprivileged Area Score in common use is based on eight variables, which were derived from a study of general practitioners' subjective expressions of social factors amongst their patients that most affected the need for primary care services and therefore their workload. Figure 1.3 shows the strong association between one of these deprivation measures (the Townsend Score) and an important cause of death.

In the world of local government, the most commonly used measure is the Index of Multiple Deprivation. This combines 37 separate indicators of deprivation into a single index for each Super Output Area and local authority area in England. The indicators are grouped into seven domains, one of which is 'health deprivation and disability', which contains four indicators that cover mortality, mental health, emergency hospital admissions and disability.

HEALTH EVENTS

There are a number of routes through which data triggered by health events are collected. A major one is the certification of cause of death when an individual dies. Although it may seem a strange starting point when considering population health, there are good reasons to suppose that mortality data are amongst the most reliable indicators of the extent and nature of ill health in a population, although clearly suffering from limitations in considering chronic and non-fatal illness.

A second route is the recording of data relating to episodes of hospital care, which continues to improve in accuracy and completeness but still relates to only a minority of ill health. The vast majority of ill health does not involve hospital referral or indeed contact with the health service at all.

A third route is the recording of primary care data, which should cover a much greater proportion of ill health (over 90% of episodes of illness that result in contact with general practitioners are dealt with entirely

in the primary care setting). However, data collection is still markedly less well developed and complete in primary care.

These three routes are discussed in more detail below.

MORTALITY

Mortality notification has the advantages that it is legally required and it refers to an event that is unlikely to be missed. Even so, some data may be unreliable. If the qualified informant is a close relative, then clearly data are likely to be more accurate than if details are given by someone more remote. However, the qualified informant may be vague about the deceased person's actual occupation or may give the most senior occupation held during life, even though they should be asked to give the last gainful occupation of the deceased. Even the medical reason given for death may be subject to uncertainty, being based largely on clinical opinion in many cases. Deaths in the elderly are often ascribed to terminal conditions such as 'bronchopneumonia' when the certifier is unsure of the precise cause, whereas a death in a young person maybe investigated more fully.

Measures of Mortality

The basic unit of measurement used in studying mortality in populations is the rate. The rate consists of three components: a numerator, which is the number of people in the population who have died; a denominator, which is the total number of people in the population; and the time period during which deaths took place. The

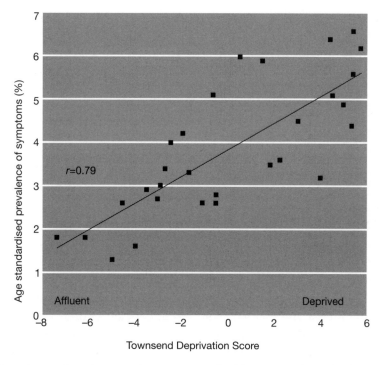

Figure 1.3 Prevalence of angina symptoms compared with Townsend Deprivation Score
Source: Payne N, Saul C. Variations in use of cardiology services in a health authority: comparison of coronary artery revascularisation rates with prevalence of angina and coronary mortality. *BMJ.* 1997; **314**: 257.

use of a rate allows a comparison between different populations, between different subgroups within the same population, and between different times for one population. A statement of absolute numbers, such as '100 deaths from coronary heart disease occurred last year in District A compared with 700 in District B', may be of value to the local undertakers in helping to assess their likely workload, but it does not tell us whether mortality from coronary heart disease is a greater health problem amongst the inhabitants of District A compared to District B, since the relative sizes of the two populations are not given.

Crude Death Rate

The simplest form of mortality measure is the crude death rate, which takes the number of deaths in a period, usually a year, and expresses that number per 1000 population at risk of dying in the middle of the year, using the mid-year population estimate described earlier.

Use of crude death rates has the advantage that mortality can be expressed in a single figure. This is helpful in comparing mortality within an area over a period of time, so long as the age and sex structure of the population does not change too much. The disadvantage of crude death rates is that they cannot be used to compare mortality experience between areas because of possible differences in age and sex structures of the populations in those areas. A new town, for example, is likely to have a lower crude death rate than a seaside retirement resort. This is because in the former there will be fewer people in age groups at risk of dying.

Specific Mortality Rates

The need to look beyond crude death rates leads to the use of specific rates. A specific mortality rate refers to the number of deaths occurring in a subgroup of the population. Age and sex together with cause are the most commonly described subgroups. Occupation, social class and ethnic group are others. Thus the annual age-specific death rate for males aged 15–24 would be expressed as number of deaths in the year amongst men aged 15–24 years divided by the number of men of that age in the population. If this value is multiplied by 1000, it gives the rate per 1000. In practice, age-specific rates are nearly always also sex-specific since important differences exist between males and females in their risk of dying from or developing certain diseases.

Death rates may be expressed for individual causes of death rather than the all-cause rates that have been described thus far. Most health problems show an effect of some kind with age, as shown in Figure 1.4, so crude death rates are inadequate to describe conditions which are heavily loaded at the extremes of life. The study of age/sex and other specific rates is by far the best way of examining how mortality or other measures vary between different populations. However, by moving away from the crude death rate in order to observe such detailed measures an attractive feature of the crude rate is lost, namely its ability to convey an impression in a single figure.

Standardised Rates

A more useful summary measure, which takes account of the different age structures of two populations so that their mortality experience can be compared directly, is provided by standardisation. In age standardisation, a single standardised death rate is calculated in which allowance has been made for the age (and usually also sex) structure of the population in question.

There are two methods of standardisation: indirect and direct. Both involve choosing a standard population (for example, the population of England and Wales in 2001 or the European standard population), which is broken down into specific age (and usually sex) groups.

In the *indirect method* of standardisation, the death rates experienced by each age group of the standard population (for example, females aged 15–24 years in England and Wales) are applied to the population of the same age groups in the study area. This shows how many females aged 15–24 years in the study area would have died if the standard population's death rate had prevailed. After the calculation has been performed for all age groups, the resulting total number of deaths is added up. These deaths did not actually occur, but are those that would have occurred if the study population had experienced the same mortality as the standard population, and hence they are referred to as 'expected' deaths.

The 'expected' number of deaths can then be compared to the actual, or 'observed', number of deaths. The most common means of comparison is the standardised mortality ratio (SMR). This is the ratio of observed deaths to expected deaths and is usually expressed as a percentage. By definition, the standard population has an SMR of 100% (i.e., observed and expected deaths are the same). SMRs over 100 (the % sign is usually not used) represent unfavourable mortality experience, and SMRs below 100 show relatively favourable mortality experience, the effect of differences in the age and sex profile of each population having been taken into account.

Table 1.2 illustrates the process of calculating the SMR for deaths in females aged 15–64 in one part of the country, compared to the standard female population of England and Wales. The SMR of 106 for the area in question indicates that the mortality rate was 6% higher than if the specific rates for the England and Wales population had applied.

In indirect standardisation, the death rates occurring in the standard population are applied to the study population. In the *direct method* of standardisation, the reverse process is used (Table 1.3). The age-specific death rates of the study population are applied in turn to the numbers in each corresponding age group of the standard population to give the number of deaths which would have occurred in the standard population if the death rates in each study population had applied. This number of deaths is divided by the total standard population to give an age-standardised death rate for the population under study.

In these examples, standardisation has been used to examine mortality in different areas. The process can be applied to any subgroups of the population where suitable data are available – for example, social class or occupational group. Although most commonly used to take account of age and sex, standardisation can also be used to adjust for differences in other characteristics. For example, perinatal mortality rates may be standardised for birth weight.

The essence of standardisation is that it holds constant and therefore eliminates the effect of the characteristic being standardised (for example, age or sex) so that the effect of other factors can be examined. Once a factor has been used in standardisation, it cannot be used to explain variation between rates. Figure 1.5 shows standardised mortality rates for circulatory disease in the regions of England. The differences cannot be explained by the fact that different regions had different age structures, since it is age that has been standardised.

Avoidable Deaths

Avoidable death is a concept that addresses deaths from those causes and in those age groups where preventive measures or better clinical management might have avoided deaths. There are complexities in this approach because of the variety of definitions used. Different approaches can be taken based on whether the definition includes conditions that are amenable to medical care or public health interventions, or to both. Similarly, the age range used in some analyses may vary between conditions – for example, one approach

Table 1.2 Indirect standardisation: worked example of the calculation of a standardised mortality ratio (SMR)

The aim is to compare the mortality experience of women (aged 15-64 years) in one part of the country (the study population) with that of all women of the same age group in England and Wales (the standard population).

Age-specific death rates for all females in England and Wales (standard population)

	Deaths per 100 000 population
15–24 years	29.7
25–34 years	44.2
35–44 years	110.7
45–54 years	290.2
55–64 years	855.4

Population of females in the study population

	Population
15–24 years	70 100
25–34 years	72 000
35–44 years	65 000
45–54 years	57 200
55–64 years	59 400

'Expected' number of deaths of females living in the study population if their experience was the same as all females in England and Wales

	'Expected' deaths	
15–24 years	29.7 × (70,100/100,000) =	21
25–34 years	44.2 × (72,000/100,000) =	32
35–44 years	110.7 × (65,000/100,000) =	72
45–54 years	290.2 × (57,200/100,000) =	166
55–64 years	855.4 × (59,400/100,000) =	508
		799

'Observed' (actual) deaths of study population   849
females aged 15–64 years

SMR (as a percentage) (England and Wales = 100)

$$\text{SMR} = \frac{\text{observed deaths}}{\text{expected deaths}} \times 100$$

$$= \frac{849}{799} \times 100$$

$$= 106$$

Table 1.3 Worked example of direct standardisation

The aim is to produce an age standardisation death rate for females (aged 15–64 years) in one part of the country (the study population) standardised to the England and Wales population.

Age-specific death rates for females in the study population

	Deaths per 100 000 population
15–24 years	25.7
25–34 years	36.1
35–44 years	103.1
45–54 years	304.2
55–64 years	949.5

Population of females in England and Wales (standard population)

	Population
15–24 years	3 631 600
25–34 years	3 852 300
35–44 years	3 500 400
45–54 years	2 873 200
55–64 years	2 631 500
Total population	16 489 000

'Expected' number of deaths of England and Wales females if their experience was the same as females in the study population

	'Expected' deaths
15–24 years	25.7 × (3 631 600/100 000) = 933
25–34 years	36.1 × (3 852 300/100 000) = 1 391
35–44 years	103.1 × (3 500 400/100 000) = 3 609
45–54 years	304.2 × (2 873 200/100 000) = 8 740
55–64 years	949.5 × (2 631 500/100 000) = 24 986
Total expected deaths	39 659

Age standardised death rate of the study population females aged 15–64 years

Deaths per 100 000 population

$$= \frac{\text{expected deaths}}{\text{standard population}} \times 100\,000$$

$$= \frac{39\,659}{16\,489\,000} \times 100\,000$$

$$= 241 \text{ per } 100\,000$$

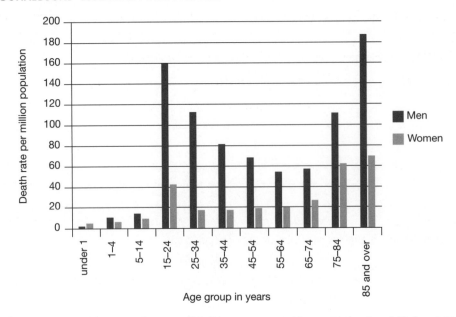

Figure 1.4 Age- and sex-specific mortality for transport accidents, England and Wales, 2005
Source: Office for National Statistics.

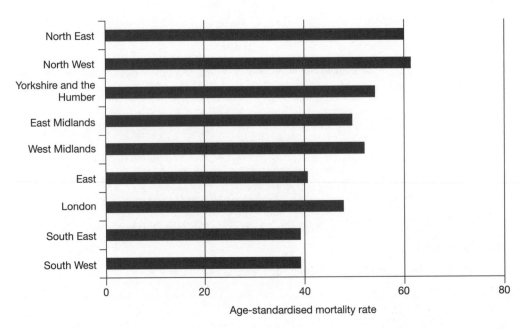

Figure 1.5 Under-75 years of age standardised mortality rate for coronary heart disease, English Regions, 2004–06
Source: National Centre for Health Outcomes Development.

only included asthma deaths below 45 years of age. Nevertheless, the avoidable deaths concept has proved valuable in providing a focus for further investigation or for targeted action. Table 1.4 shows the mortality rates for the top ten causes of avoidable mortality in men.

Another approach to assessing the scope for improvement in population mortality is the examination of deaths according to years of life lost prematurely. In a typical calculation, the number of deaths under 75 years is multiplied by the number of years of life lost (at zero age, an average of 74.5 years; at 74 years, an average of 0.5 years) to give total years of life lost. This total figure can then be expressed both absolutely and as a rate relative to the population at risk (Table 1.5). By comparing the two tables it can be seen how congenital abnormalities and perinatal death are important in terms of the years

of life lost but not when the data is ranked only on the mortality rate.

HOSPITAL SYSTEMS
MORBIDITY

The lesser reliability of mortality data as a window on illness and disease makes it important to establish and maintain systems of information that describe, more directly, the size of the pool of such morbidity in the population. Yet no single source of routinely collected health data will provide a comprehensive picture of the range of illnesses and diseases from which people suffer. Moreover, much of the information that is available is incomplete, largely because a substantial number of cases may not be counted.

The process of the health service in dealing with morbidity can be simplified into a

Table 1.4 Leading causes of avoidable mortality in men (age-standardised mortality rates), England and Wales, 2005

Cause	Rate per 100 000 population aged 0–64 years
Ischaemic heart disease	72.7
All respiratory diseases (excluding pneumonia and influenza)	22.2
Cerebrovascular disease	17.7
Malignant neoplasm of colon and rectum	13.2
Pneumonia	8.2
Leukaemia	4.0
Diabetes mellitus	3.7
Gastric and duodenal ulcer	2.3
Hypertensive disease	2.3
Epilepsy and status epilepticus	1.9

Source: Wheller L, Baker A, Griffiths C, Rooney C. Trends in avoidable mortality in England and Wales, 1993–2005. Office for National Statistics. *Health Stat Q.* 2007; **34**.

linear process (Figure 1.6) that begins with need and results in a particular outcome. There may be blocks and impediments at each stage. Some need may never translate into demand. Even if it is expressed as demand, it may not (perhaps due to waiting times) translate into health service activity. Health services are usually quite good at counting activity and the resources applied but poor at detecting and determining need and also poor at monitoring outcomes.

It is difficult to imagine a service industry in the non-health sector functioning without a clear idea of the size of various groups of customers within the population who will require, or benefit from, its services. Yet this is just the position in which the health service has traditionally been.

Mortality more or less defines itself, death being so clear-cut, whereas morbidity does not always do so. While there may be a relatively common understanding of what represents a strangulated hernia, there may be less of an understanding, even amongst doctors, about what threshold of blood pressure represents hypertension. Self-reporting

Table 1.5 Leading causes of avoidable mortality (years of life lost) in men aged 0–74 years, England and Wales, 2005

Cause	Rate per 10 000 population years
Ischaemic heart disease	69.6
All respiratory diseases (excluding pneumonia and influenza)	18.4
Cerebrovascular disease	16.9
Malignant neoplasm of colon and rectum	11.8
Pneumonia	9.3
Epilepsy and status epilepticus	6.0
Leukaemia	5.5
Congenital malformations of the circulatory system	5.2
Perinatal deaths, all causes, excluding stillbirths	4.2
Diabetes mellitus	4.2

Source: Wheller L, Baker A, Griffiths C, Rooney C. Trends in avoidable mortality in England and Wales, 1993–2005. Office for National Statistics. *Health Stat Q.* 2007; **34**.

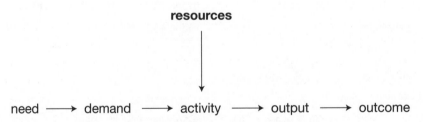

Figure 1.6 Process for need to become outcome in the health service

of illness is also enormously variable. Patients do not have common thresholds in presenting illness to a general practitioner. One person's problem may not be perceived as such if experienced by another. Similarly, changes over time may reflect changes in people's expectations of their own health, as well as changes in the incidence and duration of sickness.

A wide diversity of data about illness or disease (morbidity data) are collected, some nationally, others only locally, some routinely, others on an ad hoc basis for a specific purpose, some as a statutory requirement, others on a voluntary basis. In considering the value of such data, it is important to be fully aware of the limitations. These are best appreciated by understanding the source and method of collection of the data.

Mostly, those using morbidity data will be concerned with two issues. Firstly, they will want to understand how complete a coverage of the disease problem the data provide, and secondly, they will want to decide how valid the method of ascertaining whether disease was present or absent was. Many routinely available sources of morbidity data are deficient in both these respects. If they are based upon the collection of information about patients who have made contact with services (and many are), they will not provide comprehensive information about all cases of the disease that exist in the population.

In considering how completely a particular source of morbidity data described the disease problem in the population, it is helpful to bear in mind the 'iceberg' concept depicted in Figure 1.7. The proportion of patients who make contact with health services, and in particular with the hospital services, is often referred to as the tip of the iceberg. The process which leads people into the tip of this iceberg is complex and depends on many factors, such as: the patient's perceptions of their ill health; their own attitude and that of their family, friends and society in general to illness; the availability of medical services; and the quality of previous consultations.

A number of types of morbidity data are collected, analysed and presented on a routine basis. Examples include notifications of communicable diseases (described in detail in Chapter 9), data on hospital inpatients, notifications of foetal anomalies (described in detail in Chapter 6), abortion statistics and cancer registration. Many other types of morbidity data are available routinely or on an ad hoc basis but are less useful in assessing the health of a population on a day-to-day basis.

Hospital-based Data

Traditionally, many countries have used hospital inpatient data as an indicator of morbidity. However, such data can only take account of those conditions for which inpatient care is required. Diseases for which patients do not require hospitalisation will not be revealed by examining hospital inpatient statistics only. Many 'important' health problems (for example, the common cold, migraine, backache), at least as judged by the proportion of the population affected by them and the economic impact of working days lost, will seldom lead their sufferers to require hospital inpatient care.

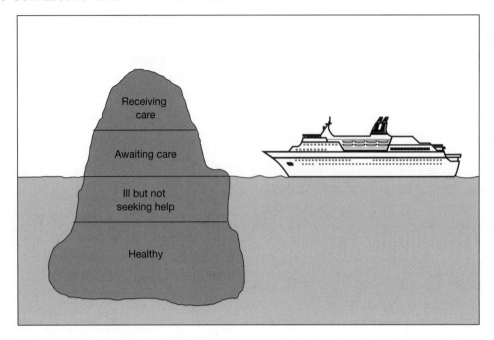

Figure 1.7 The iceberg concept of health care

For relatively serious conditions, such as asthma, hernia or arthritis, a proportion of people afflicted will not make the decision to seek health care (even though they may recognise themselves as ill). A further proportion will visit their general practitioners only. Others will come to the attention of hospital services as outpatients or inpatients. Only the very last group will be recorded in a system of morbidity data based on hospital inpatients. In some disorders where hospitalisation is virtually mandatory, such as a fractured neck of femur or a perforated duodenal ulcer, hospital rates may approximate to the total size of the disease problem in the population. These situations are so few that conclusions about incidence of disease based on hospital inpatient data should be interpreted with great caution (*see also* Chapter 2).

Hospital Episode Statistics

The Hospital Episode Statistics (HES) system of data recording seeks to capture every episode of inpatient care that takes place within a NHS hospital in England and also all care given to NHS patients by the independent sector in treatment centres. An 'episode' is defined as a period of treatment under the care of a particular hospital consultant. Patient-based inpatient and day-case events are recorded daily in every hospital through a computerised Patient Administration System (PAS). Each year, records of more than 13 million separate patient treatment episodes are collected.

The range of data collected covers items such as: hospital of treatment; area of residence; patient administrative details (for example, birth date, sex, postcode of usual address, ethnicity); admission details (for example, referring general practitioner, admission/discharge details, method/source of admission); consultant episode details (for example, consultant code, specialty); and clinical details (primary and subsidiary diagnoses, operations and procedures undertaken). For maternity admissions, details of the delivery record are entered, as are details about the baby itself. For people with mental illness, additional information is collected annually on long-stay patients (those over one year) and on patients detained under one of the sections of the Mental Health Act.

While Hospital Episode Statistics data provide a useful potential source of information on illnesses treated in hospital, in the authors' experience their value is limited for this purpose by the quality of clinical information recorded, as well as by the completeness of returns made by some hospitals – although coverage and data quality improved during the late 1990s. The quality of clinical information will continue to improve with the increased use of Hospital Episode Statistics data to measure hospital, and in particular clinical, performance. The planned extension of HES to cover outpatient care and A&E attendances will further increase the usefulness of this important data source.

Korner Data

In the 1980s and 1990s the main system for recording health service activity was the Korner aggregate returns (named after the chair of a Steering Group that reviewed health information requirements in the early 1980s). Information was collected on

a variety of types of patient activity in the hospital and community health services in England. Although many of the returns have been superseded, examples still in use include the KT31 return on family planning services, KC50 on childhood immunisation and KA34 on ambulance performance.

SYSTEMS FOR AGGREGATION OF DATA

The relatively systematic recording of morbidity data in hospitals has raised issues of how to classify the conditions that people present with and the treatment that is carried out. Statistical classifications aggregate data into a defined number of categories according to a documented framework of rules, conventions and index; for example, *The International Statistical Classification of Diseases and Related Health Problems, Tenth Revision (ICD-10)* and *The OPCS Classification of Surgical Operations and Procedures, Fourth Revision (OPCS-4)*. Groupers such as Healthcare Resource Groups (HRGs) aggregate treatment data into larger categories for the purpose of higher-level analysis; for example, resource management needs assessment, commissioning and performance monitoring.

International Statistical Classification of Diseases and Related Health Problems, Tenth Revision (ICD-10)

The World Health Organization, by international agreement, produces *The International Statistical Classification of Diseases and Health Related Problems*, or *ICD* as it is commonly known, and this is used in many countries as the principal means of classifying and coding both mortality and morbidity experience.

The most recent revision of the *ICD*, known as *ICD-10*, was published by the World Health Organization in the early 1990s. The existence and widespread use of such an internationally agreed disease classification is of vital importance. Without it, comparisons of statistics over time and between different places would not be possible in any valid or meaningful form. Through the years, the classification has moved from being disease-orientated, and primarily a means of assigning causes of death, to include a wider framework of illness and other health problems.

The tenth revision groups diagnoses, signs and symptoms, causes and other factors into 21 chapters, starting with those relating to infectious and parasitic diseases and ending with codes for factors influencing health status and contact with health services (Table 1.6).

The codes are alphanumeric and run from A00.0 to Z99.9, excluding the letter U, which is reserved for additional codes and changes arising between revisions of the classification. The first three characters of a code define a category, with the fourth character supplying extra detail. Hence K26 is the category 'Duodenal ulcer' and K26.1 is 'Duodenal ulcer – acute with perforation'. Figure 1.8 shows a short extract from the chapter on diseases of the digestive system to illustrate the range of code numbers available for a common surgical condition.

The classification is stable over time and has a fixed number of mutually exclusive, all-encompassing categories. Conditions are assigned to the categories according to defined rules, conventions and an index. In order to ensure that all conditions can be classified, a number of specialised categories exist – most notably the 'other specified' notation. These latter codes provide the stability of the classification over time, allowing new conditions a slot in which to be placed.

The OPCS Classification of Surgical Operations and Procedures (OPCS-4)

In England, the primary classification of operative procedures and other interventions is the fourth revision of *The Classification of Surgical Operations and Procedures*, known as *OPCS-4*. The codes use a similar format to those in *ICD-10* and cover procedures within anatomical systems, as well as subsidiary codes for methods (laser therapy, for example) and specific sites of operation (such as upper inner quadrant of the breast). The classification was designed specifically for theatre-based surgery. Continuing advances in the provision of treatment means that the classification requires annual review with substantial new codes being added to keep pace with clinical practice. Version *OPCS-4.4* of the classification was released in April 2007.

Healthcare Resource Groups (HRGs)

Codings of diagnoses and operations using the classification systems described in this section are essentially primary, in that they represent the finest level of detail routinely available. Increasingly, classification systems at a secondary level are being used. These take one or more of these, or other, primary

Table 1.6 Composition of chapters in the tenth revision of *The International Classification of Diseases (ICD-10)*

Chapter number and designation		Range of codes
I	Certain infectious and parasitic diseases	A00–B99
II	Neoplasms	C00–D48
III	Diseases of the blood and blood-forming organs and certain disorders involving the immune mechanism	D50–D89
IV	Endocrine, nutritional and metabolic diseases	E00–E90
V	Mental and behavioural disorders	F00–F99
VI	Diseases of the nervous system	G00–G99
VII	Diseases of the eye and adnexa	H00–H59
VIII	Diseases of the ear and mastoid process	H60–H95
IX	Diseases of the circulatory system	I00–I99
X	Diseases of the respiratory system	J00–J99
XI	Diseases of the digestive system	K00–K93
XII	Diseases of the skin and subcutaneous tissue	L00–L99
XIII	Diseases of the musculo-skeletal system and connective tissue	M00–M99
XIV	Diseases of the genito-urinary system	N00–N99
XV	Pregnancy, childbirth and the puerperium	O00–O99
XVI	Certain conditions originating in the perinatal period	P00–P95
XVII	Congenital malformations, deformations and chromosomal abnormalities	Q00–Q99
XVIII	Symptoms, signs and abnormal clinical and laboratory findings, not elsewhere classified	R00–R99
XIX	Injury, poisoning and certain other consequences of external causes	S00–T98
XX	External causes of morbidity and mortality	V01–Y98
XXI	Factors influencing health status and contact with health services	Z00–Z99

Source: Ashley J. The international classification of diseases: the structure and content of the 10th revision. *Health Trends.* 1990–91; **4**: 135–7.

classifications together with factors such as age and sex to produce broader groupings that describe clinical activity, which are called measures of case mix. Diagnosis-related groups (DRGs) were originally used by the Medicare system in the United States for reimbursement of health service charges. The most widely used version of this system had 467 groups, each defined by one or more of the following: diagnosis, surgical procedure, co-morbidities and complications, age, sex and discharge disposition.

Each case-mix group was intended to cover a clinically coherent set of conditions that carried approximately the same cost implication (so-called iso-resource groups).

Healthcare Resource Groups (HRGs) are the specific British evolution of DRGs, both for use within hospitals and more widely in other health settings. HRGs require revision on a regular basis to allow for current and anticipated developments in clinical treatments and investigations and also to make this particular aggregation tool more useful for health services management purposes. The change to the version HRG4 in 2006 saw an expansion of the groupings from 650 to more than 1400 and also saw additional coverage of specialties such as radiology and radiotherapy.

Clinical Terminologies

A relatively recent development (certainly in contrast to the long-standing diagnostic and surgical systems described above) are schemes in which terms are used to describe concepts that are arranged formally according to their meaning to produce an electronic thesaurus. These terminologies seek to cover most of the information included in a medical record (symptoms, physical signs, diagnosis, treatments, clinical procedures).

At the end of the 1990s, two such systems were in use: SNOMED, standing for Systematised Nomenclature of Medicine, which was developed in the United States, and Clinical Terms Version 3 (Read Codes), developed in the United Kingdom. Collaboration between the College of American Pathologists and the NHS has led

K35	**Acute Appendicitis**
K35.0	Acute appendicitis generalised peritonitis

Appendicitis (acute) with:
• perforation
• peritonitis (generalized)
• rupture

K35.1	**Acute appendicitis with peritoneal abscess**

Abscess of appendix

K35.9	**Acute appendicitis, unspecified**

Acute appendicitis without:
• perforation
• peritoneal abscess
• peritonitis
• rupture

K3.6	**Other appendicitis**

Appendicitis:
• chronic
• recurrent

K37	**Unspecified appendicitis**

Figure 1.8 Extract from the chapter on diseases of the digestive system within the tenth revision of *The International Statistical Classification of Diseases and Related Health Problems (ICD-10)*
Source: Reproduced, by permission, from *The International Statistical Classification of Diseases and Related Health Problems (ICD-10)*. Tenth revision, volume 1. Geneva: World Health Organization; 1992. p. 569.

to the development of SNOMED Clinical Terms, which has been adopted as the standard nomenclature and is replacing the Read Codes.

These clinical terminologies are intended to allow doctors to use their preferred clinical terms, which can then be converted automatically by computer software into codes. In this way, the detailed clinical information required to support patient care and the electronic health care record can also be aggregated into statistical classification and groupings (Figure 1.9).

GENERAL PRACTICE SYSTEMS

The primary care setting is a very important source of data. A high proportion of the population is registered with a general practitioner, and a very substantial proportion of the contacts between the public and the health service take place in primary care. A wide range of health problems are dealt with in primary care. Knowledge of the health experience of this population allows greater insight into the early stages of the natural history of illnesses, and, in the majority of cases, it is the point of entry into the hospital system. It does not, of course, tell us anything about illnesses that are unrecognised by the patient or for which the patient undertakes self-medication.

The new contract for general practitioners that was introduced in 2004 introduced a new national system of data collection and analysis that was directly linked to the remuneration of general practices. The Quality Management and Analysis System enables general practices and primary care trusts to review how they are doing against the agreed targets under the Quality and Outcomes Framework. There is, however,

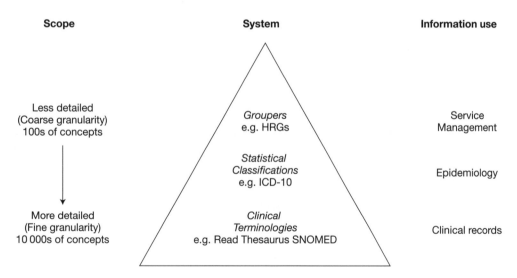

Figure 1.9 The relationship between terminologies, classifications and groupings
Source: Adapted from Read JD, Sanderson HF, Drennan YM. *Terming, Encoding, Grouping: the language of health.* Proceedings, International Medical Information Association's Eighth World Congress on Medical Informatics. Vancouver: 1995.

no national system in England for the aggregation of anonymised data from individual general practices into a comprehensive database.

The introduction of computer systems to general practice did not follow a uniform pattern, but one such system, VAMP, had a facility to collect and aggregate data from practices that were using the system. The database created using the system eventually moved to the public sector and is now run by a government agency, the Medicines and Healthcare products Regulatory Agency (MHRA). The General Practice Research Database, as it is known, is based on data supplied by almost 400 general practices and contains only anonymised patient data. It is of particular use as a research tool in the area of prescribing.

A further source of prescribing data from primary care is the information available from the recording of data from prescriptions dispensed in the community. The Prescription Pricing Division of the NHS Business Services Authority collects data from all prescriptions dispensed in England, and the data is analysed for use within primary care (by general practices interested in their use of generic drugs, for example) and also at primary care trust level. Although the major use of these data is for cost control of prescribing, they can also have uses in public health programmes. Examples might include monitoring the usage of antibiotics in the community or the rate of prescription of antipsychotic drugs.

REGISTRATION OF DISEASE

A register has four main characteristics:
1   it identifies individuals
2   these individuals each have the same particular feature in common, which is the focus of interest for the register
3   it is longitudinal in that the information held about individuals is updated in a defined systematic manner
4   it is based on a geographically-defined population.

A number of registers are currently maintained in the health field and serve a range of different purposes.

CANCER REGISTRATION

The National Cancer Registration Scheme has been operating since the end of World War II, although a system was in operation in some parts of the country in the 1920s, when radium treatment commenced. It is organised on a historic basis rather than on current regions, and information is also processed nationally by the Office for National Statistics, which maintains a National Cancer Registry for England and Wales. Each regional cancer registry collects a common set of data of the identity and type of neoplasm for each person resident or treated in the region who has been diagnosed as having cancer (certain premalignant tumours are also included). Electronic notification from histology laboratories is an important source of information. An effective cancer registry will have a very low proportion of cases where the first notification comes after the patient's death.

The National Cancer Intelligence Centre at the Office for National Statistics, through notification by each region, assembles a minimum data set. This includes patient identification details (name, previous surname, address, postcode, sex, date of birth, marital status, NHS number, date of first diagnosis, date of death) and details of the tumour (site of primary growth, type of growth, basis upon which the diagnosis was made and grade and stage – the latter two items for some cancers only). Also included are certain other details relating to the tumour and its treatment. Such data enable the incidence of cancer to be examined geographically, within subgroups of the population and over time. They also enable survival to be compared for cancer

at different sites. Such analyses can reveal improving survival for cancer at some sites due to more effective treatment (Figure 1.10).

OTHER CASE REGISTERS

Registers have been established to study other conditions such as psychiatric illness, child abuse, ischaemic heart disease, stroke and trauma. There is also a varied pattern of registers collecting data on the incidence of congenital abnormalities. It has been argued that the proliferation of such registers, accumulating large amounts of data, must incorporate checks to ensure high quality and comparability, or their cost will not be justified.

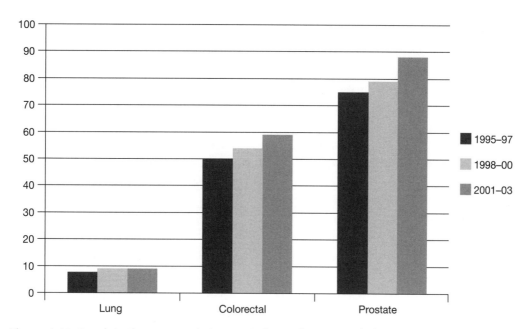

Figure 1.10 Trends in three-year relative survival rates for men with three common cancers in the North West region of England
Source: North West Cancer Intelligence Service.

ESTABLISHING AND RUNNING A REGISTER

Before a register is established, consideration must be given to why the register is required, what disease is being registered, how cases are to be identified and reported, what information will be recorded on each case, how information will be stored and communicated, who will be responsible for producing analyses and servicing requests, who will produce reports, what the financial implications will be, and how patient confidentiality and ethical and data protection requirements will be satisfied.

To be of any real value, a disease register, once established, must be maintained to a high quality. This means addressing at least two fundamental issues: completeness of case ascertainment and validity. Unfortunately, this is not always recognised, and the resources set aside to run the register may be insufficient to allow quality-control issues to be tackled. The day-to-day problems of running a case register are formidable and include searching for missing records, dealing with incomplete or inaccurate records, the elimination of duplicate entries, resolving coding queries, ironing out computing difficulties and responding to requests for analyses.

One of the main problems of any registration system is achieving comparability of diagnosis. Wherever possible, strict rules should be laid down so that there are well-defined criteria that must be present before a particular diagnosis is made. Variations in diagnostic and classification practices can give rise to problems when comparing data for different countries, for different parts of the same country, or for the same population over time. Duplication sometimes occurs, but with proper organisation it is usually possible to identify whether an incoming record belongs to an existing registration or not. However, under-coverage (cases eluding registration) is an almost intractable problem with all registers. Most registers rely on some agreed procedure of notification of cases by health workers, with varying degrees of success.

The decision to establish a register should not be undertaken lightly. It requires proper justification, skilled organisation, adequate resources and, above all, dedicated and imaginative leadership.

USES OF REGISTERS

While in practice many disease registers have a single disease focus, they also have the potential for multiple uses. In addition to measuring the amount of disease in the population, they can monitor temporal trends, be used in patient follow-up, enable comparisons of treatment outcomes, facilitate service evaluation, be used as the basis for studies of disease causation, be used for research and clinical audit, and be used to plan and organise services for patients.

MEASURES OF MORBIDITY

There are two types of measure of illness or morbidity. They are *incidence* and *prevalence*. It is important to be able to distinguish between them (Table 1.7).

Table 1.7 Measures of morbidity

• Incidence rate	=	$\dfrac{\text{number of new cases of disease in specified time}}{\text{number of person-years at risk during period}^{*}}$
• Point prevalence	=	$\dfrac{\text{number of persons with disease at a point in time}}{\text{total population}}$
• Period prevalence	=	$\dfrac{\text{number of persons with disease during specified period}}{\text{total population at mid-point of interval}}$

*Average number at risk during period x length of time.

INCIDENCE AND PREVALENCE

The incidence rate measures the number of new cases of a particular disease arising in a population at risk in a certain time period. In contrast, prevalence measures all cases of the disease existing at a point in time (point prevalence) or over a period in time (period prevalence). Although one often speaks of the prevalence rate of a particular disease, strictly speaking it is not correct to refer to prevalence as a rate. More correctly, it is a ratio, since it is a static measure and does not incorporate the idea of cases arising through time. The point prevalence measure is often compared to a snapshot of the population. It states the position at a single point in time. In measuring a particular disease, prevalence counts individuals within the whole spectrum of that disease, from people who have newly developed the disease to those in its terminal phases; whereas incidence just counts new cases. Thus prevalence results from two factors: the size of the previous incidence (occurrence of new cases of the disease) and the duration of the condition from its onset to its conclusion (either as recovery or death).

In most chronic diseases, complete recovery does not occur. Many people develop diseases (for example, chronic bronchitis, peripheral vascular disease, stroke) in middle age that they may carry until their death. The incidence of a condition is an estimate of the risk of developing the disease and hence is of value mainly to those concerned with searching for the causes or determinants of the disease. Knowledge of the prevalence of a condition is of particular value in planning health services or workload, since it indicates the amount of illness requiring care. Relatively uncommon conditions (i.e., those with a low incidence) may become important health problems if people with the disease are kept alive for a long period of time (producing a relatively high prevalence figure). An example of such a condition is chronic renal failure, which is rare; because dialysis and transplantation can keep sufferers alive, it becomes an important health problem that consumes considerable resources.

POPULATION-BASED HEALTH INFORMATION

Data that describe lifestyle and other underlying factors that influence a population's health are important in monitoring and improving the public health.

GENERAL HOUSEHOLD SURVEY/ INTEGRATED HOUSEHOLD SURVEY

One way of obtaining information on illness that does not present to the health service at all is to choose people from the general population and obtain information about their health directly. The most important of the national surveys for public health purposes has been the General Household Survey (GHS).

The General Household Survey began in 1971, and from 1988 it was on the financial year rather than the calendar year. It was a continuous survey based upon a representative sample of around 13 000 post-code addresses in Britain. Interviews were conducted throughout the year with the adult members of these households, and, in addition, parents were asked for some details of each child in the household under 16 years of age. The information collected was not restricted to health. Indeed the survey served many government departments and also included housing, employment, education and the family to make up its five core topics. The questions on health related to acute illness in the last two weeks, health during the previous year, presence of chronic illness, consultations with a doctor, visits to hospital (as an inpatient or outpatient), wearing of glasses or contact lenses, and smoking and drinking habits.

In 2008, the new Integrated Household Survey brought together five of the established surveys into a new format with a larger sample size of approximately 200 000 households. The survey covers the same topics as the pre-existing Labour Force Survey, General Household Survey, Expenditure and Food Survey, Omnibus Survey and the Annual Population Survey. Standardisation of questions, analyses and outputs combined with the large sample size are important features of the new and very comprehensive source of data. The advantage of the much larger sample size is that for the first time it allows data to be analysed and presented at the level of local authorities and primary care trusts on topics such as smoking.

The survey gathers data on self-reported morbidity and disability. Questions are asked about both acute and long-standing illness and, if present, whether they limit or restrict activity in any way. Figure 1.11 illustrates the use of such data and shows a steadily increasing trend for self-reported long-standing illness. However, such changes should be interpreted with caution in view of the subjective nature of the reported information and its possible susceptibility to rising expectation.

The main limitation of the survey method is that, since it relies on the evidence of the individual, errors may be introduced due to forgetfulness, differing perceptions of illness or withholding of certain information. Moreover, in some cases diagnostic labels are attached to the illness by the patient. Although the interviewers, who are not medically qualified, are trained to probe for as much clarifying detail as possible, diagnostic labels are unlikely to conform with the terminology or accuracy of a medical practitioner's diagnosis.

Despite these disadvantages, the survey methodology has enabled major and minor illness to be described in the population as a whole. It avoids the disadvantages of data systems that monitor contact with health services, as it seeks to count both declared and undeclared illness. Data are collected along with information on a wide range of other subjects, thus allowing associations between such variables and health indices to be explored in a preliminary fashion.

HEALTH SURVEY FOR ENGLAND

The Health Survey for England has been run annually since 1991. The survey is based on a random sample of some 6000 private households in England. Since 1995 children aged 2–15 years have also been included, and since 2001 infants under the age of two years have been included in the survey. The survey is described in more detail in Chapter 2 as an example of a prevalence study.

It has three main components: a health and socio-economic questionnaire, physical measurements and a blood or urine sample. The clinical aspects of the survey vary depending on the age group of the respondent. Key topics are repeated each year to enable comparison over time, and, in addition, there are modules on specific disease areas and health problems that are covered at periodic intervals (e.g., cardiovascular disease, respiratory disease, accidents, disability). Furthermore, in individual years specific population groups (e.g., children and ethnic minorities) may be over-sampled. The data are robust enough for analyses to

be available at regional as well as national level, and the continuity of the survey since 1991 provides valuable information on trends over time.

LOCAL HEALTH SURVEYS

Although information from national survey sources provides valuable insights into health-related lifestyles and risk factors, it cannot readily be extrapolated to populations at local level. Increasingly, local health programmes are seeking to promote health and to prevent illness and premature death. Information on the prevalence of risk factors and health-related behaviours is required for this purpose.

The gap in public health information at local level can be addressed by commissioning or conducting lifestyle assessments involving postal or face-to-face interview questionnaire surveys of the population. It is essential that such local surveys seek to adopt valid survey instruments and survey methods. Comparisons over time and with other populations are then possible. It is also important that local surveys are properly resourced so that there can be comprehensive data capture and control of quality as well as effective analysis and communication of the findings. A useful means of obtaining high-quality comparable data for a local area is to commission an enhanced sample for a particular geography from an established national survey such as the Health Survey for England.

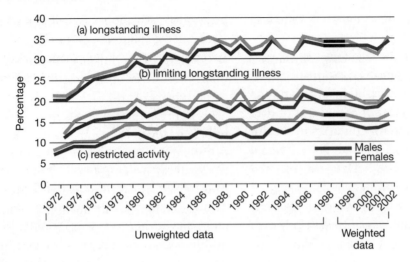

Figure 1.11 Percentage of men and women reporting long-standing illness and restricted activity, 1972–2002
Source: Living in Britain: results from the 2002 General Household Survey. London: The Stationery Office; 2004.

OTHER HEALTH STATUS MEASURES

A separate set of measures seeks to go beyond the more clear-cut health events that have been described so far. Many such measures have been developed because many existing indicators do not fully measure the effects that disease has on people's physical, social and emotional well-being. There is a need to address issues such as quality of life and the concept of health itself.

HEALTH AND DISEASE RATING SCALES

Measures that attempt to do this fall into two main categories. Disease-specific measures focus on the aspects of health that are considered to be especially important in determining the quality of life for patients suffering from particular conditions. For example, some rating scales have been developed for arthritic patients that provide summary measures of symptoms, including pain, function, range of motion of joints and the absence of deformity.

In contrast, general health scales attempt to measure the aspects of quality of life that are important to everybody, irrespective of their health status. These scales are an attempt to capture overall health status in a cost-effective and relatively simple way. Very few such measures are in regular use, but they have been widely developed in a research context. One example is the Nottingham Health Profile 3, which asks people a series of questions and assigns a score for each of six categories (physical mobility, pain, sleep, energy, social isolation, emotional reactions). Each category is scored 0 to 100, and rather than combining the scores to derive a summary health status measure, the score in each category is presented separately. Other measures that are more suitable than the Nottingham Health Profile for use in general population samples include the Short Form 36 (SF36), Health Status Questionnaire 12 (HSQ-12) and the EuroQol (EQ-5D). Even a simple question on self-rated health has been shown to predict the likelihood of subsequent death.

QUALITY-ADJUSTED LIFE YEARS

The quality-adjusted life year, or QALY, is a health measure of a different kind. The concept arises from the wish to compare the effect of different interventions across the spectrum of health care. Such comparisons are needed, for instance, to assess priorities for the use of limited resources or to identify the effectiveness of different programmes to improve health (such as, say, coronary artery surgery and smoking cessation). One obvious measure would be the number of years of life that each intervention would, on average, be expected to add, compared with the average expectation of what would happen without treatment. Thus, for example, treatment of a particular cancer might be known from follow-up studies to result in an average survival of 10 years, compared with untreated average survival of two years, resulting in an estimated gain of eight years of life per person treated.

There are two problems with this approach. Firstly, it is known that individuals do not value all years of life equally. For example, a year of life spent suffering the side effects of repeated chemotherapy would be regarded by most people as decidedly inferior to a year spent symptom-free, and survival under these conditions should

not be assessed as such a gain. Secondly, many conditions do not markedly shorten life, but they reduce its quality, and many treatments are aimed at improving quality of life rather than increasing survival, which could not be assessed simply by estimating expected additional life years.

Some mechanism therefore needs to be found to adjust life years for quality of life, and this is the objective of the QALY. Quality of life is usually measured by assessing two or more aspects of people's health, such as pain; disability; mood; or capacity to perform self-care, social activities or main activities like housework or paid employment. These assessments are then reduced to a single measure of changes in quality of life relative to a state of perfect well-being which is valued at unity. Combining this measure with information on life expectancy, by multiplying each year by its corresponding quality adjuster, gives an estimate of health improvement as QALYs gained.

Because the capacity to improve the population's health is inevitably constrained by the resources available to health care, the increase in QALYs arising from the use of health services is usually compared to the cost of treatment.

QALYs are an appropriate measure to focus on the predominant modern health problem – chronic disease. Table 1.8 shows how QALYs can be used to compare all kinds of health care, from preventive services to acute care.

However, while QALYs continue to be developed in a research context, their routine use in the health service is limited by the practical and theoretical difficulties of deriving valid single indices of quality of life and by reservations regarding the fairness and appropriateness of QALYs as a basis for assessing the need for different health services. The National Institute for Health and Clinical Excellence (NICE) uses QALYs as a means of comparing pharmaceuticals and measuring their clinical effectiveness.

Two other measures are also used to express related concepts, although neither has overtaken QALYs as a routinely used measure. Disability-adjusted life years (DALYs) is the opposite to QALYs, with DALYs representing years lived in disability rather than years of healthy living, and a further and more infrequently used measure is healthy years equivalent (HYE).

COMPENDIUM OF CLINICAL AND HEALTH INDICATORS

Data on local populations in England covering demography, fertility, morbidity, mortality and the provision of health care have been produced as the Public Health Common Data Set since the late 1980s. In 1998 its production shifted from the Department of Health to the National Centre for Health Outcomes Development, and it was retitled *Compendium of Clinical and Health Indicators*. Data are presented in more than 1000 different comparative analyses and are presented at national, regional and local levels. Although the data are generated from many of the traditional sources already described, particularly population, mortality and vital statistics and hospital activity data, its production in such a conveniently accessible form (with statistical derivations such as rates and confidence intervals already calculated) represents a major step forward.

The main groups of data that are presented in the *Compendium* are:

➢ mortality
➢ cancer incidence
➢ cancer survival
➢ cancer screening programmes
➢ Hospital Episode Statistics (HES) based indicators
➢ vaccinations
➢ infectious diseases
➢ congenital malformations

Table 1.8 Cost per quality-adjusted life year (QALY) league table

Intervention	Extra cost per QALY gained (£)
GP advice to stop smoking	270
Hip replacement	1180
Cholesterol testing and treatment (all adults aged 40–69)	1480
Kidney transplantation (cadaver)	4710
Home haemodialysis	17 260
Hospital haemodialysis	21 970
Erythropoietin treatment for anaemia in dialysis patients	54 380
Neurosurgery for malignant intracranial tumours	197 780

Source: Phillips C, Thompson G. *What is a QALY?* London: Hayward Medical Communications; 1998.

> births and infant mortality
> oral health in children
> fertility
> conceptions
> abortions
> life expectancy
> census-based indicators
> ONS area classification
> Indices of Deprivation 2004
> General Household Survey (GHS) smoking and drinking indicators
> Health Survey for England (HSE) based indicators
> Expenditure and Food Survey (EFS) fat consumption indicators

> population indicators, including ONS 2001 Census-based estimates and GP registered and resident relevant estimates
> primary care based indicators.

The *Compendium* therefore represents a major source of comparative public health data covering very many major health issues.

PUBLIC HEALTH OBSERVATORIES

Following on from the development of the Liverpool Public Health Observatory in

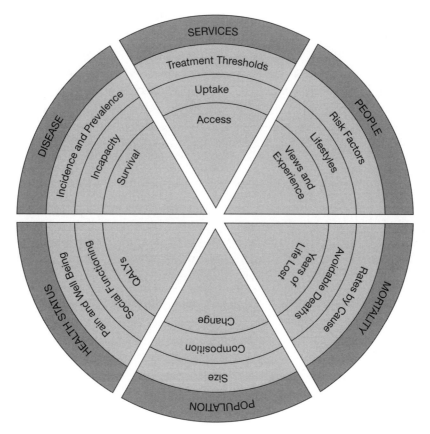

Figure 1.12 The scope of health needs assessment

the 1990s, the government's White Paper on public health published in 1999, *Saving Lives: Our Healthier Nation*, established public health observatories (PHOs) in each of the nine English regions. Further ones were established in Scotland and Wales and for the island of Ireland. The seven functions that lie at the core of their role are:

> ➤ monitoring health and disease trends and highlighting areas for action
> ➤ identifying gaps in health information
> ➤ advising on methods for health equity audits and health impact assessments
> ➤ drawing together information from different sources in new ways to improve health
> ➤ carrying out projects to highlight particular health issues
> ➤ evaluating progress by local agencies in improving health and cutting inequality
> ➤ looking ahead to give early warning of future public health problems.

The 12 public health observatories collaborate via the Association of Public Health Observatories (APHO) in their task of producing high-quality health intelligence for all of those engaged in public health action. Although not initially involved in collecting primary health-related data, there has been a trend for some observatories to merge with other public health information bodies such as cancer registries to form more comprehensive regional health intelligence organisations. The individual websites of the observatories provide a valuable portal to a wide range of population health data and are used extensively by the public health community, as well as by others seeking high-quality analyses.

CONCLUSIONS

All the sources of data covered in this chapter (and others not described) can be of value in assessing the health needs of a population. In practice, however, the needs-assessment process involves a variety of approaches, including the use of routinely available data to provide continuous surveillance of health patterns or trends; ad hoc analysis of routinely available data to answer a particular question or throw light on a particular problem; and the gathering of data that are not available routinely. The form of the needs assessment will differ according to the purpose for which the information is required. Figure 1.12 shows the main categories of information that are required to make an assessment of a population's health needs.

CHAPTER 2
Approaches to Investigation

INTRODUCTION

The investigation of health problems in populations, and of the health services that provide care for them, is a key function of public health. Anyone leading, or participating in, such investigative work should have a good knowledge of the range of routinely available data about health and health services, some of which is described in Chapter 1. It is equally important to have an understanding of the strengths and weaknesses of these data sources, because there are enormous dangers in the uncritical use of routinely available health data. Indeed, it is all too common to see analytical reports written for bodies responsible for taking major policy or resource-allocation decisions that contain conclusions far more sweeping than should be drawn given the limitations of the data.

Those involved in public health investigative work must also be familiar with, and skilled in, the methods and techniques of epidemiology. Epidemiology is one of the population sciences basic to public health. The techniques and methods of epidemiology and its general approach of a population perspective on health, disease and health services leads it to having a very widespread application throughout the field of public health. The epidemiological perspective is a key component in identifying health needs, examining the pattern of disease problems within and between populations, searching for the causes of disease, formulating health promotion and disease prevention strategies, studying the natural history of disease, and planning and evaluating health services.

This chapter deals with the way in which epidemiological techniques and methods can be used to investigate the health problems of, and the health service provided for, a population (Table 2.1).

COMPARING DISEASE PATTERNS BETWEEN AND WITHIN POPULATIONS: DESCRIPTIVE EPIDEMIOLOGY

Chapter 1 described the range of information that could be used to describe the health of a population. Having assembled the necessary information to be able to examine a particular indicator (for example, mortality under the age of 65 years from coronary heart disease or the incidence of fractured neck of femur), the next questions that will inevitably occur to the investigator involve comparisons. How does the population under study compare with other populations? How does the occurrence of the problem in the population currently compare with earlier time periods? Are different subgroups within the population affected by the health problem to a greater or lesser degree? Comparisons of this kind are the basis of hypothesis formulation and problem-solving.

The use of health information in this way, whether derived from routinely available data or assembled by special surveys, is usually referred to as descriptive epidemiology.

When using the technique of descriptive epidemiology, it is particularly important to take a cautious and stepwise approach to interpreting the findings and before drawing conclusions, no matter how tentative. This is not just good scientific practice, it is the duty of the responsible investigator to the

Table 2.1 Some reasons for carrying out a public health investigation

Defining the characteristics of a population
Assessing health needs
Describing a problem
Searching for causes
Identifying areas for improvement
Evaluating new and existing services
Planning service responses
Pointing to scope for prevention
Assisting resource allocation decisions

Source: Adapted from Donaldson LJ, Kirkup W. The public health practitioner as investigator. *Hosp Med.* 1998; **59**: 1–5.

population that he or she is studying. For example, to present information showing that the incidence of childhood leukaemia in one part of a region is higher than another without first carrying out some checks on the data in the cancer register (and other data sources) would be wrong. Comprehensiveness of ascertainment of cases, the validity of the recorded diagnoses on individual children and the accuracy of the places of residence attributed to the cases are all potential sources of misleading conclusions as well as of unnecessary public disquiet and anxiety.

It is essential that before conclusions are drawn about differences in the occurrence of health problems between different populations, or over time, consideration is given to whether the differences are real.

ARE DIFFERENCES REAL? THREE IMPORTANT QUESTIONS

In determining whether differences between populations or over time truly reflect different levels of a particular disease, it is helpful to address three questions.

What are the Criteria for Defining the Disease?

It is well known that there are variations in medical practice (between different time periods, different places and even individual doctors on different occasions) that influence the way in which a particular diagnostic label is applied to a particular condition.

An illustration of apparent variations in the occurrence of psychiatric illness that can be partly explained by variations in the diagnostic process is provided by considering a cross-national study carried out in the mid-1960s. This study, although from some time ago, is a classic in illustrating the pitfalls in equating diagnosed illness with its true occurrence. At that time it had been recognised that there were apparent differences in the frequency of certain psychiatric illnesses in the United States compared with the United Kingdom. If such differences were real, then valuable clues to the causes of certain psychiatric illnesses might have been available. These considerations gave rise to an investigation into the differences.

Table 2.2 shows the results of an analysis of two samples of patients in psychiatric hospitals in London and New York. There appeared to be a much higher percentage of people with schizophrenia and alcohol dependency in the New York sample than in the London sample. In contrast, patients with depression and mania were much more common in the London sample. Using a standardised interviewing technique, each patient in the sample was examined by a member of a team of project psychiatrists as soon as possible after admission and independently of the hospital staff.

Table 2.3 shows the results of comparing the original hospital diagnoses with the subsequent project diagnoses in the two samples. Once alcoholics and drug addicts had been excluded, the comparison of the two sets of project diagnoses showed no significant difference for schizophrenia, personality disorders, neurosis (other than depressive) and organic psychosis. This suggests that the original differences – in the hospital diagnoses – between the two centres were largely the result of variation in the diagnostic criteria used by the psychiatrists at the time.

The report concluded that the most important of these differences was that the New York concept of schizophrenia, at that time, was much broader than that used in London, and it included cases that many British psychiatrists would have called depressive illnesses, neurotic illnesses or personality disorders (*see* Figure 2.1).

Although this study is many years old, it illustrates a principle that can be a pitfall for any comparison of disease frequency. Variation amongst doctors in the choice of labels for particular clinical problems or causes of death is quite commonplace. While it may not be of paramount importance as far as the individual doctor and patient are concerned, it becomes central when data are aggregated for the purpose of producing a population count of the number of cases of a disease or the number of deaths from a particular cause. It is even more important to establish the diagnostic criteria that have been used to count cases of the disease when comparisons are made between different populations or when disease trend over time is observed. Otherwise, spurious conclusions about apparently major differences may be made (just as in the psychiatry example described above). This potential problem is applicable to all diseases, no matter how objectively the diagnosis is made.

Have all Cases of the Disease Been Identified?

False impressions about the amount of disease in one population compared to another may also be gained through a failure to take account of differences in the efficiency of case detection. For example, the observation that a particular cancer is more common in a developed country than in a developing country may lead to speculation about risk factors in the two countries. Such a line of thought would be unwise without first examining the efficiency of the two cancer registration systems. The apparently higher

Table 2.2 The hospital diagnoses of the London and New York samples

	New York percentage (n=192)	London percentage (n=174)
Schizophrenia	61.5	33.9**
Depressive psychoses	4.7	24.1**
Mania	0.5	6.9**
Depressive neuroses	1.6	8.0**
Other neuroses	2.6	5.7
Personality disorders	1.0	4.6*
Alcoholic disorders	19.8	3.4**
Drug dependence	0.0	0.6
Organic psychoses	5.2	1.7
Other diagnoses	3.1	10.9**

*Difference significant at 5% level. **Difference significant at 1% level.
Source: Cooper JE, Kendell RE, Gurland BJ. *Psychiatric Diagnosis in New York and London: a comparative study of mental hospital admissions.* London: Oxford University Press; 1972.

Table 2.3 The project diagnoses of the London and New York samples after the exclusion of alcoholics and drug addicts

	New York percentage (n=192)	London percentage (n=174)
Schizophrenia	39.4	37.0
Depressive psychoses	26.8	24.2
Mania	7.7	6.7
Depressive neuroses	9.2	15.2
Other neuroses	2.1	4.2
Personality disorders	5.6	3.6
Organic psychoses	3.5	3.6
Other diagnoses	5.6	5.5

Source: Cooper JE, Kendell RE, Gurland BJ. *Psychiatric Diagnosis in New York and London: a comparative study of mental hospital admissions.* London: Oxford University Press; 1972.

occurrence of the cancer in the developed country may simply reflect the fact that it has an efficient, well-maintained cancer registry that detects and records most cases of cancer that occur. The cancer registry of a developing country, perhaps covering a rural population that does not readily have access to medical services, may not be so efficient at detecting cases of the cancer. This does not necessarily mean that they are not occurring

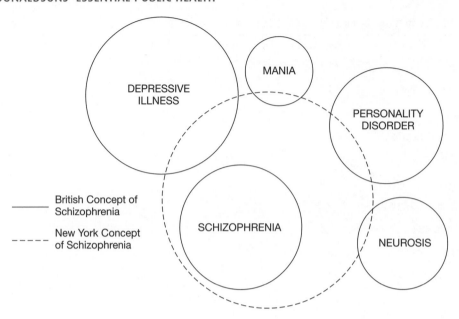

Figure 2.1 The difference between the New York and British concepts of schizophrenia
Source: Cooper JE, Kendall RE, Gurland BJ. *Psychiatric Diagnosis in New York and London: a comparative study of mental hospital admissions.* London: Oxford University Press; 1972.

as often as in the developed country, merely that they are not being recorded.

This is a rather obvious example to illustrate the importance of being aware of possible differences in disease detection rates when making comparisons. This pitfall can be encountered when comparing disease frequency from region to region, city to city, and hospital to hospital, not just between developing and developed countries.

A particularly common source of fallacious reasoning about disease differences between populations is when studies use hospital inpatient data. This is also an issue of differential case ascertainment. Because the true incidence of the condition in the population is seldom known, it must be remembered that hospital cases of the disease can only approximate incidence in

diseases where a high proportion of people who develop them are hospitalised. Since there are relatively few diseases that fall into this category, differences between populations in the occurrence of a particular disease based upon studies of hospital admission rates should be treated with great caution. They are likely to reflect differential admission rates for the condition rather than differences in the true incidence of the disease in the population (Table 2.4).

An example is the analysis depicted in Figure 2.2. This shows the rate of cataract surgery for planned episodes of care in different parts of Ontario, Canada. Thus it is describing the treatment of patients who have a disease of the eye causing impaired vision. Geographical variation between services in the different localities of Ontario was marked: the service with the highest rate performed surgery 50% more often than the service with the lowest rate.

The incidence of cataract is strongly age-related, so it is important that the comparisons in Figure 2.2 are made after age adjustment. However, the error in interpreting this variation would be to regard operation rate as a proxy for disease incidence. Someone drawing such a conclusion might start to explore theories as to why eye disease was more common in some parts of Ontario than others. There may indeed be genuine geographical variation in the incidence of cataracts, but a study based on surgical treatment rates is not the way to establish it.

Is the Population at Risk Accurately Defined?

In any measure of disease frequency, it will be necessary to relate the number of cases of the disease to the population from which they arose. A difference between two populations in the incidence of a disease or in mortality from a particular cause may be related to differences in the characteristics of the populations (such as age and sex) that affect the rate of disease. Once such characteristics are corrected for, an example being through standardisation (*see* Chapter 1), the differences in disease experience are no longer apparent. It is important to recognise this possibility at an early stage before too much interest is shown in apparent major variations in disease frequency.

It is also important to be sure that all cases of the disease or deaths are related to an identifiable (ideally) geographically-defined population for which accurate estimates are available of size and structure. Hospital catchment populations, which can change rapidly over time and may vary according to the type of diseases being examined, are notoriously unreliable in this respect.

THE APPROACH OF DESCRIPTIVE EPIDEMIOLOGY

Provided these limitations are always borne in mind when comparisons of disease frequency are being made, important

Table 2.4 Possible reasons for variations in surgical operation rates between populations

Demographic differences
Different rates of underlying illness
Random fluctuation
Availability of resources or supply
Clinical judgement varies
Different patient expectation or demand
Prevailing clinical traditions vary
Inaccuracies in data sources

Source: McPherson K. Why do variations occur? In: Anderson TF, Mooney G, editors. *The Challenges of Medical Practice Variations.* London: Macmillan; 1989.

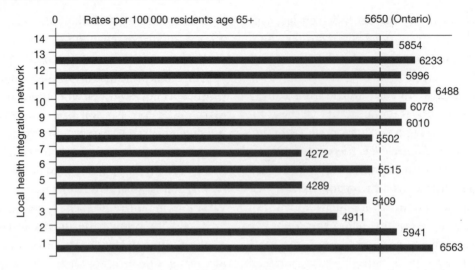

Figure 2.2 Age- and sex-adjusted rates of cataract surgery per 100 000 residents aged 65 years and older in Ontario by local area

Source: Hatch W, Cernat G, Singer S, *et al.* A 10-year population-based cohort of cataract surgery rates in Ontario. *Can J Ophthalmol.* 2007; **42**: 552–6.

observations may result from examining the pattern of diseases within populations.

Beyond simply the interest that is engendered by studying any population health problem, the process of descriptive epidemiology has three specific purposes: firstly, to identify the scope for research into the causation of diseases or other health problems that might lead ultimately to their prevention; secondly, to help plan services for the whole population; and thirdly, to highlight populations or groups within the population that are in special need of health service initiatives.

Example of a Descriptive Epidemiological Approach Yielding Clues to Causation

Figure 2.3 shows the findings of a study that used routinely available data to describe the trend over time in mortality from asthma.

The most striking observation from this trend was the rapid increase in the mortality rate from the disease that occurred in boys aged 10 to 14 years over the period from the mid-1950s to the mid-1960s.

This led the investigators to seek an explanation for the tragic apparent increase in loss of life and try to discover whether the trend might be reversible. However, before going further it was important for them to bear in mind that such a change may be artefactual rather than real. For example, was it possible that asthma was being more frequently used as an underlying cause of death by doctors completing death certificates in circumstances where previously some other terminology had been used? This was excluded by the investigators, who found no downward trend in deaths from other respiratory disease diagnoses to coincide with the apparent increase in asthma deaths.

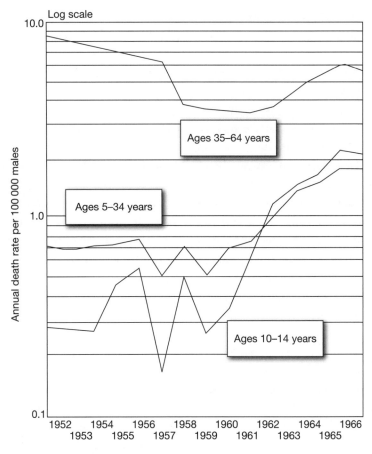

Figure 2.3 Asthma mortality in males in England and Wales from 1952 to 1966
Source: Speizer FE, Doll R, Heaf P. Observations on recent increase in mortality from asthma. *BMJ.* 1968; **1**: 335–9.

Having excluded this and other artefactual possibilities for the increase in asthma mortality, two other explanations were considered. One was that the disease (asthma) had become more common (the incidence had increased) but that the proportion of asthmatic children who died from their disease remained static (i.e., that the case fatality rate remained stable) or, alternatively, that the disease had not become more common (the incidence was stable) but that the children who developed the disease died

more often from it (the case fatality rate had risen).

The investigators in this study could find no evidence from other data sources to suggest an increase in the incidence of asthma and therefore concluded that the rise in mortality shown in Figure 2.3 was due to an increase in case fatality. There was a strong suspicion that the change was due to medications used to treat childhood asthma at that time, and the next phase of the study was to seek information from the general practitioners of the children who had died of asthma about the treatment used prior to death.

At the time, corticosteroids had been introduced into clinical practice, and one of their known side effects was suppression of the adrenal gland. Therefore there was a suspicion that this group of drugs may be implicated in causing the deaths of asthmatic children. However, the survey of general practitioners revealed that this was not the case, but that bronchodilators in the form of pressurised inhalers had been used in a high proportion of cases. A high-dosage form of isoprenaline, administered in the form of an inhaler, was the drug most commonly involved. This drug can, amongst other side effects, produce abnormal heart rhythms when taken to excess, and there was clearly a possibility that children self-administering the drug to relieve acute bronchospasm might have used it indiscriminately and excessively when symptoms were severe.

This drug had been available without a doctor's prescription. As a result of the findings of the study, it was subsequently made available only on prescription. Warnings were circulated to all doctors about these side effects, and printed warnings were also included in the instructional material for patients using these pressurised inhalers. As a result, mortality from asthma declined. Similar epidemics of asthma deaths occurred in Scotland, Ireland, Australia and New Zealand. The drug was not sold in the Netherlands (a point that becomes relevant in the description that follows).

This is a classic example of descriptive epidemiological investigation leading to successful preventive action. Usually, however, it would first be necessary to move from the suggestion of causation created by the descriptive approach to investigate the presumed causal factors using more specialised epidemiological methods before drawing firm conclusions and taking action. In this case, however, the findings were of sufficient importance that immediate action was justified.

The subject of preventable deaths in asthma continued to be controversial. While the trend in Britain, and in some other Western countries, declined following the 1960s, a further increase subsequently occurred in New Zealand, and the cause of this has not been fully elucidated. Studies strongly suggested that another inhaled beta agonist drug – fenoterol – may have been associated, and a health warning was issued in New Zealand. Fenoterol was then effectively withdrawn in New Zealand by removing it from the Drug Tariff, and this was accompanied by an immediate fall in the asthma death rate. Unlike in England and the Netherlands, this drug was available without prescription in New Zealand.

Other experts have disagreed with the assertion that these trends in asthma mortality are treatment-related. This shows that descriptive epidemiology does not provide proof of causation, only pointers to further investigation. Nevertheless, the time trends represent a fascinating epidemiological story and a challenge to public health in identifying a source of potentially preventable death (Figure 2.4).

PATTERNS OF DISEASE: TIME, PLACE, PERSON

The technique of descriptive epidemiology traditionally examines disease patterns across three main dimensions: in relation to time, in relation to place, and in relation to person.

DESCRIBING DISEASE IN RELATION TO TIME

When describing the way in which the occurrence of a disease varies with time, there are three common methods of examining the relationship: seasonal variation, epidemic curves and long-term (secular) trends. However, any temporal cyclicity may be studied (for example, diurnal rhythms or patterns).

Seasonal Variation

Many diseases exhibit seasonal variations in their occurrence: peaks in the frequency of these diseases occur regularly at particular times of the year. Respiratory infections, for example, are more common in the colder months. In some non-infectious conditions, seasonal variations have been clearly demonstrated, but no satisfactory explanation has, as yet, indicated why they should occur. For example, Figure 2.5 shows apparent seasonal variation in the onset of insulin-dependent diabetes mellitus in children. The data are derived from a large study in Sweden. There was a peak occurrence in the autumn and winter. Data were published in the early 1960s that showed a greater incidence of childhood acute lymphoblastic leukaemia in the summer months. This has led to the idea that these diseases in children maybe caused or precipitated in genetically susceptible

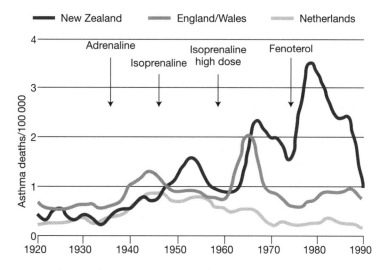

Figure 2.4 Time trends in asthma mortality (aged 5–34 years) in three countries in relation to introduction of inhalation therapies

Source: Blauw GJ, Westendorp RGJ. Asthma deaths in New Zealand: whodunnit? *Lancet.* 1995; **345**: 2–3.

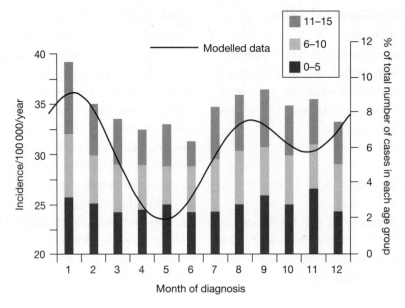

Figure 2.5 Seasonal variation of type 1 diabetes mellitus in south-east Sweden
Source: Samuelsson U, Carstensen J, Löfman O, *et al.* Seasonal variation in the diagnosis of type 1 diabetes in south-east Sweden. *Diabetes Res Clin Pract.* 2007; **76**: 75–81.

individuals by an infectious agent, possibly a virus.

Such findings must be interpreted cautiously because they raise questions about the extent of detection of cases and the way in which the onset of the disease is determined. Even if such a seasonal pattern is established, it is not proof of a causal link. However, it is a further example of how examination of the pattern of disease can provide a clue that may prompt further investigation of the relationship between genetic and environmental factors, which in turn may lead to a greater understanding of the causal mechanism.

Epidemic Curves

The increase in the frequency of a disease above its baseline level of occurrence over a relatively short period of time is termed an epidemic.

Sometimes the term is also used to describe increase in frequency, over a period of years, of diseases that have had a stable (and lower) level of occurrence for decades. Coronary heart disease and lung cancer are often referred to as the modern epidemics. Trends over years, or decades and longer, however, are usually described as secular trends.

Secular Trends

The study of the pattern of diseases over long periods of time, years, decades or even centuries, highlights many changes. Major diseases of the past have faded from importance, while others have become increasingly prominent.

As will be clear from the discussion earlier

in the chapter (particularly the asthma mortality example), there are many pitfalls in interpreting secular trends in the frequency of a disease. Its true frequency may not have changed over time, but improvements in methods of detection and diagnosis, fashions in diagnosis and changes in the criteria used to define or classify it may suggest that it has.

Some of the most spectacular secular changes in the pattern of disease in industrialised countries have involved the decline in the importance of the infectious diseases as major health problems and causes of death. The decline in infant and childhood mortality, largely as a result of general measures (sanitary reforms, improvements in living standards and nutrition) that reduced the impact of the infectious diseases, improved life expectation for modern Britons compared to their Victorian counterparts. These changes are discussed in detail in Chapter 8 in relation to population ageing. This secular change in mortality from infectious diseases in turn, therefore, had wider implications beyond its immediate impact for the size and structure of the population.

Tuberculosis was one of the great scourges of the recent past, often referred to as the 'white man's plague'. Bunyan, in his writings, gave it the chilling and evocative title 'Captain of the men of death'. In 1855, for example, 13% of deaths from all causes were attributed to tuberculosis. Although the disease is now a much less common cause of mortality and morbidity, it is becoming an important health problem again worldwide – particularly in ethnic minorities in the United Kingdom, where it has begun a resurgence (*see* Chapter 9).

The decline in mortality from tuberculosis (Figure 2.6) had begun before the advent of specific medical measures. This highlights another principle in interpreting secular trends. If the frequency of a disease is already declining, it must not be assumed that the introduction of a particular measure has brought it about.

Examining time trends in health service usage can also provide important insights. Figure 2.7 shows changes over only a six-year period in treatments for coronary artery disease. In the 1980s, the only real option for achieving 'revascularisation' for someone with obstructed coronary arteries was a coronary artery bypass graft, a surgical operation in which blood vessels taken from other parts of the body are used to bypass diseased coronary segments. An alternative to this open-heart surgery emerged with the advent of angioplasty – a procedure in which a balloon is inflated within the vessel so as to widen it. With stents (cylindrical meshes to hold open a vessel once it has been widened), angioplasty became a true alternative to bypass surgery in some (but not all) types of coronary artery disease. Figure 2.7 shows the clinical popularity of this less invasive technique compared with bypass surgery. In some parts of the United Kingdom, immediate angioplasty is being used for patients with acute heart attacks, transforming the management of this condition. It is an aspiration to make this service widely available within the NHS.

DESCRIBING DISEASE IN RELATION TO PLACE

Description of the pattern of disease in

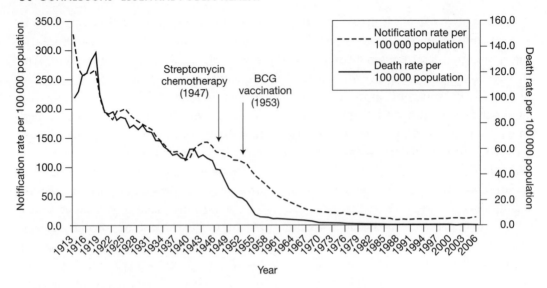

Figure 2.6 Tuberculosis notification and death rates, England and Wales
Source: Office for National Statistics, 2008.

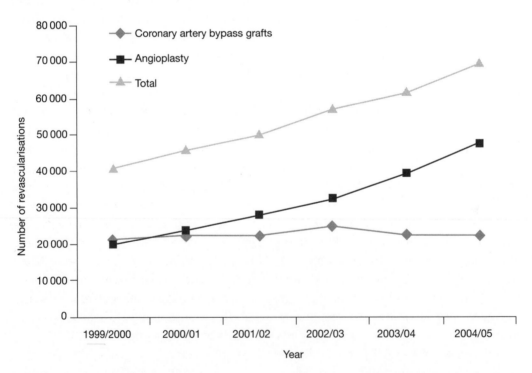

Figure 2.7 The growth in interventions to treat coronary artery disease has been entirely in angioplasty rather than open heart surgery
Source: Chief Medical Officer. *On the State of Public Health 2005*. London: Department of Health; 2006.

geographical terms can be undertaken in a number of ways, although there are three main aspects: national variation (within a country), international variation (between countries) and smaller area variation (for example, urban/rural).

National Variation

For many diseases in Britain, there is variation in morbidity and mortality rates between different geographical areas. Chronic bronchitis, for example, is more common in the urban industrial areas of northern England than in the rural areas of the south. Other diseases are also distributed in a similar way. The overall result is that general mortality within Britain is lower for the population of southern England and

East Anglia and higher for parts of northern and northwestern England, Wales and Scotland.

The mortality from chronic liver disease (including cirrhosis) illustrates this geographical variation. This disease is a marker of alcohol consumption and its hazardous effect on health. Men in the North West and North East of England had significantly higher death rates than the national average, while those in the East of England and South East fared significantly better. The north–south divide was not so pronounced for females, although women in the North West of England died significantly more often than the national average from chronic liver disease (Figure 2.8).

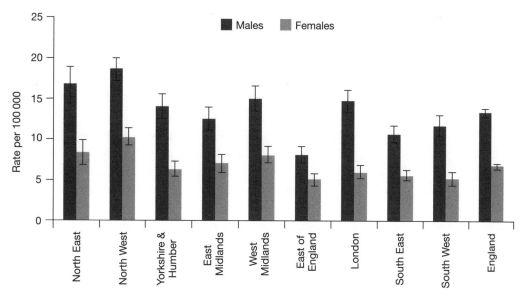

Figure 2.8 Rate of mortality (directly standardised rate) from chronic liver disease including cirrhosis per 100 000 population, 2004–06
Source: Association of Public Health Observatories, England.

International Variation

Many diseases vary in frequency between different countries, and on occasions this may give clues to causation. Table 2.5 shows the variation in the prevalence of neural tube defects (spina bifida, anencephaly and encephalocele) between populations in European countries. Registers of congenital malformations had been established to monitor the occurrence of such birth defects and enable comparisons to be made.

As Table 2.5 shows, there was considerable variation between the different populations. Moreover, rates were generally higher amongst births occurring in the British and Irish centres than those in many other European countries.

The reasons why some countries show a higher prevalence of neural tube defects than others is not known, but the observation emphasises the need for studies to elucidate causation. Until it becomes possible to prevent all cases of neural tube defect, reducing its impact requires folate supplementation preconceptually and successful antenatal detection programmes, coupled with the offer of termination of affected pregnancies (see also Chapter 6).

Smaller Area Variation

Mesothelioma is a cancer of the outer lining of the lungs (pleura). About eight in every 10 cases of mesothelioma are caused by exposure to asbestos dust. This cancer has a long latent period and develops between 15 and 30 years (sometimes longer) after exposure to asbestos.

The data in Figure 2.9 show variation in the occurrence of mesothelioma cases in towns and cities in the South West region of England. The greatest numbers of cases are in local authorities with a history of shipbuilding (Plymouth, Portsmouth, Southampton and Bristol).

Another interesting feature of this analysis is the striking difference in male to female ratios in the incidence of the disease between Plymouth (25:1), Portsmouth (9:1), Southampton (8:1) and Bristol (3:1). Investigations have suggested that in Plymouth, males with mesothelioma predominantly worked in shipyards that provided onsite laundry services for workers' clothing. This is in contrast to Portsmouth and Southampton, which did not have onsite laundries, so workers there brought their overalls home for their wives to wash. These women were then also exposed to asbestos dust, and this explains the higher occurrence of mesothelioma amongst women. This is just an hypothesis, but it again illustrates how descriptive epidemiological data can be a first step to exploring disease causation.

DESCRIBING DISEASE IN RELATION TO PERSON

There are many more ways of examining the pattern of disease in relation to the characteristics of people than by either time or place. Most diseases show a distinct pattern when looked at by age, sex, occupation and social status. In addition, there are diseases that vary with ethnic origin and with marital status. Some examples of patterns of disease in relation to some of these variables are described in this section, though there are many others.

Table 2.5 Prevalence of neural tube defects (including live births, foetal deaths/still births from 20 weeks' gestation and termination of pregnancy for foetal anomaly) in 17 EUROCAT registries, 1980–2006

Registry	N	Rate per 10 000
Glasgow (UK)	633	25.10
Sofia (Bulgaria)	76	19.87
Mainz (Germany)	117	19.70
Ukraine	99	18.27
Dublin (Ireland)	1049	18.05
CARIS Wales (UK)	466	16.13
Wessex (UK)	452	13.25
Cork and Kerry (Ireland)	80	12.70
Paris (France)	1176	12.42
Malta	110	11.12
Netherlands (NL)	424	9.97
Antwerp (Belgium)	221	9.33
Barcelona (Spain)	140	9.21
Styria (Austria)	217	8.50
Hungary	406	7.23
Tuscany (Italy)	336	6.69
Zagreb (Croatia)	75	5.20

Source: EUROCAT Working Group, www.eurocat.ulster.ac.uk/pubdata/tables.html.

Age and Sex

Almost all diseases show a marked variation with age. Indeed, mortality rates from all causes show a distinctive pattern (Figure 2.10). Once the first few years of life have been passed, there are relatively few deaths per unit of population until the age of about 35 years, when death rates begin to increase sharply with each successively higher age group.

There are differences, too, in the importance of various causes of death at each age. Figure 2.11 shows that in the younger age groups, accidents and violence are a more important cause of death than diseases, while in the older age group, cancer and diseases of the respiratory and circulatory systems come to the fore.

Figure 2.12 shows that even within a disease category there can be marked age and sex patterns. In a study of fracture incidence, the risk increased rapidly with age amongst males until aged 15–24 years, after which it declined until there was a second peak at 85 years and older. This reflects a higher participation in sports, other activities and violence amongst boys, teenagers and young adult males than amongst their

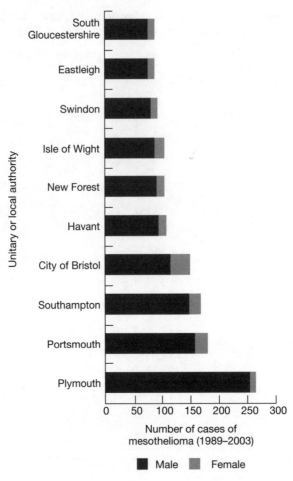

Figure 2.9 The 10 unitary and local authorities in the South West, Hampshire and Isle of Wight with the highest number of cases of mesothelioma over a 15-year period
Source: Chief Medical Officer. *On the State of Public Health 2005.* London: Department of Health; 2006.

female counterparts. For girls and women, there is a peak in early childhood but no early adult peak, and there is a sustained earlier rise in incidence from 55 years onwards (Figure 2.12).

Figure 2.13 is derived from the same study of fracture incidence, but this time compares the size of the male and the female incidence rate at each site in two broad age groups: people over 55 years of age and people under 55 years of age. The incidence rate for males and females in each age group is compared by means of their ratio. The purpose of analysing these data in this way was to try to throw light on the possible influence of menopausal changes on fracture incidence.

There was a male fracture preponderance for the under-55s and a female excess for the over-55s. The effect was most marked

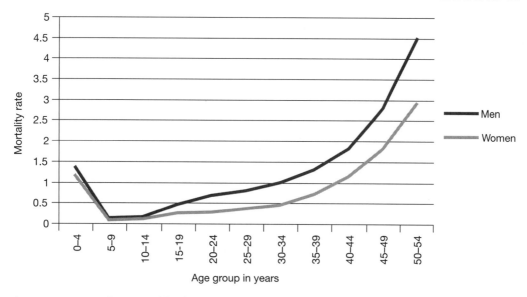

Figure 2.10 Mortality rates (deaths per 1000 population) in England and Wales, 2006
Source: Office for National Statistics.

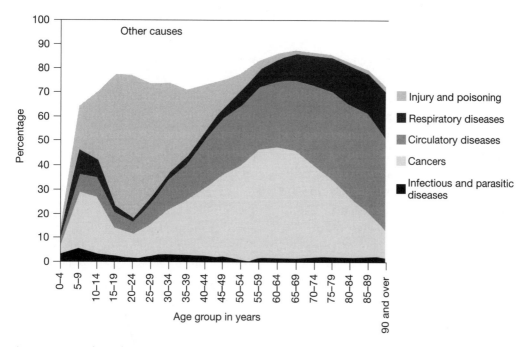

Figure 2.11 Selected causes of death by age, England and Wales, 2006
Source: Office for National Statistics.

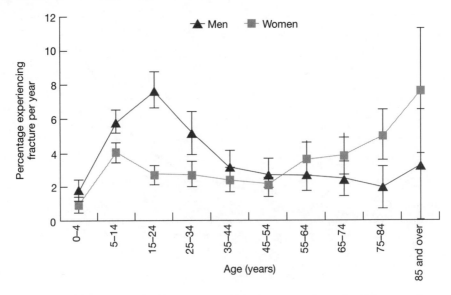

Figure 2.12 Annual fracture incidence per 100 people, by age and sex, English general population, 2002–04
Source: Donaldson LJ, Reckless IP, Scholes S, *et al.* The epidemiology of fractures in England. *J Epidemiol Community Health.* 2008; **62**: 174–80.

for fractures of the trunk (which included vertebral fractures) and long bones (which included hip fractures).

This age and sex pattern in fracture incidence at different sites points to a number of possible explanations: osteoporotic fall in bone mass around the time of the menopause; a greater propensity to falls amongst older women; and neuromuscular deterioration with age, which may reduce the degree of skeletal protection when trauma occurs.

As with any descriptive epidemiological data, these interesting age and sex differences do not provide direct evidence of causal association, but they do point the way for further epidemiological studies aimed at elucidating causation and possibly provide scope for prevention of an important public health problem.

Occupation and Social Status

The study of mortality in groups of workers in particular occupations or industries has a long tradition, and through the years it has uncovered particular risk factors for particular diseases that have arisen in the working environment.

In 1911, the Registrar General in Britain first used a hierarchical classification of social class based on occupation. The move to collect and present data in this way was prompted by the concern expressed by many of the social reformers of the time – such as Charles Booth (1840–1916) and Seebohm Rowntree (1871–1954) – about the high rates of mortality amongst the poor; in particular, infant mortality. The classification grouped people according to the skill required for, and the social standing carried by, their particular occupation.

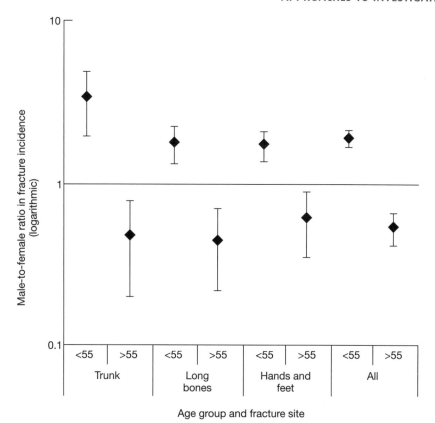

Figure 2.13 Male-to-female fracture incidence ratios (age-standardised) by age group and fracture site, English general population, 2002–04
Source: Donaldson LJ, Reckless IP, Scholes S, *et al.* The epidemiology of fractures in England. *J Epidemiol Community Health.* 2008; **62**: 174–80.

Data on occupation continue to be used to produce various methods of social and economic classification. Broadly, the assumption underlying this approach is that someone's occupation is a good guide to his or her position within society.

A very wide range of approaches to defining social status have been used by research workers or governmental agencies in different countries. Most measures take, either singly or as a composite measure, three aspects about the person: occupation, education and income.

In Britain, occupation remains the main basis for social and economic classifications. Detailed data about occupation are collected at birth, marriage, death, at the time of the census and in responses given to government social surveys.

Two major classification systems were used in the twentieth century. The first is the allocation of people into one of (usually) five social classes based on their occupation. This was first used in the Registrar General's Annual Report for 1911. The second is the classification of people based on employment status, size of employing organisation and occupation into one of 17 categories (usually collapsed into six categories) called socio-economic groups. This was first used in 1951. It is important to be aware of these classifications. While they have now been replaced by a single National Statistics Socio-economic Classification (NS-SEC) (see below), historical reports and studies, as well as presentation of trends, often refer to the old classifications of social class and socio-economic groups.

The National Statistics Socio-economic Classification (NS-SEC) was introduced in 2001. It is occupationally based but covers the whole adult population, including students, those who have never worked and the long-term unemployed. It is usually presented in eight categories (Table 2.6).

Most analyses of death or disease by these social groups show an adverse trend moving down the social scale.

Figure 2.14 shows the familiar gradient in mortality, while Figure 2.15 shows that self-reported illness or disability were very much higher for people in routine occupations than those in higher managerial and professional groups. Those who had never worked or were long-term unemployed had even poorer levels of self-reported health.

Ethnic Origin

The pattern of health of migrant groups in Britain became clearer during the 1980s and 1990s when ethnicity was a more commonly recorded variable. However, most studies of mortality still rely heavily on country of birth, and therefore second-generation migrants are often excluded. Valuable understanding of the generational effects on immigrant health has been gained from the Office for National Statistics Longitudinal Survey, which is based on the tracking of the health experience of a one percent sample of the 1971 census of the whole population of England and Wales.

In relation to all adult men, all-cause

Table 2.6 The National Statistics Socio-economic Classification analytic classes

1	Higher managerial and professional occupations
	1.1 Large employers and higher managerial occupations
	1.2 Higher professional occupations
2	Lower managerial and professional occupations
3	Intermediate occupations
4	Small employers and own account workers
5	Lower supervisory and technical occupations
6	Semi-routine occupations
7	Routine occupations
8	Never worked and long-term unemployed

Source: Office for National Statistics.

Rate per 100 000

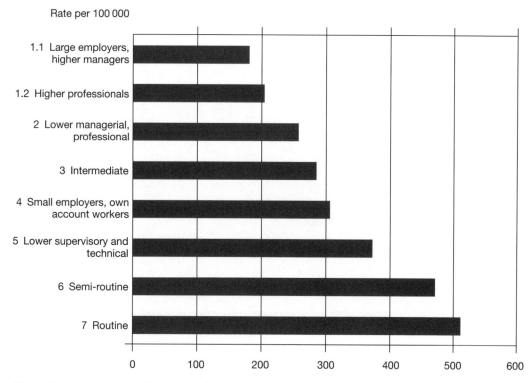

Figure 2.14 Age-standardised mortality rate by NS-SEC: men aged 25–64 years, England and Wales, 2001–03
Source: Office for National Statistics.

mortality is generally higher for people born outside England and Wales. When specific causes of death are examined, particularly striking is the relatively high rate of death from circulatory disease amongst men born in the Indian subcontinent (Figure 2.16).

The study of disease and mortality in populations of different ethnic origin can provide important clues to disease causation. There is a particular tradition in descriptive epidemiology of studying the disease and mortality experience of migrant populations to see whether their disease experience remains as in their country of origin or changes to match that of their new country of residence.

The study of an ethnic minority population that retains distinct cultural traditions and practices in comparison to a long-standing indigenous population can also yield clues to disease causation. Figure 2.17 compares the occurrence of cancer at different sites for Asians (defined as people not of United Kingdom descent who originate from India, Pakistan or Bangladesh or people of Indian or Pakistani descent who originate from East Africa) and non-Asians living in Leicestershire, England.

A relatively complex statistical approach was necessary to compare the incidence of cancer in the two populations, because, at the time of the study, concurrent denominator

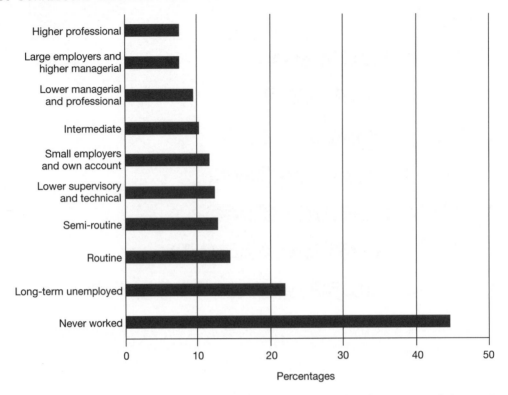

Figure 2.15 Age-standardised rates of long-term illness or disability that restricts daily activities by NS-SEC: England and Wales, April 2001
Source: Office for National Statistics.

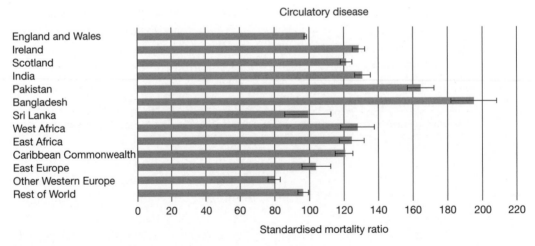

Figure 2.16 Standardised mortality ratios for circulatory disease by country of birth, residents of England and Wales, aged 20–69 years, 1999–2003
Source: Office for National Statistics.

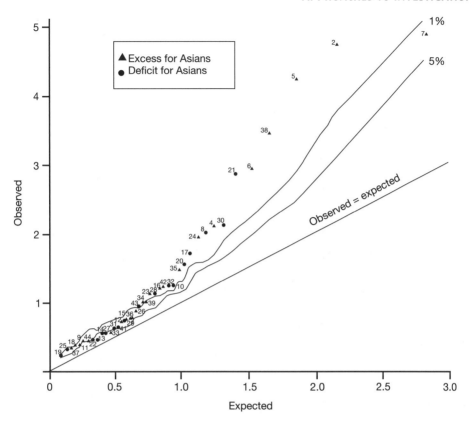

Site of cancer: 1 lip; 2 tongue; 3 salivary glands; 4 gum, floor of mouth, other mouth; 5 oro-, naso-, hypopharynx; 6 other oral cavity; 7 oesophagus; 8 stomach; 9 small intestine; 10 colon, rectum; 11 liver, bile ducts, gallbladder, extrahepatic bile ducts; 12 pancreas; 13 peritoneum; 14 other and ill-defined (digestive organs, and peritoneum); 15 nasal cavities, etc; 16 larynx; 17 trachea, bronchus, lung; 18 pleura, thymus, heart; 19 bone and cartilage, connective tissue; 20 malignant melanoma; 21 other skin; 22 breast; 23 uterus unspecified; 24 cervix; 25 placenta; 26 body of uterus; 27 ovary and tubes; 28 other female genitalia; 29 prostate; 30 testis; 31 penis and other male genital; 32 bladder, kidney, ureter; 33 eye; 34 brain, other nervous system; 35 thyroid; 36 other endocrine; 37 other ill-defined sites; 38 lymph nodes, other and unspecified; 39 secondary of respiratory and digestive system and other site, unspecified site; 40 lymphosarcoma and reticulosarcoma; 41 Hodgkin's disease; 42 other lymphoid; 43 multiple myeloma, and 44 leukaemia.

Figure 2.17 Contributions of each cancer site to the overall chi-squared test with stimulation envelopes for 1% and 5% levels of significance (log units)

Source: Donaldson LJ, Clayton DG. Occurrence of cancer in Asians and non-Asians. *J Epidemiol Community Health.* 1984; **38**: 203–7.

data on the Asian population were not available (the study was before the time of the 1991 Census, when ethnic origin questions enabled much more reliable information on the size and structure of the ethnic minority populations to be made available).

It is not necessary to understand the details of the methodology for the purpose of this illustration, merely to note (as is shown in Figure 2.17) the apparent excess (over the 'expected' occurrence) amongst Asians of cancers of the tongue, oral cavity, pharynx and oesophagus and of some other sites.

It is, of course, important to exclude spurious explanations of the kind discussed earlier and particularly to consider the possibility that the findings might be due to selective immigration. In this case, could Asian people have come to Britain because they were already suffering from cancer (for example, to obtain treatment)? This is always an important potential explanation to consider in studies of immigrant populations. However, it was considered implausible in this particular example.

Of particular relevance to the excess of Asian cancer cases at the particular sites found in the study shown in Figure 2.17 is the habit of betel chewing. In countries where betel is chewed, its common accompaniment in the chew, tobacco, has been implicated in the causation of cancerous and precancerous lesions of the oral cavity. It has further been suggested that elements in the betel chewing habit other than tobacco – that is, the areca nut, the betel leaf, or the lime additive – may be causally linked to oral cancer, as well as to pharyngeal and oesophageal cancer.

The Asian population, one of the main ethnic minority populations of present-day Britain, is still relatively young in its age structure. Chronic diseases such as cancer are less common. This will not always be so. As the population ages, there will be a need to be able to anticipate the main health problems of this community. Observational studies, such as the one illustrated here, can never prove cause and effect, but they do provide important pointers to areas where further epidemiological inquiry is required. They also indicate a need to establish the prevalence within the ethnic minority population of traditional practices and behaviours that may be of public health importance.

THE VALUE AND LIMITATIONS OF DESCRIPTIVE EPIDEMIOLOGY

The previous sections have given examples of the use of descriptive epidemiological data. When such data are used to highlight a disease problem, health trend or a major difference in disease occurrence between or within populations, important insights can be generated about disease causation. As has been explained, interpretation must be made with caution – understanding the limitations of such studies and the potential for fallacious conclusions must always be uppermost in the investigator's mind.

Observational epidemiology is often criticised or denigrated when compared to other more formal methods of epidemiological research. However, even brief reflection brings to mind many important findings that originally stemmed from description of disease patterns and subsequently led to greater understanding of disease causation,

Table 2.7 Examples of important causal associations uncovered by descriptive epidemiology

Smoking and cancer
Radiation exposure and cancer
Lipids and coronary heart disease
Blood pressure and stroke
Sleeping position and sudden infant death
Folate and neural tube defects
Late circumcision and HIV infection
Aspirin use and colorectal cancer
Hormone replacement therapy and breast cancer

Source: Rothwell PM, Bhatia M. Reporting of observational studies. *BMJ.* 2007; **335**: 783–4. (See paper for original reference to each causal association.)

public health action or treatment interventions (Table 2.7).

In response, others[1] have pointed out that some conclusions from observational studies alone have been seriously flawed. For example, in cardiology, the protective effects of female hormones and the advantage of dual over single chamber pacing seemed to demonstrate a benefit and influenced practice, only to be 'disproved' by subsequent randomised controlled trials.

The lesson is that observational studies can sometimes prove a causal link or a benefit, but they should usually be the starting point for further analysis and formal evaluation, rarely the definitive conclusion.

CROSS-SECTIONAL OR PREVALENCE STUDIES

The previous sections have dealt with the techniques of descriptive epidemiology in which comparisons are made in mortality or the occurrence of disease between populations, within groups of the same

population and over time. Most of the examples given derived the information for making such comparisons from routinely available health data.

Quite often, it will be important to describe the size of a health problem within a population but routinely available data are not adequate to fulfil this task. For example, a primary care trust wishing to establish the prevalence of dementia within its population would not readily be able to do so from available sources of data. Leaving aside problems with the quality of death certification in the elderly, mortality statistics would completely underestimate the problem because only a relatively small proportion of people with the disease at any one time are dying from it. Similarly, statistics derived from hospital admissions (whether to psychiatric or general wards) would also underestimate the problem because a high proportion of people with dementia might be expected to reside within the community and not be in contact with hospital services. It is in such circumstances that consideration may be given to carrying out a survey to gather data directly about members of the population to gain a more accurate estimate of the prevalence of the disease in question.

If such a special study is to be carried out, it will also usually be widened to include the gathering of other relevant information on the population under study, other than purely the disease of interest. Thus a prevalence study of the extent of dementia in the population would be unlikely to limit itself to assessing elderly people for the presence or absence of dementia: it would also gather data on factors such as their domestic circumstances, their capacity for self-care and their physical status.

Surveys in which information is gathered directly from members of a population can be carried out for reasons other than to establish the prevalence of a disease, and this section describes the general approach to such surveys and why they may be carried out. Notwithstanding the precise purpose of a particular population survey, two general terms are often used to describe them: prevalence studies and cross-sectional studies. Both terms emphasise a key feature of such surveys – that they describe the population at a point in time, like a snapshot.

AIMS OF CROSS-SECTIONAL SURVEYS

One purpose in carrying out a cross-sectional survey is to establish the prevalence of a disease in the population. Another is to describe the characteristics of the population when there are no routinely available data to do this. This may be to establish a particular aspect of the population's need for health or social services or to establish the prevalence of risk factors (for example, intravenous drug abuse, cigarette smoking, obesity), which can be the basis of health promotion programmes. A population may also be surveyed to establish people's views on health or health services, thereby yielding information not otherwise available that may also be of major importance in planning and developing services. Whatever the aims of a cross-sectional study, many of the aspects of the methodology will be broadly similar.

OUTLINE OF METHODOLOGY

The cross-sectional study is a type of epidemiological investigation that seeks to gather data on one or more aspects or characterics of individuals resident in that population at a particular point in time. Because it will seldom be feasible or necessary to gather such data about every member of the population, usually a sample is chosen to be studied. On the basis of the findings within the sample, general conclusions are drawn about the population.

CHOOSING THE STUDY POPULATION

Assembling the population for this kind of study involves gaining access to a representative list of members of the population and then applying the technique of sampling to this list.

Sampling

A number of important considerations should be borne in mind when choosing a sample. Uppermost is the need to appreciate that, in taking a sample, the underlying objective is to make true statements about the population itself.

The technique of drawing a sample has an important bearing on this process. There are two main ways of obtaining a sample of people: firstly, by the quota method and secondly, randomly.

Quota Sampling

The quota sample is often employed by market research organisations. This method involves the interviewer seeking a specified number of people to fit into a pre-agreed sample configuration. Men or women of particular ages or social backgrounds may be sought out, for example, by approaching people in the street. This type of sampling is generally unsatisfactory because it is unlikely to result in a sample that is representative of the whole population. For instance, a sample of middle-aged men, drawn by quota sampling in a shopping centre in mid-morning, would be unlikely to be truly representative of all middle-aged men in the particular town. Groups such as the unemployed or shift workers would tend to be over-represented.

Random Sampling

The basic and most commonly used sampling method in survey research is the random sample. There are a number of different ways of obtaining a random sample, but all have the following in common: the results can be generalised to the total population from which the random sample was drawn and the precision of the estimates derived from the sample can be calculated statistically.

Choice of a Sampling Frame

The first step in drawing a random sample is to construct a suitable sampling frame. A sampling frame is merely a list (actual or notional) of the population. The nature of the sampling frame will vary according to the purposes of the survey. A sample for a survey of infant feeding practices might be drawn from all birth registrations in a particular area. In a survey of occupational diseases, the sampling frame might be the employment records of particular firms.

Many population surveys in public health will aim to conduct an investigation in a sample of the population of a geographically defined area, say a strategic health authority. Obtaining a suitable sampling frame (i.e., a list of the residents of that authority) from which to draw a suitably sized sample survey is not a straightforward proposition. A traditional approach is to use the electoral roll, which supplies a list of people qualified to vote listed by the street within the different electoral wards of a town or city. As a sampling frame representative of the general population, however, this has serious limitations. The most obvious is that people below voting age are excluded. In addition, the rolls often become out of date as people move into or out of the area.

As more general practitioners have combined into large group practices, the potential for the use of age-sex registers as representative sampling frames has increased. It is important here, too, to realise that the register may be inflated by people who have died or left the area but whose names have not yet been removed from it.

Having obtained a suitable sampling frame, there are a number of different approaches to obtaining the random sample. The most direct is to choose people at random from the sampling frame until the required sample size is achieved (simple random sample).

A simple 10% random sample of a population of 1000 people would involve picking at random 100 names from amongst the 1000 listed. It is absolutely essential, however, that each time a name is chosen, every individual has an equal chance of being picked. One technique for ensuring that this is the case is through the use of a table of random numbers. In the example above, the people in the population are numbered from 000 to 999. Using a special table of random numbers, 100 numbers are then picked, and the people corresponding to the numbers listed become the sample. Modern computer technology can be used to generate a random sample if the sampling frame is held on a computer database.

Another approach is to draw a systematic random sample in which individuals are picked from the sampling frame in sequence. A 10% random sample drawn in this way would involve choosing every tenth name on the list (a 1-in-10 sample), only the first selection being made from the table of random numbers. This is often a much more convenient way of drawing a sample. Systematic sampling is usually a perfectly satisfactory method, but it depends on people or items listed on a sampling frame being arranged in a way that does not introduce bias. For example, a 1-in-10 systematic sample drawn from a list of married people in which the husband's name always came first would result in either every person chosen being female or every person being male.

Stratification

This may be used to ensure adequate representation of different sections of the population. The population is divided into sections or strata, such as age groups or places of residence. A random sample is then drawn from within each stratum. Stratified sampling has the additional advantage that it allows a different size of sample to be taken from each stratum to reflect the varying size or importance of the different strata.

Multistage Sampling

This is often a convenient technique in large surveys. For example, a survey of lung disease in steel workers might take as its first-stage sampling frame a list of all towns with steelworks. Having chosen an appropriate number of towns randomly, a second-stage sampling frame consisting of the names of employees could be drawn from the towns that had initially been chosen. The workers for examination would then be drawn at random from the second frame. The advantage of having adopted a two-stage sampling technique is that the need to draw up a named list of steel workers in the whole country was bypassed, thus saving time and avoiding difficulty and cost to the investigators.

GATHERING DATA ON THE SAMPLE

The information to be gathered on members of the sample, once it has been drawn, will depend on the aims of the population survey. However, a number of general principles apply.

Definition of What to Collect

At the outset, decisions need to be taken about the information that is required to address the aims of the study and how it is to be collected. There will be some types of information that address the central research question (for example, a person's blood pressure in a population survey of hypertension), while other information will be gathered because it provides important background on the characteristics of the sample or because it may be relevant to the analysis of the main factors under study.

Consideration must next be given as to how best to obtain the data in order to provide the required information. This may sound like a simple matter, but it seldom is. Consider a seemingly straightforward variable such as socio-economic status, which might be collected as an important piece of information in a population survey of mothers' infant-feeding practice. Interviewers questioning members of the sample could not simply ask the mothers 'What is your socio-economic status?' The responses to such a general question by a population with varying perceptions of what was meant by the concept would yield data from which no valid conclusions could be drawn about the respondents in relation to the Office for National Statistics definitions. A proper approach would involve the construction of a question that would provide the elements necessary to categorise the respondent by the National Statistics Socio-economic Classification. Ideally, such a question should be derived from established survey work in the field and be of proven validity.

There are two general ground rules that are helpful to bear in mind when addressing these issues about information gathering. The first is always to take a pedantic approach to considering the way in which each piece of information, even the simplest, is to be derived. For example, to derive age, should respondents be asked their precise age, should they be asked to place their age in a banding or age group, or should they be asked their precise date of birth? This needs to be discussed in the planning stage of the survey, and a decision needs to be taken on what seems appropriate, bearing in mind the aims of the study and the method of data collection. The second ground rule is to use, wherever possible, established and validated measures or questions. For example, in a questionnaire survey of lifestyle that seeks to establish levels of alcohol intake in the population, rather than the investigators thinking up their own question to elicit information, they should make use of the format of questions used in well-respected previous studies in this field.

Special and more difficult judgements have to be made when gathering data to provide information about the prevalence of a disease. The first step is to agree on an operational definition of the disease under study and the method by which it is to be measured or detected. Even a formally stated definition of a disease may be of little practical value in conducting a survey

Table 2.8 1987 revised American College of Rheumatology criteria for rheumatoid arthritis

Criterion no.	Criterion description
1	Morning stiffness of at least one hour's duration
2	Arthritis of at least three joint groups with soft-tissue swelling or fluid observed by a physician
3	Arthritis involving at least one of the following joint groups: proximal interphalangeal, metacarpophalangeal, and wrists
4	Symmetrical arthritis
5	Subcutaneous nodules
6	Positive rheumatoid factor test
7	Radiographic changes typical of rheumatoid arthritis

Source: Hochberg MC, Spector TD. Epidemiology of rheumatoid arthritis: update. *Epidemiol Rev.* 1990; **12**: 247–51.

to determine its prevalence. It is necessary to agree and lay down strict criteria that must be fulfilled in order for a person to be counted as having the disease.

Table 2.8 shows an approach that has been used in obtaining a list of criteria to define a chronic disease. It illustrates the contrast with the clinical situation, where the features of an illness that are taken as the basis for attaching a particular diagnostic label may vary markedly between different doctors. The reasons underlying those decisions may not always be apparent. In planning a population study to determine the prevalence of a disease, it is essential to resolve and adhere to a working definition, or the results collected will have no meaning outside the context in which they are collected.

Method of Data Collection: The Survey Instrument

The choice of the method through which the data necessary to address the aims of the study will be derived is another important decision in planning a population survey. To a certain extent, this will also depend on the aims of the investigation.

The term used to describe the method of data collection is the survey instrument, and sometimes it can literally be an 'instrument' (for example, a sphygmomanometer used to measure blood pressure in a population survey of hypertension). More often, however, the survey instrument is the document in which survey data are recorded – for example, a questionnaire to be administered by trained interviewers or a pro-forma used to extract data in a standardised format from various clinical records.

A detailed consideration of questionnaire design is beyond the scope of this book, but there are a number of important aspects to be considered, such as the structuring of questions (including the relative merits of closed versus open), the order in which questions should be asked, the avoidance of questions likely to lead to ambiguous or biased answers, the layout of the questionnaire and the coding of responses to facilitate analysis.

Questionnaires are of two broad kinds: postal questionnaires and those that are administered face to face by an interviewer. Although postal questionnaires have the advantage that they allow a much larger sample size, they can have serious disadvantages because of the restricted range of topics that can be covered and the generally higher levels of non-response that tend to occur with this method of questionnaire administration.

Whatever survey instrument is chosen, it is important that before the full-scale survey is undertaken, a pilot study is carried out on a small number of people within the sample. This allows difficulties with the questionnaire or other aspects of the survey to be ironed out or corrected before the survey proper is commenced.

Standardisation of Measurement and Interview Technique

Variation between measurements is another important consideration in a population survey, and as the example of the measurement of blood pressure shows (Table 2.9), it can have a wide variety of sources. The main concern is with systematic variation or bias.

Some variation can be reduced by standardising the procedures in the study as, for example, when physical examinations are being carried out. This will best be ensured by training examiners and checking their technique (for departure from the standard) at intervals during the conduct of the study.

If interviewers are being used to elicit information from members of the study population by questionnaire, they must be trained. This can be done by recording pilot interviews on videotape. Thus the interviewers and the study organisers can assess the results together and correct any faults in technique.

These are only some aspects of the process of preparing and monitoring interviewers who are responsible for gathering the survey data. There are many others, including agreeing rules to be adopted when the respondents are reluctant to answer the questions posed, what to do when other family members seek to participate in answering questions on the respondent's behalf, and the extent to which interviewers should react to (or make observations on) responses made to the questions.

A lack of clarity on these and many other aspects of interviewing can risk the results obtained being invalid or biased in ways that may be impossible to detect or eliminate from the analysis. This is why the choice of interviewers is particularly important, as is their training and experience in both the general techniques of interviewing and the issues that are specific to the particular investigation.

Variation arising from scientific instruments used in surveys can be reduced by introducing strict quality control. In studies using laboratory measurements, test solutions or reagents can be employed to ensure standardisation.

The Problem of Non-response

A major difficulty when gathering data in population surveys is the problem of non-response or non-cooperation.

Table 2.9 Factors that influence indirect blood pressure readings

Related to the patient
'White coat' effect
Resting time
Diurnal variation
Seasonal variation (changes in temperature)
Pain, anxiety
Acute smoking or ingestion of alcohol or caffeine
Postprandial state
Distended bladder
Talking
Degree and type of activity
Between arm differences
Paretic arms
Special factors (arrhythmia, 'silent gap', soft Korotkoff sounds)
Related to the observer
Training
Terminal digit preference
Expectation bias
Impaired hearing
Related to the instruments and technique
Instrument accuracy (manufacture errors, maintenance, defects)
Noisy room
Cuff length and width
Tight, thick clothes under the cuff
Body posture (sitting, supine, standing)
Arm level with respect to the right atrium
Arm/wrist/finger cuff
Arm, back and feet support
Inflation and deflation rate
Parallax error

The planning and organisation of the study should be geared to obtaining the highest possible recruitment of the sample under investigation. Key factors for success in minimising non-response will include the nature of the initial approach made to members of the sample, the wording of a letter of introduction, the institution on the notepaper heading and who the signatory is. These are factors that can make the difference between a very high rate of participation in the subsequent interview and a disastrous level of refusals or non-response.

It is inevitable, however, that some degree of non-response will remain, even after the most careful planning and the most strenuous efforts to reduce it. The main concern with non-response is that the non-responders are unlikely to be typical of the remainder of the sample. Depending on the circumstances, they may be more (or less) likely to suffer the disease or other subject of the investigation, and hence their omission is likely to lead to bias when drawing conclusions from the results of the sample. Aside from initial attempts to keep non-response to a minimum, when it does occur the first approach is to make extra efforts to gain this group's cooperation. Where this fails, a second strategy is to obtain as much indirect evidence as possible about the non-responders so as to make an estimate of the kind of bias that may be introduced by their omission.

Sometimes it is asked what level of response rate is acceptable. This question is almost impossible to answer in general terms because it depends on the nature and aims of the study. The concept to be borne in mind, however, is a simple one. Unless data on the sample (originally chosen) are fully captured, then the findings will not be truly representative of the whole population from which the sample was drawn. This is, after all, the purpose of the prevalence survey.

Some degree of non-response is, however, a feature of nearly all population surveys. The aim should be to achieve a response rate in the 95 to 100% range. Some surveys do manage to do this, although it would seldom be expected in postal surveys. However, it is more common to see reports of surveys with response rates in the mid to upper 70% range. This is far less satisfactory but can still yield valuable findings, particularly if some data are available on the non-responders and if conclusions are drawn more cautiously than would be the case with higher response rates.

A further problem in interpreting data from population surveys to establish disease prevalence is the need to be fully aware that the population being dealt with is a survivor population. If the disease has an appreciable mortality, the most severe cases will have died and any cross-sectional study will not include the entire spectrum of disease.

EXAMPLE OF A PREVALENCE STUDY: THE HEALTH SURVEY FOR ENGLAND

A health survey of private households in England is carried out annually and includes interviews and some examinations and tests of children (over two years old) and adults in each household surveyed.

The sampling frame for the Health Survey for England is the Postcode Address File (PAD), which contains 720 postcode sectors (a description of the components of the postcode in Britain is given in Chapter 1). The method of sampling is a multistage stratified technique – a number of stratification factors are used to ensure that the eventual sample is broadly representative of the whole population of England. Sampled addresses are sent an introductory letter, which is then followed by initial contact with an interviewer. At each household that agrees to cooperate, an interviewer-administered questionnaire is first completed with the head of household or partner, and then an individual questionnaire interview is carried out with each household member. Height and weight are also recorded at this first interview. Interviewees are then asked to agree to a second-stage visit at which a nurse carries out certain measurements and takes a blood sample.

Detailed sampling rules govern which members of the household (particularly children) are to be included. Explanatory leaflets describe the purpose of the survey and help to gain compliance. Quality-control measures include training of interviewers and nurses, checking of interview and measurement quality, and protocols for interviewing and measuring children. There are rules to govern what to tell people if abnormalities are found and what action needs to be taken. Some information is gathered on non-responders and reasons for non-response.

The health survey's methods are worthy of careful study as an example of how a well-conducted prevalence study is planned, executed and analysed. Valuable information about the health of the population can be derived from it, including general health,

long-standing and acute illness, limitation of function, respiratory disease and certain other specific illnesses, experience of major and minor accidents, smoking and drinking, obesity, blood pressure, lung function, blood haemoglobin and use of health services.

An example of the kind of information that is yielded by this prevalence study is shown in Figure 2.18. The public health importance of this finding is striking: high blood pressure is a risk factor for coronary heart disease and stroke. Yet just under half of the people with high blood pressure were not being treated, and 40% of those who were being treated did not have their blood pressure under control.

STUDIES TO INVESTIGATE DISEASE CAUSATION

One of the most important areas of investigation in public health is the exploration of hypotheses involving factors that may be responsible for causing disease. It is of particular importance because, if such links can be established, then there may be scope for prevention by intervening against causal agents.

A causal hypothesis may spring from clinical impression, from laboratory observations or from examining descriptive data in populations in relation to time, place or person, as was described earlier in this chapter. Table 2.10 gives some ways in which ideas about causation emerge.

Thereafter, the testing of the hypothesis that the factor or factors under examination may be responsible for causing the disease is a matter for carefully designed studies using epidemiological methods, each of

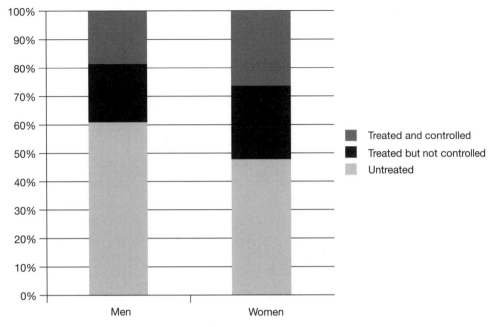

High Blood Pressure is systolic BP ≥140 mmHg or diastolic BP ≥90 mmHg.

Figure 2.18 Control of high blood pressure in adults
Source: Health Survey for England.

Table 2.10 Common ways in which ideas about causation emerge

Laboratory study
Clinical impression
Clusters of rare disease
Descriptive epidemiological studies
Cohort and case-control studies

which has its own special characteristics governing its use.

The previous section of this chapter has demonstrated that the techniques of descriptive epidemiology require a clear understanding of the sources of available data, the ways in which they can be used to make comparisons and, particularly, the limits that must be placed on any conclusions that can be drawn. This is even more important when using the more specialised study methods of epidemiology, two of which (cohort and case-control studies) are described in detail in this section.

One of the principal reasons for the existence of such study methods, and their complexity, is the fact that the investigator of causal relationships in human populations is denied the experimental approach. If the laboratory scientist wishes to investigate whether or not a suspected cause results in a particular outcome or effect, he frequently does have at his disposal the experimental approach. Suppose, for example, that a particular chemical is suspected of causing breast cancer in white mice. The investigator could take a strain of white mice and allocate them at random into two groups. One group would receive the presumed causal chemical and the other group would be treated identically in all ways, except that the mice would not receive the chemical. The investigator would then observe the occurrence of breast cancer in the two groups of animals and draw conclusions. In the laboratory experiment, the investigator is in control of the events and as a result has an extremely powerful and direct method at his disposal.

Similar experiments to test the effect of a suspected causal factor in groups of humans are usually quite unacceptable. Thus if the same chemical that caused breast cancer in the white mice was suspected of causing breast cancer in human females, an experiment could not be carried out in which one group of women was given the chemical and the other was not. Experiments may sometimes be performed on groups of people where removal of a suspected causal factor or addition of a supposed beneficial factor could result in an improvement in health, although the ethical aspects of such studies need the most careful consideration. The most usual experiment carried out in human subjects is the controlled clinical trial in which new therapies are tested out on people with particular diseases.

Sometimes, fortuitously for the investigator but often to the great misfortune of the population concerned, natural experiments take place that allow conclusions to be drawn about causation. Examples of this are the observations on the incidence of cancer following the exposure to radiation from the Hiroshima bomb and the Chernobyl nuclear accident, the observation of the association between Burkitt's lymphoma and Epstein-Barr virus infection and the observation of the incidence of vaginal tumours in the female offspring of women treated during pregnancy with diethylstilboestrol.

Usually, however, the experimental approach is ruled out for ethical reasons when investigating the effects of causes in human populations. Instead, the search concentrates on associations between the factor, or set of factors, and a disease. This 'observational' approach (to distinguish it from the 'experimental') involves comparing the disease experience of two or more groups of people in relation to their possession of certain characteristics of exposure to a suspected factor or factors.

There are two main approaches to investigating causal hypotheses: cohort and case-control studies (Figure 2.19). Each has its own specific design features. Both involve comparisons being made between different groups of people, but the basis of this comparison is entirely different in the two types of study.

In the cohort study, the comparison is being made between people who have been exposed to the hypothesised risk factor and people who have not been exposed to it; each group is then studied to see whether they develop the disease. In the case-control study, the disease is already present in one group (the 'cases') and absent in another

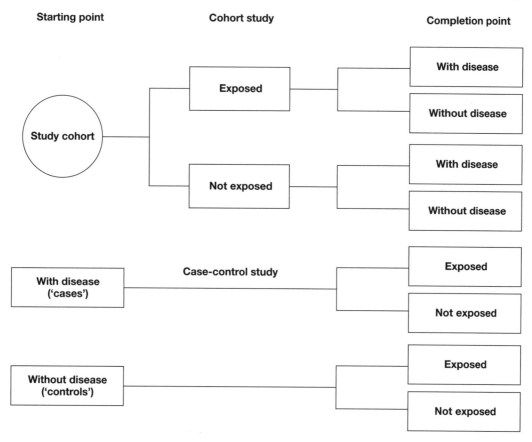

Figure 2.19 The main features of cohort and case-control studies

(the 'controls'); the two groups' previous exposure to the hypothesised risk factor is then compared.

Before each of these methods is described in more detail, two important points should be borne in mind. Firstly, most health professionals, managers and students, even those specialising in the public health field, will never themselves carry out a cohort study or a case-control study (except when investigating outbreaks of infectious disease). However, some of the decisions that they take will be based upon the evidence of such studies undertaken by others. This is why it is important to have a good understanding of each methodology, when it is appropriate to apply it, what its potential limitations are and where the possible sources of bias lie. Whole texts have been written on these study methods, particularly dealing with the statistical analysis of the data that are produced, but it is not essential to have an understanding of these matters to an advanced level. It is much more important to grasp the basic principles of both cohort studies and case-control studies.

The second point to be borne in mind is that the decision to make use of these specialised methods cannot be undertaken lightly. Their use is a matter for careful deliberation and would usually only be undertaken by a team of researchers or investigators, including (or with the advice of) a statistician skilled in the design and analysis of such studies. The next sections describe the main features of the two methods.

COHORT STUDIES
Outline of Methodology

The cohort study is a type of epidemiological investigation in which a population apparently free of the disease under study (or a sample of such a population) is assembled and each individual is categorised according to whether they have been exposed to the risk factor(s) of interest. The cohort is then followed up to see whether individual members of it develop the disease under study (or other diseases). Comparisons are then made between the occurrence of the disease in the 'exposed' compared to the 'non-exposed' groups within the cohort. If the intention is to test the hypothesis that smoking causes lung cancer, the initial step is to classify the study cohort into smokers and non-smokers. The cohort is then followed up over time, and cases of lung cancer are detected as they occur. The results would then be analysed to show what proportion of the smokers developed lung cancer compared to the proportion of non-smokers.

A cohort study may be conducted prospectively or retrospectively. In a prospectively conducted cohort study, the initial exposure data are collected on the members of the cohort and the investigators then wait for cases of the disease to crop up over time.

This is the commonest type of cohort study, so much so that the terms 'cohort study' and 'prospective study' are sometimes used synonymously.

It is possible, however, to conduct a retrospective cohort study where data on the cohort's exposure, as well as its disease experience, are already available. This can only really be contemplated where good past records exist to define a historical cohort. For example, suppose that a very large general practice had maintained very comprehensive records on medications prescribed to the practice population over a long period of time. If, in the present day, a particular drug became suspected of causing a type of cancer, the records of such a practice may allow a retrospective cohort study to be carried out. In such a study, a cohort would be assembled at some notional past date from the old practice population records, and the people within it would be classified according to whether they had been prescribed the drug of interest or not. Their past and present medical records would then also be examined to record their disease history and particularly whether they developed the cancer that was under study.

This is a simplified description of a complex methodology, but in the relatively unusual situation where past data are available comprehensively on a large population, the retrospective cohort study has advantages of speed and lower cost compared to the more common prospective approach.

Choice of a Study Population

A cohort is a group of people who share a similar experience at a point in time. A birth cohort is people born on a particular day or in a particular year, and a marriage cohort is those married in a given year. People residing in a particular geographical area or workers in an industry at a certain time also constitute a cohort.

In a cohort study investigating a causal hypothesis, the precise choice of cohort will depend on the nature of the disease under investigation. The cohort might be a group of people who have been exposed to a particular hazard (for example, a serious water pollution incident), a large workforce in a particular industry (for example, asbestos workers) or the population of a geographically defined area (for example, a small town).

Characterising the Cohort

The way in which data are assembled to characterise the initial cohort of people to be followed up will very much depend on the aims of the study. In a cohort study examining the risk of cancer arising from an industrial hazard, it is likely that quite detailed information would be gathered on the employment history of the workers concerned and their likely exposure in the workplace to quantified levels of the presumed risk factor, as well as whether they had other habits or characteristics which might influence the possibility of them developing the disease (for example, cigarette smoking). In a cohort study examining the risk of development of heart disease in a population, a sample of the population might form the study cohort and each member might be assessed by questionnaire, as well as by clinical and biochemical examination to determine

their baseline status in terms of the risk factors under investigation.

The Follow-up Phase

The follow-up phase of a cohort study, conducted prospectively, requires very careful planning and preparation. Particularly in studies where a long follow-up period is required, the difficulties in keeping track of members of the cohort who move away from the area can be very great and the process can be expensive. Considerable stability is also required in the investigative team, particularly amongst its leaders, if the study is to be brought to a successful conclusion.

A number of decisions need to be made when this phase of the cohort study is being designed. One important decision is how, and at what intervals, reassessments of the original members of the cohort will be made. This decision is somewhat easier when the outcome under study is a clear end-point such as death. In such circumstances, sources of mortality data can be kept under constant review, and the records of members of the original cohort can be flagged as the deaths occur to denote the outcome. Where the study is examining less dramatic outcomes, such as the progress of children whose mothers were exposed (and not exposed) to a particular hazard in pregnancy, it would be necessary (in this example) to decide on the time periods at which the children in the original cohort would be given further developmental assessments. Clearly, it would be quite impractical to undertake this with great regularity on the very large numbers of children who would be involved.

CASE-CONTROL STUDIES

The main attraction of a case-control study, especially when compared to a cohort study, is that it is relatively quick and cheap to undertake. Gathering data does not involve a long period of follow-up of the study population. That is not to say that the methodology is free of problems, and these, along with the main features of these studies, are described in this section.

Outline of Methodology

The case-control study is a type of epidemiological investigation in which an assessment is made of the extent to which people with an established disease ('cases') and a comparable group who do not have the disease ('controls') have been exposed to a risk factor believed to be responsible for causing the disease.

For example, if it is the intention to investigate the hypothesis that smoking causes lung cancer, the investigation begins by taking people with lung cancer and suitable controls who do not have lung cancer. Enquiries are then made to discover how many of the lung cancer patients were smokers and how many of the control patients were smokers. The method of investigation in a case-control study is, almost without exception, retrospective. The investigator looks back in time on the exposure history of present-day cases of the disease and of the controls.

Choice of a Study Population

In practice, the design of a case-control study is much more difficult than this broad outline of the methodology implies. One of the key initial decisions for the investigator is the way in which the cases and controls that make up the study population will be chosen. If wrong decisions are made at this stage of the investigation, the sources of bias that are introduced could render the results of the study invalid and useless.

Selection of 'Cases'

The choice of 'cases' should start with the formulation of a clear operational definition of what constitutes a case of the disease under study. Decisions will need to be taken on whether to study a broad diagnostic category (for example, adult acute leukaemia) or a more homogenous diagnostic grouping (adult acute myeloid leukaemia). This decision depends on the nature of the investigation, but, in general, the more heterogeneity in the diagnostic group, the less likelihood of being able to link a specific risk factor to the disease causation. On the other hand, the narrower the category of disease for inclusion of 'cases' in the study, the less general applicability the findings will have. For example, a case-control study to investigate possible risk factors in osteoarthrosis that took as 'cases' people with disease of the metacarpal joints and yielded a finding of an apparently new risk factor for the disease would have thrown light on the causation of osteoarthrosis. However, general conclusions could not necessarily be drawn about osteoarthrosis of other joints in the body, because the 'cases' were limited to people with disease at one particular site.

Having established a 'case' definition, it is most important to identify a source of all cases so that all eligible cases can be recruited into the study.

Selection of 'Controls'

The choice of an appropriate 'control' group is the issue that will usually cause the greatest discussion amongst investigators planning a case-control study. While the issues involved in selecting 'controls' are complex, and often particular to the circumstances of the study, it is important to keep in mind the central purpose of the 'control' group. This is to provide an indication of the level of exposure to the risk factor in a 'healthy' population, to which the exposure experienced by the people who have developed the disease can then be compared.

Put in the simplest terms, suppose that a case-control study was carried out to test the hypothesis that regular consumption of a particular kind of herbal tea led to the occurrence of pancreatic cancer. If 40% of cases were found to be drinkers of the herbal tea, such a finding would be of much less interest if 40% of the general population were regular herbal tea drinkers than if only 2% were. In this example, the controls are there to represent the same types of people as the cases and allow an estimate to be made of the 'normal' pattern of herbal tea drinking.

In practice, to find controls that are representative of a general population from which the cases are presumed to have arisen can be extremely difficult. For example,

some case-control studies using hospital cases take as their control group patients who attended the hospital for the treatment of diseases other than the one that is the subject of the study. This approach has advantages in that access to controls is usually relatively easy and information can be gathered in a similar fashion to the cases. It is also open to a number of potential sources of bias. For example, the hospital may have different catchment populations for the disease that is the subject of the study (the cases) and for the disease from which the control group patients were suffering. In such circumstances, the controls may not be representative of the general population from which the cases were drawn, so the degree of their exposure to the risk factor may be an unreliable basis for comparison with the cases.

Controls that are drawn from the general population do not suffer from this drawback but are less easy to identify and to gain cooperation from. The way in which they provide information may also be different to the cases in ways that may introduce bias.

The relative advantages and disadvantages of different numbers and types of controls requires the most careful consideration before final decisions are taken.

Matching Cases and Controls

A great deal of emphasis is often placed on the question of 'matching' in case-control studies. This is the process whereby controls are matched to cases on the basis of certain characteristics that are also known to be present in the cases. The purpose of matching is to eliminate the effect of so-called 'confounding' variables. Confounding can occur in other types of epidemiological investigation and is a term used to describe circumstances where there are factors, in addition to the risk factor under study, that may influence whether the disease occurs. If such confounding factors are unevenly distributed between study groups, they can distort the comparisons that are being made (and hence the conclusions that are drawn).

One of the commonest confounding variables is age. The occurrence of many diseases is strongly associated with age. If, in a case-control study, there are major differences in the age structure of cases and controls, this may distort other more important comparisons between the two groups. In descriptive epidemiological studies, standardisation (described in Chapter 1) is the method through which the confounding effect of age is reduced.

The technique of matching should be used very sparingly because there are serious problems that can result from over-matching. With modern statistical analytical techniques, the matching of characteristics of cases and controls can also be undertaken during the analysis stage. The tendency in case-control studies now is to take account of confounding variables (except age and sex) in the analysis of results rather than eliminate them at the study-design stage of matching.

Assembling Data on the Exposure

Data on the exposure to the hypothesised risk factor(s) amongst cases and controls is usually obtained retrospectively by one or both of two main methods. Firstly, it is obtained by abstracting information from medical or other records pertaining to the cases and the controls, and secondly, from the cases and controls (or where there have been deaths, their relatives) by interview.

Inherent in these approaches are further potential sources of bias. Records may not provide enough comprehensive or detailed information to fully satisfy the requirements of the investigation. This is hardly surprising, because such records seldom will have been created in the knowledge that they would be needed for a study. For example, when retrospectively obtaining data on exposure from medical records of lung cancer patients and hospital patients with other diseases (used as controls), it would be more likely that a smoking history would be recorded in the lung cancer patients because of the known association between that disease and cigarette smoking.

A further potential source of bias arises when exposure data are obtained retrospectively by interview. A person with the disease may be more likely to remember or report an exposure (perhaps because he or she is trying to rationalise the presence of the disease) than would be a disease-free person serving as a control. For example, a surgeon notices that many female patients presenting at his outpatient clinic with breast lumps give a history of localised trauma. To investigate this further, he takes two groups of women: one group comprises those who have presented to the outpatient clinic with a breast lump; the other comprises a sample of healthy women of similar ages. Each group of women is asked if they can recall having any bang, knock or bruise of the breast during the previous 12 months. A much higher occurrence of such trauma is found in the group with breast lumps than in the control group of healthy women. Should it then be concluded that localised trauma predisposes to the formation of breast lumps? This is possible, but unlikely. Women who have developed a breast lump are often in a very anxious state, and their principal fear is that the lump is malignant. They will often cling to any alternative explanation of the origin of the lump. Hence when such women are questioned about a history of trauma, they are far more likely to remember and volunteer some trivial occurrence than are those women without breast lumps.

Since data are obtained retrospectively on the exposure, whether by abstraction of case notes or by interview survey, the serious problems arise when there are differences in the completeness of information or selectivity between the two groups (cases and controls). The investigator may not be aware of it and may draw misleading conclusions – such as in the examples given above. It is not possible to fully guard against this, but an additional measure that may help is to ensure that the person gathering the data (whether abstracting it from records or questioning patients) relies on a structured format and is 'blind' to whether the individuals are cases or controls.

There is evidence to show that recall bias can be influenced by the seriousness of the condition being studied (cancer vs. an infection), the perceived importance of the event in the life of the individual (childbirth vs. drug exposure), the respondent (patient vs. proxy), the length of time since the event and the phraseology used either in the questionnaire or by the interviewer.

MEASURES OF RISK

Measures of risk are derived from epidemiological studies of causation. Such measures express how many more times the disease (or outcome) occurs in the group that was exposed to the risk factor than in the group that was not (i.e., the relative risk). Aside from the relative risk, it is possible to calculate other measures of risk when examining associations between possible risk factors and diseases.

RISK RATIO

In a cohort study, the relative risk of the disease or outcome is calculated from the ratio of incidence rates in the exposed group and the non-exposed group:

Incidence of the disease in the exposed group = I_e

Incidence of the disease in the non-exposed group = I_n

Relative risk = $\dfrac{I_e}{I_n}$

If no association, relative risk = 1

ODDS RATIO

In a case-control study, incidence rates cannot be calculated, because the subjects do not necessarily represent the population as a whole. However, an estimate of the relative risk is produced by the odds ratio.

This ratio is constructed by dividing the odds of the case group having been exposed to the risk factor by the odds of the control group having been exposed (Table 2.11). The calculation of these indices and the statistical theory underlying them is beyond the scope of this book, but they have been introduced in outline to give an insight into the way in which the results of these more specialised epidemiological studies may be presented and interpreted.

ATTRIBUTABLE RISK

An alternative approach is to examine the difference in disease occurrence between the exposed and unexposed groups rather than the ratio. Such an approach is used to construct the attributable risk.

Data from a cohort study could thus be analysed as so:

Incidence of the disease in the exposed group = I_e
Incidence of the disease in the non-exposed group = I_n
Attributable risk = $I_e - I_n$
If no association, attributable risk = 0

The attributable risk is useful in examining the absolute additional risk that individuals experience as a result of their exposure.

POPULATION ATTRIBUTABLE RISK

Another measure, the population attributable risk, is a measure of the extent to which the amount of the disease that occurs in the population is due to the risk factor. The population attributable risk is useful in terms of assessing the public health impact of a risk factor and hence the benefits which could be obtained by preventive action.

It is calculated by multiplying the attributable risk by the prevalence P of the risk factor in the population:

$$(I_e - I_n) \times P$$

A relatively small excess (i.e., attributable) risk of developing a disease where a large number of people are exposed to the risk factor would yield many additional cases. The benefits of preventive action could be great. Alternatively, an attributable risk that was large but where relatively few people were exposed to the risk would not produce a large burden of disease in the population, and the scope for major preventive action would be limited.

ANALYSIS OF CASE-CONTROL STUDY DATA

Table 2.12 shows data from one of the earliest case-control studies ever carried out – an investigation in the 1950s into the possible causes of childhood cancer. One of the factors investigated was whether irradiation of the foetus by abdominal X-ray examinations of the mother during pregnancy was associated with childhood cancer.

The data are shown to illustrate the way in which such an analysis can be presented (not to describe the study in detail). As Table 2.12 shows, there was a significantly elevated odds ratio of childhood cancer in children who were irradiated in utero. The authors concluded that foetal irradiation by diagnostic X-raying of the pregnant mother was a risk factor for childhood cancer.

ANALYSIS OF COHORT STUDY DATA

Table 2.13 is an example of a different way in which data from a cohort study can be analysed. This is because it is only a comparison

Table 2.11 The findings of a case-control study

Exposed to risk factor	With the disease 'cases'	Without the disease 'controls'
Yes	a	b
No	c	d
Total	a+c	b+d

The odds ratio is a measure of the association between the risk factor and the disease and is calculated:

Step 1: Odds of a person in the case group having been exposed to the risk factor
= a/c

Step 2: Odds of a person in the control group having been exposed to the risk factor
= b/d

Step 3: Ratio of odds = $\dfrac{a/c}{b/d}$ = $\dfrac{ad}{bc}$

Table 2.12 Analysis of data from a case-control study

	Cases	Controls
Abdominal X-ray of pregnant mother (exposed)	141	81
No abdominal X-ray of pregnant mother (unexposed)	1125	1204
Total	1266	1285

Odds ratio 1.86; 95% confidence interval 1.40–2.47

Source: Adapted from Stewart AM, Webb J, Hewitt DA. A survey of childhood malignancies. *BMJ.* 1958; **1**: 1495–508.

Table 2.13 Analysis of data from a cohort study investigating the association between oral contraceptive usage and the occurrence of chronic inflammatory bowel disease

Use of oral contraceptives	Woman-years of observation	Ulcerative colitis		Crohn's disease	
		Number of cases	Incidence/1000 woman-years	Number of cases	Incidence/1000 woman-years
Never used	75 950	8	0.11	6	0.08
Ex-user	67 319	8	0.10	4	0.06
Current user	61 116	16	0.26	8	0.13
Total	204 385	31	0.15	18	0.09

Source: Vessey M, Jewell D, Smith A, *et al.* Chronic inflammatory bowel disease, cigarette smoking, and use of oral contraceptives: findings in a large cohort study of women of child-bearing age. *BMJ.* 1986; **292**: 1101–3.

of incidence and there is no calculation of risk. However, the risk calculation is added to the table. The data are from a large study in which married women using different forms of contraception were followed up and information was gathered on a range of health outcomes. The aspect of the study shown in Table 2.13 examines the relationship between use of oral contraceptives and the subsequent development of two inflammatory bowel diseases (ulcerative colitis and Crohn's disease).

There was a higher incidence of both ulcerative colitis and Crohn's disease in current oral contraceptive users than in women who had never used the pill or had given up using it (Table 2.13). While the difference did not achieve statistical significance for Crohn's disease, it did for ulcerative colitis. Incidences in those who had stopped using oral contraceptives were similar to those who had never used them.

The authors concluded that while the associations between oral contraceptive use and chronic inflammatory bowel disease could not be regarded as established, they provided important clues to its causation.

ESTABLISHING A CAUSAL RELATIONSHIP

Both cohort and case-control studies are observational in nature. To investigate hypotheses of cause and effect, they rely on observing real life events: people who are exposed (or expose themselves) to risk factors and those people who develop disease. If an association is found, it is probable that the relationship between exposure and disease is not, in fact, one of cause and effect.

It is important, therefore, to consider the possible explanations for any association between a risk factor and a disease, whether the association has arisen as a result of a descriptive epidemiological study or from carrying out a cohort or a case-control study.

Three possible alternatives for such an association should be reviewed before detailed consideration is given to establishing whether it could be causal. The three are either that the association has arisen by chance, or that it may be spurious, or that it may be a secondary association.

Association is a Chance Occurrence

The association between the factor and the disease may be a chance occurrence that would generally not be found on another occasion. Statistical tests exist, however, to allow a statement to be made of the probability with which the observed association would have arisen by chance on the hypothesis that there is, in fact, no association between the factor and the disease.

Association is Spurious

The apparent association between causal factor and disease may not be real; it may be a product of the way in which the investigation was carried out. For example, suppose that it was intended to investigate the association between place of delivery (cause) and perinatal mortality (effect). A comparison of two groups of women might show that the perinatal mortality for those delivered in consultant obstetric units was higher than for women delivered in general practitioner maternity units. It might be concluded that general practitioner units were safer places in which to have a baby. Such a conclusion is almost certainly fallacious, however. In general, consultant obstetric units, because of their special expertise and equipment, deliberately select women at high risk for delivery in their units. Thus the consultant unit might have a higher perinatal mortality rate than the general practitioner unit because of this fact alone, not because the quality of care was inferior. This source of bias (selection bias), where like is not being compared with like, is very important. Other sources of bias (such as those described in the section on case-control studies) can also yield spurious associations between risk factors and diseases.

Association is Secondary

A factor and a disease may appear to be associated in a causal fashion when in reality the reason for their association is that both are related to a third factor. Thus an association is found between countries with a high proportion of television owners and the frequency of coronary heart disease. The fact that these two factors are strongly associated does not mean that they are causally related and that television causes coronary heart disease. A more reasonable explanation is that television ownership is an indicator of societies with lifestyles that themselves are causally related to coronary heart disease.

Criteria that Infer a Causal Association

If an association between a factor and a disease is found that probably did not occur by chance, is not spurious and is not due to a secondary association, then this does not prove that the association is causal. However, six criteria, if present, help to infer that the association is causal:

1   *Plausibility*. Greater weight is given to a possible causal factor if it seems to fit in with what is known about the pathology of the disease.

2   *Consistency*. The association would, if causal, be expected to persist when studies were carried out by different investigators working in different populations at different times.

3   *Temporal relationship*. Clearly, to assess causality it is necessary to show that the factor preceded in time the development of the disease.

4   *Strength*. A causal relationship is more likely to be present when there is a marked difference in frequency of the disease in people who have been exposed to the factor compared to those who have not. An additional piece of evidence that is strongly indicative of causality is the presence of a dose-response relationship: with increasingly greater exposure to the risk factor the incidence of the disease rises.

5   *Specificity*. An ideal finding would be that the postulated causal factor was related to the disease in question and no other. This is, however, not always the case, since a factor may be causally related to more than one disease.

6   *Change in risk factor*. If the factor is removed or reduced and the incidence of the disease falls, this strongly indicates that the factor is causal.

RANDOMISED CONTROLLED TRIALS

Another type of study is the so-called 'intervention' design. This usually takes the form of a randomised controlled trial (RCT).

In it, two or more groups are assembled. They receive defined interventions (for example, treatments, health education messages, dietary modification) that are controlled by the investigator, and they are then monitored to detect events that are hypothesised to result from these actions (for example, relief of pain, improvement in health, loss of weight). The best-established context is the clinical trial in which new therapies are assessed in comparison with old methods of treatment or with placebos ('dummy' treatments).

OUTLINE OF METHODOLOGY

The main feature of the interventional method that sets it apart from observational studies is the aim of producing groups of patients comparable in respect of features known to affect the outcome except for the different planned interventions. Other unknown differences between such groups may, of course, still be present, but the usual means of negating their effects and enabling valid inferences to be made is through introducing randomisation. This process involves dividing the group of subjects (or any subgroup or subgroups with particular characteristics) into two parts: one part becoming the 'experimental' or 'intervention' group and the other the 'control' group. The outcome or end-point of the study is then assessed as the two groups are followed up in an identical way.

Clinical trials of therapies are much more commonplace than randomised controlled trials evaluating preventive measures. This is, in part, because of the difficulty involved with large numbers of subjects being required for the latter and the necessity of a long time span to await the appearance of outcome measures. The most common type of preventive trial is of vaccines. However, there have been randomised controlled trials of coronary heart disease preventive measures and presymptomatic screening (for example, bowel and breast cancer screening).

CHOICE OF A STUDY POPULATION

An early decision must be made on the number of people who will comprise the study population. This in turn will depend on the number of interventions to be tested and the expected differences in outcome between the interventions. These parameters will determine the statistical power of the study to prove the hypothesis to be tested. In the simplest form of randomised controlled trial, there will be two groups: one that receives the intervention and one that does not.

Having made this decision, the first stage in assembling the study population will be to identify a base population from which the study groups can be drawn. The choice of this base population will influence the extent to which the findings of the investigation can be generalised to other populations.

This is a factor that is sometimes overlooked in the eagerness of investigators to eliminate other (albeit equally important) sources of bias in designing the randomised controlled trial. However, it can be extremely important in determining the value of the findings of the investigation. In the evaluation of a therapy, it is commonplace to draw the study group from amongst the admissions to a hospital. If, for example, the hospital is a centre of excellence and admits only the most complex cases within a particular diagnostic category (say patients with hypertension), then the findings on the effectiveness of the therapy under study would not be generalisable to all patients with the disease (in this example hypertension) – only to those with the same degree of complexity.

Eligibility

The next step in the process of assembling the study population is to decide upon criteria for eligibility. These will include a precise operational definition of the disease status of the patients (for the disease under study); age, sex and possibly other characteristics; and the presence or absence of other clinical features (such as complications of the disease or associated conditions).

Randomisation

Once patients have been found to be eligible for the trial on the basis of diagnostic and other criteria previously laid down, then, and only then, does randomisation take place. It is an essential requirement that, after eligibility for the trial has been confirmed, no further influences can be brought to bear on whether patients are allocated to particular groups. Anything other than random choice (for example, the deliberate placing of very

ill patients in a non-treatment group) will introduce bias.

There are various techniques through which randomisation can be accomplished: for example, computer randomisation, the use of random number tables or the opening of sealed envelopes containing the treatment category.

The process of randomisation thus involves placing individuals from amongst the eligible population into either intervention or control groups in such a way that they have an equal chance of ending up in either of the groups. Its purpose is to eliminate the effect of confounding factors that can influence the outcome of the study independently of the intervention. Randomisation probably never truly eliminates the effects of confounding, but it does minimise the potential effect, and it is a more effective technique than those used in observational studies (for example, matching in case-control studies) to eliminate confounding.

SPECIFICATION OF THE INTERVENTION

A very precise specification of the nature of the treatment or other measures to be used is also necessary, together with rules for the method of administration or the conditions under which the treatment should be administered. For example, in the evaluation of a preventive measure, criteria might be laid down as to who is to administer, say, a health education message, whereas with the treatment, the route of administration of a drug must be specified.

Placebo Effect

A further element of the investigation is to specify the conditions of the 'non-intervention' group, and it is here, in trials of clinical therapies, that the 'placebo' is brought into play. The so-called 'placebo effect' is the change in a patient's outcome or health status that can be achieved simply by being given an inactive therapy or through being a participant in a study. The psychological processes involved in this phenomenon are not fully understood.

It is easier to correct for this influence in trials of therapies. In such cases, both groups of patients (the intervention and the non-intervention groups) are given tablets; one set contains the active treatment under investigation, and the other is pharmaceutically prepared to look, smell and feel like the active treatment but is, in fact, inert as far as the disease under investigation is concerned.

Patients are therefore 'blind' as to whether they are receiving the real treatment or the placebo. It is also better to keep the investigators in ignorance so that they do not use their knowledge of the patients' treatment category consciously or unconsciously to influence their assessment of the patients' status following intervention (a 'double-blind' study).

It is much more difficult to use a placebo process in randomised controlled trials other than those evaluating drug therapies. For example, in a trial to test the effectiveness of an intra-abdominal surgical technique, it would almost certainly be unethical (as well as inappropriate) to anaesthetise patients in the control group, then open and close their abdomens as a placebo operation.

ASSESSMENT OF THE OUTCOME OR END-POINT

Very clear study rules need to be laid down to ensure that outcomes for the patients in the two groups of the trial are clearly defined, assessed and recorded in a standard way. The outcomes (or end-points) that are the subject of the investigation will vary according to its aims but might include: (in a trial of a new therapy) improvement or worsening in a patient's condition, death, length of survival; or (in a preventive trial) the onset of disease, death, change in physical or physiological characteristics such as weight, serum cholesterol, fitness.

There is a danger of bias when the patient, the clinician or the investigator (who is responsible for assessing outcome) is aware of which groups have received the intervention as opposed to the non-intervention (control) measures. This source of bias can be minimised (as described above) by ensuring that neither the patient nor the investigator is aware of which experimental group is the intervention group. This is called a 'double-blind' study. The code identifying the two groups is only broken at the end of the study unless some major risk or side-effect of the therapy emerges during the study.

It is important to ensure that if patients drop out of the study or fail to complete their treatment (non-compliance), they are included in the analysis according to the randomised group to which they were originally allocated (on the basis that there was an intention to treat). To do otherwise would be to introduce potential bias.

ETHICAL ISSUES

In the conduct of a study involving human populations, a strict ethical code must be obeyed. A number of organisations have laid down codes of practice or guidelines for the conduct of research investigations involving people. Of particular importance are those that have been produced by the Helsinki Declaration (1964), the World Health Organization and the Royal College of Physicians of London.

Within the NHS is a network of research ethics committees (RECs) to which application must be made for approval of research to be undertaken on NHS patients or for use of their records or NHS premises in the area. Since 2007, the National Research Ethics Service has provided ethical guidance and management support to RECs in England. Special arrangements address the requirements of the European Union Clinical Trials Directive.

The committees satisfy themselves that due regard has been taken for the safety of the participants in a study, that proper arrangements for consent are in place, that appropriate information on the trial and its aims is available for participants and that the trial is scientifically valid – capable of coming to conclusions and likely to yield important information that could not be obtained by other means.

INVESTIGATING HEALTH SERVICE PROBLEMS IN PRACTICE

The two major epidemiological methodologies (cohort and case-control studies) are infrequently used in day-to-day practice (aside from the use of the case-control method in the investigation of infectious disease outbreaks). However, their strengths and weaknesses must be fully appreciated to evaluate the published work of others. This is especially important if decisions about health care priorities and programmes are to be based upon such studies.

This section of the chapter contains a description of the kinds of investigation that might be carried out by those playing a part on a day-to-day basis in identifying the health problems within a population and ensuring an appropriate range and quality of health services is available to address them.

There is a great deal of misunderstanding about this area of public health practice. Firstly, this field of investigation is seldom debated and certainly is not the subject of texts such as those written about case-control and cohort studies, which deal with the possible approaches and methodologies systematically and in-depth. Secondly, health service problem investigation is often denigrated as flawed or unscientific, particularly by those investigators used to undertaking studies using the more formal epidemiological methods. Thirdly, the investigation of a health service problem usually leads to a report that is presented to a health service policy-making board or as an aid to decision-making at an operational level within the management structure of the service. All energies are usually deployed to this end, and it is less common for the investigator to set aside the time to write up his study separately for submission to a journal.

The approach of investigators based in academic institutions is very different. A report will always be produced (or internally published) for the funding body and for wider circulation, but major emphasis will also be placed on identifying those aspects of the study that can be written up for submission to journals. This will often result in one or more publications in major peer-review journals, all of which adds to the standing of this type of investigative work.

This debate is epitomised by the phrase that is sometimes used to describe the type of investigative work undertaken within the health service: 'quick and dirty'. As with any catchphrase, it is easy to see why it has gained widespread usage, but the juxtaposition of the terms 'quick' and 'dirty' when applied to any form of bona fide public health investigation is both inappropriate and unfortunate. The term 'dirty' is intended to convey the impression of crudeness or unreliability in either the study methods used or the findings. It is only necessary to think of a cohort study of disease causation, taking many years to carry out, with consequent consumption of resources, having had a seriously flawed design at the outset to realise that 'dirtiness' can equally apply to large-scale investigation using methods traditionally associated with scientific purity.

The importance of this issue cannot be over-emphasised, because it draws attention to fundamental principles that should apply equally to the investigation of a circumscribed and urgent problem in a health service as to the study of possible risk factors for the genesis of a disease that poses a large-scale public health problem.

Whether using routinely available data on an ad hoc and limited data-gathering exercise, conducting a population survey, or conducting a case-control or cohort study,

the investigator should have a clear view of the aims of the investigation and the questions that need to be answered by it. He or she should choose the appropriate method to carry out the investigation (bearing in mind the prevailing constraints, including time and money). He or she should be aware of the strengths and weaknesses of the approach chosen and, most importantly, should present the findings of the study in a way that makes clear the extent of the conclusions that can be drawn from them.

Thus some studies are more limited in scope than others because of time constraints, the availability of resources or the quality of available data. Even in such circumstances, however, good investigations can still be carried out, provided that it is made clear precisely what conclusions can be drawn from them (bearing in mind the limitations of the data). This does not make them 'dirty'.

It is also worth bearing in mind that decisions about health service priorities and the allocation of resources are being made on a daily basis and, sadly, too often on purely subjective grounds. Even a limited investigation, if carefully carried out, potentially can improve the quality of decision-making. Some practical pointers to the use of public health investigations are shown in Table 2.14.

EXAMPLES OF INVESTIGATIONS OF HEALTH SERVICE PROBLEMS

This section of the chapter describes a small number of examples of investigations of health service problems that have been carried out as part of the practice of departments of public health. Each was the subject of a comprehensive report with presentation of data, and while they are too extensive to be described in full here, the main features of each, together with some illustrative data, are included.

It is important to bear in mind that any investigation, no matter how small-scale, must be carefully planned; the first stage of which is to clearly set out the aims or questions the investigators are seeking to address or answer. It is always surprising in reading reports of investigations in public health, even those submitted to editors of journals for publication, to see that the aims of the investigation were not identified at the outset.

The main purpose of the examples, however, is not to describe investigations from start to finish in exhaustive detail. Rather it is to give the reader an understanding of some of the practicalities of designing and executing such investigations and, particularly, to show how they can be used to provide insights into, and solutions to, health problems and the working of health services.

A SURVEY OF THE HEALTH AND SOCIAL STATUS OF ELDERLY PEOPLE IN AN ETHNIC MINORITY GROUP

This investigation set out to describe certain aspects of the health and social status of people aged 65 years and over belonging to the Asian population of a city in the East Midlands area of England. An Asian person was defined as a person not of United Kingdom descent originating from India or Pakistan, or of Indian or Pakistani descent originating from East Africa.

Context and Problem Definition

The population in which the study was carried out was Leicester, where at the time approximately one in four people belonged to ethnic minority groups. The largest group of old people in the population of Leicester who belonged to an ethnic minority group were those born in India (mainly in Gujarat or the Punjab), although the majority had come to Britain via East Africa.

At the time of the investigation, a great deal of service provision work was being undertaken within the Asian community of Leicester by health, social care services and voluntary organisations, but there was little objective information on the pattern of health and social need.

Carrying out the Investigation

The first step in this study of elderly Asians was to gain the cooperation of the local community. The Asian community has strong networks and relatively well-defined leadership, so it was possible to gain agreement and support for such a large study by discussing it with a small number of people who then took on the responsibility to inform the local community.

It is important at this stage in planning an investigation to strike a balance between keeping the population to be surveyed properly informed and conveying only so much information about the detail of the survey that their responses to particular questions will not become prejudiced by prior thinking about what responses are needed. Thus in the Leicester survey, the community leaders offered to publicise the forthcoming fieldwork by a series of radio programmes.

Table 2.14 Pointers to use of investigations in public health practice

Be clear about objectives.
Do not be drawn into impossible tasks.
Follow the general principles of purer methods (e.g., sampling, defining criteria for inclusion of cases, maintaining high response rates, avoiding bias).
Do not try to do too much.
Be aware of the limitations of your data.
Pay particular attention to the presentation of results.
Decide how to disseminate conclusions and recommendations.
Make every effort to make full use of the data.

Source: Donaldson LJ, Kirkup W. The public health practitioner as investigator. *Hosp Med.* 1998; **59**: 1–54.

This offer was declined in favour of a more low-key dissemination of information to the community.

The next stage in the planning of the survey was to select a suitable sampling frame. A number of alternatives were considered. It was felt that the electoral roll could not provide satisfactory coverage of the elderly Asian population. The possibility of identifying elderly Asians by door-knocking in known Asian areas was seriously considered, but informal discussions within the Asian community indicated that this approach might run into serious difficulty. Asian people are often initially wary of enquiries that seem to be of an official nature, and it was feared that the response of relatives on the doorstep might be to seek to protect the elderly by denying the interviewer access. A further factor was that there had been recent reports in the local newspaper of people posing as survey workers in order to try to rob Asian people. On balance, it was felt that the greatest degree of cooperation could be achieved if the individuals to be approached were identified in advance so

that they could receive a personal letter that explained the aims of the survey before an interviewer called to see them.

The sampling frame eventually chosen was the central register of the Family Practitioner Committee (now a function of primary care trusts), and agreement was reached on this by seeking the permission of the Committee and its advisers.

The next major stumbling block was that the sampling frame did not categorise patients' records by ethnic status (nor is this even now a routine variable recorded in health information systems). However, experience had been gained in using the Asian naming system to identify and classify Asian people into broad cultural and religious groupings. In this way, all the names of Asian appearance occurring amongst people of 65 years and over (the elderly, for the purposes of this investigation) were extracted from the sampling frame by trained staff and used as the basis for drawing the sample.

It is well documented that general practitioner registers are inflated above their true value by people whose names appear on them but who are no longer strictly members of them, having died or moved away. The Asian population was also a relatively highly mobile group that added to sampling frame inflation and made it particularly important to eliminate errors (which was done by checking against individual general practitioners' records when individuals could not be traced).

Those identified as members of the sample were written to in the Asian languages in order to seek their cooperation and to indicate that an interviewer would be calling. Data were collected using a questionnaire that was administered by Asian-language speaking fieldworkers in the homes of the elderly people.

The areas of enquiry included demographic details (sex, date of birth, country of origin, religion, current and past employment status); family life and social contact; aspects of lifestyle; level of physical capacity; language and communication; and knowledge and use of health and social care services.

Findings and Implications

Three illustrative examples from amongst the range of information yielded by this investigation are shown in Tables 2.15 to 2.17. Table 2.15 shows that while 5% of elderly Asians lived alone and 13% with someone of their own generation, the most frequent household configuration for these old people was multigenerational. Overall, as Table 2.12 shows, 82% lived in a household with two or more generations and the most common type of household was that in which there were three generations (usually the elderly person, their children and their grandchildren). There was little variation in household composition between religious groups.

Further analysis (not shown in Table 2.15) revealed that of those old people who lived in multigenerational households, about one-fifth, whether they were married or widowed, shared a bedroom with someone else, most commonly grandchildren. This pattern of household structure of the elderly Asians was in marked contrast to that of the

Table 2.15 Composition of households in which elderly Asians lived (by religion percentages)

Household composition	Hindu	Sikh	Muslim	All religions
Lived alone	5	4	4	5
One generation	13	19	9	13
Two generations	23	17	31	24
Three generations	56	56	49	55
Four generations	3	4	7	3
With non-relatives	>1	>1	>1	>1
All households N (100%) =	100 (510)	100 (73)	100 (138)	100 (721)

Source: Donaldson LJ. Health and social status of elderly Asians: a community survey. *BMJ.* 1986; **293**: 1079–82.

indigenous elderly, where, for example, 46% of old people lived alone.

These data had major policy implications. Participation and acceptance within the family remained a key feature of old age in the Asian community of Leicester (this was confirmed by other findings of the investigation, not just those relating to household structure). While elderly Asians were at an advantage in having the immediate help and support of other household members, the implication for services was that the situation would be very sensitive to changes in kinship patterns. Furthermore, within existing households the opportunities for privacy were diminished, and there was no way of knowing how harmonious life was within these large multigenerational households. Organisations in Leicester providing sheltered accommodation at the time were seeing instances of family conflict leading to rejection of elderly members, and it was possible that this would become a larger problem.

Another very important aspect of the investigation related to the language skills of the old people. It was common for respondents to report that they could speak more than one language. Overall, half of the sample could speak a second language, and almost a third could speak a third language. Almost all Hindus spoke Gujarati, and a substantial minority spoke Hindi, Swahili or English. Sikhs nearly all spoke Punjabi, with English and Hindi being the languages next most commonly spoken. Muslims were the most diverse linguistically: after Gujarati, they were likely to speak Urdu, Kutchi and English.

It was for English-speaking ability that particularly important findings were made. As Table 2.16 shows, a fifth of the sample could speak English, but the proportion speaking it was very low amongst elderly women (only 2%). Moreover, it was also found (not shown in Table 2.16) that 63% of women could not read in any language.

Even for the old people who said that they could speak English, in three of six common social situations more than half considered that they would have had difficulty making themselves understood without an interpreter (Table 2.17).

The investigation's findings in relation to language indicated the extent to which the old people were dependent on others for contact outside their community – particularly in health settings. The finding that nearly two-thirds of Asian women were illiterate in all languages was of immediate

Table 2.16 The percentage of elderly Asian men and women who said that they could speak, read or write English

English ability	Males (n = 389)	Females (n = 337)	Both sexes (n = 726)
Spoke English	37	2	21
Read English	24	<1	13
Wrote English	21	<1	11

Source: Donaldson LJ. Health and social status of elderly Asians: a community survey. *BMJ.* 1986; **293**: 1079–82.

importance in that it implied that simply translating leaflets on health education or welfare benefits would not be adequate.

A useful alternative to the conventional approach to posters and leaflets was Asian-language radio programmes (which were listened to a by a high proportion of the old people interviewed) and home videos (ownership of rental video recorders was also relatively high in the Asian community of Leicester).

The language findings of the investigation also emphasised the need for interpreters as an integral part of health and social care provision.

Comment and Overview

The investigation yielded valuable information for policy-makers and planners in the health, social services and voluntary sectors. As a type of investigation in public health, the study was of the cross-sectional type and the techniques adopted were generally those described in the section of this chapter dealing with such studies. However, as with any other such investigation carried out in practice, its design and conduct had a number of special features that were variations on the textbook account of the study methodology concerned. This was particularly so because there had been relatively few surveys that had set out to gather data directly from people belonging to this ethnic minority group. It was important to seek the cooperation of community leaders to ensure success in the fieldwork and to ensure that there were people skilled in interviewing in the Asian languages if valid information was to be obtained.

AN INVESTIGATION INTO THE POPULATION'S ACCESS TO SPECIALIST SERVICES PROVIDED IN A LIMITED NUMBER OF CENTRES

The Northern Region was one of 14 health regions into which the NHS in England was

Table 2.17 Elderly Asians' assessment of their own ability to use English in a range of everyday situations, expressed as a percentage

Situation	Ability to make themselves understood			
	Easily	With difficulty	Only with interpreter	Total (n = 145)
Asking for cost of fare on bus	68	22	10	100
Asking for goods in an English shop	64	27	9	100
Returning faulty goods to an English shop	47	31	22	100
Telephoning to rearrange an outpatient appointment	43	23	34	100
Giving directions to an English person	52	31	17	100
Explaining a problem to a doctor	41	21	38	100

Source: Donaldson LJ. Health and social status of elderly Asians: a community survey. *BMJ.* 1986; **293**: 1079–82.

divided for administration and planning purposes at the time. It had a population of approximately three million and stretched from the border with Scotland in the north down to Yorkshire in the south, over to Cumbria in the west and Cleveland in the east. The region was made up of health districts with resident populations of varying sizes.

Many services were present in every district general hospital, but some, because of their high cost or highly specialised nature, were provided in one or a small number of hospital centres within the region. At the time of the investigation, heart surgery was provided in only one centre in the Northern Region. Patients who were thought to require coronary artery surgery (and other open-heart procedures) were referred to the specialist centre by general practitioners or consultants in other parts of the region. This was before angioplasty was widely used to treat coronary artery disease. Ophthalmology and some other specialist surgical services were provided at a number of hospitals (but not all), so that a patient requiring cataract surgery, for example, would be treated by one of these services.

The investigation aimed to describe the extent to which patients in different parts of the region, particularly those outside the district in which the regional or sub-regional centres were located, received treatment.

Context and Problem Definition

The regional health authority – the statutory body accountable at the time for services in the region (regional health authorities were abolished in 1996) – had been concerned to examine the extent to which the population in different places received access to services that, though located in only some centres, were funded on the basis that they would be available to the whole population.

Carrying out the Investigation

Data were assembled from routinely available hospital inpatient data. Patients treated by services provided on a regional (for example, cardiothoracic surgery) and a sub-regional (for example, ophthalmology) basis were classified according to health district of residence and to the smaller local government districts of residence. The extent to which residents of these different populations were treated as inpatients or day cases by each of these regional or sub-regional services was then calculated.

A small number of local government districts were omitted from the analysis because they were served by hospitals in a neighbouring health region and therefore all possible hospital admissions from within the population could not be captured in the analysis.

Data were analysed in two main ways. Firstly, simple hospitalisation rates were produced for different operations in relation to the populations living in health or local government districts. This enabled the number of operations per 1000 (or 10 000) population to be examined and compared.

Secondly, standardised hospitalisation ratios (SHRs) were produced. The concept is similar to the standardised mortality ratio (SMR) that is described in Chapter 1. It allows for differences in the age and sex composition of the resident populations and hence enables a more valid comparison to be made. For example, a district with a young age composition could be expected to record low rates for cataract operations (cataracts being more common in the elderly). SHRs enable a comparison of this district's operation rates with other districts' rates to be made, allowing for the different age compositions. In the investigation described here, the regional SHR for each specialty was, by definition, 100, and SHRs for individual resident populations were compared to this regional average value. A figure above 100 denoted more hospital discharges and a figure below 100 denoted fewer hospital discharges amongst residents of a particular area than might have been expected given the experience of the region as a whole.

Findings and Implications

Two examples illustrate the findings and show the kinds of issues that were raised by the investigation. The first relates to cataract operations, the second to coronary artery bypass operations.

Table 2.18 shows the SHRs for cataract surgery in relation to local government district of residence, together with information on the location of the sub-regional ophthalmology services that were undertaking the surgery. There was a two-fold variation in the likelihood of a person being admitted for cataract surgery according to where they lived. To some extent, the likelihood of being admitted was higher in resident populations with greater geographical proximity to the service, but some local government districts with a service within

their boundaries appear to have substantially lower admission rates than others. These lower rates often apply to adjacent local government districts predominantly served by this same service.

Table 2.19 displays the data for coronary artery bypass operations and clearly shows that the highest admission rate was for residents of the host district, with the lowest for a district (South Tyneside) some eight miles away. Other districts further from the host district (for example, North Tees, 36 miles away) had higher resident access rates.

The interpretation of data on the use of health services is made difficult by the absence of any general understanding of what constitutes need. Thus when comparing admission rates to a particular hospital service from two or more populations, there is no way of knowing, in any of the communities concerned, the size of the pool of patients requiring treatment. Therefore, it is not possible to say what level of hospital admission would have been appropriate in the investigation described.

Demographic differences can account for some variation in admission rates when diseases are more common at certain ages. For example, coronary heart disease is more common in older males; if one district contains more older males than another with the same total population, then it is to be expected that they will record higher admission due to this disease. This was tested as a possible source of variation in Table 2.19, where unstandardised rates are used, but it was found to be a very minor source of variation. It cannot be responsible for any of the variation documented in Table 2.18 however, because there the data are presented

Table 2.18 Extent to which residents of local government districts in the Northern Region received cataract surgery operations

Place of residence	Standardised hospitalisation ratio (inpatients and day cases)
Castle Morpeth	128
Durham	127
Darlington	123*
Newcastle	122*
Gateshead	112
Derwentside	109
Stockton	107
North Tyneside	106
Blyth	103
Wansbeck	103
Sunderland	98*
Carlisle	96*
Copeland	95
Middlesbrough	93*
Tynedale	92
Sedgefield	88
Wear Valley	88
Berwick	85
Allerdale	81*
Alnwick	81
Easington	78
South Tyneside	76
Langbaurgh	75
Eden	71
Hartlepool	61
Chester-le-Street	60
Region	100

* Local government districts that had, within their boundaries, an ophthalmology unit.

as SHRs, which allow for any demographic differences between the districts.

Why were SHRs not also the method of presentation of the data for the coronary artery bypass surgery analysis? They could equally well have been. The reason SHRs were not used was the potential impact of the presentation of the findings on a health authority that included lay members. SHRs (or SMRs for that matter) are usually quite well understood by people without a background in public health if the concept is simply explained as part of the presentation of data. Their power of impact is as a comparative measure, showing the extent of variation between populations. Used alone, however, they can sometimes have reduced impact with the lay person because of the abstract nature of a relative measure. Therefore, it is sometimes important to give the target audience a feel for absolute values. There is additional impact in being able to picture the number of people being admitted for every 1000 or 10 000 in the population.

While such data must be interpreted

Table 2.19 Extent to which residents of district health authorities in the Northern Region received coronary artery bypass surgery (1984–85)

Place of residence	Inpatient discharges per 1000 resident population
Newcastle	0.27*
North Tyneside	0.22
Northumberland	0.20
North Tees	0.17
East Cumbria	0.16
Durham	0.16
Darlington	0.15
Gateshead	0.12
North West Durham	0.12
South Tees	0.12
Hartlepool	0.11
West Cumbria	0.11
South West Durham	0.11
South Cumbria	0.10
Sunderland	0.09
South Tyneside	0.07
Region	0.15

*District health authority with cardiothoracic unit.

cautiously, it is unlikely that differences in the size in the examples described could have resulted from limitations in the data (considerable validity checks were in any case carried out).

As was indicated earlier, broad knowledge of the population and its pattern of disease and mortality does not suggest that the variation could have arisen from differences in morbidity and demography. The cataract data were in any case standardised to eliminate the effect of differences in age structure, the strongest correlate with incidence. Mortality rates from coronary heart disease in the Northern Region were amongst the worst in the country, and districts such as South Tyneside (with low access to coronary artery bypass surgery) were amongst the worst within the region. There was no evidence either that Newcastle's population was being overtreated (another theoretical explanation for the differences).

Thus the investigators felt it a fair assumption that the variations represented the differing extent to which need was being recognised and acted upon by patients and doctors.

The underlying factors that determine the extent to which a given level of need is translated into inpatient care include patient consultation rates (with general practitioners), general practitioner referral rates (to hospital consultants), availability and accessibility of hospital facilities, thresholds for admission and treatment (by individual consultants) and secondary referral rates (from one hospital consultant to another).

Tentative ideas about the main sources of the variation in the investigation described here were that the differential coronary artery bypass admission rates may have partly been explained by the availability, in district services, of physicians with expertise in cardiology who were able to recognise and refer appropriate cases. This certainly seemed to fit with existing knowledge of the pattern of district service. For example, in Newcastle a specialist cardiology team was in place, and many general practitioners would refer cases to them as a first choice. The North Tees physicians also had expertise in the specialty, which may explain higher access rates in a more geographically remote population.

The data for rates of cataract extraction seemed to be more closely related to geographical proximity to a service-providing centre. Beyond this, descriptive data like these can only be used for discussion and exploration of issues, not to draw conclusions.

Comment and Overview

This investigation used routinely available data and hence was relatively rapidly carried out and limited in its scope. Nevertheless, it stimulated a debate at the time at the highest policy-making level within the region. The debate ranged across issues such as the siting of specialist services, the level and distribution of consultant posts in particular specialties, resource-allocation policy, general practitioner referral patterns and the prioritisation of patients on waiting lists. It led to the establishment of a second cardiothoracic centre in Middlesbrough – in the southern part of the region. Towards the end of the first decade of the 21st century, this second centre was well established and dealing with a large workload of revascularisation procedures. The strong clinical impression of the cardiologists and cardiothoracic surgeons appointed to the new service was that it was dealing (in its first few years of operation) with very severe coronary heart disease in much younger people than they had seen in other centres where they had worked.

A STUDY OF SURVIVAL OF AN ELDERLY POPULATION ACCORDING TO THE LEVEL OF FUNCTIONAL CAPACITY
Context and Problem Definition

The entire population of people aged 65 years and over who were in any type of institutional care (hospitals or residential homes) in Leicestershire was enumerated on a single day. Amongst other information gathered on each elderly person at the time was an assessment of his or her functional capacity expressed as basic activities of daily living. This institutional elderly population was then followed up over a three-year period. The aim of the study was to examine survival against different levels of incapacity and independence in each type of care.

Carrying out the Investigation

A total of 4490 people aged 65 years and over had been enumerated in a one-day census in the full range of institutional care provided by the public sector (NHS and social care services) and the independent sector (private and voluntary) in the health district. Hospital beds, nursing homes and residential care places were all covered. A range of data was gathered on each patient or resident, but included in the original survey was an assessment of their functional capacity (mobility, urinary incontinence, faecal incontinence, washing/dressing and feeding). The scale used had been validated.

Copies of death returns were then gathered over a three-year period, and details of deaths amongst any of the original population were recorded. A life-table analysis of mortality was then carried out to produce survival times from the time of the initial assessment. The basis of this standard life-table approach was that exposure to the risk of death was grouped into a number of person-years of observation. For each patient or resident, it was known whether or not they died and the time from initial enumeration. The exposure time then ran from the starting date to the date of death, or if they did not die, to the end of the corresponding follow-up period. Confidence intervals were calculated for the proportion surviving. A regression analysis of the life-table allowed differences in survival in different groups to be compared, taking account of other factors that appreciably affected survival. The statistical methods are referred to here in general terms in order to allow an understanding of the principles of the analysis (a more detailed account is in the original paper).

Findings and Implications

The rate of survival at all time periods after assessment fell with increasing incapacity. For example, two years after having been assessed as 'bedfast', 36% of old people were still alive, compared to 73% in the group who had been 'fully ambulant'. A similar pattern was observed for people falling into different categories of urinary incontinence. Table 2.20 illustrates the pattern, which was similar for each 'activity of daily living'. In all these activities, the differences in the rate of survival between incapacity groups remained highly statistically significant, even after adjustment for differences in age, sex and duration of stay using regression analysis.

The analysis for the different types of care (Table 2.21) showed what would have been expected given the much higher levels of dependency in some settings compared to others. What was more surprising was that when differences in levels of functional capacity (and also age and sex) between the different types of care were allowed for in the statistical analysis, most of the differential survival disappeared. This was true of the three types of NHS care and the homes for the elderly.

The findings demonstrated the power of this relatively simple measure of incapacity in an elderly population to predict survival. Moreover, it seemed to be an important core characteristic of health status almost irrespective of where an elderly person was being cared for.

Comment and Overview

This investigation established that gathering data on functional capacity of an elderly population can provide an important basis for summarising its health status. The approach does not require complex procedures and has a range of other potential uses, including planning services and rehabilitation policies, evaluation of the components of care and assessing the impact of individual institutional regimes. The importance of such measures to the concept of healthy life expectancy is discussed further in Chapter 8.

Table 2.20 Percentage survival (with 95% confidence limits in brackets) from time of assessment by degree of urinary incontinence

Time from assessment	Not incontinent	Needed raising or sending	Incontinent once	Often incontinent	All degrees
6 months	90.7 (89.4–91.9)	85.1 (80.8–88.6)	82.3 (78.0–86.0)	73.5 (70.4–76.4)	85.4 (84.2–86.5)
1 year	84.1 (82.5–85.7)	74.1 (69.1–78.7)	70.1 (65.2–75.0)	61.1 (57.7–64.4)	76.5 (75.1–77.9)
2 years	69.6 (67.6–71.6)	56.5 (51.0–61.9)	48.2 (43.0–53.3)	41.1 (37.8–44.5)	59.6 (58.0–61.2)
3 years	57.3 (55.1–59.5)	43.3 (38.0–48.8)	35.9 (31.1–41.0)	28.9 (25.9–32.1)	47.3 (45.6–48.9)

Source: Donaldson LJ, Jagger C. Survival and functional capacity: three year follow-up of an elderly population in hospitals and homes. *J Epidemiol Community Health.* 1983; **37**: 176–9.

Table 2.21 Estimated percentage survival (95% confidence limits not shown here) to various times after admission to different types of care

Time from admission	NHS geriatric beds	NHS psychiatric beds	NHS acute beds	Homes for the elderly	Private nursing homes	All types of care
6 months	61.9	77.2	75.0	81.0	80.4	72.3
1 year	49.5	64.4	67.4	68.8	64.4	60.9
2 years	37.2	49.2	59.9	53.9	53.4	48.4
3 years	27.4	38.7	53.2	43.3	40.0	38.5
5 years	10.6	21.8	49.8	27.0	23.5	22.5

Source: Donaldson LJ, Jagger C. Survival and functional capacity: three year follow-up of an elderly population in hospitals and homes. *J Epidemiol Community Health.* 1983; **37**: 176–9.

AN INVESTIGATION INTO THE REASONS FOR THE DELAYED DISCHARGE OF PATIENTS HOSPITALISED WITH FRACTURED NECK OF FEMUR

Fractured neck of femur is a common injury in the elderly and one that is responsible for a high proportion of admissions to acute orthopaedic hospital inpatient services. In the past, many patients were treated conservatively through traction, with the consequent high mortality and morbidity associated with prolonged bed-rest in elderly people. Today, the approach to clinical management is based upon early surgical intervention to allow rapid mobilisation and to give the greatest chance of returning the elderly patient to his or her pre-fracture level of independence. Nevertheless, the high volume of cases and the underlying frailty and associated medical problems that many elderly people have, together with the fact that the fracture often brings to light unsatisfactory home and social circumstances, means that hospital stays can easily become prolonged.

The investigation described here set out to examine the factors that were leading to extended hospital stay in patients admitted to the major hospital dealing with trauma cases in a large health district in the East Midlands part of England.

Context and Problem Definition

An acute orthopaedic ward may not be the best environment in which to meet the continuing care needs of an elderly person who is not able to return home, nor may it be the most appropriate use of scarce acute-sector resources. The issue is encapsulated in the emotive and even hostile term 'blocked bed'. This is sometimes used to describe the occupation of a bed in an acute hospital by an elderly person, judged not to be acutely ill or whose stay is longer than what is perceived as being within the normal confines of an acute illness.

The investigators wanted to understand what specific stages of care account for the hospital stay (for example, preoperative stabilisation, postoperative complications, placement problems). Routinely available hospital data provided details of the total length of stay but not its components.

The Leicestershire Health District was a large urban and rural population, with approximately 850 000 residents at the time of the investigation, of whom about 15% were aged 65 years and over. The organisation of trauma and orthopaedic services was such that a high proportion of injuries (including fractured neck of femur) occurring in the population of Leicestershire were treated at one large centrally placed hospital.

Carrying out the Investigation

The investigators began by formulating an operational definition of fractured neck of femur. The study entry criterion was: 'the presence of an intracapsular or extracapsular fracture of the femur down to 1 cm below the lesser trochanter'. There were no exclusions.

The study population was a consecutive series of admissions to hospital over a 20-week period from October to February. The choice of this time period was dictated by the resources available to undertake the study and the need to produce a result reasonably quickly.

A system was established whereby a member of the investigative team visited the wards of the hospital daily to identify the patients who had been admitted and who met the entry criterion. While time-consuming, such an arrangement was preferable to ensure completeness of capture of the study population rather than relying on busy nursing or medical staff to notify cases.

Each of the patients had a stage of care identified for each day of the hospital stay using a methodology adapted from one developed by North American investigators. This was based on the application to each day of care of the question 'Why is this patient in hospital now?'

After discussion with the clinical team, each day of each patient's stay was assigned to one of the following categories:

a preoperative, no perceived problems, awaiting surgery

b preoperative, awaiting medical assessment or therapy before surgery

c postoperative, condition improving, no complications

d postoperative, complications of surgery have developed and are prolonging the stay

e postoperative, medical difficulties have developed which would have required hospital admission regardless of surgery

f medically and surgically fit for discharge, but hospital stay continues for other reasons (e.g., awaiting geriatric assessment or bed, arrangements being made for domiciliary services, arrival of caring relatives awaited)

g receiving conservative therapy, no operation.

As Table 2.22 shows, almost all the bed-days were spent by the patients awaiting a theatre session (10%); recovering from surgery without complications (51%); or waiting to leave the orthopaedic ward, despite being medically and surgically fit to do so (28%). Other analyses (not presented here) were performed on the number of days spent in each stage.

It was calculated that if all patients who were fit for surgery had been taken to theatre without delay, 492 hospital-days could have been saved. Moreover, if it had been possible to discharge or transfer patients when they no longer needed to remain in hospital for medical and surgical reasons, 1437 hospital-days could have been saved.

It was further estimated that by combining both of these strategies, the average duration of stay could have been reduced by eight days.

Comment and Overview

The methodology contained elements of the cohort study approach, the study population being a consecutive group of patients admitted to hospital and then followed up during their stay. While the period of the year chosen to recruit the cohort could have been unrepresentative of all patients'

experience (for example, if there had been strong seasonal differences), there was no evidence that overall length of stay varied markedly at different times of the year. The use of caring staff to contribute to the classification of the days of care is open to the criticism that through the knowledge of being studied they could have modified their assessment of each patient. However, one of the senior investigators was in active clinical practice and had made his own baseline assessment of the patients and review of the medical records. Thus a more independent judgement was also available.

The investigation provided a focus for policy discussion. It pinpointed and addressed the problem of extended hospital stay in this group of elderly patients and provided the focus for in-depth review of the whole issue, including the timing of surgery (with implications for out-of-hours staffing of operating theatres and the availability of on-call radiographers) and arrangements

Table 2.22 Number of patient-days spent in each stage of acute hospital care by people with fractured neck of femur

Stage of care*	Number of patient-days	Percentage of total stay
a	492	10
b	141	3
c	2690	51
d	59	1
e	56	1
f	1437	28
g	292	6
Total	5167	–

*See text for definition of stages.

Source: Robbins JA, Donaldson LJ. Analysing stages of care in hospital stay for fractured neck of femur. *Lancet.* 1984; **1**: 1028-9.

for assessment, rehabilitation and future placement (with implications for greater involvement of geriatricians and social workers earlier in the acute hospital stay).

AN INVESTIGATION TO DESCRIBE RAPIDLY AN EMERGING PROBLEM FOR WHICH LITTLE INFORMATION WAS AVAILABLE

From time to time, a health problem will suddenly come to the attention of the public through critical comment in the local or national media in such a way that there may be a high level of disquiet or a loss of confidence in services. Just such a major crisis was caused when a sudden increase in the number of children suspected of having been sexually abused were taken into local authority care in Cleveland, a county in the North East of England, over a three-month period in the summer of 1987.

Little information was available to be able to define the size or nature of the problem so that it could be discussed rationally and objectively. This example describes an investigation that was carried out very rapidly to provide such contextual information.

Context and Problem Definition

The Cleveland crisis came about because of a number of factors. Firstly, there was a sharp rise in admissions of children with a diagnosis of suspected sexual abuse to one of the main hospitals in the county (Middlesbrough General Hospital). Many of these children were then made the subject of court orders (under the then child protection legislation), which led to them being retained in the hospital as a 'place of safety' for further assessment and investigation.

The presence of these additional children, who were physically active, boisterous and in some cases behaviourally disturbed, placed enormous pressure on the physical facilities available and on the nursing staff, who were also trying to care for acutely ill children. The Social Services Department (as the lead agency in child protection services) did not have the skilled social-work staff, to respond to this rapid increase in cases referred to it.

The presence of high numbers of parents whose children were being kept largely in one place focused parental anger and led to involvement of members of parliament, who publicly and effectively articulated the collective sense of indignation and concern. Finally, the open airing of professional differences of opinion on the validity of the diagnoses led further to the impression of confusion. In the first few weeks of the crisis, the services underwent a period of major instability and perceived loss of public confidence.

Much of the prevailing media comment led the public to believe that the number of cases being diagnosed was large and unprecedented (amounting to one in 10 of the population). This added to the sense of incredulity and the impression that a wholesale mistake had been made by the professional staff involved.

At this stage, however, no firm data were available on the numbers of children involved. Therefore, numbers could not be related to the population of origin or valid comparisons made with elsewhere in the country or with other countries. In addition, many professionals expressed public disquiet at the frequency of anal abuse diagnosed – particularly in very young children and in girls. Thus part of the initial controversy resulted from a failure to be able to quantify and describe the problem in population terms. Coupled with this, the perception that parents were being denied their rights, that social workers and paediatricians had acted over-zealously (apparently seeking out abuse where it did not exist) and that undue reliance had been placed on an unproven diagnostic technique (the reflex anal dilatation test) added to the sense of public concern and turmoil.

A judicial inquiry was established by the Minister for Health, for which evidence was prepared on a wide range of aspects of the background to the problems in Cleveland. As part of this evidence, information was gathered to describe the population of children who were the subject of the diagnosis of suspected sexual abuse.

Carrying out the Investigation

All records of cases of sexual abuse or suspected sexual abuse in children coming to the attention of paediatric services or the Social Services Department over the three-month period were assembled. These cases were identified by searching hospital records of all paediatric admissions (sexual abuse was not a diagnosis recorded in routinely available hospital inpatient data) and the cases referred to the Social Services Department over the same period.

A pre-coded structured pro-forma was designed to record data extracted from the children's records. The main areas of data recording were demographic and administrative, mode of presentation, main clinical findings, subsequent management, and details of referral for other medical opinion (where this occurred).

High standards of confidentiality were observed when extracting the data. Medical staff undertook the work personally. Analyses were carried out on an aggregated and anonymised basis only so that no children or families could ever be identified.

Cases were classified into three categories according to the way in which they came to light:

a   index case – the child in a family (or group of children) who, on presentation, first gave rise to the suspicion that sexual abuse may have occurred

b   sibling of index case – brother or sister of index case, who was examined because of the suspicion of child sexual abuse in the index case

c   contact of index case – a child connected with the index case (but not a brother or sister), who was examined because of the suspicion of child sexual abuse in the index case.

Findings and Implications

Figure 2.20 shows the time at which children were diagnosed over the three-month period. The crisis broke publicly following the peak of diagnoses in the week commencing 15 June 1987.

Table 2.23 shows the overall rate for the three-month period was 9.8 per 10 000 population, which is equivalent to approximately one case in 1000 children (aged 0–14 years). The rate for girls of all ages was approximately twice that for boys, and the highest rate was in girls up to the age of four years.

Table 2.24 shows an analysis of anal or vaginal physical signs recorded by the doctors following their examinations of the children.

The figure and the two tables show only a small selection of the analyses. Nevertheless, they illustrate the role that simple descriptive data can play in throwing light on a problem. In this investigation, they illustrated that the problem was far less common than some of the exaggerated early impressions had suggested. Furthermore, they emphasised that part of the numerical problem arose from children who had been examined because they were siblings or contacts of children suspected of being sexually abused. On the other hand, the doctors' findings of signs of anal abuse even in very young children emphasised the centrality of these physical signs to the debate and demonstrated the need to address issues of 'normality' and 'abnormality'. Many of these issues were the subjects of extensive scrutiny by the judicial inquiry.

Comment and Overview

The study could not, and did not purport to, provide a definitive estimate of the size of the problem of sexual abuse in the population concerned. Neither did it set out to examine the validity of the diagnoses made. It also used a retrospective method of enquiry whose primary source of data – medical and social services records – was not created specifically for investigative purposes. Nevertheless, a prospective study

would probably have proved impossible in the light of the attention that had been focused on the issue; circumstances would have certainly influenced the way in which information was recorded.

However, given that its limitations were made clear (which they were at the time), the investigation fulfilled a useful purpose in helping to correct a misleading anecdotal impression. This can be an important and useful role for investigations in public health medicine in a situation where absolutely no data are available, and when decisions are being made and conclusions drawn on purely subjective grounds. The investigation also proved invaluable in designing a conceptual framework for categorising the cases (index, non-index) so that the size of the problem that arose from children being diagnosed at presentation could be distinguished from the extent to which children contributed who were only included by virtue of their association with other cases. This approach was subsequently adopted by the judicial inquiry in its own case analysis.

The investigation also highlighted the need for further study: in particular for population-based studies of the size and distribution of sexual abuse using agreed criteria for their case definition. It also highlighted the need for improvement of the quality of routinely collected statistics held on child protection registers.

AN INVESTIGATION TO EXAMINE THE IMPLICATIONS OF THE PHASING OUT OF LARGE MENTAL HOSPITALS

It has been long-established policy of British governments in the field of services for peo-

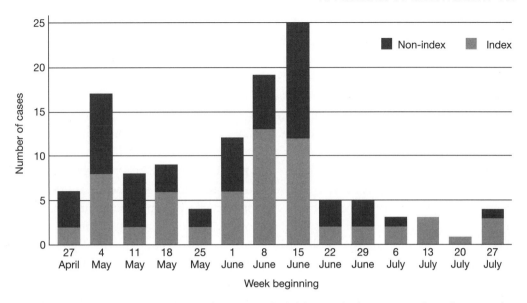

Figure 2.20 Time at which cases of suspected child sexual abuse were first diagnosed in Cleveland

Table 2.23 Age- and sex-specific rates of occurrence for cases of suspected child sexual abuse per 10 000 population during the three-month period from May to July 1987 in Cleveland

Age group (years)	Male	Female	Both sexes
0–4	5.4	19.2	12.2
5–9	8.9	17.7	13.2
10–14	4.4	4.2	4.3
0–14	6.2	13.7	9.8

Source: Donaldson LJ. Evidence given to the Judicial Inquiry into Child Abuse in Cleveland, 1987.

ple with mental illness to shift the balance of care from hospital to community. An important element of this policy has been to provide care for mentally ill people in need of hospital care in facilities that are integrated within district general hospitals.

The most visible manifestation of these policies has been the closure (or redesignation), in many parts of the country, of the past cornerstone of care for the mentally ill: the large mental hospitals, many of which are buildings that housed Victorian asylums.

The investigation described here set out to identify some of the practical problems of implementing these policies by assessing the levels of physical, mental and social functioning of mentally ill people in institutional care within a large health district in the East Midlands part of England.

Table 2.24 Presence of anal and vaginal signs in all cases of suspected child sexual abuse diagnosed in Cleveland May/June 1987 (percentages)

Physical signs	Male	Female	Both sexes
Anal only	100	28	51
Vaginal only	N/A	9	6
Both	N/A	60	41
Neither	0	2	2
Not stated	–	1	1
Total	100 (n = 38)	100 (n = 82)	100 (n = 120)

N/A = Not applicable.
Source: Donaldson LJ. Evidence given to the Judicial Inquiry into Child Abuse in Cleveland, 1987.

Context and Problem Definition

One of the key determinants of the success of the policies described above was the ability of local psychiatric services to satisfactorily reduce the number of patients requiring nursing care on a longer-term basis. In practice, this was (and still is) an issue about suitability for discharge of patients who have already spent much of their life in a psychiatric hospital setting. It is also about preventing the accumulation of a 'new' long-stay group arising from younger patients who are admitted for what are intended as short spells of hospital inpatient care.

Further key factors for policy success were, and also still are: the adequacy of community-based psychiatric services to care for mentally ill people who would previously have ended up in hospitals; and to have effective ways of helping elderly, severely mentally ill people whose physical and mental frailty make it extremely difficult for them to be returned from hospital to the community.

The investigation set out to evaluate each patient within psychiatric inpatient hospital care facilities in the health district of approximately 850 000 population and to assess their level of physical, social and mental capacity relevant to care requirements.

Carrying out the Investigation

The method was a one-day census in which each patient was identified and the assessment carried out. With over 1000 beds or hospital places in psychiatric facilities in the district, the investigation was a very major exercise and required careful planning and detailed preparatory work in advance of the date that was agreed for the census.

Nursing and medical staff completed a 47-item assessment schedule on each patient in their care, the assessment covering eight main areas: demographic and administrative; current diagnoses; ward behaviour and nursing problems; current treatment; employment status and occupational therapy; contact with the outside world; rehabilitation prospects; and family dependants.

In many of these areas of assessment, standard scales or measures that had been validated in earlier studies were used.

Findings and Implications

At census point, there were 1086 inpatients, of whom 1052 (96%) were resident in two large mental hospitals. Table 2.25 shows that the largest group of psychiatric inpatients was the very elderly. Thirty-seven percent of patients were 75 years or older, a much greater proportion than the very elderly population of the health district as a whole (5% were aged 75 years and over). The table also indicates that while the proportion of very elderly people was lower amongst those who had been resident for the shortest and longest times, even in these length-of-stay groups it was still very substantial.

Comparing the bottom row of figures in Table 2.25 gives an impression of the relative sizes of the different length-of-stay

groups. While the largest proportion (413 out of 1086, or 38%) of patients had been in hospital for less than one year, 26% were inpatients of more than 10 years' standing, and more than half this latter group were elderly (65 years of age or older). The remaining group of patients, whose stay had extended beyond a year but was less than 10 years, made up 36% of all inpatients; a third of these were under 65 years of age.

Dementia was the most common diagnosis in patients of all lengths of stay, except the very long-stay group, amongst which schizophrenia predominated.

The social withdrawal rating scale used in the investigation provided an indication of patients' level of social functioning within the hospital and gave an indication of their chances of discharge. The possible score derived from this rating scale ranged from a minimum of zero to a maximum of

Table 2.25 Cumulative percentages of psychiatric patients in different length-of-stay groups who were a given age or older

| Age (years) | Length of current stay (years) | | | | | |
	<1	1–2	2–5	5–10	10 and over	All lengths of stay
85 and over	8	17	19	15	7	11
75 and over	29	56	51	39	31	37
65 and over	45	70	70	57	59	56
55 and over	58	82	80	78	82	72
45 and over	67	88	88	88	92	81
35 and over	78	92	96	94	98	89
25 and over	88	97	100	100	100	95
15 and over	100	100	100	100	100	100
(n =)	(413)	(174)	(92)	(121)	(286)	(1086)

Source: Levene LS, Donaldson LJ, Brandon S. How likely is it that a district health authority can close its large mental hospitals? *Br J Psych.* 1985; **147**: 150–5.

16 points. A score in the 0–4 range had been shown from previous studies to indicate that psychiatric inpatients have the potential for discharge.

Overall, more than half of all patients had scores above the 0–4 range. However, the patterns were so different for elderly patients, compared to younger patients, that data are presented for the two groups separately (Tables 2.26 and 2.27).

Of patients under the age of 65 (Table 2.26), almost three-quarters, regardless of length of stay, had low social withdrawal scores, but less than half of those with a duration of stay of 1–2 years had such scores. Furthermore, another finding of the study (not tabulated here) showed that one-quarter of patients aged under 65 years with a 1–2 year length-of-stay were not fully continent of urine. These findings strongly suggest that disability in this group was intrinsic to the disorder, rather than a consequence of institutionalisation, and that major efforts at treatment, rehabilitation or training would need to be directed at these patients.

The patients under 65 years of age with a length of stay of 10 years or more (comprising a quarter of all patients aged under 65 years) were people in the main with low social withdrawal scores, but it is this group who are most used to institutional life and therefore potentially the most difficult to return to the community.

Three-quarters of all residents in the over-65 age group (Table 2.27) had substantial social withdrawal, and two-thirds were not fully continent of urine.

The group of patients aged over 65 years who had been in hospital for less than one year had lower social withdrawal scores overall and therefore seemed to have greater potential for discharge.

Overall, the investigation clearly showed that the presence of large numbers of elderly patients was the most important feature of the short-, intermediate-, and long-stay groups of patients in psychiatric hospitals. Those elderly patients who had been in hospital for longer than 10 years were less incapacitated, both socially and physically, than their shorter-stay counterparts, though they clearly exhibited much higher levels of incapacity than younger patients. Nevertheless, it seemed possible that for a proportion of this group of very long-stay elderly patients some alternative less-dependent form of care could have been provided. However, prolonged exposure to an institutional way of life, coupled with advancing years, made it likely that this care would need to continue to be provided in a very protected environment.

It was noted that while the elderly group amongst the long-stay patients would dwindle (because of deaths), this could be a slow process, and optimism about reduction of numbers in this category needed to be tempered by the observation that there were substantial numbers of elderly mentally ill people in the intermediate-stay groups. Moreover, the continuing demand for hospital places from patients in the community and the possible development of a younger long-stay group would create further pressure on the same facilities.

Comment and Overview

The findings of the investigation could not

Table 2.26 Percentage of psychiatric inpatients aged under-65 years with different social withdrawal (SW) scores, by length of stay

SW score*	Length of current stay (years)					
	<1	1–2	2–5	5–10	10 and over	All lengths of stay
0–4	81	46	61	86	65	72
5–9	12	28	28	10	28	198
10–14	4	20	11	4	6	7
15–16	3	6	0	0	1	2
All scores	100	100	100	100	100	100
(n =)	(220)	(50)	(28)	(51)	(117)	(466)

*Higher scores denote more severely incapacitated patients.
Source: Levene LS, Donaldson LJ, Brandon S. How likely is it that a district health authority can close its large mental hospitals? *Br J Psych.* 1985; **147**: 150–5.

Table 2.27 Percentage of psychiatric inpatients aged 65 years and over with different social withdrawal (SW) scores, by length of stay

SW score*	Length of current stay (years)					
	<1	1–2	2–5	5–10	10 and over	All lengths of stay
0–4	28	14	19	15	41	26
5–9	37	30	31	29	37	34
10–14	28	44	34	30	20	30
15–16	7	12	16	26	2	10
All scores	100	100	100	100	100	100
(n =)	(185)	(122)	(64)	(69)	(168)	(608)

*Higher scores denote more severely incapacitated patients.
Source: Levene LS, Donaldson LJ, Brandon S. How likely is it that a district health authority can close its large mental hospitals? *Br J Psych.* 1985; **147**: 150–5.

provide a blueprint for future services, but they did identify several key issues.

Firstly, the large existing number of elderly disabled patients, together with the expectation of a further increase in their numbers, presented the most serious obstacle to hospital closure. It was noted that alternative facilities would take time to develop and were likely to consume even more resources than were currently being expended. If admission and treatment facilities were to be transferred to general hospital units while the existing mental hospitals remained open, they were in danger of becoming repositories for the disabled elderly, with consequent major problems in maintaining staff morale and high standards.

A second issue identified by the investigation was the high disability scores amongst patients with a duration of stay exceeding one but less than two years. This suggested that services were focused upon the acute episode or on the rehabilitation of long-stay patients. The needs of medium-stay patients were being comparatively overlooked. The transition from acute admission to long-term resident is often insidious. Concentration on treatment may delay efforts at social rehabilitation.

The findings on aspects of physical disability were also of major policy importance. Incontinence, for example, is a significant impediment when alternative accommodation is being sought. The substantial number of patients, even in the younger age groups, who were incontinent of urine suggested this as a target symptom demanding special attention. It also pointed the way for studies to examine the role of medication in causing and reducing incontinence, the development of behavioural programmes in incontinence management and the criteria for more vigorous intervention with this problem.

The investigation as a whole exposed a wide range of policy issues relevant to the organisation of psychiatric services in the health district concerned.

CONCLUSIONS

This chapter has described an important facet of public health, namely the study methodologies and investigative approaches that must be mastered if the full range of health and health service problems are to be addressed. The practice of clinical medicine is often compared to a series of detective stories in which the clues to the diagnosis of a patient's clinical problem are investigated. In population medicine, the mysteries of health and disease in entire populations, some extremely complex, are also very challenging. The benefits of solving these problems in delaying death, preventing disease and improving the quality of health care are enormous. To develop the analogy, while the clinical detective is pursuing the ordinary criminal, the public health investigator is on the trail of the Godfathers of syndicated crime.

REFERENCE

1 Glasziou P, Chalmers I, Rawlins M, *et al*. When are randomised controlled trials unnecessary? Picking signal from noise. *BMJ*. 2007; **334**: 349–51.

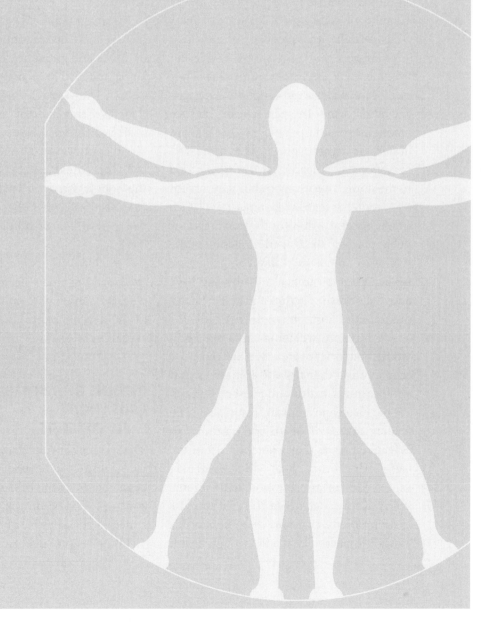

CHAPTER 3
The Promotion of Health

INTRODUCTION

As the twenty-first century progresses, concern amongst the population living in Britain and other industrialised countries about health and its relationship to individual lifestyle and to the environment has never been greater. This is evident not just in the behaviour of individuals but also in shifts in societal attitudes as reflected, for example, in the response of major manufacturers to consumers' wishes and expectations, as well as in the increasing preoccupation of mass media with health issues.

Examples that illustrate this greater health consciousness are numerous. They include the widespread adoption of jogging and other forms of regular aerobic exercise amongst the adult population, the growth in sales of organic foodstuffs and the success of box schemes delivering organic food to the door. The strong public support for legislation has seen environmental tobacco smoke become a thing of the past in indoor public places in the United Kingdom. In the workplace, more and more companies are paying attention to health issues and have adopted stress-reduction and other health programmes for their employees.

All these are welcome signs that individuals and societies are now more receptive than at any other time to initiatives that will promote health and prevent disease. Yet the challenges remain formidable. The leading causes of death and disability in Britain remain as they were for most of the twentieth century: heart disease, stroke, cancer, chronic bronchitis and unintentional injury. Knowledge about the causation of these problems provides the potential for a major impact to be made through health promotion programmes. Despite this, consistent success in reducing the burden of illness and premature death from these causes has remained elusive. In particular, inequalities in disease experience between different social strata are as great as ever, and addressing their wider determinants – physical and social environment, education, employment and reduction of relative poverty – remains fundamental to successful action.

The major aims of health services should be to reduce the amount of illness, disease, disability and premature death in the population and also to increase the numbers of people who spend a high proportion of their lives in a state of health rather than in ill health. Health services do not have direct control over all the factors that can influence these aspects of the health of the population, so it is vital to emphasise multisectoral approaches at local level and pan-governmental coordination at national level.

This chapter describes the main strategies available to promote health and prevent disease, beginning with an historical account of the development of thinking about the causation of disease.

ORIGINS OF DISEASE AND ITS CAUSATION
EARLY CONCEPTS

The writings and teachings of Hippocrates had an impact far beyond his lifetime, which began on the island of Cos, near the Ionian coast of Asia Minor, about 460 BC and ended (legend has it) when bees swarmed on his grave, producing a special honey: the cure for stomatitis in infants. Hippocrates is regarded by many as the father of medicine, although medicine was practised before this time. Indeed, writings on such matters date back to the earliest civilisations. In Hippocrates' time, however, there were no boundaries between medicine, art, religion or philosophy.

One of the main contributions of the Hippocratic school lay in focusing intellectual attention on medicine in its own right, as a science founded on the observation of facts and the recording of clinical experiences. One of the major teachings was that the body contained four humours: blood, black bile, yellow bile and phlegm. In health, the humours mingled together and were in harmony or balance; in disease there was a derangement of this mixture.

Hippocrates was the first to seek to explain the origins of disease, and in so doing he put forward many observations that do not seem out of place even today. He distinguished between diseases that were endemic (always present in a given area) and those that at times become excessively common (epidemic). In suggesting a role for exercise, diet, climate, water and the seasons, he foreshadowed modern views of the importance of the interrelationship between man and his environment in the causation of disease.

Many of his aphorisms resonate with modern causal thinking, for example:

> 'Those naturally very fat are more liable to sudden death than the thin.'

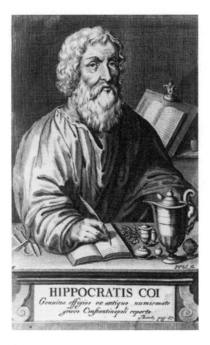

Figure 3.1 Hippocrates. Engraving, 1665
Source: The Wellcome Institute Library, London.

During the time of the Roman Empire, which eclipsed its Greek predecessor, it is the name of another Greek, Galen, which stands out in the history of medicine. Galen, who lived in the second century AD, is said to have cured the emperor Marcus Aurelius of abdominal pain. While his observations on the nature and cause of disease added little to the Hippocratic writings, he did much to advance knowledge in relation to anatomy and physiology. It was also the Roman Empire that introduced sanitation and domestic water supplies, thereby making a significant contribution to public health.

Throughout the Dark and Middle Ages, Europe was ravaged by disease and pestilence: the plague, smallpox, diphtheria, tuberculosis and leprosy. Millions of lives were lost to these scourges of mankind. It is clearly apparent from reading about the measures that were adopted at the time to combat these diseases that they were understood to be contagious. For example, sufferers from leprosy were isolated and required to carry bells to warn of their approach. However, there was no suggestion at this time of a contagious agent; rather, such diseases were held to be caused by changes in the composition of the atmosphere ('bad air') arising from stagnant or decaying organic matter.

Fracastorius (1478–1553), a Veronese poet and physician, is best remembered for writing a long poem about syphilis, or the 'French disease'. His views on the general nature and cause of infectious diseases were, however, remarkable and were expressed some 200 years before such ideas were embraced as new and revolutionary.

Fracastorius compared contagion in disease to the putrefaction that passes from one fruit to another when it rots. Moreover, when he referred to the essential nature of infection he suggested that minute particles or seeds were conveyed from person to person and propagated themselves. This first mention of the possibility that diseases are caused by specific germs attracted little attention at the time it was published.

THE MIASMA

Thomas Sydenham (1624–89) was essentially a practical physician who regarded experimental physiology, so much in vogue at the time, with contempt. His philosophy was to set aside all theory and begin by observing and recording symptoms and signs and their progression (march of events) in the sufferer from the particular ailment. He is greatly revered for his classical descriptions of diseases such as gout, measles, scarlet fever and pneumonia. He is often called the English Hippocrates because his observational method had many similarities with his distant Greek predecessor. Yet despite his genius in this respect, Sydenham added little to the understanding of why people became ill. Because of his stature, his miasmic theory of the causation of disease – little more than a re-expression of earlier ideas – was much more influential than it deserved to be. The miasma was an unidentified vapour believed to result from mysterious changes in the air. It is easy now to scoff at such an apparently preposterous suggestion. Nonetheless, as recently as the second half of the nineteenth century many medical officers of health in their annual reports still related epidemics of infectious diseases to bad odours arising in a locality.

However, the fact that the true nature of infectious disease had not been revealed did not impede progress. This was largely due to sanitary interventions, such as sewage disposal and clean water, that were necessary to remove the foul-smelling air, as these were very similar to what is needed to remove and avoid infections.

BILLS OF MORTALITY

An important, though less spectacular, contribution to this progress was the start of mortality data gathering. Before causes of disease can be investigated or preventive measures initiated, it is essential to have an indication of the size of the problem. Statistics that would allow the various outbreaks of infectious diseases to be traced originated from the work of a man who died in impoverished circumstances towards the end of the seventeenth century. This man, John Graunt (1620–74), analysed the statistics that he gleaned from the Bills of Mortality. These Bills were broadsheets issued weekly, which listed, for the London parishes, the numbers and (in a crude fashion) causes of death. They were purchased by well-to-do people who could forewarn themselves of an outbreak of the plague and forsake the city for less hazardous surroundings.

Graunt laid the foundation for the work of his illustrious successor, William Farr (1807–83), whose statistical writings from the office of the Registrar General served as the basis for the great sanitary reforms.

THE BROAD STREET PUMP

There is one episode on the road to the discovery of the true nature of infectious disease that has assumed almost romantic proportions for students and practitioners of public health: that of the investigation of the London cholera outbreak of 1854. John Snow (1813–58), apprenticed as a doctor in Newcastle upon Tyne, could justifiably have settled for one claim to immortality when he became the first man to introduce anaesthesia in childbirth. He used chloroform in the delivery of two of Queen Victoria's children. Yet it was his interest in cholera and his painstaking investigation of an outbreak of this disease that earned him a further place in medicine's hall of fame.

Cholera is a major infectious disease that spreads rapidly and causes death by the gross fluid depletion that results from the intense diarrhoea produced by the infection. It is rare today in the Western world, but it is still a serious cause of mortality in some developing countries. During the early nineteenth century, epidemics of cholera swept through London killing thousands of people.

Snow's own words best describe the outbreak in 1854:

> The most terrible outbreak of cholera which ever occurred in this kingdom is probably that which took place in Broad Street, Golden Square and adjoining streets, a few weeks ago. Within two hundred and fifty yards of the spot where Cambridge Street joins Broad Street, there were upwards of five hundred fatal attacks of cholera in ten days. The mortality in this

limited area probably equals any that was ever caused in this country, even by the plague; and it was much more sudden as the greater number of cases terminated in a few hours. The mortality would undoubtedly have been much greater had it not been for the flight of the population.

By plotting the geographical location of each case, Snow deduced that the deaths had occurred amongst people living in close proximity to the Broad Street pump (many families at this time had no water supply in their own homes, instead using a communal supply). There were one or two pieces of evidence, however, which did not at first seem to fit Snow's theory of the complicity of the pump. Firstly, a workhouse with 535 inmates in a street very close to the Broad Street pump experienced only five deaths from cholera

amongst its population. Secondly, a brewery in Broad Street itself had no fatalities amongst its workforce. Snow investigated these differences and found that the workhouse had its own pump on the premises, and the workers in the brewery never frequented the Broad Street pump. Finally, Snow turned his attention to a woman and her niece living at a considerable distance from Broad Street who, nevertheless, died of cholera during the epidemic. As a result of his interview with neighbours and next of kin, Snow ascertained that the woman had a particular liking for the flavour of the water of the Broad Street pump and sent her son to it every day for a bottle to drink.

On completing his inquiries, Snow sought an interview with the Board of Guardians of St James' Parish (who were in charge of the pump), and as a result of his representations the pump handle was removed and

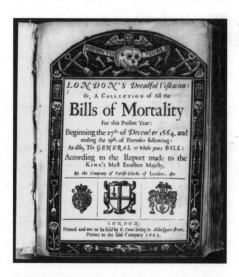

Figure 3.2 Company of Parish Clerks of London. *London's Dreadful Visitation, or a Collection of all the Bills of Mortality for the Present Year.* London: E Coles; 1665
Source: The Wellcome Institute Library, London.

the epidemic, which was already declining, came to an end.

The importance of the removal of the pump handle was symbolic of a new understanding of the nature of the disease, for Snow had demonstrated that disease can be conveyed by water and specifically that cholera is a water-borne disease.

In a less dramatic but similarly painstaking series of investigations, Snow further clarified the mode of transmission of cholera. In London at that time, a number of private companies supplied water to residents, and Londoners paid for their supply. Snow turned his attention to the water supplies of two of these companies: the Lambeth Waterworks Company and the Southwark and Vauxhall Water Company, which both supplied similar areas of London. In some cases, the pipes of both companies went down the same street, so it was possible to identify individual households supplied by one or the other. The death rate from cholera in the areas of London supplied by these two water companies was much higher than it was in places supplied by other companies. Both companies obtained their supply from the lower part of the Thames, which was the part most greatly contaminated by sewage.

A chance occurrence in 1852 provided Snow with a marvellous opportunity for a natural experiment. In that year the Lambeth water company changed its intake to another source, which was free from sewage. Snow obtained the addresses of all people dying of cholera and sought information on the source of the water supply to each household. During the epidemic in the year 1853, Snow found that there were 71 fatal attacks of cholera per 10 000 households supplied by the Southwark and Vauxhall company, compared with only five per 10 000 in those supplied by the Lambeth company. In other words, people getting their water from the polluted part of the Thames had 14 times more fatal attacks of cholera than those getting their supply from the purer source.

Snow's theory of the mode of transmission of cholera then appeared to be vindicated. He considered that cholera was spread from person to person, from the sick to the healthy, rather than by contact with any miasma or similar substance. Moreover, he deduced that this spread took place via morbid material from the alimentary canal of the sufferer, which was then swallowed by other people and had the power of multiplication in the body of the person it attacked.

Even so clear an explanation, backed by Snow's careful scientific observations, failed to convince the many doubters who still categorically rejected the idea of a specific contagion in the cause of disease.

THE GERM THEORY

The invention of the microscope around 1670 had allowed living organisms to be seen for the first time. Leeuwenhoek (1632–1725), a Dutchman, examined a range of materials such as saliva, blood, water and faeces and made drawings of micro-organisms, including what are now clearly recognisable as bacteria. No attempt was made, however, to associate these living organisms with disease in man. For example, there is no evidence that Snow saw them as the morbid material

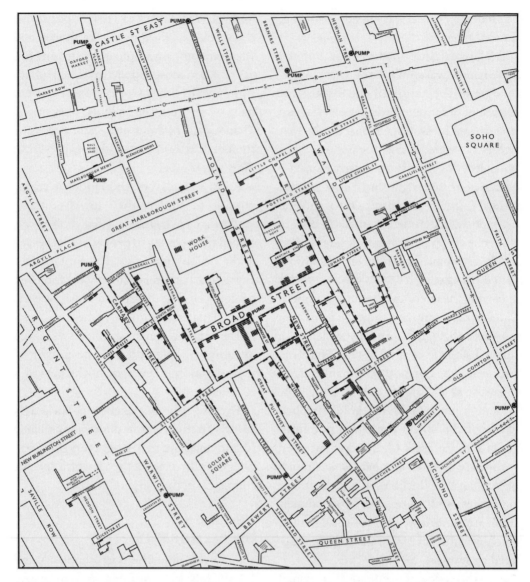

Figure 3.3 Snow's map of Soho with black units indicating deaths from cholera from 19 August to 30 September 1854
Source: The Wellcome Institute Library, London.

he suggested as a cause of cholera. Indeed, a separate controversy existed as to the origins of these micro-organisms themselves. Some scientists believed that they arose de novo (by spontaneous generation) from the fluids in which they were discovered.

Two names stand out as transforming causal thinking and finally giving birth to the germ theory of disease that had been so slow in its gestation: Louis Pasteur (1822–95) and Robert Koch (1843–1910).

Pasteur firmly rejected the idea of spontaneous generation, a long-standing theory holding that tiny particles, which were present in the air, formed into living material. He believed that micro-organisms came from the air and settled on the culture media in which they were found. To prove his theory, he conducted an experiment in which he filled two flasks with suitable culture medium. These flasks were then heated to kill any organisms that were likely to be present in the medium; one was covered and the other left open. Bacteria quickly appeared in the uncovered flask but not in the covered one, thus firmly refuting the idea of spontaneous generation.

Development of preparation and staining techniques allowed Robert Koch, a doctor working in the town of Wollstein, Germany, to isolate the tubercle bacillus (1882) and the cholera vibrio (1883). In a very short period of time a wide range of organisms were identified and linked to disease in man: *Bacillus anthracis* (anthrax), *Corynebacterium diphtheriae* (diphtheria), *Mycobacterium leprae* (leprosy) and *Salmonella typhi* (typhoid fever). The practical applications of the work were not slow to be realised. Joseph (later Lord) Lister took up Pasteur's ideas and using carbolic acid during surgery founded the modern methods of antisepsis

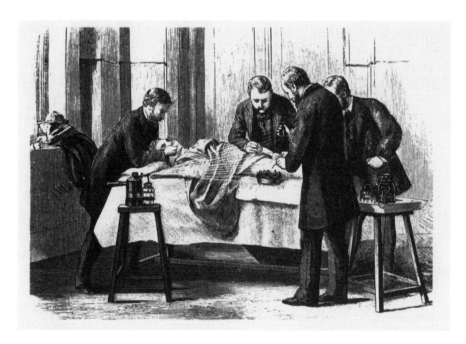

Figure 3.4 Lister carbolic spray in use. Engraving from WW Cheyne, *Antiseptic Surgery*. London: Smith and Elder; 1882
Source: The Wellcome Institute Library, London.

that transformed hospital wards from places where virtually every postoperative case became septic and developed fever.

There are many other examples of the growing understanding of the ways of combating sepsis. Ignaz Philipp Semmelweis (1818–65) was born in Hungary, trained as a doctor in Vienna and became an obstetrician. In his early career he took an intense interest in the high rates of sepsis in the lying-in hospitals. Many women in these times died from puerperal fever.

Semmelweis conducted careful epidemiological research in which he observed the incidence of puerperal fever in different settings. He noted that medical students came from the dissecting room and, with only a cursory washing of hands, examined the women in labour. Semmelweis made his students scrub up carefully, and as a result mortality in the labour wards fell dramatically.

Such was the enthusiasm with which the medical establishment now embraced the germ theory of disease that attempts were made to link virtually every known disease to a specific causal contagious agent. Claim and counterclaim abounded. It was left to the Nobel laureate Robert Koch, who had begun his career as a general practitioner in Germany, to impose a scientific discipline to check this bandwagon effect in which the hunt for micro-organisms in diseases led to causal inferences being made on very flimsy grounds.

Koch's postulates, sometimes also referred to as the Henle–Koch postulates (Koch was Henle's pupil), may be summarised as follows:

1 The organism should be isolated in pure culture from each case of the disease.

2 It should not occur in any other disease as a fortuitous and non-pathogenic occurrent.

3 Once isolated it should be grown in a series of cultures.

4 This culture should reproduce the disease on inoculation into an experimental animal.

It is clear today that Koch's postulates, if interpreted literally, are too rigid and would exclude most viral diseases and also many bacterial diseases from having a proven causative agent. Nevertheless, they served as an important landmark at the time.

THE SEARCH FOR OTHER CAUSATIVE AGENTS

Almost at once, the germ theory of the causation of disease dispelled myths, superstitions and ill-conceived quasi-scientific theories that had stood for centuries. It should be remembered that, at that time, the infectious diseases were the major killing diseases, so the excitement produced by the revelation of the causative role of micro-organisms was quite understandable. Nevertheless, there were other landmarks in causal thinking in which specific agents other than micro-organisms were linked with diseases.

The possibility that factors in one's occupation could be a cause of illness and disease was largely ignored in ancient writings, despite the grim and inhuman working conditions that often prevailed, such as those endured in the quest for valuable metals in the mines of ancient Egypt, Greece or Rome. After the Renaissance, there emerged a man who is generally regarded as the father of occupational medicine: Bernardino Ramazzini (1633–1714). His *De Morbis Artificium*, published about 1700, was a systematic study of diseases arising from occupational factors. When he recommended in his writings that, in addition to other questions and examinations the doctor should ask the question 'What is your occupation?' he could scarcely have realised the enormous importance of his words.

Subsequently, occupational medicine has had a long and distinguished history. Discoveries such as Percival Pott's observation in 1775 of the occurrence of scrotal cancer in chimney sweeps as a result of persistent contact with soot, or of the cerebral effects of mercury poisoning in the hat-making trade (the basis of Lewis Carroll's Mad Hatter), opened new vistas when considering possible causes of disease.

Another field of study in disease causation is to be found in those conditions that arise because of lack or excess of some specific substance in the diet. A classic account is to be found in the work of James Lind, a surgeon in the Royal Navy at a time when long voyages were commonplace and provisions taken on board were those that could withstand such voyages without perishing. Sailors were afflicted after a time at sea by a strange malady: lethargy and weakness, pains in the joints and limbs and swelling of the gums. This was scurvy, and it cost many thousands of lives on the great sailing ships of the time. In 1747 Lind performed an experiment in which he added different substances to the diet of 12 sailors on such a voyage. He divided his patients into pairs and supplemented the diets of each pair with either cider, elixir vitriol, vinegar, sea water, a mixture of nutmeg, garlic, mustard and tamarind in barley water, or two oranges and one lemon daily. Only the sailors given oranges and lemons recovered. Thus, long before vitamin C was isolated, Lind had determined the cause of scurvy and instituted preventive measures to redress the dietary deficiency. Sailors on long voyages took supplies of fruit juice, and the tendency to use limes led to the nickname 'limeys' for British sailors.

THE IMPORTANCE OF THE HOST

In parallel with the development of the concept of a contagion in the cause of infectious diseases, attention was also being directed to the capacity of the person to resist infection. It had been known since ancient times that people who had suffered from certain diseases and survived rarely contracted the same disease a second time.

This observation led to the practice in smallpox of deliberate inoculation with material from a diseased person, in the belief that a milder infection would ensue than from a natural infection. The risks were great, since the people being inoculated were acquiring a real attack of smallpox. Smallpox was one of the major scourges of the past, often called the 'minister of death'. It is estimated that during the eighteenth century 60 million people died from the disease in Europe alone. The practice of inoculation spread across Europe but was not completely effective, as a small proportion of those inoculated would go on to develop a virulent form of the disease and die.

Towards the end of the eighteenth century, Edward Jenner (1749–1823), a country physician in Gloucestershire, decided to investigate a piece of local folklore relating to the disease. It was well known by country people that milkmaids often acquired, from infected cows, a disease called cowpox that gave rise to a pustule on the finger or crop of pustules on the body. It was believed that girls who contracted this mild disease would not contract smallpox when they were exposed to it. This observation is probably the origin of the following rhyme:

'Where are you going my pretty maid?'

'I'm going a-milking, Sir', she said.

'What is your fortune my pretty maid?'

'My face is my fortune, Sir', she said.

In 1779, Jenner took material from the sore of Sarah Nelmes, a milkmaid who had cowpox, and scratched it onto the arm of a boy, James Phipps. In an experiment that would be considered completely unethical today, the boy was later inoculated with smallpox. He did not develop the disease, and Jenner's experiment was repeated on others with similarly successful results. Thus the practice of vaccination became widespread, although it was a very different procedure from that practised today. Material was scratched from arm to arm amongst vaccinees without any antiseptic precautions, and complications were thus common.

Despite its obvious historical importance and success in retrospect, Jenner's discovery was not universally accepted at the time. In many quarters of the medical establishment, he was bitterly denounced as a charlatan. Jenner had earlier been elected to the Royal Society as a Fellow following the publication of a treatise on the natural history of the cuckoo. Yet the Royal Society showed little interest in his cowpox discovery, and it was many years before Jenner received his just professional and public acclaim for a discovery that effectively began one large element of preventive medicine – immunisation.

Almost a century later, a further great advance was made in knowledge of how to protect the host against disease. On this occasion, Louis Pasteur – who had

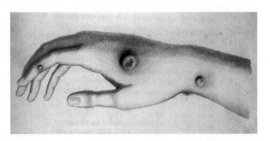

Figure 3.5 Hand of Sarah Nelmes. Cowpox pustule. From Jenner's *An Inquiry into the Causes and Effects of Variolae Vaccinae*, 1798
Source: The Wellcome Institute Library, London.

developed techniques for immunisation of animals against anthrax – turned his attention to rabies in humans. Rabies, frequently a disease of dogs, was one of the most feared diseases because of its universal fatality. At different periods in history, it had been attributed to the sun, the weather or the 'Dog Star'. Although existing technology meant that he could not see or produce a free culture of the rabies virus, Pasteur reasoned that it existed in the saliva and nervous system of infected animals and was the mode of transmission of the disease. He attenuated material from infected animals by desiccation and then injected the material into other animals.

In July 1885, a nine-year-old boy from Alsace, Joseph Meister, was brought to Pasteur's laboratory by his mother. The child, while walking to school alone, had been pounced on and bitten 14 times by a mad dog. Pasteur was a chemist, not a physician, and he consulted with his medical colleagues as to whether his success in the immunisation of animals against rabies justified using it on a human being. It was decided that the child faced almost certain death, and thus a 10-day course of immunisation was begun. The child survived, and Pasteur allowed himself the following excess of emotion when he wrote to his family:

> . . . perhaps one of the great medical facts of the century is going to take place; you would regret not having seen it!

Pasteur had further success with another celebrated case. A shepherd boy, Jean-Baptiste Jupille, had fought off a rabid dog that had been terrorising a group of children. He had been badly mauled. Six days after the attack,

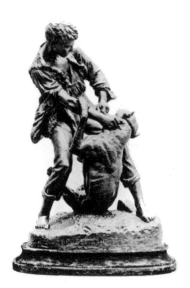

Figure 3.6 Jean-Baptiste Jupille (b. 1871) being attacked by a rabid dog. Statue in the Institut Pasteur, Paris
Source: The Wellcome Institute Library, London.

Pasteur treated him with his new vaccine. The 14-year-old shepherd boy survived.

Pasteur was the subject of criticism from many sections of the scientific and medical establishment who did not accept his claims. But as with Jenner, Pasteur's contribution to public health would turn out to be lasting and immense. A new era in preventive medicine had dawned.

Despite the attention that was directed towards producing specific immunity in the host to allow a person to resist disease, concern with other more general factors was singularly absent. Apart from the investigation of specific dietary problems like scurvy, the relevance of nutrition to health was largely ignored. This was despite the fact that the majority of the population at most periods of history was seriously undernourished. Such a state limits the individual's ability to resist infection and compounds the sequelae of the disease. Even so, this was not recognised and measures against under nutrition were not taken until well into the twentieth century.

THE MULTIFACTORIAL CONCEPT OF CAUSE

The concept of cause embodied in the germ theory is of a one-to-one relationship between causal agent and disease. It was soon realised, however, that a more complicated relationship existed for most diseases. For example, it is only possible to develop pulmonary tuberculosis by being infected with the tubercle bacillus. Yet not everyone who is exposed to it becomes infected, and only a minority of cases will proceed to pulmonary tuberculosis. Thus the realisation

that some people developed the disease because of their nutritional status or their genetic make-up led for a time to a 'seed and ground' model of causation, in which there was seen to be an interplay between causal agent and host. This was quickly superseded by the modern view of cause, which is the multifactorial one. It is now recognised that a disease is rarely caused by a single agent alone, but rather depends on a number of factors that combine to produce the disease. These factors may be grouped together under three main headings:

➤ Agent – a specific agent may be recognised or presumed depending on the level of current knowledge. It may be a micro-organism, a chemical or physical agent, or the presence or absence of a particular dietary substance.

➤ Host – the involvement of the host in the causation of disease is today a much wider concept than it was in the past. Constitutional factors such as genetic make-up and general nutritional status are still important. More recently, however, the behaviour or lifestyle of an individual is seen to be of growing importance. A true understanding of the causes of many diseases means appreciating the complexity of factors (such as education, family and social background, occupation and economic status) that lead people to behave in a particular way.

➤ Environment – similarly, the concept of environment does not merely encompass physical, chemical and biological elements that have a bearing on health; it also involves the socio-cultural milieu in which the person lives. In this way, many factors can be seen as implicated in the causal pathway of many of the common diseases. On the larger scale, the political and economic climate can have a distinct bearing on health. Moreover, the general attitudes and expectations of society, apparent through stress and many other manifestations, can become part of the web of causation.

This classification considerably simplifies what for many diseases is a highly complex interrelationship. For example, the causation of lung cancer is amongst the most straightforward, with about 90% of cases attributable to the effects of smoking. However, while prevalence of smoking is a good indicator of the risk of lung cancer in a population, it is difficult to predict lung cancer in individual smokers. It still remains unclear why some people can smoke heavily for most of their lives and not develop the condition, leading to the challenging thought that if the whole population smoked we would probably regard lung cancer as caused by a genetic predisposition.

THE LIFE-COURSE APPROACH

The concept that early life experience can produce profound effects in later life is not new. The understanding that antenatal care and early childcare could have both important short- and long-term effects led to the development of health visiting and community midwifery services. In the second half of the twentieth century, the rapid development of chronic disease epidemiology tended to concentrate on studies based on recruitment from adult populations and examine current or relatively recent effects. The emerging approach of 'life course epidemiology' studies the long-term effects on health in later life of a range of physical, environmental or psychosocial exposure during gestation or early life.

The stimulus for this developing field came from studies in the field of cardiovascular disease by David Barker, which concluded in the hypothesis that antenatal 'insults' had an important effect on the development of cardiovascular disease in later life.[1] This 'biological programming' approach was a counterpoint to the emphasis on current risk factors in causation of disease. Life-course epidemiology seeks to study risk-producing and protective factors both in early and later life and to examine their combined effects across the whole life course.

HEALTH PROMOTION STRATEGIES

Extensive debates have taken place and a great deal has been written about the concept of health and how it should be defined. A formal definition was produced in 1946 by the World Health Organization (WHO) in the preamble to its constitution:

> Health is a state of complete physical, psychological and social well being and not simply the absence of disease or infirmity.

Over the years that followed the promulgation of this concept of health, the definition was considered too idealistic and just too difficult to convert into operational goals upon which action could be based. However, the World Health Organization's post-war definition is seen as being increasingly in harmony with a modern concept of health. Programmes to improve health have become much more wide-ranging. They have placed greater emphasis on individuals' perceptions of their own health status and have stressed the importance of psychological, social and environmental measures in achieving true health improvement in populations.

This more profound view of health, while acknowledging the importance of improving lifestyles, health services and environment, sees even more fundamental conditions as needing to be met if high levels of health in populations are to be achieved (Table 3.1).

A modern public health movement began to take shape in the early 1970s based upon ideals of improving health and tackling some of the seemingly intractable problems of chronic disease and its consequences.

Probably the main turning point in focusing attention on prevention, after many years of relative neglect, and introducing the concept of health promotion, was the publication in 1974 of a report by the Canadian government.[2] This report, *A New Perspective on the Health of Canadians*, written by the Canadian Minister of Health (Marc Lalonde), can be viewed in retrospect as a major international breakthrough that placed health promotion high on the agenda of governments across the world. In Lalonde's 'health field concept', health was recognised as being a function of lifestyles and the environment, as well as being influenced by human biology and health care provision.

Of particular significance to health worldwide was the Declaration of Alma Ata, which was the product of a joint conference between WHO and the United Nations International Children's Emergency Fund (UNICEF). The conference was held in 1978 in the city of Alma Ata, in the former USSR,

Table 3.1 Prerequisites for health

• Peace
• Shelter
• Education
• Food
• Income
• A stable ecosystem
• Sustainable resources
• Social justice
• Equity

Source: Ottawa Charter for Health Promotion, 1986.

and it identified primary health care as the key to improving health worldwide. The definition of primary health care used in the Declaration was very broad-based and went well beyond the provision of first-line health care services to unwell individuals. It included promotion, prevention, curative and rehabilitative approaches and services. Notably, it included food supply and sanitation in the definition and thus provided a link to the approach taken to the improvement of public health in the late nineteenth century.

In 1977, at its annual Assembly, WHO had declared that:

> The main social target of governments and of the World Health Organization (WHO) in the coming decades should be the attainment by all citizens of the world by the year 2000 of a level of health that will permit them to lead a socially and economically productive life.

The adoption of the 'Health for All by the Year 2000' (HFA2000) theme led to many initiatives around the world and was further developed by the WHO European Region, of which the United Kingdom is a member state. This resulted in the formulation of targets across a broad range of health promotion and disease prevention fronts, addressing two main issues: firstly, to reduce health inequalities between and within countries and, secondly, to strengthen health as much as to reduce disease.[3] Four principal areas of action were identified as part of the HFA2000 process:

1   Ensure equity in health by reducing the present gap in health status between countries and groups within countries.

2   Add life to years by ensuring the full development and use of people's integral or residual physical and mental capacity to derive full benefit from and to cope with life in a healthy way.

3   Add health to life by reducing disease and disability.

4   Add years to life by reducing premature deaths and thereby increasing life expectancy.

THE DEVELOPMENT OF POLICIES ON PREVENTION AND PUBLIC HEALTH IN THE UNITED KINGDOM

The first significant publication reflecting government policy on public health was *Prevention and Health: everybody's business*, published by the Department of Health and Social Security under the then secretary of state, Barbara Castle, in 1976. It took the form of a discussion paper rather than a programme of action and proposed some positions that now look remarkable. For example, it argued against compulsory wearing of front seat belts: 'The difficulty here, of course, is that some people do not like wearing seat belts and to force them to do so would be an infringement of personal liberty.'

The publication by the British government in the early 1990s of a public health White Paper called *The Health of the Nation* further raised the profile of health improvement as a national priority. It identified areas of action and set targets and was thus seen as the first attempt to put a national strategy in place. It had an important symbolic role, as it gave a significant degree of recognition to public health within the health care system.

The Labour Government that came to power in the spring of 1997 set out a new policy direction in *Saving Lives: our healthier nation*, restricting the number of targets to manageable numbers, emphasising the wider determinants of ill health (e.g., poverty, employment, education, the environment), acknowledging the importance of reducing inequalities in health and emphasising the importance of partnership in achieving goals.

In one of two important reviews undertaken for the Treasury, the former banker Derek Wanless turned his attention to public health. In his report, which was published in early 2004 and entitled *Securing Good Health for the Whole Population*, Wanless noted that previous public health policies had been successful at identifying key public health problems and proposing how they might be tackled. He was, however, critical of the successive failure to rigorously implement the identified solutions.

Later in 2004, a further public health White Paper was produced by the government. *Choosing Health* was published and represented an updated public health policy for the country – one that laid considerable emphasis on enabling individuals to make healthy choices for themselves.

THE THREE (OR FOUR) LEVELS OF INTERVENTION FOR HEALTH IMPROVEMENT

The generally used classification of the realms of intervention to achieve improvement in health status outlines three separate, but not necessarily isolated, areas of activity: individual, interpersonal and community.

At the level of the individual, the focus is on health knowledge, beliefs, attitudes and motivation. Because the individual is the basic building block of groups and communities, many public health practitioners concentrate their efforts at the individual level. Health education had its traditional base in the provision of information to individuals, but it has evolved guided by theoretical approaches such as the health belief model. This evolved in the 1950s as an explanation of why people were reluctant to participate in programmes aimed at detecting early stages of diseases. Efforts based on this model deal with issues such as individual perception of susceptibility, perceived severity of the illness and perceived benefits of taking action. Further development of the theoretical model has included the 'stages of change' model, which holds that individuals alter their behaviour in an evolutionary way rather than in a single event.

The second realm that is relevant to health promotion is the interpersonal. Individuals are influenced by their social interactions, whether that is with family, friends, fellow workers or health professionals. Social cognitive theory is one of the approaches used to understand health promotion in the interpersonal realm. It emerged from understanding that individuals learn not only from their own experience and knowledge acquisition but also from observing and interacting with the experiences of others.

The third is the community or organisational realm. Community-level approaches emphasise the importance of various forms of social organisation in dealing with health problems, whether it be in their prevention or in intervention to reduce harm from established problems. Examples can range from local communities taking action to enable their children to play safely by blocking cars from driving through their streets, to legislators promoting laws to prevent environmental tobacco smoke in the workplace. 'Communities' can be geographically based or be based on populations of common interest – on gender, race or disability, for example. Theoretical models such as those dealing with the diffusion of innovation, community organisation and change management have a role to play in this realm.

A fourth and emerging realm is that of so-called 'e-health'. The use of new methods of information transfer has had a major effect on the process of delivering health care and on the availability of information direct to individuals. The growth in access to the Internet has been matched by greater availability of health content on the World Wide Web. This is sometimes unmediated and of uncertain scientific validity, but it has the possibility of significantly affecting how individuals regard their health. There are some instances of how health promotion has used new technology and the development of new e-communities (or 'electronic commons', as they have been termed) to target health messages at specific groups, and the future possibilities are substantial. Content of health messages can be targeted to meet individual need and achieve more intense engagement. There are, of course, risks that the most marginalised people, who will probably have the poorest access to the Internet, will be left behind in this developing area.

PREVENTION

It is a popular misconception that efforts directed at promoting health and preventing disease have a limited overall impact on health care. Some argue that they merely create a larger number of elderly people who then require expensive forms of care. This overlooks the fact that many diseases caused by preventable factors do not lead to sudden death, but they do produce a chronic lingering state of ill health during which time the person involved will be a major consumer of health and social care. An important aim should be to secure a maximum period free of ill health. This could enable individuals' levels of health and functional status to be improved considerably in their later years, so that the elderly do not become dependent until much nearer the ends of their lives. This approach of aiming for healthy life expectancy (or more negatively, the 'compression of morbidity') is fundamental to modern public health policy (Figure 3.7). It is also discussed in Chapter 8 in relation to older populations.

Reducing the risk of disease, premature death, illness or disability or any other undesirable health event is the orientation of preventive activity within the health promotion process. Traditionally, prevention has been classified into three types (Table 3.2).

a *Primary prevention.* This approach seeks to actually prevent the onset of a disease. The ultimate goal of preventive medicine is to alter some factor in the environment, to bring about a change in the status of the host, or to change behaviour so that disease is prevented from developing. Many of the triumphs of public health in the past, relating to the infectious diseases, were brought about by primary prevention.

b *Secondary prevention.* This level of prevention aims to halt the progression of a disease once it is established. The crux, here, is early detection or early diagnosis followed by prompt, effective treatment. Special consideration of secondary prevention aimed at asymptomatic individuals is necessary. This subject is covered later in the chapter in the section on screening. Whilst it may seem to be merely a logical extension of good clinical practice, careful evaluation is necessary before early disease detection is carried out on a population scale.

c *Tertiary prevention.* This level is concerned with rehabilitation of people with an established disease to minimise residual disabilities and complications. Action taken at this stage aims at improving the quality of life, even if the disease itself cannot be cured.

A preventive component of a population-based health promotion programme can involve specific interventions or procedures to reduce the risk of disease occurrence. Immunisation and vaccination programmes are an example of a primary preventive approach to reducing or eliminating the infectious diseases of childhood (such as whooping cough, measles, rubella, poliomyelitis and mumps), which can still have serious consequences. In practice, specific preventive techniques will often be used in combination with another element of health

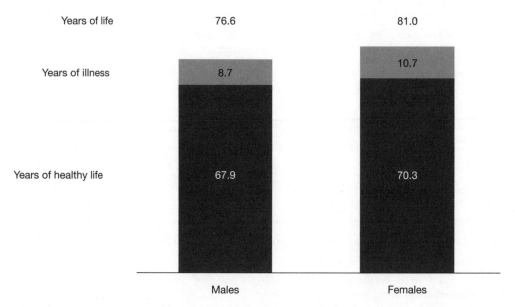

Figure 3.7 Life expectancy and healthy life expectancy at birth in the United Kingdom, 2004
Source: Office for National Statistics; Government Actuary's Department.

promotion. In this example, health education would be an essential element in order to raise parents' awareness of the benefits of immunisation, to give a balanced account of any risks and to encourage them to bring their children into the programme.

The field of secondary prevention is an important one for health services and public health practice and is therefore dealt with at greater length in the remainder of this section on prevention.

SCREENING: THE DETECTION OF DISEASE IN ITS PRE-SYMPTOMATIC PHASE

In its widest sense, the term 'screening' implies the scrutiny of people in order to detect the presence of disease, disability or some other attribute that is under study. There are a number of kinds of screening, each of which is carried out for a particular purpose. These can be summarised as follows.

Protection of the Public Health

This type of screening has its origins in long-established methods to control infectious diseases. For example, people entering a country have sometimes been subjected to tests or examinations designed to detect the presence of infectious diseases or a carrier state. An immigrant in this category would be judged as a potential risk to the indigenous population and might be refused admission altogether or only admitted after appropriate treatment. Mass chest radiography was originally introduced in Britain to identify cases of tuberculosis, which could then be isolated from the rest of the population.

Prior to Entering an Organisation

It is a universal requirement that all potential recruits to the armed forces should undergo screening by medical examination. This practice dates from the time of the Boer War, when a similar screening exercise revealed the high levels of ill health that so shocked the government and resulted in a wide range of measures aimed at improving the health

Table 3.2 Spectrum of health and disease with the main strategies for prevention at each level

		Stages			Outcomes	
	Health	Asymptomatic	Symptomatic	Disability	Recovery	Death
Intervention strategies	Health education*, immunisation, environmental measures and social policy	Presymptomatic screening	Early diagnosis and prompt effective treatment	Rehabilitation		
Levels of prevention	Primary	◄──── Secondary ────►		Tertiary		

* Some of these strategies, particularly health education, can also operate at other levels.

of the nation. In addition to the armed forces, industry may use an occupational health questionnaire as a screening tool in the pre-employment context. In some cases, this may also serve to protect the public (for example, in the case of airline pilots or train drivers), but its essential purpose is to benefit the organisation so that it recruits a healthy workforce.

Protection of Workforce

In addition to the pre-employment occupational health assessment that is compulsory in certain occupations, many industries have a statutory obligation to screen their workforce. This is usually for the protection of workers in industries that have a high risk of disease due to hazards in the working environment (for example, ionising radiation).

For Life Insurance Purposes

Most life insurance companies screen prospective policy holders, either by a questionnaire about their health or by direct medical examination. Their aim in so doing is to allow them to distinguish between low- and high-risk clients so that premiums can be weighted accordingly.

The Early Diagnosis of Disease

This form of screening is concerned with the detection of disease in its early stages so that early treatment for that disease may be started. It can be defined as:

> . . . the systematic application of a test or inquiry to identify individuals at

sufficient risk of a specific disorder to warrant further investigation or direct preventive action, amongst persons who have not sought medical attention on account of the symptoms of that disorder.

With chronic degenerative disorders like late-onset diabetes mellitus, often first seen in their later stages, this may seem to be a logical extension of clinical practice. This argument, coupled with the fact that many population surveys showed a high frequency of previously unrecognised abnormalities, led in the early 1960s to the advocacy of pre-symptomatic screening for disease on a large scale.

It is important to draw the distinction between proactive screening of the kind described so far, in which members of a geographically defined population are called by invitation to be offered screening (for example, a cervical cancer test), and opportunistic case finding, in which people attending a health facility – such as a general practitioner's surgery or a clinic – for one purpose may be offered a screening test (e.g., a blood pressure measurement).

It does not follow that population screening should be carried out whenever technology allows a disease to be detected in its pre-symptomatic phase. A number of criteria first drawn up by Wilson and Jungner for the World Health Organization in 1968 have been used extensively in the past to judge whether to screen.[4] They are described below.

> *Is the disease an important health problem?* Before channelling resources on a large scale, the problem must

be deemed to be a serious one. Nevertheless, importance is, of course, a relative concept. Some health problems may be important because they are very common. Others, although rare, may have serious consequences for the individual or society as a whole.

➤ *Is there a recognisable latent or early symptomatic stage?* In order to detect a disease in its early stages, there must be a reasonable time period during its natural history when symptoms are not manifesting themselves.

➤ *Are facilities for diagnosis and treatment available?* If a screening programme were to reveal large numbers of patients with a particular disease, facilities to provide the necessary follow-up investigation and treatment would have to be available.

➤ *Has the cost of the programme been considered in the context of other demands for resources?* At no time in the foreseeable future are there likely to be unlimited resources that would permit every proposal to be followed through. Proposed expenditure on any one health option must, therefore, be weighed against other proposals.

➤ *Is there an agreed policy on whom to treat as patients?* This brings in the question of borderline cases. In any population, disease exists in a spectrum of severity. At the less severe end of the spectrum, there is a problem of differentiating people with the disease from normal people. Strict criteria must be laid down, therefore, about

what constitutes the particular disease, before screening is carried out.

➤ *Does treatment confer benefit?* This is perhaps the most important consideration of all, and it raises fundamental ethical principles. The pre-symptomatic screening of people for the presence of disease differs from normal medical practice. In the usual situation, patients make contact with a doctor because they have recognised that they are ill and in need of medical care. The doctor attempts to formulate a diagnosis and give the best treatment available to the patient, based on the doctor's experience and current medical knowledge. In the screening situation, the 'patients' have not recognised that they are ill. In fact, they probably believe themselves to be healthy. The doctor (or screener), in offering patients the opportunity to be screened, implies that a health benefit will result, i.e., the early treatment of the disease (if present) and favourable outcome. The reality is that only in a few diseases is there any convincing evidence that striving for early diagnosis on a total population basis, and hence early treatment, affects the outcome for the patient. Thus it is essential, before embarking on a screening programme for a particular disease, to review all the evidence and decide whether early diagnosis and treatment will truly benefit the person being screened. Or whether, on the other hand, the outcome is no different for a person detected through screening than for someone who is treated at such time as the condition manifests itself clinically. The phenomenon by which a screening test simply makes evident at an earlier stage a disease without actually affecting its course (but apparently leads to longer survival because of the earlier detection) is known as lead-time bias.

The Wilson and Jungner criteria have subsequently been developed further and a new list of criteria is shown in Table 3.4.

RUNNING A SCREENING PROGRAMME
Identifying, Inviting and Informing

The first stage in a screening programme is the identification of the population to be offered screening. Decisions about the age at which screening should start or stop have huge resource consequences. Having agreed the population, individuals have to be identified, bearing in mind that those most in need may be most difficult to identify (for example, because they are homeless). Members of the public also need to be clearly informed not only about the possible benefits of screening but also about the risks and limitations.

Choosing the Screening Test

Having decided to embark on a programme to screen for the presence of a particular disease in a population, the next issue centres on which test to choose for the purpose. Usually those proposing to carry out the screening will have a particular method in mind for detecting the disease, whether it is a blood test, a urine test, an examination or a questionnaire. When making the choice, however, a number of general criteria should be borne in mind. The test should be *economic* and one that can be carried out *rapidly* by trained non-medical personnel. It should be *acceptable* to the majority of people, and this usually rules out very painful or time-consuming procedures. The test should be *reliable*; in other words, the same result would be expected if it was repeated by a different observer altogether or by the same observer on a number of occasions.

Finally, and most importantly, the *validity* of the test must be known. By validity is meant the test's ability to measure or discover what the investigator wants to know. How good is the test at discriminating between people who have the disease and people who are healthy? Validity is usually expressed in terms of *sensitivity* and *specificity*.

Applying a screening test to a population may divide people into four possible types (Figure 3.8). Firstly, there may be people who have the disease and give a positive result on screening (*true positives*); secondly, there are people who are healthy, or non-diseased, and give a negative result on screening (*true negatives*). If a screening test was ideal, these are the only categories of people who would exist. No test is perfect. So, two further categories are possible: people who, despite having the disease, are classified as healthy by the screening test (*false negatives*) and healthy people who are classified by the screening test as diseased (*false positives*).

The concepts of sensitivity and specificity take account of these problems (Figure 3.9). The sensitivity of the test is a measure of its ability to detect the disease when present. A

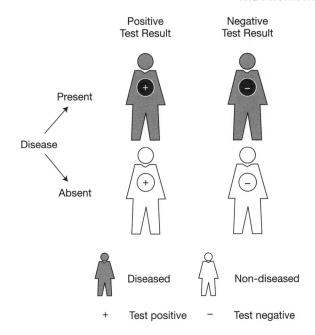

Figure 3.8 Possible outcomes of a screening test

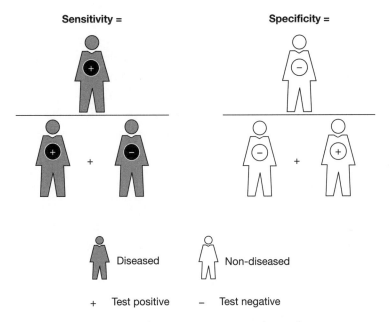

Figure 3.9 Results of a screening test showing sensitivity and specificity

very highly sensitive test would have no (or very few) missed cases (false negatives).

The specificity of the test is a measure of its ability to identify healthy people as non-diseased. A test of high specificity would have no (or few) people wrongly labelled as diseased (false positives). It is seldom possible to have a test that is 100% sensitive and 100% specific. Usually a compromise level must be agreed. Figure 3.10 shows (diagrammatically) different levels of sensitivity and specificity.

Clearly, a level of 60% would be unlikely to be acceptable. A level of 90% might possibly be, depending on the disease in question, but a higher level than this would usually be sought. In making a decision on what levels of sensitivity and specificity will be accepted, the practical implications of the choice must be realised. A sensitivity below 100% means that some people with the disease will be missed, and the consequences of this depend on the particular disease concerned. A specificity below 100% means that some healthy people will be told that they might have the disease, with the ensuing anxiety that might result from this. It is important to stress that screening tests cannot be regarded as diagnostic, and those people with positive results must undergo further examination and investigation to establish a definitive diagnosis.

Two measures of effectiveness of a screening test previously described, sensitivity and specificity, are estimates of the probability of particular test results in individuals who either have, or do not have, the condition in question. Thus, sensitivity is the probability of a positive result given that the individual has the condition, and specificity is the probability of a negative result given that they do not. This is the complete reverse of the situation in reality, where a clinician will know for an individual patient whether the test result is positive or negative, but not whether they actually have the condition being tested for – because of the occurrence of false positive and false negative results. The positive predictive value estimates the probability, given a positive test result, that the individual in question will turn out to have the condition. In practice, what clinician and patient want to know is: given that we have a positive test result, how likely is it that the disease is really present? Positive predictive value is therefore a useful summary of the effectiveness of a screening test. It depends on both the sensitivity and specificity of the test, as well as the prevalence of the underlying condition, as an example will demonstrate.

Suppose that a screening test has a sensitivity of 90% and a specificity of 98%; suppose that the prevalence of the condition being screened for is 2% in the population to be tested. Now consider a typical group of 1000 of that population. From the prevalence, 20 of them will have the condition, and 980 will not. Of the 20 with the condition, the sensitivity tells us that on average 18 will yield a positive test result, and two will be false negatives. Of the other 980, the specificity tells us that on average about 960 will generate a negative test result, while about 20 will be false positives. In total, then, there will be 38 (18 plus 20) positive results, of which 18 are true positives. Hence the probability that an individual testing positive actually has the condition is 18 out of 38, or 47%. This is the positive predictive value

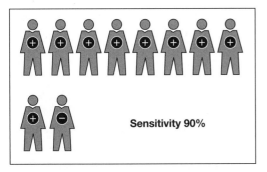
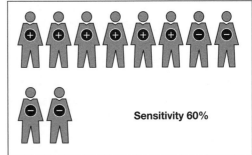
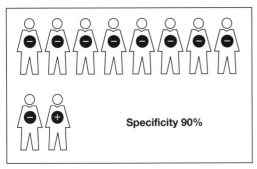
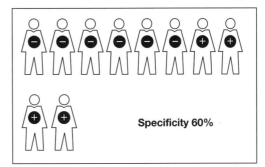

Figure 3.10 Differing levels of sensitivity and specificity tests

of the test, and a little reflection should confirm that the higher the sensitivity, specificity and prevalence, the higher will be the positive predictive value. However, the numbers quoted are not untypical of real examples, showing how the diagnostic value of screening tests may be very limited even where sensitivity and specificity are quite high. This is because of the effect of a typical prevalence value, where those without the condition greatly outnumber those with it.

The question of the validity of a screening test, as expressed in sensitivity, specificity, and positive predictive value, is thus an extremely important issue. Knowledge of these principles is, however, of value far beyond the arena of screening. Great benefit would result to the patient, to the standard of medical practice and to the health service if such a scientific approach were taken to many of the diagnostic tests and examinations in common use today. For example, if we are told that colonic cancer is diagnosed by barium studies, we might not accept that at face value without asking 'How good are barium studies at diagnosing colonic cancer? How do they compare with other diagnostic techniques? How many cases of colonic cancer do I fail to identify if I only investigate them by doing a barium study?'

The Diagnostic Phase of a Screening Programme

The screening test by itself usually identifies a subset of the population that requires more detailed investigation. Some screening programmes (for example, screening programmes to reduce the risk of stroke by lowering blood pressure) proceed straight from the screening test to the intervention, such as advice on lifestyle and drug treatment. However, most screening programmes have a further diagnostic stage (for example, colposcopy and cervical cone biopsy in the Cervical Screening Programme).

The Treatment Phase of a Screening Programme

Once a diagnosis is made, there are two options. One is to refer the person for usual care. The second is to offer treatment within a service particularly aligned with the screening programme. Many screening programmes have taken this extra step to ensure that the quality of treatment service offered meets accepted standards for two reasons. Firstly, it is felt that if individuals are invited to come for screening, there is a greater responsibility on the health service to ensure that treatment is of high quality. Secondly, the introduction of a screening programme based on systems thinking allows those who pay for or manage health care to involve clinicians providing treatment in a review of the service they offer, and this provides a stimulus for more explicit measurement of quality, and therefore the introduction of steps to improve it.

Evaluation and quality assurance

It is obviously essential for screening programmes to be evaluated, but many screening programmes have made the jump from evaluation to quality assurance. Evaluation implies measurement to ensure that performance improves continuously against explicit standards and that those standards are themselves reviewed regularly to set higher challenges for the screening programme when performance improves to a level at which the previously set standard becomes inadequately challenging. Quality assurance must permeate all aspects of the programme.

Many screening programmes in health services around the world have been introduced in the past before there was a proper understanding of the basis upon which they should be evaluated. Policy on population screening is not just concerned with whether to introduce new programmes, but with the attitude that should be taken to existing programmes (Table 3.3). This is a difficult area because stopping a programme would be portrayed by sections of the media as withdrawal of a service and may produce adverse public reaction. Moreover, in countries that do not have national health systems, it is less easy to regulate the offering of screening tests to healthy populations by private sector providers.

Calls for the introduction of new screening programmes have become increasingly common as technological advances have produced relatively cheap, non-invasive diagnostic tests that provide early markers of the presence of disease. Within the United Kingdom, this issue was addressed by the establishment in 1996 of a National Screening Committee (NSC) to advise on the case for implementing new screening programmes and modifying or withdrawing existing ones. The NSC keeps the case for screening in a wide variety of conditions

Table 3.3 Broad public health policy options when taking an evidence-based decision about a population screening programme

- The proposed programme should not be introduced.
- The proposed programme should be introduced, provided that the skills and resources are available to ensure adequate quality standards.
- The programme that is currently being offered to the population should be stopped.
- The policy for a programme currently being offered to the population should continue (with modification as appropriate).

Source: First Report of the National Screening Committee. London: Department of Health; 1998.

under regular review. The number of conditions where it has been considered but not recommended far outweighs those conditions where a screening programme has been put in place.

Many of the criteria to be taken into account when evaluating the case for a population screening programme have been described in the foregoing sections of this chapter, but the main areas that must be addressed are set out in Table 3.4.

EXAMPLE OF A POPULATION SCREENING PROGRAMME IN CURRENT USE: PRE-SYMPTOMATIC BREAST CANCER SCREENING

Breast cancer is one of the leading causes of premature death amongst women in many Western countries. In the absence of individual risk factors on which to base a strategy of primary prevention, the main issue in this disease relates to pre-symptomatic screening. An early important study on the impact of screening apparently healthy women for breast cancer was a randomised controlled trial of women enrolled in the Health Insurance Plan of New York.[5] Two groups of 31 000 women were assigned either to annual screening (in the form of breast palpation and X-ray mammography) or to routine medical care with no such annual screening. Follow-up over a number of years showed a lower mortality from breast cancer in the screened group, but only amongst older women. There was no apparent benefit from screening women aged under 50 years.

Introduction of a National Breast Cancer Screening Programme in Britain

In 1988 the British government established a national programme to detect breast cancer in its early stages. The decision to adopt a population screening approach to reducing the impact of this disease was taken after consideration of the report of an expert committee on breast cancer screening under the chairmanship of Sir Patrick Forrest, then Regius Professor of Clinical Surgery at the University of Edinburgh.[6] The committee, having evaluated the evidence for and against screening, recommended that a national programme should be established and laid down an organisational model.

The roll-out of the programme was not completed until the mid-1990s, and it was

Table 3.4 Evaluation of a proposed screening programme: summary of aspects to consider (do not rely on this table in isolation – see text for fuller description)

Aspect	In particular
Research evidence	Of benefits and risks
Priorities and other strategies	Importance of the health problem, whether other control strategies (e.g., primary prevention, treatment) are more appropriate
Properties of the test	Validity (false positives, false negatives), positive predictive value, convenience, safety, acceptability
Clinical consequences	Effectiveness, acceptability, cost, side effects of diagnosis and treatment following screening positive
Resources	Costs of testing, organisation of the programme, diagnosis and treatment of the cases of disease detected
Quality assurance	System needed to monitor, assure and improve quality if programme established
Ethical and moral	Confidentiality of data

initially targeted at women between 50 and 65 years of age. The programme is estimated to cost approximately £75 m per year and in 2006–07 screened over 1.6 million women. The organised programme has now been extended to women up to 70 years of age everywhere in the United Kingdom (with the exception of Northern Ireland), and in England the target is to extend routine screening to women aged 47 to 73 by 2012. The programme is open to all women over the age of 50 on request, but it is only those in the 50 to 70 age group who are the subject of an organised system of regular invitations to be screened.

The method of screening has also been developed since the programme was initiated, with the introduction of two-view mammography, instead of the previous single view. The introduction of digital mammography is in its early stages but promises higher specificity than traditional X-ray mammography. The cancer detection

rate has increased since the inception of the programme, and in 2006–07 in England, it stood at 7.1 per 1000 women aged 50 to 64 who were screened. Coverage is best described using the 53 to 64 age group, since women may be invited for the first time at any point between their 50th and 53rd birthdays. In England, of the women aged 53 to 64 who were invited for screening, 74% took up the invitation.

The acid test of the programme, however, is whether it is effective in achieving a reduction in mortality. This is particularly true in respect of mammographic screening, where the low level of radiation delivered during screening does carry with it a tiny but measurable risk of inducing cancer. The outcome of the screening programme is heavily dependent on the quality and effectiveness of the arrangements for treating woman who have had tumours detected. The highly developed and regionally organised quality assurance programme that is an integral part of the breast screening programme (and is mirrored in the cervical screening programme) monitors and peer reviews the operation and performance of local screening services, including their surgical and counselling components.

The International Agency for Research on Cancer (IARC) has concluded that breast screening results in a 35% reduction in breast cancer mortality for women who are screened regularly. It is estimated that the NHS breast screening programme saves approximately 1400 lives annually in England, at a cost of £3000 per year of life saved. It is, however, very difficult to separate the effect of screening from that attributable to improvements in treatment and underlying changes in incidence through changes in risk factors.

MODIFYING THE ENVIRONMENT

Another way in which policy changes can influence the health of individuals and the community is by action taken to adjust the environment. For example, measures that control atmospheric pollution and noise levels or those that limit the effect of radiation and other environmental hazards are contained within a legal framework that acts to modify the environment in such a way as to meet health aims. These issues are discussed fully in Chapter 10, but it must be remembered that this is not just an issue of ecology in the sense that it is usually understood. The home, the workplace and places where the public gather are linked to health in a complex range of ways. Designs for safety, policies on matters such as smoking and drinking, and the prevalence of product

advertising can affect people's outlook and influence the choices they make.

The health service alone is relatively limited in influencing these matters within the general population, but in its own premises and workforces it has considerable influence. The NHS in a typical region counts for approximately 10% of gross domestic product. The scope for the health service working in a concerted way with other public bodies and other sectors, including business and commerce, is enormous and, as yet, largely unexploited.

An emphasis on multisectoral collaboration is likely to be a common feature of successful health promotion programmes in the future. For example, in the area of health risk-taking amongst young people, which is discussed in other sections of this chapter, there could be important roles for the food and beverage and leisure industries in creating and promoting attractive and acceptable alcohol- and drug-free environments and in extending the range of recreational and leisure opportunities available to young people.

INEQUALITIES IN HEALTH

Why some individuals are more or less prone to ill health than others is a recurring theme of epidemiology and has obvious practical implications for public health. One aspect that has attracted a great deal of attention and debate is the relationship between deprivation and poor health.

The observation that those less well-off in a society experience much higher levels of premature death has a long history and has been found consistently across a range of measures of deprivation. More recently, the findings have been extended to include various causes of acute and chronic illness as well as mortality. A relatively early example of a systematic analysis is due to THC Stevenson, a registrar-general who, in 1911, grouped occupations into 'social classes' to demonstrate a gradient in standardised mortality ratios, rising steadily from lowest in social class I to highest in social class V (*see also* Chapter 2). The persistence of three- or four-fold variations in health and mortality between groups in society has remained a consistent finding, despite improvements in the overall health of the population evident through the twentieth century.

The subject of inequalities in health related to deprivation came to national prominence in the 1980s through the report of a government-appointed working group generally known after its chairman, Sir Douglas Black, as the Black Report.[7] The group had been established in 1977 when Sir Douglas was chief scientist at the Department of Health and Social Security. By the time the report was complete, in 1980, there was a new government, which did not endorse the group's recommendations. However, the report, originally made available in limited numbers for discussion and subsequently published independently as a paperback, stimulated wide-ranging debate and considerable further research into the topic.

The Black Report confirmed again the gradient of mortality from social class I to V, both for total deaths across age and gender groups and for a very wide range of specific causes of death. Although data were less complete, the same findings were evident for morbidity, and the report also looked at time trends and international comparisons. As a whole, and despite subsequent criticism of its reliance on social class as a measure of deprivation, the report stands as a striking testimony to the degree and consistency of inequalities in health.

The report suggested possible explanations of the observed differences. They might be artefactual (social class V consisting of fewer and fewer individuals as time goes by, who may be unrepresentative of any real group in society); due to natural and social selection (healthier individuals will prosper while unhealthier people will 'drift', by reason of their actual or latent incapacity, to lower social classes); materialist or structuralist (due to the direct effects of poverty and material deprivation); and cultural or behavioural (due to adoption and maintenance of unhealthy lifestyles, including smoking, poor diet, physical inactivity and alcohol).

Subsequent reaction focused largely on often heated debates about the relative contributions of these mechanisms to the observed health differentials. Concern that the true role of material deprivation was being obscured by the focus on alternative explanations led Peter Townsend, a member of the Black Group with co-workers Peter Phillimore and Alastair Beattie, to adopt a different approach to the investigation of health differentials.[8] They looked at the populations of 678 local authority wards in the Northern Health Region of England, a region that included some highly disadvantaged areas. Rather than relying on social class, they constructed a 'social index', deliberately intended to reflect material deprivation, from four census variables: unemployment, non-car ownership, non-owner housing occupation and over-crowding. When they ranked the wards according to this index (based on the 1981 census), there were remarkable correlations with premature death rates, chronic ill health, low birth weight and a composite health indicator made up of all three. If the health experience of the 136 wards with the best health record had applied to the 788 000 people in the worst 136 wards, there would have been significant benefits: fewer prema-ture deaths, less sickness and disability and fewer low-birth-weight babies at high risk of complications.

In the mid-1990s, the same investigators repeated the investigation using 1991 census data. They found that the health gap had widened between the most deprived and least deprived ward populations, principally due to a decline in the relative health of the most deprived wards. Overall, there was a four-fold difference in health index between the lowest fifth of wards and the highest. Townsend's work showed the strength of the association between material deprivation and poor health and led to behavioural and lifestyle explanations being challenged.

In North America and Britain, one focus has been on low income as a predictor of morbidity and mortality. The same gradi-ents of ill health and premature mortality have been evident, but a new twist has been added to the story. This is the suggestion, largely associated with Richard Wilkinson, that the degree of variation in income levels in a society may be as important, or more important, than an individual's absolute income.[9] This depends on the repeated

observation that measures of the spread of income within populations are better correlated with poor health than are the aver-age levels of income. Those favouring the hypothesis point out in support that a large spread in income levels would be expected to reduce the cohesiveness of a society (and there is evidence that this is so from locality-based studies), that less cohesive societies lead to more social isolation and that social isolation may lead to poor health.

This view that the degree of dispersion of income levels may be more important than the absolute level has been challenged by some observers. It is argued that if the effect of income on health is most pronounced at low income levels and becomes less so at higher levels, so that a 'law of diminishing returns' applies and the relationship is cur-vilinear rather than straight-line, then this alone could explain the observed effects at population level. This is because the most 'efficient' way to distribute income in a population would be evenly, since the effect of adding additional income is greatest at low levels; a move towards a more uneven distribution would, in effect, remove income from those at low levels, where it is doing most to improve health, and redistribute it to those at higher levels, where it would have a smaller effect. Whichever view may turn out to be correct, the overall implication remains the same: the greater the discrep-ancy between those least well-off and those best-off in a society, the higher the overall levels of ill health and premature death.

Other important factors are relevant to the relationship between social inequalities and health. Education has repeatedly been found to be a significant predictor of health status, whether this is at an individual level (progress to higher education, academic qualifications) or at a population level (proportion in higher education, spending per capita on education). It is not known whether the effect operates because individuals are better informed and equipped to make positive lifestyle choices or because educational achievement leads in general to higher income, less likelihood of unemployment and better living conditions.

There has been a change in the way that stress is seen as a cause of ill health. In the past, attention focused on occupations that were considered to generate high stress levels and on personality types that were thought to be prone to stress (or to an 'unhealthy' response to stress). More recently, it has been recognised that a range of social, economic and workplace circumstances operate in concert to generate a long-term psychological state that ultimately predisposes to poor health and mortality. In particular, a wide range of forms of social disadvantage create the circumstances in which people's health experience has been found to be very affected (Table 3.5).

This issue of which programmes can be effective to reduce inequalities in health has been widely debated, and at the end of the 1990s, possible approaches were summarised by expert groups (Table 3.6).

The health inequalities debate was given fresh impetus in 1998 when the report was published of the *Independent Inquiry into Inequalities in Health*, led by Sir Donald Acheson, formerly the government's chief medical officer. The report made many wide-ranging recommendations for reducing health inequalities that had implications for government generally and for a broad range of local agencies. Sir Donald identified as priorities:

> the importance of evaluating government policies for their impact on health inequalities
> policies affecting the health of families with children
> steps to reduce income inequalities and improve the living standards of poor households.

In 2003 the government published a policy document specifically aimed at tackling health inequalities. *Tackling Health Inequalities: a programme for action* had four themes:

> supporting families, mothers and children
> engaging communities and individuals
> preventing illness and providing effective treatment and care
> addressing the underlying determinants of health.

In a progress report published by the Department of Health in 2005, it was noted that although there had been an encouraging fall in the mortality rates for heart disease and stroke and a narrowing of the absolute gap, there had been no reduction in the social class inequalities gap in relative terms. The 2008 policy statement *Health Inequalities: progress and next steps* reaffirmed the importance of the goal of reducing inequalities and sought to scale up efforts to make significant reductions building on the experience and knowledge gained in recent efforts.

Table 3.5 Some forms of social disadvantage that adversely affect health

- Having few family assets
- Social exclusion
- Insecure employment or unemployment
- Lack of control over one's work
- Poor housing
- Poorer education during adolescence
- Weak social support
- Bringing up a family in difficult circumstances
- Slow growth and development in utero and early childhood.

Source: Wilkinson R, Marmot M, editors. *The Solid Facts: social determinants of health.* Copenhagen: WHO Regional Office for Europe; 1998.

Table 3.6 Recommendations for policies to tackle inequalities in health

Income maintenance policies that provide adequate financial support for people who fall into poverty
Education and training policies that help prevent poverty in the long-term
More equitable taxation and income-distribution policies
Targeted investment in new and improved housing
Investment in community development
Expansion of childcare and pre-school education, particularly for children living in disadvantaged circumstances

Source: Benzeval M, Judge K, Whitehead M, editors. *Tackling Inequalities in Health: an agenda for action.* London: King's Fund; 1995.

INEQUALITIES IN HEALTH ACROSS THE GLOBE

The recognition that gross inequalities exist both between and within countries worldwide has led to a number of responses. These have included the formation of organisations such as the Global Fund to Fight AIDS, Tuberculosis, and Malaria, which has been established to tackle major killers, and the adoption of Millennium Development Goals by the United Nations in the year 2000, which are designed to tackle poverty.

The World Health Organization recognised that the social determinants of health inequalities went wider than poverty. As its contribution to policy development on the reduction of health inequalities, in 2005 the World Health Organization established the Commission on Social Determinants of Health. The Commission reported in 2008 on the situation worldwide. It noted that a girl born in some countries can expect to live to more than 80 years of age but in others has a life expectancy of less than 45 years, and it stated that 'social injustice is killing people on a grand scale'. The Commission made three overarching recommendations: firstly, improve daily living conditions; secondly, tackle the inequitable distribution of power, money and resources; and thirdly, measure and understand the problem and assess the impact of action. The Commission pointed to examples where health inequalities had been reduced as a result of concerted effort and called for action to reduce the health gap within a generation.

SOME SIGNIFICANT HEALTH PROBLEMS

To illustrate the public health challenges faced by those concerned with promoting health, some examples of health problems relevant to the population of the United Kingdom are discussed in the sections that follow.

CORONARY HEART DISEASE AND STROKE

Circulatory disease is the most common cause of death amongst the population of the United Kingdom and much of the developed world. Approximately one in four people die from circulatory disease, which has two major components: coronary heart disease (also referred to as ischaemic heart disease) and cerebrovascular disease. Coronary heart disease is more frequent as a cause of death in men than in women and cerebrovascular disease a more frequent cause of death in women than in men (Figure 3.11).

Coronary heart disease is responsible for more than 100 000 deaths every year in the United Kingdom. It results from total or partial occlusion of the coronary arteries. This is brought about by deposits of a fibrofatty substance called atheroma in the inner part of the coronary arteries, which become thickened as a result so that the space through which the blood flows is narrowed. This process of narrowing of the coronary arteries can be added to by deposits of blood clot. These changes in the coronary vessels produce a number of main clinical manifestations: sudden death, heart attack (acute myocardial infarction), angina pectoris, heart failure and abnormal heart rhythms.

The impact on the population is substantial and not only in deaths. Coronary heart disease is a major cause of years of life lost prematurely, hospital bed-days used, major surgical procedures performed and working days lost to the economy. Coronary heart disease is considerably more common in males than it is in females until late middle age, when the male excess gets smaller.

The second element of circulatory disease is stroke or cerebrovascular disease, which results from reduction in the supply of arterial blood to the brain. The pathological basis of stroke is more diverse than that of coronary heart disease. Atheroma of the cerebral arteries with thrombus formation is one of the common underlying processes. Haemorrhage from a cerebral vessel either associated with atheroma or with a ruptured aneurysm is a second mechanism. A third is through an embolism lodging in a cerebral artery and obstructing it.

The clinical manifestations of a stroke are often devastating: loss of consciousness (from which the person may not recover); weakness or paralysis (usually) of one side of the body (arm, leg, face); loss or impairment

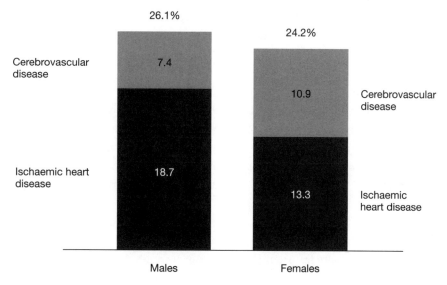

Figure 3.11 Percentage of deaths attributed to ischaemic heart disease and cerebrovascular disease, England and Wales, 2007
Source: Office for National Statistics.

of speech; emotional lability; and loss of other functions (such as continence of urine or faeces). Cerebrovascular disease can also result in loss of function without the acute occurrence of a stroke. Of particular importance is its role in the causation of one of the forms of dementia. Dementia varies in the way in which it affects mental, physical and social functioning, but (as is discussed in Chapter 8) it can affect all three.

As with coronary heart disease, stroke has a major impact on the person concerned and on the family. If the person survives, he or she will often be seriously impaired and unable to function independently. A spouse or a middle-aged son or daughter (with children of their own) may then have to assume the burden of care.

The impact in population terms is also considerable. The large number of deaths, the demand for hospital care during the

acute episode, the need for rehabilitation and longer-term residentially-based care and the pool of chronic disability created make stroke a major public health problem.

Circulatory disease, combining coronary heart disease and cerebrovascular disease, has declined substantially as a cause of death in recent decades (Figure 3.12). The decline has been particularly marked in coronary heart disease: between 1981 and 2000 there was a reduction in mortality rates in England and Wales of 62% in men and 45% in women aged between 25 and 84 years. Substantial though this decline has been, it has not been as rapid as in some other countries, such as Australia. An academic analysis of the decline in England and Wales attributed 58% of the decline to reductions in population risk factors, particularly smoking.[10]

Rate of death from stroke has declined in Britain and some other countries, particularly during the 1970s and 1980s, though it remains an important cause of death from middle-age onwards. Internationally, the United Kingdom tends to be in the middle range of countries in Europe for mortality from both ischaemic heart disease (Figure 3.13) and cerebrovascular disease (Figure 3.14). The mortality rates for both these conditions are particularly high in the countries of eastern Europe.

Risk Factors for Coronary Heart Disease

The causation of coronary heart disease has been the subject of extensive epidemiological investigation over many years, and the evidence relating to markers of risk is well established. While it is clear that the causation of the disease is multifactorial, it is possible to identify and quantify individual risk markers. The known risk factors explain a substantial proportion of disease incidence, but there remains a significant amount of risk that is not currently explained. The major known factors associated with coronary heart disease include:

- smoking
- blood pressure
- serum cholesterol
- diet
- physical activity
- alcohol
- psychosocial factors, including stress
- overweight and obesity
- diabetes.

These factors are of course not independent of each other, and several are closely linked. Neither are the factors always simply additive. Smoking, for example, has a multi-plicative effect on risk when it operates in conjunction with some of the other factors that are associated with the occurrence of stroke.

While coronary heart disease and stroke have many of the same risk factors in common, there are a number of risk factors that are particularly associated with the occurrence of stroke. These include carotid artery disease, atrial fibrillation and sickle cell anaemia.

In 2000 a national service framework was published in England that laid out a programme for a NHS response to the burden of coronary heart disease. In 2005 an additional chapter was published that dealt specifically with cardiac arrhythmias.

Cigarette Smoking

The main data regarding smoking and coronary heart disease is summarised in the points that follow.

- Autopsy studies have shown that cigarette smoking increases the extent of atheroma formation in the coronary arteries.
- Cigarette smoking is a major risk factor in the genesis of acute myocardial infarction (AMI) in both sexes, and the risk is dose-related (i.e., risk increases with the amount smoked). The greatest risk of AMI in smokers compared to non-smokers is in the youngest age groups; the differences decrease in the older age groups. This age-related effect could be due to the elimination (by death) of susceptible individuals at younger ages or probably, more importantly,

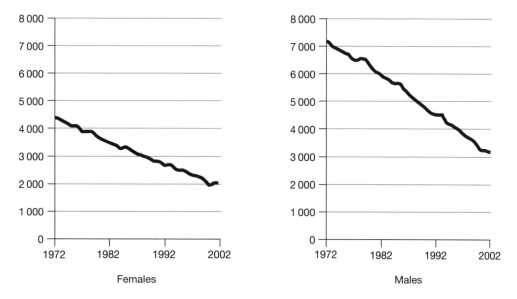

Figure 3.12 Decline in mortality rates from circulatory disease in the United Kingdom (rates per million population)
Source: Office for National Statistics.

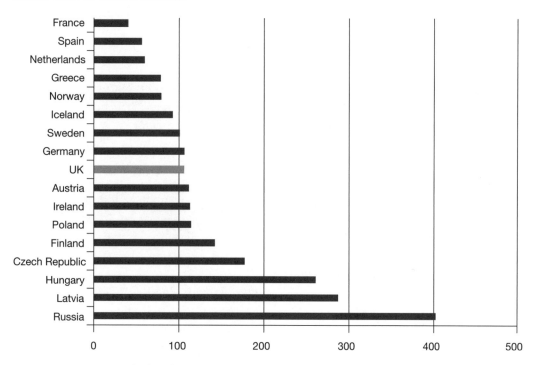

Figure 3.13 Age-standardised mortality rate from ischaemic heart disease per 100 000 population, selected European countries, 2005
Source: World Health Organization Regional Office for Europe. European Mortality Database, 2008.

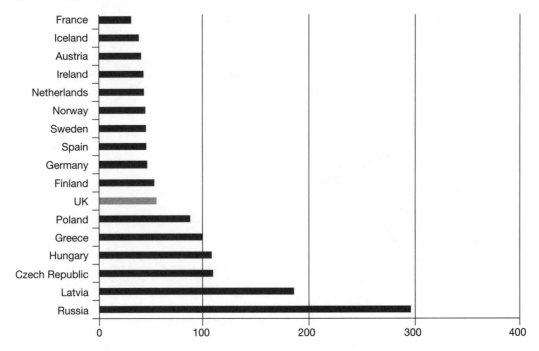

Figure 3.14 Age-standardised mortality rate from cerebrovascular disease per 100 000 population, selected European countries, 2005
Source: World Health Organization Regional Office for Europe. European Mortality Database, 2008.

the greater influence of risk factors other than smoking in the older age groups. Although cigarette smoking is an independent risk factor in AMI, it may also act in a synergistic fashion with the other major risk factors.

➤ The occurrence of sudden death is strongly related to cigarette smoking, and though the risk for smokers compared to non-smokers decreases with age, it persists even into the older age groups.

➤ Studies point to a number of ways in which smoking damages the cardiovascular system. Smoking causes reduced transport of oxygen, increased blood clotting, increased LDL (bad) cholesterol, reduced

HDL (good) cholesterol and vascular dysfunction.

Thus smoking is a major risk marker for coronary heart disease in both men and women. Coronary heart disease mortality is lower in ex-smokers than in those who continue to smoke.

Raised Blood Pressure (Hypertension)

Increased levels of the systolic and the diastolic components of blood pressure are both strong independent predictors of coronary heart disease risk. Those who have high levels of blood pressure have three to four times the chance of developing coronary

THE PROMOTION OF HEALTH

heart disease when compared to those with normal blood pressures.

Raised Blood Cholesterol

There is little doubt about the importance of raised serum cholesterol as a risk marker at population level. Higher average blood cholesterol levels lead to higher mortality from coronary heart disease in comparisons of populations. Conversely, populations with very low cholesterol levels, such those in the rural areas of Japan, have very low rates of coronary heart disease.

It appears that there is a continuous curvilinear relationship between blood cholesterol and coronary risk throughout the range. This has important implications. Firstly, as there is no cut-off level above which risk begins to rise, there is no such concept as the 'normal' level that confers only a baseline risk – 'lower is better', whatever the level. Secondly, because blood cholesterol follows a roughly normal distribution in the population, there are many more people in the central part of the distribution than in the upper tail, and although their risk is more modest than those with very high levels, they contribute the great majority of the incident cases. This is sometimes known as the 'Rose paradox' after the epidemiologist who pointed out the phenomenon in relation to coronary heart disease. Thirdly, the implication of the Rose paradox is that much more improvement in population health will result if the whole curve is shifted to the left (everyone reduces their cholesterol level a little) than if the relatively few in the upper tail reduce their cholesterol to the mean. Strategies that reduce the mean and those that address high-risk individuals are complementary and need not be mutually exclusive.

The level of cholesterol in a group of people is clearly related to risk of developing coronary heart disease, but because many other factors are also involved, it alone is not a good predictor of subsequent mortality from the disease for individuals. In addition, the relation is complicated by the different classes of lipids in blood. Cholesterol is carried in the plasma-attached proteins. Two main classes of these protein-lipid complexes (lipoproteins) are low-density lipoprotein (LDL) and high-density lipoprotein (HDL). The level of LDL cholesterol is the major component of total plasma cholesterol and is directly related to coronary heart disease risk. HDL cholesterol, on the other hand, is inversely related. Recent research suggests that LDL cholesterol may only become harmful when it is oxidised, so low dietary intake of antioxidants (e.g., vitamin E and substances in fruits and vegetables) may contribute to coronary heart disease risk. There is as yet insufficient evidence to identify any particular nutrient, but increasing consumption of fruit and vegetables is prudent advice. The effect of blood lipids on coronary artery disease is only one part of the pattern. It appears that this factor interacts with others such as smoking, hypertension and physical inactivity, and its overall contribution in any individual is hard to distinguish.

There is a strong international correlation between high levels of intake of saturated (mainly animal) fat and high rates of coronary heart disease. Similarly, high average saturated fat intakes are strongly correlated with national average serum cholesterol levels. This relation is more difficult to identify within populations because of the large intra- and inter-individual variation both in plasma cholesterol and in dietary intake. In addition, dietary assessments are notoriously imprecise. However, clinical studies show clearly that, on average, higher intakes of saturated fat (of carbon chain lengths C12–C16) reliably increase plasma cholesterol, while polyunsaturated fat reduces it, though to a lesser extent. There is considerable inter-individual variation in this response, but the mechanics for this are not clear. A number of intervention studies using diet or drugs have now clearly demonstrated that reduction of plasma cholesterol reduces risk of coronary heart disease not only in people who have had a previous coronary heart disease event but also in those at risk.

Other nutritional factors that may influence coronary heart disease risk include total dietary fat (high intakes of which predispose to obesity and increase the tendency of the blood to clot); fruit and vegetable consumption (probably due to their content of antioxidants); dietary sodium (which increases the likelihood of high blood pressure); folic acid (inadequate intakes of which increase blood levels of homocysteine, which is an independent risk marker for coronary heart disease); and obesity (which increases blood pressure and plasma cholesterol).

There are two other major strands to aetiological research on diet and coronary heart disease. The first puts forward evidence of influences in early life being a determinant of coronary heart disease in adulthood and the second postulates a role for an insulin resistance syndrome (syndrome X). Diet and metabolism will remain an important area for research into coronary heart disease causation.

Physical Inactivity

Regular vigorous physical activity confers protection against coronary heart disease. Physical inactivity strongly increases the likelihood that a person will develop coronary heart disease. If other adverse factors are present, the beneficial effect of exercise may be lost.

Obesity

Risk of coronary heart disease is higher amongst individuals who are above the average weight for their height. While obesity is a marker for coronary heart disease, it is often present with other risk markers such as hypertension and raised serum cholesterol. When these and other factors are controlled for during analysis of survey data, obesity is not identified as an independent marker of risk. Nevertheless, it is a marker that is amenable to preventive action, even though its effect on risk is indirect.

Genetic Predisposition

The increased occurrence of coronary heart disease in close relatives, particularly of a person who has developed the disease at a young age, is well recognised. Much of the association is explained by inheritance of two risk factors: hypercholesterolaemia and hypertension.

Stress

In the minds of the public and in media coverage, stress often seems to be a major risk marker for coronary heart disease. There is little evidence of such a simple relationship between risk factor and disease. Stress is difficult to define and measure, and thus studies to elucidate its role have been inconclusive. There is some evidence that particular personality types have an excess risk. When explaining risk to the public, it is important that discussion of stress does not obscure the importance of the major risk markers (such as cigarette smoking).

However, the role of stress resulting from long-term social disadvantage and the workplace is increasingly being seen as important (see previous section on inequalities in health). An important new role for stress has been defined through studies of social, economic and work-related influences on coronary heart disease mortality. Thus factors such as high-demand jobs coupled with low control appear to put people at high risk. Low levels of social cohesion in a community are also associated with high levels of coronary heart disease mortality. These psychosocial and social determinants appear to be mediated through a form of 'social stress', the biological processes of which are not yet elucidated.

Diabetes Mellitus

The presence of diabetes mellitus increases a person's risk of developing coronary heart disease.

Risk Factors for Stroke

The predominant risk marker for the development of stroke is raised blood pressure. Linear increases in the frequency of stroke occur with rises in both systolic and diastolic blood pressure. Numerous controlled trials of hypertension have shown that a reduction in the occurrence of stroke can be achieved in treated, compared to control, groups. As a consequence, factors that contribute to hypertension (such as obesity) are also risk markers in stroke. Risk is also increased with pre-existing heart disease, diabetes mellitus and previous stroke or transient cerebral ischaemic attacks. Alcohol intake above recommended safe levels increases the risk of stroke. Serum cholesterol and cigarette smoking are associated with increased risk of stroke, though the relationship is not as strong as for coronary heart disease. People with sickle cell anaemia are also at increased risk of stroke.

Prevention and Control

Strategies to reduce the impact of coronary heart disease as a public health problem must be based largely on primary preventive measures aimed at the principal risk factors. It remains to be seen what the impact will be, in population terms, of the therapeutic approaches such as thrombolytic therapy administered immediately after an acute myocardial infarction or the revascularisation techniques (coronary artery bypass graft and angioplasty).

Experience has shown that, certainly as far as acute myocardial infarction is concerned, people do not interpret the symptoms and summon medical help immediately, so a substantial proportion of fatalities occur before patients are in a position to receive therapy. Some element of public health education should be devoted to raising people's awareness of the early symptoms of heart attacks so that they present more quickly and to providing people with the skills for cardiopulmonary resuscitation. In many developed countries, the use of primary angioplasty (balloon dilation of the coronary arteries in the acute phase of a heart attack) is increasing. It is not suitable in all situations, but, when possible, it is likely to be the preferred treatment in the next decade.

Health promotion strategies directed at the principal risk markers for coronary heart disease are discussed in other parts of this chapter. The key determinants of chronic diseases can be identified at a variety of levels (Figure 3.15), and it is important to emphasise the multifaceted nature of programmes for their prevention and control – in particular, the need for coordination and the key role for multisectoral collaboration. The approach necessary at a very local level is typified by programmes such as the Heart of the Community Project established in 2004 and working with the people of the Ogmore and Garw Valleys near Bridgend in South Wales. Their activities have encompassed all ages and take place in a variety of community settings, including schools and workplaces.

Scope for the prevention of stroke lies with reducing risk factors that are important in the production of hypertension (including the reduction of obesity), smoking cessation policies and strategies to increase safer levels of drinking in the population.

Aside from these primary preventive measures, the other major control measure in stroke is to recognise and effectively treat established hypertension. Rapid advances have taken place since the 1960s in the development of antihypertensive drugs that are effective without having the severity of side effects of earlier drugs. The step from clinical trials, demonstrating control of hypertension and hence reduction of stroke, to advocating population detection on a wide scale is not a straightforward one. Many complex issues are raised. First is the question of screening an apparently healthy population to detect abnormality (and the principles of this are discussed fully earlier in this chapter). In the case of hypertension, the benefits of reducing or delaying death and disability from its sequelae must be balanced against the physical, social and psychological impact of putting a sizeable proportion of the population on therapy for life. This is in addition to the direct financial consequences. Secondly, there are other important practical issues raised by the population approach. Even if cases of hypertension are detected, to bring their blood pressure under control would not be easy to achieve across a whole population. Non-compliance with therapy by patients, particularly those with mild hypertension, is an important cause of failure of antihypertensive therapy. It may be difficult to persuade people who do not experience symptoms to remain diligently on therapy over a period of many years. Similarly, some individuals may experience side effects that may lead to them discontinuing therapy.

For these reasons, identification and treatment of hypertension on a case-finding

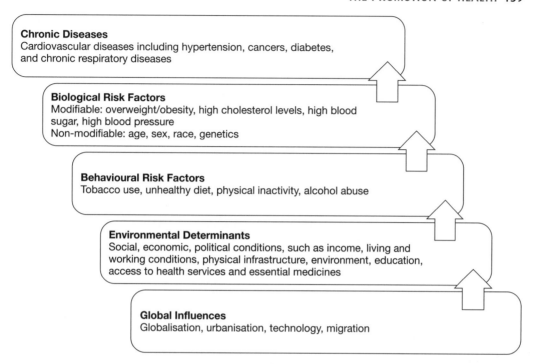

Figure 3.15 Key determinants of chronic diseases
Source: Pan American Health Organisation. *Regional Strategy and Plan of Action on an Integrated Approach to the Prevention and Control of Chronic Diseases.* Washington, DC: PAHO; 2006.

rather than a population basis is the preferred strategy. Such an approach can be carried out effectively in general practice with the backup of hospital specialist departments in the management of the patients detected.

UNINTENTIONAL INJURY

The terminology applied to this area of health experience has changed in recent times, with the word 'accident' being replaced by 'injury' and a distinction being drawn between unintentional and intentional injuries. The term 'accident' has been used in the past to imply an event that happens purely by chance, and sometimes the term also suggests a fatalistic approach. This is suggested by the phrase 'accidents do happen'; but injuries do not occur at random. Some groups of the population – for example, children, the elderly or those in particular occupational groups – are at much greater risk than others.

Age is a powerful influence in determining the risk of unintentional injury in a number of ways. Firstly, it influences the degree and nature of exposure to particular hazards. Secondly, it is related to skills, competence and attitudes in particular activities. The young child and the elderly person, although for very different reasons, are at greater risk as pedestrians and fall more often than do others in the population. Young children are still developing physically, mentally and socially and are poor judges of dangers such as speed or distance; in addition, their attention wanders easily. The elderly person may have limited mobility and failing vision or eyesight. Thirdly, age may influence the ability of a person to withstand the forces involved and thus the likelihood of sustaining an injury.

The World Health Organization regards injury (both intentional and unintentional) as a major global health problem that spans developed and developing countries. It estimates that injury results in the loss of five million lives annually. A 2004 World Health Organization report on road injury surveillance estimated that road traffic injuries accounted for 1.2 million deaths annually worldwide and that as many as 50 million suffer non-fatal injury. In England and Wales each year there are just over half a million deaths that are attributed to the category of 'accidents, poisoning and violence'.

Injuries account for approximately 13% of years of life lost under the age of 65 years, and they are a particularly important cause of preventable death and incapacity in the younger age groups. There are also substantial numbers of non-fatal injuries each year, leading to considerable health service expenditure. Causes of injuries include road traffic collisions, falls, poisoning, drowning and fires. They occur in the home, on the roads, in a variety of outdoor locations and in the workplace. Particular categories of road users (for example, pedestrians, motorcyclists, pedal cyclists, car drivers) have differing risks of dying or being injured.

Injury as a cause of death in Britain has declined in recent decades. Motor vehicle traffic deaths are at lower levels than in many other countries (Figure 3.16) but still represent an unacceptably large public health problem.

For many young people, car driving and motorcycle riding represent two ways in which they can experience the thrills of risk-taking. Most studies of young motorcyclists have found that excitement and adventure are the prime motivating forces behind their behaviour on the road, and this is often reinforced by motorcycle manufacturers' advertising. The risk of serious injury or death from motorcycling is estimated to be 100 times greater than from the safest form of travel by road (bus) and 25 times greater than from driving a car.

At the same time, car advertising reflects an increasing concern about safety features. Rigid passenger compartments and front and rear crumple zones are almost standard, while seatbelts fitted both in the front and back of new cars are now a legal requirement in Britain. Furthermore, even more sophisticated safety features are appearing, such as anti-lock brakes, collapsible steering columns and inflatable driver crash airbags. However, despite improvements to car design, travelling in motor vehicles still accounts for a substantial number of deaths each year. The largest proportion of these deaths occur to those between 15 and 24 years of age and are probably connected to young people's relative lack of driving experience and also to the element of risk-taking. An additional and extremely worrying aspect of this behaviour by young people on the roads is the incidence of joy-riding in stolen cars – sometimes with fatal consequences.

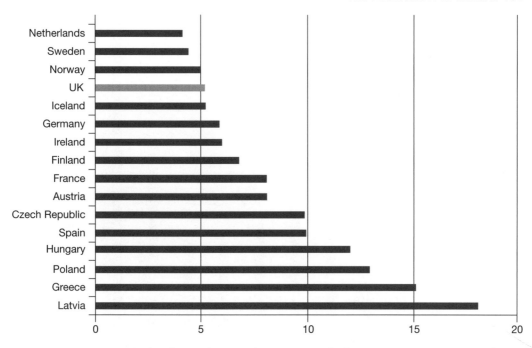

Figure 3.16 Age-standardised mortality rate from motor vehicle injuries per 100 000 population, selected European countries, 2005
Source: World Health Organization Regional Office for Europe. European Mortality Database, 2008.

The importance of road traffic collisions as a cause of death and serious injury in childhood is emphasised by the fact that they account for about a quarter of all deaths of children under the age of 15 years. While the rate of deaths and serious injuries on the road is lower in Britain than in most other European countries, the rate of pedestrian deaths amongst children is relatively high in Britain. Indeed, pedestrian road collisions are the single commonest cause of injury related death in children, accounting for 40% of all injury related deaths in the 5–14 age group and over 20% of injury related deaths in the younger and less mobile children from one to four years of age.

While the numbers of transport-related deaths are greatest amongst young males aged between 15 and 24 years, the age-specific rate of mortality is slightly greater in males aged 85 years and older (Figure 3.17). The increased frailty of elderly people and their reduced ability to recover from serious injury means that they are more vulnerable in the case of a collision.

An important aetiological factor in road injuries is alcohol. It is present in about a quarter of fatal injuries involving car users and pedestrians. Misuse of alcohol is also implicated in other types of injuries, such as falls, fires and drowning. Smoking is an additional important factor in fires that start in the home. Data on the true occurrence of home injuries that do not result in death

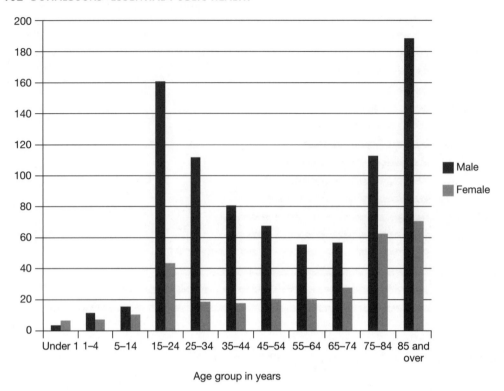

Figure 3.17 Age-specific death rates per million population from transport injuries, England and Wales, 2005
Source: Office for National Statistics. *Mortality Statistics: injury and poisoning.* Series DH4, no. 30. London: ONS; 2007.

cannot be routinely obtained. Many such injuries are self-treated or are treated in primary care.

Prevention and Control

As a public health problem, injuries have been the subject of detailed study internationally, particularly in North America, where a great deal of work has been undertaken to develop ways of classifying them in a form that helps consideration of how they can be prevented. Fundamental to this is the view that the agent that produces an injury is energy in one of its five forms, that

is, mechanical, chemical, thermal, electrical or various forms of radiation (for example, ultraviolet rays or X-rays). It is the sudden and harmful transfer of these types of energy to human beings that causes the injury (Figure 3.18). For instance, a teenager might get on a friend's motorcycle without any lessons or instruction and crash into a parked car, breaking his leg (mechanical energy); a toddler might open and drink from a bottle of turpentine that his mother is using for decorating and be poisoned (chemical energy); an elderly woman might drop a smouldering cigarette into her lap after she has fallen asleep in her chair and sustain a

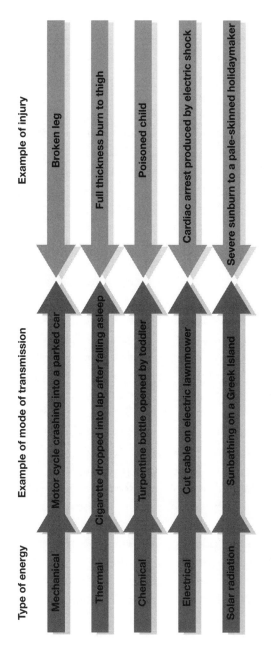

Figure 3.18 A concept of unintentional injury based upon the exchange of one of five forms of energy with the human body

Source: Haddon W. The changing approach to the epidemiology, prevention, and amelioration of trauma: the transition to approaches etiologically rather than descriptively based. *Am J Public Health*. 1968; **58**(8): 1431–8.

deep burn on her thigh (thermal energy); a middle-aged man might cut through a cable on his lawnmower and receive an electric shock (electrical energy); the pale-skinned holidaymaker from Britain, with little previous exposure to the sun, might sunbathe on a Greek island beach and be seriously sunburned (solar radiation). The size of the transfer of energy, its duration, its distribution and the body's ability to resist it are all factors that determine the type and severity of the resulting injury. In each case, the energy source has caused the injury to the person concerned through a transmitting agent or vector. In the examples given here, the agents were the motorcycle, the turpentine, the smouldering cigarette, the electrical cable and the sun's rays.

The individual's susceptibility to being injured by the transmission of the energy is always an important factor. Everyone, every day, is in contact with or is using many forms of energy. If the energy source is under control, it is not usually harmful. However, when it exceeds the ability of its user to control it, an injury can be caused to that person or to others. The balance between an energy source and the person controlling it is therefore a crucial one. The balance can be tipped in favour of the energy source when it suddenly becomes stronger or more difficult to control. For example, a car skidding on an icy road risks causing the driver or the passengers injury as the mechanical energy source becomes uncontrolled. The balance can also be altered if the person controlling the energy source lacks sufficient skill, the necessary physical attributes or the relevant experience to exert full control over it. An elderly woman with arthritic hands

who picks up a heavy frying pan full of hot oil risks a scald injury due to her reduced capacity to exert full control over a source of thermal energy. A young, physically able person would not have such difficulty.

This description of injuries as interchanges of energy between their source and a man, woman or child is not just an interesting theoretical idea. It has proved to be an excellent basis for planning comprehensive action to minimise the unfortunate consequences of such impacts.

Many of the approaches used in the past to prevent injuries, which are often still used today, are based upon the concept of injuries arising from acts of carelessness or stupidity. Successful solutions are therefore seen as those that ensure people take a much greater degree of personal responsibility for their actions and adopt behaviour that appears less likely to result in unintentional injury to themselves and others. Education, particularly of young children, regarding individual behaviour and safety still remains an important component of injury-control strategies. Yet, additionally, today's thinking places greater emphasis on safer products and planning and construction of the built environment, drawing upon methods of research, innovation and design from within fields such as science, engineering and psychology. This stems from recognition that if a major proportion of crashes, for example, cannot be prevented, structural modifications to reduce and distribute impact forces might at least minimise injuries and enhance the chances of survival.

This approach has been developed to identify three critical stages to an injury: pre-event, event and post-event. The factors that determine what will occur and what its impact will be are influenced by the interplay between a diversity of elements at each of these stages. This concept has been developed into a matrix that can help in understanding the causes of unintentional injuries and, even more importantly, can assist in designing prevention and control measures.

These ideas can be illustrated by considering such a matrix when it is applied to a car crash (Figure 3.19). The pre-event stage (in this example, 'pre-crash') involves all the influences that determine whether the collision will occur in the first place, including the human factors (for example, how good the driver's eyesight is, how experienced and skilled a driver he or she is and whether he or she has been drinking alcohol). Other important pre-crash factors will include the functioning state of the vehicle, as well as aspects of the physical and socio-cultural environment (for example, tyre pressure and tread, effectiveness of brakes, provision of zebra crossings and adequacy of road surface).

Once the collision has taken place, its seriousness and the severity of injuries sustained by those people involved through the transfer of mechanical injury to their bodies will also be determined by the same groups of influences: human (for example, whether a seatbelt was worn); vehicular (for example, how crash-resistant the car body shell was);

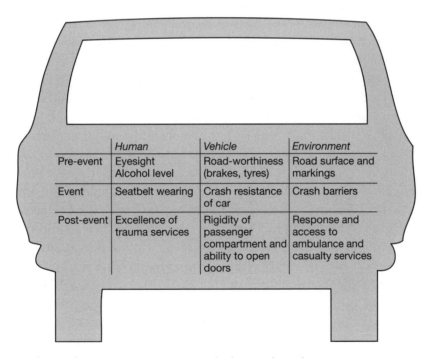

	Human	Vehicle	Environment
Pre-event	Eyesight Alcohol level	Road-worthiness (brakes, tyres)	Road surface and markings
Event	Seatbelt wearing	Crash resistance of car	Crash barriers
Post-event	Excellence of trauma services	Rigidity of passenger compartment and ability to open doors	Response and access to ambulance and casualty services

Figure 3.19 The accident prevention matrix applied to road accidents
Source: Adapted from Haddon W. Advances in the epidemiology of injuries as a basis for public health policy. *Public Health Rep.* 1980; **95**: 411–21.

physical environment (for example, whether crash barriers were present alongside the road) and socio-cultural environment (for example, attitudes to seatbelt wearing).

Post-crash, a range of factors will determine whether those injured survive the crash and, if they do, how well they recover or are free of long-term disability. It is here that vital issues such as rapid response by the trauma services come into play.

It will be clear from this illustration that a comprehensive strategy to reduce the toll of injury, disability and premature death arising from car crashes should not just involve measures directed at drivers themselves. It should also include targets for improved vehicle construction and design so that, as far as possible, drivers and passengers are 'packaged' to withstand the mechanical energy released if the car should crash. Similarly, roads that permit clear visibility and have well-constructed surfaces, good signposts, clear lane markings and adequate crash barriers are also factors that, if targeted in an injury prevention programme, would contribute to the saving of lives and serious injuries.

Teaching children road safety procedures and imparting knowledge about the dangers are important components of strategies to reduce injuries to children in traffic. There have also been important, though limited, efforts to ensure that children are separated from fast-moving traffic. The development of the Safe Routes to School programme in the 1990s was an attempt to create an environment around schools that not only reduced the likelihood of injury but also encouraged children to walk or cycle to school. This has had the health by-product of increasing levels of physical activity and reducing air pollution and congestion caused by cars.

Legislative measures in Britain have included the mandatory wearing of crash helmets by motorcyclists, compulsory wearing of front and rear seatbelts by drivers and passengers in cars and making driving a car while using a mobile telephone an offence. These measures have sometimes been controversial at their inception, since they have been said to reduce individual liberty.

A major problem in road injury prevention is alcohol. The Road Safety Act 1967 made it an offence to drive with more than the prescribed limit of alcohol in the blood. During the 1980s, the number of deaths on the roads associated with drinking and driving fell substantially. The introduction of the roadside breathalyser test and its use by the police initially received widespread media attention and has done so periodically since then. The original legal limit was 80 mg of alcohol per 100 mL, and it has remained at this level, but a number of countries subsequently introduced lower legal limits. The problem of alcohol in pedestrian injuries is often overlooked. It is difficult to envisage any acceptable legislative measure similar to the breathalyser being used in pedestrians, though existing legal provision for dealing with drunk and disorderliness has little impact on this problem.

A similar multifaceted approach is required to prevent non-transport injuries. For example, in domestic injuries, improvements in the design of buildings and products can reduce the risk of injury. In some areas, this may be backed up by legislation or by voluntary codes of practice agreed with manufacturers. Public awareness of these hazards has helped to encourage action to prevent the sale of such things as dangerous toys and to introduce the childproof medicine container. The role of local authorities and their trading standards officers is an important element is ensuring that the goods available for purchase by people at a local level do not put them at risk of injury. Local authorities have also been at the forefront of offering 'homecheck' schemes, particularly to the elderly, with the goal of advising people about hazards in their own homes of which they might be unaware or which they might be unable to rectify without assistance.

Strategies to reduce deaths and injuries in the workplace rely on a strong legislative framework. Appropriate training is an important element in workplace safety. Unlike health education aimed at the general public to prevent injuries in the home or on the roads, education of the person at work can be a mandatory component of training programmes in which knowledge and skills are formally assessed. As such, it has the potential to be more effective than population health education programmes. Factory design, operating procedures and adequate maintenance of machinery are also important measures in preventing injuries in the workplace. Special measures are required for occupations or processes where there are particular hazards. The most successful programmes are undoubtedly those where an organisation's management demonstrates a strong commitment to occupational health and safety.

The transfer-of-energy idea has been used to provide a comprehensive injury prevention framework. In it there are 10 types of strategy for intervening to control the release or impact of energy (Table 3.7). This approach is extremely valuable, not necessarily in applying all measures to every injury prevention programme but in allowing all options to be carefully thought through prior to designing the particular programme.

THE MISUSE OF SUBSTANCES

One of the most important influences on health is behaviour associated with the use and misuse of substances such as alcohol, drugs and tobacco. While the use of these substances occurs at all stages of life, their adoption in childhood and adolescence poses a particular problem to the health of young people. Moreover, such patterns of behaviour established early in life can carry forward into adult life, with long-term consequences in terms of dependency, illness and premature death.

Alcohol

Alcohol has a profound effect on the health of individuals and communities. In 2005 there were 6517 deaths in England directly attributed to alcohol. This figure represents a 19% increase since 2001. In addition, alcohol was estimated to result in more than 207 000 admissions to hospital in England in 2006/07 with a diagnosis directly or indirectly related to alcohol. There are three main spheres of behaviour associated with alcohol misuse: intoxication, excessive use and dependence (Figure 3.20). A spectrum of

Table 3.7 Accidents as energy forces: Countermeasures to prevent injury

	Countermeasure	Accident type	Example
1	Prevent the creation of a form of energy in the first place	Poisoning caused by a chemical agent	Stop production of the agent
2	Reduce the amount of energy marshalled	Hot water scald	Limit temperatures in hot water systems
3	Prevent the release of the energy	Mauling by wild animals	Caging tigers
4	Modify the rate of release of energy from its source	Fire started by electric kettle boiling dry	Shut-off valve on the kettle
5	Separate in space and time the energy source from the individual who might be harmed	Burn from hot fat in frying pan	Keep toddlers out of the kitchen when cooking
6	Interpose a barrier between the energy source and the susceptible individual	Child poisoned by tablets	Child-proof medicine container
7	Modify the basic structure of the hazard	Strangulation of baby in cot sides	Narrow space between bars in cots
8	Strengthen the resistance of the susceptible individual	Head injury in child cyclist	Widespread use of cycle helmet
9	Counter the damage done by the energy source	Lacerating wound due to broken glass	Apply first aid to stop further loss of blood
10	Stabilise and rehabilitate the person damaged by the energy	Multiple injuries in car crash	Rapid transfer to major accident and emergency department and provision of care

Source: Adapted from Haddon W. On the escape of tigers: an ecologic note. *Am J Public Health.* 1970; **60**: 2229–34.

health and social consequences is associated with each.

Drinking patterns vary greatly internationally (Figure 3.21). Within Europe, the United Kingdom is amongst the countries with a high level of per capita alcohol consumption. Within England, there is also considerable variation between regions in the proportion of those aged 16 years and older who drank alcohol on five or more days in the last week (Figure 3.22). There is an apparent disparity in the United Kingdom between self-reported alcohol consumption and the significantly higher quantities of alcohol on which duty is paid to the Revenue and Customs authorities. It is suspected that self-reporting of alcohol consumption is prone to underestimation.

There is also an enormous variation between communities in the death rates associated with alcohol, depending on the prosperity or otherwise of the community. Death rates are up to three-fold higher for women and five-fold higher for men in the

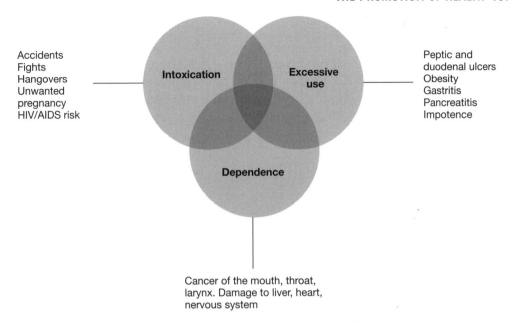

Figure 3.20 Drinking alcohol and its effects

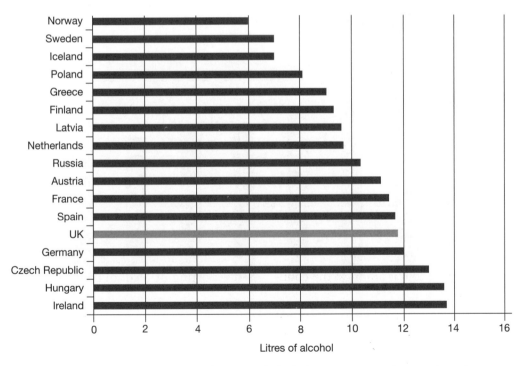

Figure 3.21 Recorded per capita adult (≥15 years) alcohol consumption in litres, selected European countries, 2003
Source: World Health Organization. Global Information System on Alcohol and Health, 2007.

most deprived areas compared with the least deprived.

The United Kingdom is unusual amongst countries in Europe in placing an emphasis on the concept of drinking at 'sensible' levels in the forefront of its public campaigning on alcohol (Table 3.8). The concept of 'sensible drinking' was first introduced in 1981, and the introduction of the concept of 'units' of alcohol and 'sensible limits' in terms of the number of units per week was introduced in 1987. The emphasis has therefore been on individuals to monitor their own consumption. In the United Kingdom a unit is 10 mL or 8 g of pure alcohol. Some of the difficulties facing individuals in monitoring their own consumption include variation in the size of glasses used in serving wine in pubs and restaurants and the gradually increasing strength of many of the wines

and beers that are commonly sold.

While there has always been a concern about the long-term effect of alcohol consumption and the immediate consequences of undertaking various activities (such as driving) after drinking, more recently there has been growing attention paid to the rise in what is termed 'binge drinking'. This is a term used to describe the consumption of a substantial amount of alcohol over a short period of time, such as an evening. Binge drinking is associated with street disorder, including assault, and also with unwanted pregnancy and sexually transmitted diseases. This has led to the production of guidelines recommending that a man should not drink more than three or four units of alcohol in a single day and a woman should drink no more than two or three.

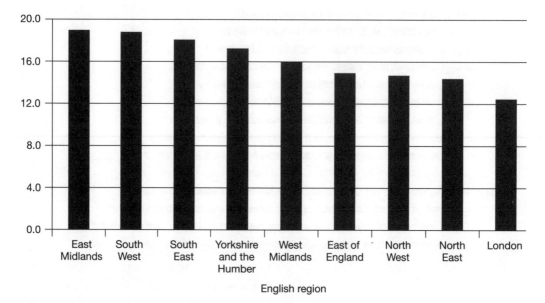

Figure 3.22 Percentage of population aged 16 years or over drinking on five or more days in the last week
Source: Office for National Statistics.

Alcohol is related to deaths from injuries, violence and disease, more so in men than in women (Figure 3.23). However, for men over the age of 40 years and for post-menopausal women, low levels of alcohol consumption have a protective effect against coronary heart disease and stroke.

Of particular concern in relation to

Table 3.8 The three types of drinking

Sensible drinking

Sensible drinking is drinking in a way that is unlikely to cause yourself or others significant risk of harm.

Harmful drinking

Harmful drinking is drinking at levels that lead to significant harm to physical and mental health and at levels that may be causing substantial harm to others.

Binge drinking

Binge drinking is essentially drinking too much alcohol over a short period of time, e.g., over the course of an evening, and it is typically drinking that leads to drunkenness. It has immediate and short-term risks to the drinker and to those around them.

Source: Department of Health, Home Office, Department for Education and Skills, Department for Culture, Media and Sport. *Safe. Sensible. Social: the next steps in the National Alcohol Strategy.* London: DoH; 2007.

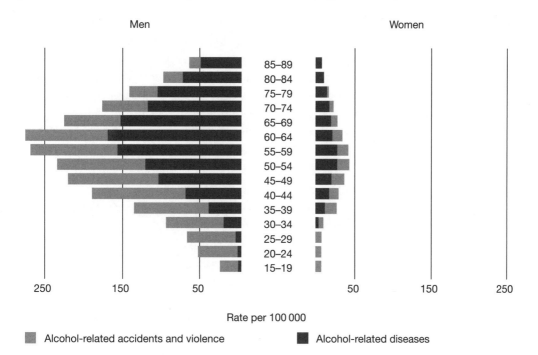

Figure 3.23 Alcohol-related mortality per 100 000 person-years
Source: Makela P. Alcohol-related mortality by age and sex and its impact on life expectancy: estimates based on the Finnish death register. *Eur J Public Health.* 1998; **8**(1): 43–51. By permission of Oxford University Press.

alcohol is the level of drinking taking place amongst the very young. The concern is not only that the physical and psychological damage of drinking at a very early age is likely to be greater than amongst mature adults but also that establishing a pattern of harmful drinking at an early age may be associated with addiction throughout subsequent life. Based on survey data of school pupils in England, there is a notable upward trend in the amount of alcohol being consumed by those who do drink, and there is also a closing of the gender gap in consumption (Figure 3.24).

Much attention has been paid recently to the approach to drinking in the United Kingdom. In contrast to many of the countries of the Mediterranean, where consumption of alcohol is closely associated with the consumption of food, in the United Kingdom drinking alcohol is frequently seen as a separate activity from eating. One of the elements of thinking behind relaxation in the licensing hours governing the sale of alcohol in 2005 was that more relaxed approaches would encourage the development of a café culture in the United Kingdom in which eating and drinking were more closely associated.

Action at national policy and governmental level can play a part in the reduction of alcohol misuse (Table 3.9). There is a close, observable relationship between the price of alcohol relative to personal disposable incomes, alcohol consumption and alcohol-related harm indicated by deaths from chronic liver disease. Put simply, if people have more disposable income and there is a fall in the price of alcohol in real terms, it is likely that consumption of alcohol will rise

and there will be a corresponding increase in the harm produced by it. Alcohol is not expensive to produce, and the price of alcohol is largely determined by the amount of tax the government decides to put on it.

In addition to the enormous burden placed upon health services by the short- and long-term effects of alcohol, there is also an important role for health services and other organisations in the identification of serious alcohol problems and intervention to resolve them. This is a particularly important role for primary care services, where an approach based on the 'brief interventions' model is possible. A review of the cost-effectiveness of alcohol treatment published in 2006 concluded that investment in evidence-based alcohol treatments could save £5 for each £1 spent.

The provision of help for people who have become dependent on alcohol or who are suffering serious effects because of excessive use can include the creation of day centres in which skills training, counselling and befriending services can be provided. Help also includes treatment services (inpatient, residential, outpatient, day care) that can provide detoxification programmes, family therapy and other specific treatment and support services.

Few local services are based upon health service initiatives alone. The most successful are those in which the emphasis is on close collaboration between health, local authority and voluntary organisations skilled in these areas of service. Self-help groups can also be very effective, and some benefit from support and encouragement from statutory agencies.

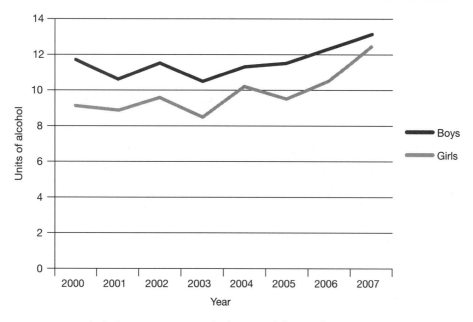

Figure 3.24 Mean alcohol consumption in the last week by pupils ages 11 to 15 who had drunk, 2000–07

Source: Fuller E, editor. *Drug Use, Smoking and Drinking Among Young People in England in 2007.* Leeds: The Health and Social Care Information Centre; 2008.

Table 3.9 Key features of the alcohol strategy for England

- Sharpened criminal justice for drunken behaviour
- A review of NHS alcohol spending
- More help for people who want to drink less
- Toughened enforcement of underage sales
- Trusted guidance for parents and young people
- Public information campaigns to promote a new 'sensible drinking' culture
- Public consultation on alcohol pricing and promotion
- Local alcohol strategies

Source: Department of Health, Home Office, Department for Education and Skills, Department for Culture, Media and Sport. *Safe. Sensible. Social: the next steps in the National Alcohol Strategy.* London: DoH; 2007.

Other Substances

The predisposition to drug misuse lies in a wide range of influences. Deprivation, unemployment, social exclusion and poor educational status are all important factors in creating conditions where children and young people are more likely to misuse drugs. But all social groups are at some risk, including well-educated young people. Particularly high-risk groups are young people who are in care, homeless or involved in truancy from school. Generally, family and peer group influences are also important. It is noteworthy that drug misuse can be the cause of deprivation and unemployment, not just the result.

The proper initial focus for consideration of the problem of the misuse of drugs in the population is on young people. For them, there are many paths leading to experimentation. A first offer of drugs most commonly comes from a friend or member of their peer group and not, as is popularly imagined, from the stereotypical drug pusher skulking by the school gates or in a darkened alley.

Of particular concern amongst young people is misuse of volatile substances. This habit came to prominence in the 1970s, when it became commonly known as 'glue-sniffing'. Volatile substance misuse is the inhalation of gases and vapours with the intention of getting a pleasurable sensation from their effects. The major hazard is sudden death, and more deaths commonly occur amongst young people under 16 years of age from volatile substance inhalation than from other forms of drug misuse.

The 1990s saw a major rise in so-called 'recreational drug use' – in young people, this is often in the context of visiting nightclubs. This issue captured wide public attention in the mid-1990s with media coverage of the deaths of a number of teenagers who had been supplied tablets of ecstasy at 'raves'.

The scale of substance misuse in the United Kingdom, and the level of personal and social consequences resulting from it, is substantial in both adults and young people. In 2005 there were 1608 deaths related to drug misuse in England and Wales. Data on population levels of drug misuse are difficult to obtain, as the possession and supply of drugs is illegal. Therefore, responses of individuals to population surveys are likely to be cautious and to underestimate the extent of the problem. The British Crime Survey, which provides population data on the use of drugs in society, reported that in 2005 some 10.5% of adults had used one or more illicit drugs during the last year. Substantial gender differences are present, with almost twice as many men as women reporting drug-taking. The school-based survey of young people in 2006 on the subjects of smoking, alcohol and drugs reported that 17% of young people aged 11 to 15 reported drug use over the preceding year. Drug use was linked to ethnic origin, age, smoking and alcohol use. It was also linked to truanting or school exclusion. In 2007/08 the British Crime Survey reported that the proportion of the population aged between 16 and 59 years that used illicit drugs was 9.3%, and this was the lowest level recorded since the survey started in 1995.

The Lisbon-based European Monitoring Centre for Drugs and Drug Addiction, which began operation in 1995, compiles data from across the European Union (EU). Its 2006 report shows that the United Kingdom has levels of drug usage that place it at the top end of the scale of the problem within Europe. However, the data are complicated by differing collection methodologies.

In England, the regionally-based National Drug Treatment Monitoring System provides data on the use of treatment services. These data are collected from a range of service providers in the statutory and voluntary sectors. In the year 2006/07, there were over 195 000 people receiving drug treatment, of whom more than 80 000 commenced treatment during that year.

One of the interesting contrasts is between the drugs used by those in the general population who misuse drugs and those used by people who are in contact with drug-treatment services. In the general population, and particularly amongst younger people, most drug misuse is associated with cannabis, but amongst those in contact with the treatment services, heroin is by far the main drug that is misused.

Prevention and Control of Substance Misuse

The overall approach to the control of the drug problem in the United Kingdom is to combine prevention of the development of drug misuse with the goal of getting the maximum proportion of those addicted to drugs into the treatment system. Specific goals to reduce the rate of drug-related deaths and curb the spread of blood-borne viruses are also important components of the strategy. Wider social goals concerning crime reduction have also had a major influence, with programmes developed specifically to provide rapid access to drug treatment for those drug misusers who come into contact with the criminal justice system.

The main responsibility for tackling drugs at a local level in England rests with Drug Action Teams (DATs), which are partnerships between agencies operating at a local level. They are usually based on the geographical boundaries of local authorities and involve the primary care trusts as their key NHS partner. Drug Action Teams have a major role overseeing the commissioning of drug-treatment services for their population. In many areas, they operate within the overall framework provided by the Crime and Disorder Reduction Partnership.

Confidential counselling, advice and information services should be available and easily accessed by drug users and their relatives and friends. Detoxification programmes, maintenance schedules and other prescribing regimes to reduce the effects of dependency can be provided in the community with close cooperation from general practitioners. Heavily dependent individuals and those with poly-drug problems need access to specialist services and may require inpatient admission and extended support through rehabilitation and aftercare.

In many parts of Britain, a key role is played by voluntary organisations with expertise in the drug misuse field, and it must be acknowledged that many people who have problems are more comfortable in using these informal, non-statutory services. Most residential rehabilitation services are provided by this sector. Moreover, voluntary organisations and their staff may also have more credibility with young people in relation to relevant health promotion and disease prevention programmes.

There is very substantial overlap between alcohol abuse, drug misuse and mental illness. Very often patients coming forward for treatment will have two, or sometimes all three, of these problems with which to contend. It is very important that services develop in an integrated and coordinated way, making use of the expertise of health, local authority and other statutory services and of the substantial number of voluntary organisations.

Tobacco

Cigarette smoking is the commonest preventable cause of death in Britain. Over 10 million adults in the United Kingdom smoke tobacco, and it is estimated that smoking was responsible for 120 000 premature deaths in Britain each year by the end of the 1990s. On a global level, the World Health Organization estimates that tobacco is responsible for 4.9 million premature deaths annually, and because of the increase in smoking across the world, they predict that this death toll may double by the year 2020.

Smoking is implicated in the causation of coronary heart disease; stroke; peripheral vascular disease; diseases of the lung (such as bronchitis and emphysema); and cancer of the lung, larynx, oesophagus, pharynx, oral cavity, pancreas and bladder. Women who are smokers have more low-birth-weight babies and more thromboembolic disease (particularly if they are taking the oral contraceptive pill). There are potential risks to non-smokers through passive smoking (inhalation of the components of cigarette smoke in the environment). Apart from the smoking-related diseases described above, there is an increased risk of upper-respiratory disease in children living in a household where the adults smoke.

In 2006 approximately 22% of adults smoked, a proportion that has shown a decline from the level of 27% in 2000 (Figure 3.25). There is a marked difference in levels of smoking between people in different economic and social circumstances, with those in routine and manual socio-economic groupings having levels of smoking substantially higher than those in professional and managerial groupings (Figure 3.26). Many more men than women used to smoke, but the gap has narrowed considerably. Amongst young people (aged 11 to 15 years) the gender balance is reversed, with more girls than boys smoking at least once a week.

It is increasingly recognised that a comprehensive approach is needed if society is to dramatically reduce the use of tobacco. The terminology has altered in response to this more developed understanding, shifting from 'anti-smoking' to 'tobacco control'. The key goals and content of a tobacco control programme approach are outlined in Table 3.10.

As economic measures are used to reduce tobacco use and the price of tobacco products rises, there is an increasing concern about the smuggling of tobacco products. It has been estimated that one-quarter of all cigarettes and two-thirds of all rolling tobacco smoked in the United Kingdom have avoided domestic taxes and duties. The availability of very cheap tobacco means that a major incentive for smokers to quit is removed.

Important measures adopted in the United Kingdom to reduce both tobacco use and the effects of environmental tobacco smoke have included the landmark legislation in all parts of the United Kingdom that made virtually all enclosed public places and workplaces smoke-free. This represented the biggest campaigning success for anti-tobacco interests for many years. Other

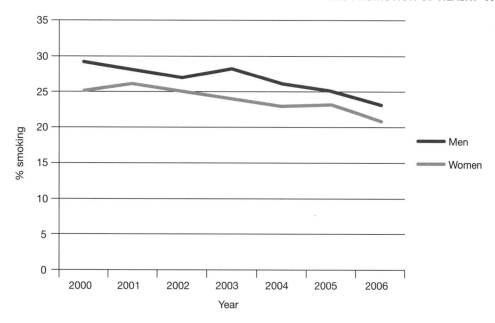

Figure 3.25 Prevalence of cigarette smoking, 2000–06
Source: Office for National Statistics.

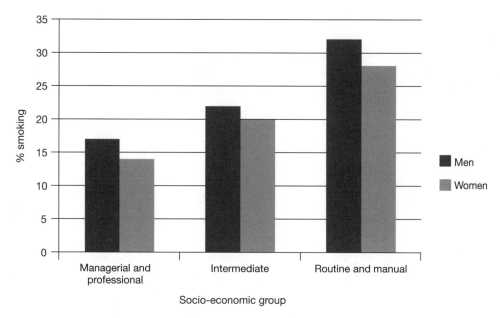

Figure 3.26 Prevalence of cigarette smoking by socio-economic classification
Source: Office for National Statistics.

Table 3.10 Tobacco control

The key goals for tobacco control are:

- preventing initiation among young people
- encouraging quitting among adults and young people
- eliminating exposure to environmental tobacco smoke
- reducing tobacco-related inequalities among population groups.

The key elements of a tobacco control programme can include:

- economic measures, such as increased taxes
- prohibition of advertising and promotion
- restriction of availability, such as licensing outlets
- social marketing campaigns
- young people's peer education programmes
- services to assist smokers in quitting
- surveillance, evaluation and research

hard-hitting measures have included steadily more potent messages and graphic images on cigarette packaging and raising the age at which tobacco can be sold to young people from 16 years to 18 years.

The NHS has developed smoking cessation services based on the evidence on effectiveness, and targets for achieving numbers of quitters have been made part of the performance management approach for primary care trusts.

There are good examples from elsewhere of success in tackling smoking. California is notable for having reduced adult smoking rates from 22.7% in 1988 to 13.3% in 2006. On a global level, the World Health Organization has led the fight against tobacco and brought into existence the Framework Convention on Tobacco Control. This legally binding international treaty contains provisions aimed at reducing both the supply of and demand for tobacco. The Convention entered into force on 27 February 2005 following its ratification by the requisite 40 member states (which included the United Kingdom). From that point on, all the countries that have ratified the Convention are legally bound by its provisions.

NUTRITION

Any consideration of the relationship between nutrition and health in an industrialised country like Britain must begin by setting the problem in an international context. In many developing countries of the world, large sections of the population are in a state of chronic malnutrition caused by the lack of adequate amounts of food. At times of war and natural disaster, as is all too evident from the widespread media coverage such events receive, situations rapidly turn to famine and large numbers of people die.

In many developing countries, protein-energy malnutrition, particularly amongst children, is present to some degree in the population all the time. In famine or other circumstances of acute food shortage, the severe forms of protein-energy malnutrition, marasmus and kwashiorkor, become common. Often there is also failure of sanitation, poor hygiene and lowered resistance to infection (which accompanies malnutrition). This leads almost inexorably to outbreaks of communicable diseases, which then contribute to the high loss of life.

While public health practitioners in the Western world grapple with a set of nutritional problems mainly associated with dietary excess and imbalance, their counterparts in Third World countries are confronted with public health problems related to nutrition that are of an awesome magnitude.

This section is concerned with nutrition in industrialised countries such as Britain, where the dietary issues concern the balance of nutrients in the diet and whether they are present in sufficient quantities. In such countries, therefore, the issues in nutritional policy concern the measures necessary to avoid dietary deficiency diseases as well as those necessary to promote health and proper growth and development in childhood.

The importance of diet in the causation of chronic disease has been considered earlier in this chapter as part of the discussion of risk markers for coronary heart disease and stroke. Diet may also be related to the causation of a number of other major chronic diseases, such as hypertension and some forms of cancer. The government obtains advice from the Scientific Advisory Committee on Nutrition (SACN), which replaced the Committee on Medical Aspects of Food and Nutrition Policy (COMA) in 2001.

Obesity

The rapid increase in the prevalence of obesity is a serious cause for concern in the United Kingdom and in many developed countries. Indeed obesity can be regarded as the major nutritional disorder in the industrialised world. It is an important cause of premature death and is associated with the development of a number of chronic diseases, including cardiovascular disease, stroke, type 2 diabetes mellitus and hypertension.

In 2007 the United Kingdom government published its report *Tackling Obesities: future choices*. This authoritative report, which was part of the government's Foresight Programme, brought to prominence the term 'obesogenic environment'. The term describes the collection of environmental factors that contribute to the imbalance of energy intake and expenditure and result in the population-wide problem of obesity.

The most commonly used measure for assessing the prevalence of overweight and obesity in individuals and in the population is the body mass index (BMI). This is calculated by dividing the person's weight in kilograms by the square of their height expressed in metres. This measure can be used to construct a definition of 'obesity' and 'overweight' and then to assess the status of the population in relation to their weight against these defined concepts. Although other measures, such as body fat, can be of more direct correlation with risk, they are less easily measured on a population basis. The World Health Organization defines 'overweight' as having a BMI equal to or over 25 and 'obesity' as having a BMI equal to or over 30.

The World Health Organization estimates that in 2005 over 1.6 billion adults were overweight worldwide and more than 400 million were obese. On the basis of current trends, it projects that these numbers will reach 2.3 billion and 700 million by 2015. Direct international comparisons can be made, but their reliability is questionable since the method of data capture varies between structured weighing and measuring and self-reported height and weight.

The trend of obesity in England, as shown by data from the Health Survey for England, shows a very clear upward trend in both adults and children (Figure 3.27). It is estimated that by 2050, based on current trends, 60% of males and 50% of females could be obese.

The basic causation of obesity in an individual is an imbalance between energy intake and energy expenditure. At a population level, the causative factors are more complex. For example, in relation to physical activity, the decline in manual labour in developed countries has had an important effect. People's working lives are no longer dominated by physically demanding jobs, and in the domestic setting, the development of labour-saving devices has reduced individual energy expenditure in the home.

A major contributor to the energy imbalance has been the change that has taken place in transport with the growth of car ownership. The resulting decline in walking and cycling has affected both adults and children. While the total distance travelled in Britain has grown by 62% between 1980 and 2005, the bulk of that growth has been in car travel, which has grown by 75%. In contrast, travel by pedal cycle has fallen by 22% over the same period. The recommended amount of moderate physical activity for adults is 30 minutes a day on at least five days per week. This could easily be obtained by walking and cycling, but in Britain between 1995/97 and 2005 the amount of time spent cycling and walking declined by 9%, from 12.9 minutes on average every day to 11.7 minutes.

A major element in strategies to achieve goals in nutrition and health is to ensure that the public is well informed about the issues, the risks and of ways of reducing risks through dietary modification. There is a clear generational dimension to obesity, with the strongest predictor of childhood obesity being parental obesity. This is the result of a mixture of social, biological and environmental factors, but it does point to there being an important role for parents in introducing their children to healthy eating alternatives and helping them to realise the importance of patterns of eating to their future health and well-being. There is a clear life-course component to the development of obesity, and basic interventions such as good maternal nutrition, breast-feeding and healthy weaning have all been linked to healthy weight later in life.

A number of programmes have been developed to support healthy eating. A

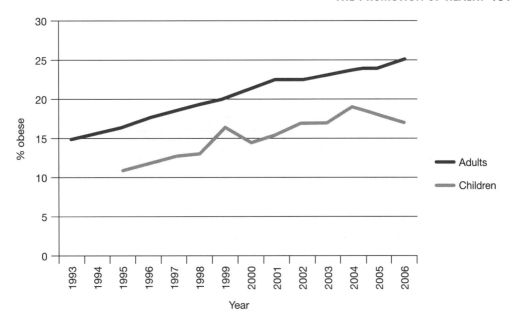

Figure 3.27 Trend in levels of obesity amongst adults (16 years and over) and children (2 to 15 years) in England
Source: Health Survey for England 2006. London: The Information Centre for Health and Social Care; 2008.

fundamental component of this has been a healthy eating message aimed at encouraging everyone to eat at least five portions of fruit or vegetables per day. A notable innovation has been the School Fruit Scheme, which provides daily fruit or crunchy vegetables to the youngest group of primary school children. There is some evidence that the proportion of the population reaching the five-a-day target level is increasing (Figure 3.28).

The achievement of fundamental population change will, however, require much broader and concerted action. People's patterns of eating and their choice of food is governed by a wide range of factors, such as family income, access to different types of food, the behaviour of other members of their social network and the powerful forces

of product marketing and advertising. For children in particular, what their parents can afford and choose to give them to eat is an important part of their early dietary experience.

To create a culture within Britain where healthy food choices are widely available and are adopted by a large proportion of the population poses a formidable challenge. Health services can play an important part by setting targets and gathering appropriate information about current dietary patterns. They can also take the lead in those areas where health care professionals are in a position to assess and advise people about their present food intake and provide information and assistance that will help them to make beneficial modifications. This is particularly important in the primary care

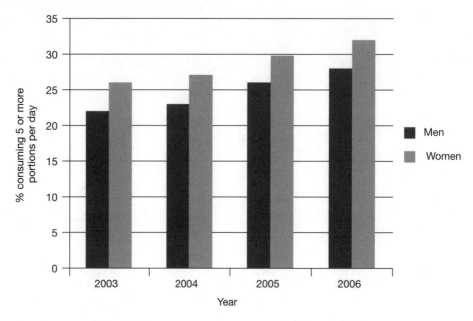

Figure 3.28 Fruit and vegetable consumption amongst adults in England
Source: Health Survey for England 2006. London: The Information Centre for Health and Social Care; 2008.

setting, where a relatively high proportion of the population is in regular contact with the health service. There are particular responsibilities for doctors and nurses assessing the growth and development of the youngest children to ensure that their daily nutritional requirements are being met and to ensure that under-nutrition is recognised early and corrected.

Health care professionals also have an important part to play in counselling the smaller number of people who come into contact with the hospital service as patients. It is important that the health service ensures that adequate skills and expertise in this field exist amongst their professional staff, notably that sufficient skilled dieticians are available.

Schools have a particular responsibility to introduce nutrition and health issues in the health education curriculum. They can also create catering policies that help children to develop positive attitudes towards eating for health and enable them to become used to healthier food. Starting in 2006, primary schools in England have been engaged in an annual weighing and measuring programme designed to provide accurate data on the BMIs of school children.

The food industry in all its diversity is another key element in population-based nutrition and health strategies. Industry is influenced by government, which can enjoin it at national level. It is also influenced by consumer demands and expectations. Increased labelling of food with nutritional information has been an important step forward in educating consumers about nutrition and health. A greater availability of healthier options (for example, containing less saturated fat) in processed food is still required. Similarly, such options are still in the minority amongst the choices offered by restaurants and fast-food catering outlets.

The growth of vegetarianism in young people has also been important in opening up the issue of food and health to public debate (though the prime motivation behind the movement is concern for animal welfare, not health consciousness per se). Similarly, the substantial growth in demand for organic produce and the development of home-delivery 'box schemes' is evidence of a growing desire amongst many people to improve the quality of the food that they eat.

As with many other lifestyle-related issues, the greatest challenges are with the most deprived social groups within the population, in which behaviour has proved intractable to change. The issue of poverty, the extent to which a limited household budget is spent on food (particularly for its younger members) and the presence of 'food deserts' in many disadvantaged communities are major concerns when considering the public health problems of some parts of the population in Britain. The differential adoption of healthy eating and exercise amongst better-off groups in the population has the potential to further increase health inequalities in the future.

Clinical Treatment of Obesity

While there is a good evidence base for lifestyle interventions involving dietary change and increased physical activity, not everyone will benefit, and maintaining weight loss is difficult for many people. Pharmaceutical interventions have been developed that are based on either suppressing appetite or reducing the absorption of food through the bowel wall. The development of surgical treatment has concentrated on bariatric procedures, which reduce the size of the stomach. The development of clinical services offering a range of weight-management treatments, including pharmaceutical, surgical and behavioural approaches, is highly variable. However, the sheer scale of what has been described as the obesity epidemic makes it highly inappropriate to rely on clinical treatment of obesity as making any substantial contribution to the reduction of population levels of this major health problem.

PHYSICAL ACTIVITY

While physical activity is an important component of any strategy to combat obesity, it is also connected with a wide spectrum of other conditions. Physical inactivity has been connected with mental illness, colorectal cancer, coronary heart disease, osteoarthritis, osteoporosis and low back pain. The relative contribution of physical inactivity is sometimes greater than more obvious factors. For example, in one study 37% of coronary heart disease deaths were attributed to physical inactivity, compared to the 19% attributable to smoking.

The benefits of physical activity in combating chronic physical disease are more commonly appreciated than the clear benefits associated with mental health. The positive effects of regular physical exercise include reduction in the symptoms of depression and anxiety as well as improvements in self-esteem and self-perceived positive body image. These positive effects on psychological well-being appear to result from the positive effects of the exercise itself combined with the cultural and social aspects of participation in physical activity. While the health sector can play a role in increasing levels of physical activity, the contribution of other sectors of society is extremely important (Table 3.11)

CONCLUSIONS

This chapter has described the background and approaches used in one of the main aspects of public health practice – the promotion of health. Many of the health problems in a population are capable of major reduction, if not elimination, through these health promotion measures. Similarly, the promotion of health as a positive state to be attained by as many people in a population as possible is another important goal for this aspect of public health practice.

The potential for change is enormous if ways can be found to modify risk factors on a population scale and to help people adopt and sustain lifestyles that are supportive to health rather than harmful and injurious. However, the underlying influences on

Table 3.11 Examples of action from different sectors on determinants of physical activity

Determinant type	Action from key sectors		
	Health	*Sport and leisure*	*Transport and urban planning*
Macro environment	Providing stewardship for multidisciplinary action Delivering public health programmes to increase opportunities for physical activity for people on low incomes	Planning and delivering strategies for sport for all that reduce the cost of participation for people on low incomes and celebrate cultural diversity	Developing regional spatial plans that maximise public health and opportunities for active living
Micro environment	Representing the health sector on multidisciplinary planning committees Promoting physical activity among health-sector employees and service users	Improving access to sport and leisure opportunities for pedestrians and cyclists	Prioritising access by pedestrians and cyclists in urban planning and designing communities conducive to walking
Individual	Delivering counselling for physical activity in primary care	Delivering targeted community sport programmes	Delivering targeted social marketing programmes for walking and cycling

Source: Cavill N, Kahlmeier S, Racioppi F, editors. *Physical Activity and Health in Europe: evidence for action.* Copenhagen: WHO Regional Office for Europe; 2006.

health – for example, poverty, lack of educational opportunity and social exclusion – are powerful, and reducing their impact is an enormous challenge.

One of the keys to success lies in shaping the behaviour and values of children and young people. It lies in enabling them to lay the foundations for a life that will achieve the maximum of the biological span and in which most of those years will be characterised by health rather than illness, chronic disease or disability.

If these challenges can be met in the twenty-first century, the scale of public health achievement will be as great as the historical discoveries whose descriptions began this chapter and which transformed the health landscape of the past.

REFERENCES

1 Barker DJP, editor. *Fetal and Infant Origins of Adult Disease.* London: BMJ Books; 1992.

2 Lalonde M. *A New Perspective on the Health of Canadians: a working document.* Ottawa: Information Canada; 1974.

3 World Health Organization. *Targets for Health for All: targets in support of the European Regional Strategy for Health for All.* Copenhagen: World Health Organization Regional Office for Europe; 1985.

4 Wilson JMG, Jungner G. *Principles and Practice of Screening for Disease.* Geneva: WHO; 1968.

5 Shapiro S, Venet W, Strax P, *et al. Periodic Screening for Breast Cancer: the Health Insurance Plan project and its sequelae, 1963–1986.* Baltimore, MD: Johns Hopkins University Press; 1988.

6 Forrest APM. *Report to the Health Ministers of England, Wales, Scotland and Northern Ireland by a Working Group Chaired by Sir Patrick Forrest.* London: HMSO; 1987.

7 Department of Health and Social Security. *Inequalities in Health: report of a research working group.* London: DHSS; 1980.

8 Townsend P, Phillimore P, Beattie A. *Health and Deprivation: inequality and the North.* London: Routledge; 1988.

9 Wilkinson RG. Income distribution and life expectancy. *BMJ.* 1992; **304**: 165–8.

10 Unal B, Critchley JA, Capewell S. Modelling the decline in coronary heart disease deaths in England and Wales, 1981–2000: comparing contributions from primary prevention and secondary prevention. *BMJ.* 2005; **331**: 614.

CHAPTER 4
The National Health Service

INTRODUCTION

As the first decade of the twenty-first century has progressed to its end, governments throughout the world have critically examined their health care systems and asked fundamental questions about how best they can serve their citizens. The driving force for health care reform has been how to meet ever-increasing demand for health services while containing costs to ensure that scarce resources go further. There has also been a desire to make services much more patient-centred and less producer-driven than they were in the past. In many countries this has led to new ways of organising and allocating funds for health services.

Change has created a new environment: health care organisations have increasingly become managed rather than being led by professional staff as in the past; health service workforces have had to adapt rapidly to ever-changing roles and responsibilities; the rights of patients as consumers of health care have created a new balance in the relationship between clinicians and their patients; and traditional notions of clinical freedom have been reassessed as responsibilities at the bedside and to the boardroom have become intertwined. This process of change has inevitably been accompanied by tensions as well as major benefits as traditional attitudes and practices have been challenged.

This chapter describes the factors that influence the demand for health services, the historical development of the National Health Service (NHS), its present structure and the way in which it functions.

HISTORICAL PERSPECTIVE
THE POOR LAW

The development of services for the sick, aged and infirm in Britain is inextricably linked to the attitudes of society towards the poor at various points in history, for it is often the case that sickness and old age are states that coexist with poverty.

Much of the responsibility for the poor, aged and sick in medieval Britain fell on the Church and on parishes, which often levied local taxes to assist them in providing relief. The dissolution of the monasteries and religious fraternities by Henry VIII created considerable hardship, leaving large numbers of elderly and sick people with no means of support. Many individual items of legislation passed during the reign of Elizabeth I were rationalised in 1601 with the passage of the Elizabethan Poor Law (most commonly referred to as the 'Old Poor Law'). Under this law, the 'impotent poor' (for example, the old or sick) were to be cared for in poorhouses or almshouses, whilst the able-bodied paupers were provided with work in houses of correction.

From the 1760s, purpose-built workhouses began to be provided, financed by the poor rate. Much of the responsibility for the administration of the Old Poor Law rested with individual local parishes in the form of parish overseers. While tyranny undoubtedly existed, there were also many examples of caring parishes, and by the early nineteenth century the Poor Law was seen as 'the largest branch of public administration'.

Dissatisfaction with the Old Poor Law mounted for two main reasons. Firstly, the Law was proving an increasingly costly exercise. The system of 'outdoor relief', which gave payments in cash or kind to the poor, was becoming widespread in many parishes. However, because of the economic problems of the time, the size of the pool of such needy individuals and their families had grown. Secondly, some critics considered that the regimes in houses of correction were too comfortable for their inmates. This climate of opinion led ultimately to the establishment of a Royal Commission of Inquiry into the Poor Law and to the subsequent Poor Law Amendment Act 1834 (the 'New Poor Law'). Many commentators regard this resulting legislation as being strongly aligned to the utilitarian philosophy of Jeremy Bentham (1748–1832) and his follower Edwin Chadwick (1800–90), the latter being intimately involved in the framing and implementation of the legislation. Chadwick had made detailed calculations in the early nineteenth century of various costs of crime, disease and poverty that society had to bear. It was this economic motivation that helped to persuade parliament of the need for legislation.

It was believed that the old system of poor relief and the condition of the houses of correction might actually encourage idleness and pauperism. The New Poor Law of 1834 was intended to abolish pauperism by measures based on deterrence. The system of outdoor relief for the poor was abolished. Those in need of support had to apply for it and were offered the workhouse. The workhouse regime was harsh and austere, deliberately designed to pose a very unattractive prospect for those applying for poor relief. By this central tenet of 'less eligibility' (the person receiving poor relief could not

be better off than the worst-paid independent worker), it was reasoned that only those who were truly needy would accept poor relief in the form of the workhouse.

Under the New Poor Law, responsibility was taken out of the hands of individual parishes, which were grouped together as Poor Law Unions (administered by boards of guardians) and placed under the control of a central body headed by three poor law commissioners, the aim being to introduce a uniform process of administration. Although separate provision was laid down for the sick and aged, in practice few Unions allowed themselves the expensive luxury of separate workhouses, and in many mixed workhouses the able-bodied pauper rubbed shoulders with the sick, the old and infirm, children and the mentally handicapped.

Gradually, many workhouses set aside annexes or 'wards' for the care of the sick pauper. In a few individual workhouses, infirmaries were to be found, and the rudiments of a domiciliary service for the sick poor were also present. Although the Poor Law authorities stipulated that each Union had to employ a properly qualified medical practitioner, they were poorly paid and under the control of the lay administrators, who decided on all applications for medical relief. Standards within workhouses were pitifully inadequate, with overcrowding and unsanitary conditions prevailing. 'Nursing' was carried out by other inmates. Moreover, the crux of the problem was still that the law implied poverty was a result of idleness or waywardness on the part of the individual. Florence Nightingale commented that these civilian hospitals were just as bad as, or worse than, the squalid military hospitals that she so strongly condemned in the Crimean War. Towards the end of the nineteenth century, conditions had become so appalling that parliament authorised the building of separate infirmaries with trained medical and nursing staff.

THE LOCAL AUTHORITY HOSPITALS

In addition to the Poor Law medical service, the major local authorities (county and borough councils) provided a separate publicly owned system of hospitals that had its origins in the isolation hospitals for infectious diseases constructed from the 1860s onwards and in the asylums for the mentally ill and handicapped. By the early part of the twentieth century, in many regions of the country, local authority (municipal) hospitals were also treating other, more general illnesses. Following the transfer of the powers and responsibilities of the Poor Law to local government by a further act of parliament in 1929, the local authorities were allowed to take control of and administer the Poor Law infirmaries. The local authority hospitals fell mainly under the jurisdiction of the medical officer of health, who delegated his responsibility in each hospital to a medical superintendent. This achieved some degree of unity in hospital services, although many local authorities were slow to take up this opportunity.

VOLUNTARY HOSPITALS

The main alternative to the publicly owned hospital system was the voluntary hospital movement. Some of the earliest hospitals, such as St Thomas' Hospital in London,

began life as religious institutions in the Middle Ages. However, there was a surge in hospital building from the middle of the eighteenth century, financed from donations, charitable funds and subscriptions. Mostly these were established to cater for the 'deserving' poor, with the 'undeserving' poor continuing to look to their local poorhouse for care. It is important to stress that the bulk of medical care before the twentieth century took place outside institutions.

Over time, great variation developed in the size and function of the voluntary hospitals as they became one of the main foci for medical practice. They often provided a standard of care that was far above that provided by the state and indeed served as a model that the latter strove to attain. Each voluntary hospital had its own committee of lay governors, and originally they decided which patients deserved to be admitted. Medical care was provided by visiting physicians and surgeons, who were almost always in private practice and provided their services to the voluntary hospitals free of charge, as the prestige of a hospital affiliation enabled them to build up their practices.

The voluntary hospital system encompassed a wide variety of funding and administrative arrangements. Patients who could afford to pay were often asked to do so, while others provided themselves with some security for illness by making weekly payments to one of the hospital contributory schemes. As the involvement of the medical profession in the voluntary hospitals grew with the flourishing of teaching and research, so their function began to alter. Admission policies were selective, with an emphasis on patients with illnesses that were of a short-term or acute nature, thus ensuring a rapid turnover, or those with diseases that were of particular interest. There was little place for the elderly or chronically sick. Children, the mentally ill, those with infectious diseases and pregnant women were usually refused entry. Although some charitable specialist hospitals were formed in the late nineteenth century to meet these demands, this emphasis of traditional voluntary hospitals on acute medicine was partly responsible for the extension of the publicly owned hospital service to fill the gap.

Voluntary hospitals were hard hit by the economic depression of the period between the World War I and World War II. Many were brought to the brink of insolvency by the increasing salaries paid to resident medical and nursing staff despite falling revenue and more demand for expensive services. Means-testing for patients brought in some additional income, as did the Hospital Saturday and Sunday Funds. By the late 1930s, the voluntary hospitals were increasingly relying on income from treating patients funded by local authorities.

Hospitals became safer places in which to be treated following the introduction of anaesthesia and antiseptic practices in the nineteenth century. The development of new medical technology such as X-rays meant that middle- and upper-class patients were increasingly required to have their treatment in hospitals rather than in their homes. Many of the voluntary hospitals responded to this new demand by creating 'private beds', where patients paid fully for their treatment. By the inter-war period, hospitals were beginning to lose the social stigma they once held and were increasingly seen as resources for the whole population.

THE EMERGENCY MEDICAL SERVICE

As part of the preparation for the anticipated receipt of military and civilian casualties during World War II, a hospital service was created in 1938 to be administered directly by the Ministry of Health (which had been formed in 1919). The number of beds in some hospitals was increased, temporary buildings were erected or premises were extended and some of the former Poor Law institutions were renovated or upgraded. Some centres were created with specialist facilities, such as rehabilitation, plastic surgery and neurosurgery, and the Ministry laid down what the functions of the existing hospitals should be on a regional basis.

The Emergency Medical Service is of considerable importance in the development of the Health Service. Although its influence was short, in the context of the long period of evolution of the Service it represented a watershed for the hospital service. It resulted in the review and classification of all hospitals provided by the wide variety of agencies, and it brought their administration for the first time under a central authority, the Ministry of Health. This laid the foundation for the unified hospital service when the National Health Service came into being in July 1948, three years after the war had ended.

PRIMARY CARE

Medical services for those who did not receive care in hospital were slower to evolve. Under the Poor Law, domiciliary care or treatment by the Poor Law medical officer existed in some parts of the country, but the standard was very variable and care generally very basic. Other forms of care were provided by a variety of other agencies, such as free dispensaries run on charitable lines or outpatient departments within voluntary hospitals. Dispensaries performed a vital medical service from the early nineteenth century. As well as dispensing medicines, they offered basic diagnostic and medical treatment for poorer people. The medical officers attached to dispensaries carried out home visits, and they were an important source of information on the prevalence of infectious diseases in communities. Other developments during the nineteenth century provided private panel systems or clubs where, by paying a retention fee, the patient could claim the services of a doctor in time of need. Friendly societies and a few industries operated similar schemes.

The National Health Insurance Act 1911 (the Lloyd George Act) was the most influential development in primary care. The scheme was directed at relieving hardship amongst working men during periods of illness. When it was implemented in 1912, it was confined to workers earning less than £160 per year and it was based on contributions from the employee, the employer and the state. It entitled the insured man to choose his own general practitioner from a local panel of doctors (hence the term 'panel system') and to secure treatment (including prescribed drugs) and other consultations free of charge on demand. The exclusion of dependant wives and children from the scheme, together with the denial of the

right of insured people to receive free hospital inpatient care, meant that considerable hardship was left untouched. Moreover, a sizeable proportion of the population still paid a fee to their general practitioner for advice or treatment.

This system continued (although the eligibility was subsequently increased) until the National Health Service was established in 1948. Until then, general practitioner services were administered throughout the country by a network of insurance committees responsible for making available these services for all insured people in their locality, representing almost half of the population.

OTHER LOCAL AUTHORITY SERVICES

The new industrial towns, which were the products of the industrial revolution, forced the consideration of health problems on a population or community-wide basis. As a growing proportion of the population came to live in towns and work in factories, their circumstances came to be characterised by scarce and overcrowded housing of a very poor standard, pollution, inadequate sanitation, a contaminated water supply and limited diet. Such conditions were ripe for the infectious diseases such as cholera, typhus and tuberculosis to flourish, ravaging the population and taking a high toll in mortality, particularly amongst the young. This phenomenon of urban growth through inward migration rather than natural growth has been termed the 'urban penalty'.

Once again, the impetus for change was the doctrine of the utilitarian philosopher Jeremy Bentham. The great milestones along the path to reform were the public health reports and legislation in the middle of the nineteenth century that bore the mark of Edwin Chadwick, this time in the guise of public health reformer, and his champion Thomas Southwood-Smith (1788–1861), who, like Chadwick, had been Bentham's secretary.

Chadwick promoted 'the sanitary idea', and his efforts led to a sanitary commission in 1839, which reported in 1842. *The Sanitary Conditions of the Labouring Population* was a landmark in public health in pointing to the importance of increasing the provision of a pure water supply, effective sanitation, drainage and disposal of sewage and improved standards of housing. The Public Health Act of 1848 followed. It established a new national body, the General Board of Health, and permitted the establishment of local sanitary authorities. The first medical officer of health was appointed in Liverpool in 1847, and other local authorities followed suit. However, the 1848 Act was fundamentally flawed because it was essentially permissive, with very few coercive powers. Many towns ignored this call for sanitary reform until forced to pay attention to it by the later Public Health Acts of 1872 and 1875.

These developments all contributed to the reduction in mortality in the last quarter of the nineteenth century and in the early twentieth century. There was also a shift in cause-specific mortality. As the 'filth' diseases were increasingly conquered, attention became focused on chronic diseases such as cancer, heart disease, tuberculosis and sexually transmitted diseases. Thus by the end of the nineteenth century, local authorities turned their attention to personal

health services for a major feature of their work during the twentieth century. Part of the stimulus for this move from sanitary reform to the focus on the health of the individual came from the rise of bacteriological laboratories following the development of the germ theory of disease in the 1880s (described more fully in Chapter 3). It was now possible to test for some specific diseases, and this soon led to the development of customised drug treatments.

Although the Poor Law had provided a form of community health service (for example, for expectant mothers and children), it was patchy and inadequate. During the first 20 years of the twentieth century, the health-visitor system was developed and maternity and child-welfare clinics were opened. This was welcomed at a time of increasing public and governmental concern about 'national deterioration' – the suggestion that the British were becoming unfit through inherited health conditions and lack of proper health education. It stemmed from a lack of physically fit men amongst recruits to the Army at the time of the Boer War. These concerns were examined in the 1904 report from the government's Interdepartmental Committee on Physical Deterioration. Thus by 1948 the local authorities not only had responsibility for a large part of the hospital service but also for a whole range of community services. When the National Health Service was established, they continued to be responsible for community services but lost responsibility for hospitals.

The personal social services, which were provided by the local authorities for groups such as the elderly, children and the physically and mentally handicapped, also had diverse origins. In a few cases, services arose from voluntary or charitable organisations; in most others they arose from the structure of the Poor Law, with its strong orientation towards institutional care. The Liberal Government that came into office in 1906 passed a number of important acts, which taken together can be seen as a 'welfare state in embryo'. Their innovations included free school meals and school medical inspections. Although local authorities subsequently assumed responsibility for certain services, it was not until the implementation of the National Assistance Act 1948 that they became responsible for providing comprehensive welfare services.

THE WELFARE STATE AND THE NATIONAL HEALTH SERVICE

In the summer of 1941, the government appointed Sir William (later Lord) Beveridge (1879–1963) to chair a committee of senior civil servants charged with undertaking a survey of existing national schemes of social insurance and allied services and then making recommendations. The Beveridge Report, published a relatively short time later in December 1942, contained a series of sweeping proposals and recommendations that laid the foundation for the modern welfare state. The White Paper *A National Health Service*, which was published in February 1944, ambitiously moved beyond the initial brief for a national hospital service and provided instead a plan for a comprehensive national health service. Beveridge based his proposals for a compulsory social security scheme on three assumptions: that there would be a policy for the maintenance of

employment, a system of children's allowances and a comprehensive health service.

The medical profession was initially reluctant to participate in Beveridge's plan, which required work within a state-managed system and restriction on their capacity to determine their own incomes. The election of a Labour Government in 1945, which appointed Aneurin Bevan minister of health, created new difficulties and resulted in a breakdown of negotiations with the British Medical Association (BMA). Bevan exploited existing divisions in the medical profession between generally wealthy consultants and comparatively poorly paid general practitioners to achieve their eventual agreement to work within the National Health Service.

Beveridge's original report and the 1944 White Paper formed the basis for five main acts:

1 the Family Allowances Act (1945) provided for cash allowances to the second and subsequent child

2 the National Insurance Act (1946) established a comprehensive contributory national insurance scheme

3 the National Insurance (Industrial Injuries) Act (1946) made provision for insurance against accidents, injuries and prescribed diseases due to a person's employment

4 the National Assistance Act (1948) finally replaced the Poor Law, placing on local authorities the responsibility for the elderly, the handicapped and the homeless and setting up a scheme for financial assistance on a national basis to those in need

5 the National Health Service Act (1946)

created a comprehensive health service available to all citizens.

With the commencement of the National Health Service on 5 July 1948, the minister of health became statutorily responsible for providing a comprehensive health service for the population of England and Wales. All hospital property, whether it had been in the voluntary or municipal sector, came under the control of the minister, including all but a small number of privately owned hospitals. Thus the minister inherited a wide array of buildings and accommodation with varying origins, traditions and functions, and with differing levels of upkeep, which were spread unevenly throughout the country. However, the administrative merging of these made it possible to plan a hospital service for a locality, to begin to rationalise the distribution and to make arrangements for the training of medical, nursing and technical staff.

England was originally divided into regions with regional hospital boards whose chairmen and members were appointed by the minister of health. These regional boards appointed hospital management

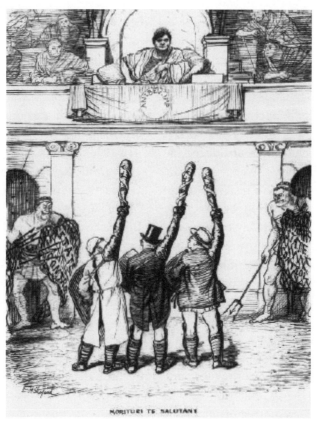

Figure 4.1 Members of the British Medical Association, represented as gladiators, conceding the introduction of the National Health Service to Aneurin Bevan, represented as Nero
Source: Drawing by EH Shepard (194–). © Punch Ltd.

committees to be responsible for the day-to-day running of individual hospitals or groups of hospitals. Teaching hospitals had separate arrangements, being administered by boards of governors appointed by the minister and responsible directly to him rather than being administered through the regional hospital boards.

The National Health Service also provided general medical, general dental, ophthalmic and pharmaceutical services under a national contract through local executive councils. Thus with the advent of the National Health Service, primary medical care was also provided free and as a right for all who wished to request it. However, Bevan's vision for a completely free National Health Service did not last long. The original estimated cost of the NHS was £176 million (for 1948–49). The actual cost was £225 million, grossly in excess of the tight post-war budget. As a remedial measure, charges for dental work and optical services were reluctantly introduced in 1951 in conjunction with a stricter financial regime. This led to Bevan's resignation as minister of health. Prescription charges were introduced by the Conservative Government in 1952. However, by 1960 it was clear that the NHS required substantial investment, and expenditure was once again allowed to rise, enabling a major hospital building programme to be started in 1962.

Health centres were seen as a major focus for primary care for the local authorities at the time, but they were very slow to gain acceptance with general practitioners. As early as 1920, the Dawson Report had recommended that local authorities provide, equip and maintain health centres where groups of doctors and other health care staff could work together. One of the most widely praised was the Finsbury Health Centre in London, which was constructed to an award-winning design in 1938. Yet by 1966 only 28 purpose-built group-practice premises, housing about 200 general practitioners, had been established.

The first experiments with local authority nursing staff attached to practices occurred in the late 1950s and early 1960s. General practice at this time was experiencing problems. There was a common perception that general practitioners were failed hospital doctors. General practitioners' income was wholly dependent on the number of patients registered with them, and they received no assistance from the government towards the provision of adequate premises or supporting staff. In consequence, morale amongst general practitioners was low. Many United Kingdom graduates emigrated to North America.

In 1966, as a result of the *Charter for the Family Doctor Service*, a new contract for general practitioners introduced major change. A three-part payment system of basic practice allowances, capitation fees and item-of-service payments was supplemented by group-practice allowances and incentives for doctors to work in under-doctored areas. Partial reimbursement of the salary costs of practice clerical and nursing staff was instituted, and funds were made available for the building or upgrading of premises.

These steps encouraged a trend towards group practices, the employment of ancillary staff, the imaginative development of premises and an expansion in the range of services offered to patients. Attachment of district nurses and health visitors developed steadily, and practices progressively sought to accommodate these staff in their premises. These positive developments were accompanied by the expansion of vocational training for general practitioners, which became mandatory in 1982, and the establishment of academic departments of general practice in the medical schools.

Local Authority Health Responsibilities

Aside from therapeutic services that were based in hospitals or general practice, the National Health Service laid down a range of other services concerned with the health of the population that were delivered mainly by major local authorities (counties and county boroughs). This was the only part of the new service that had specific responsibility for the prevention of disease. However, little detail was specified, giving considerable scope for innovation by individual local authorities. The authorities discharged their functions through health committees whose chief officer was the medical officer of health. There was ongoing competition between the medical officers of health and the general practitioners, who also saw preventive medicine as their professional remit.

In addition to the general responsibility for developing a preventive function, local authorities were charged with providing a range of supportive services. These included a wide variety of 'community' services (such as health visitors, home nurses, domiciliary midwives and home helps) to provide care, support and advice to people in their own homes; a responsibility for the control of infectious diseases, including immunisation and vaccination; the care of expectant moth-

ers, infants and young children; the provision of an ambulance service; and the provision of health centres.

Following the heyday of public health in the inter-war period, the formation of the NHS made for an awkward and relatively unfocused development of the public health profession. Many authorities adopted new duties without fully considering their strategic public health function. Public health doctors attempted to reinvent their discipline as 'community medicine' in the late 1960s with limited success. Medical officers of health were replaced with community physicians, but they found it increasingly difficult to balance their commitments to epidemiology and NHS resource management.

A major blow to local authority public health came in 1968 with the publication of the Seebohm Committee report, which recommended the removal of social workers from public health departments to new independent units. This was implemented in 1971. Sanitary inspectors had already made the break in 1956, when they were renamed public health inspectors and were no longer under the line management of the medical officer of health.

REORGANISING THE NATIONAL HEALTH SERVICE: 1974 AND AFTER

Between 1948 and 1974, the health service was organised in a so-called 'tripartite' fashion, whose three components were:

1 the hospital service (administered by regional hospital boards and a network of hospital management committees at a local level) and teaching hospitals (administered by boards of governors)

2 the family practitioner services (with contracts held by executive councils)

3 the local authority health services (which operated within the sphere of local government administration to provide public health services in the form of infectious disease and environmental hazard control, preventive services and community-based services).

A Unified Health Service: 1974

The first major administrative reorganisation of the National Health Service took place in 1974. Its aim was to provide a better, more sensitive and more coordinated public service. Before 1974, it had never been the responsibility, nor had it been within the jurisdiction, of any single named authority to provide a comprehensive health service for the population of a given area. As a result, it had not been easy to balance needs and priorities rationally and to plan and provide an integrated service within the resources available. From 1974, local authority health services were brought within the National Health Service, along with hospital services. The service was organised geographically around 14 regional health authorities, and below them were area health authorities.

The Introduction of General Management

A further reorganisation took place in 1982. This attempted to solve further problems by removing one administrative tier (area health authorities) and devolving from the centre the responsibility for providing the service within available resources. District

health authorities were left to decide on the type of organisational structure most suited to local needs. Before the impact of the 1982 restructuring could be fully realised, further major changes in the organisation of the service were stimulated by a National Health Service Management Inquiry in 1983. The most noticeable consequence of this 'Griffiths Report' was the introduction for the first time of general managers at various levels within the health service.

Sir Roy Griffiths had criticised the consensus style of administration in the NHS at that time, which gave each member of a team of equal partners (administrator, nurse, doctor and treasurer) in effect a right of veto over decisions; he wondered who could tell a latter-day Florence Nightingale who was in charge of the wards and other services. He recommended that a single general manager should be appointed to each district health authority, accountable to the board and responsible for unit general managers at operational level. In this way, for the first time since 1948, there was (in theory) a clear line of accountability, with a single nominated individual at each point. In practice, there were considerable tensions, particularly between the new general managers and the professionals providing services, and the 1980s were marked by a series of clashes over financial targets and service responsiveness.

The Creation of an Internal Market: 1990

The next significant shift in thinking about the structure and functioning of the National Health Service came as the end product of a review undertaken by the Thatcher

Conservative Government. This followed unwelcome publicity in the winter of 1987 that had focused on two perceived shortcomings:

1 incidents of hospitals closing beds, deferring or redirecting admissions or sending doctors on extended leave to limit workload in order to stay within budget, despite continued real increases in health service funding

2 the existence of 'perverse incentives', whereby extra workload in the most efficient, effective and sought-after hospitals was not matched by extra funding, and these hospitals were the first to have to limit their services.

The proposals ended the conflicting roles of the then district health authorities, in which operational responsibility for health care provision (in local hospitals) within their geographical boundaries was coupled with serving the needs of the resident population. The proposals also ended the system of funding, which was seen as offering no incentive to hospitals to treat more patients, to improve quality or to provide a wider range of services.

The 1990 reforms introduced a number of new features to the way in which the National Health Service functioned. The principal thrust of the 1990 reforms was to separate responsibility for purchasing health care from its provision. District health authorities and general practice fund-holders became service purchasers, funded according to the health needs of their population. Fund-holding general practices could use their budgets to purchase some hospital and community services, to cover prescribing costs and to employ practice staff. By the middle of the 1990s, some 15% of the population was served by fund-holding general practitioners.

Under the internal market arrangements, hospitals and other provider organisations were free to concentrate on improving the effectiveness and efficiency of health care in order to win service contracts, the means of agreeing service delivery between purchasers and providers. National Health Service trusts were created as a new and more autonomous kind of provider of NHS services. These were described in the *Working for Patients* White Paper (and for some time afterwards in the media) as 'self-governing hospitals', which reflected the philosophy of the time: to free hospitals from bureaucratic interference by management tiers above them. They had their own trust boards directly accountable to the secretary of state and significant freedom in the way they could employ staff and invest in capital infrastructure. Trusts were dependent upon contracts with purchasers for most of their income, keeping services provided in line with the requirements of the populations they served.

Despite all the reassurances that were given, many health service staff and sections of the public in Britain seemed to hold to the view that these reforms concealed a hidden agenda to privatise the National Health Service. In addition, where problems did occur – as they do from time to time in any health service – the media and the public were quick to attribute them to the organisational changes introduced in 1990. Moreover, the managerialism that swept into many public services in the late 1980s and early 1990s was also unpopular. The idea of salaries that were more competitive with the private sector and of employee benefits (such as 'company cars') was anathema to those for whom the National Health Service was a cherished institution sustained by the taxpayer. Money not used very directly for patient care was readily portrayed as money squandered.

Looking back on this important period in the history of the NHS, it is difficult to assess fully the benefits of the changes. It must be remembered that, at the start of the decade, many other countries were also experimenting with health care system reform. The changes in Britain to separate purchasing from provision of service were in keeping with an international philosophy towards the public sector. Undoubtedly, the discipline of being explicit about the cost and quality of health services was long overdue. However, the central concept of an internal market – bringing the perceived benefits of competition to a publicly funded system – increased bureaucracy and set up significant transaction costs. This could only be justified as an indirect cost of service if the overall system led to greater efficiency and drove up quality. The incoming 1997 Labour Government initially judged that it had not been successful and abolished the internal market, replacing the philosophy of competition with one based on partnership and collaboration. The next section of the chapter describes how this policy evolved and deals with the structure and function of the present health service.

THE PRESENT STRUCTURE AND FUNCTION OF THE NATIONAL HEALTH SERVICE

The Labour Government that first came to power in Britain in the summer of 1997 initially ended the experiment with competition within an internal market. Therefore, new policies and legislation were introduced in the late 1990s. The internal market was dismantled. The separation of planning (or commissioning) and provision of care was retained, as was the devolution of management responsibility for running local health care organisations. However, a new emphasis was placed on collaboration and partnerships rather than competition.

The main elements of the modernisation programme, were:

1 clear national standards
2 devolution of responsibility for delivery of services to the local level
3 local planning mechanisms to draw together all relevant parties to establish how to meet health needs and how to improve health in the population served
4 grouping general practitioners and other health professionals in primary care organisations to deliver primary and community health services and to commission hospital services for the local community
5 a greater emphasis on improving the health of communities through public health programmes, addressing national and local targets to reduce mortality, increasing healthy years of life and narrowing health inequalities
6 improved local partnership working (especially between health and local

authorities) to create a 'whole system' approach to planning and delivering care, particularly for groups with multiple needs, such as older people

7 a duty of quality placed on all local health organisations and implemented through clinical governance programmes

8 a stronger framework of accountability for performance of local services, to be monitored, managed and independently inspected.

To strengthen the modernisation programme, the government published a 10-year NHS Plan in 2000. This followed a commitment by the then Prime Minister, Tony Blair, to invest more in the NHS (to European Union average funding levels) and to address public concerns resulting from a small number of high-profile service failures and from prolonged waiting times for treatment. This plan reaffirmed the commitment to the principles of an NHS free at the point of need. Emphasis was put on encouraging local solutions and redesigning existing services to meet the needs and convenience of patients. At the same time, the government published its Neighbourhood Renewal Strategy, which required primary care and public health practitioners to play a leading role in addressing health inequalities and regeneration with local authorities and other agencies through local strategic partnerships.

The NHS Plan provided a clear national vision of the need for rapid improvement in the health service. Linked to additional investment was a range of centrally set targets, including scaled increases in the number of doctors and nurses, building

up additional technology for diagnosis and treatment, and further reductions in access times for patients.

The pledge to increase the level of the United Kingdom's spending on health to the European Union member-state average (about 9% of gross domestic product) was linked to the goals of the NHS Plan. The extra investment actually came after an independent report by the former banker (now Sir) Derek Wanless,[1] which argued the need for it and also argued the importance of reform not just in the delivery system but also in preventing more ill health, conceptualising this as a 'fully engaged scenario'. Wanless later produced a second report, specifically on public health.[2]

The NHS Plan was initially widely welcomed by health service staff, professional bodies and external commentators, as it recognised long-standing funding shortages and the way in which the infrastructure of the National Health Service had fallen behind that of many other developed countries.

The approach was initially successful. For example, long waits in accident and emergency departments were largely abolished, waiting times for cancer care rapidly fell and waiting times for planned operations in many parts of the country became very much shorter.

These changes came at the expense of criticism of the way that the service operated. Too many 'top down' targets were seen as stultifying and oppressive to local discretion in meeting health care needs and in pursuing innovation. At the same time, the government remained concerned that the pace of change and improvement was too slow and was not meeting public expectation, especially given the extra public funding that had accompanied implementation of the ambitious NHS Plan.

From 2002 onwards, a series of structural changes and incentives were introduced to speed up change, improve services and secure greater value for money. The five key components of this reform programme were:

1 *choice* – guaranteeing patients needing planned operations a choice of provider

2 *payment by results* – a system of fixed national tariffs for treatments to ensure that money followed patients and to encourage efficiency and competition based on quality of service, not price

3 *independent sector treatment centres* – central procurement of facilities for surgery and diagnostic services to add capacity as well as to put competitive pressure on traditional NHS services

4 *NHS foundation trusts* – a new, more autonomous form of NHS provider with a membership and board of governors, still part of the NHS but with more freedoms, expected to move further and faster to achieve levels of excellence

5 *commissioning* – strengthening the role of primary care trusts and general practitioners to shape and improve services.

Towards the end of the first decade of the twenty-first century, the National Health Service stands part way through a period of tumultuous change. The incoming Labour Government of 1997 had initially abandoned the previous Conservative Government's unpopular internal market design for the health service. Gradually, however, elements of this were readopted, modified and developed further in a quest to create a health system that could meet the needs of patients in an efficient and effective manner while still relying largely on the tax-funded approach that has been the hallmark of the British system since the National Health Service was created in 1948.

An initial phase of change was driven by centrally imposed targets, major structural reorganisation, greater investment and performance management. This has gradually been replaced by processes and incentives to encourage reform, improvement and higher-quality services. The intention is to create more local decision-making, greater diversity in provision, greater choice and personalisation of services for patients, stronger emphasis on treatment in primary and community settings and more focus on population health and prevention of disease and illness.

THE NHS NEXT STAGE REVIEW

In the summer of 2008, the government published the report of a review of the NHS carried out by the practising surgeon and health minister Lord Darzi of Denham. This was a landmark report. Firstly, it was undertaken with very wide participation from patient groups and large numbers of frontline clinicians. Secondly, it drew attention to the need to remedy the lack of clinical involvement in the design, planning and management of the NHS. Thirdly, it sought to move the NHS on from a focus on 'quantity' of care to quality of care. More important even than the specific proposals was the emphasis on making quality the organising principle of the NHS at every level and placing clinicians at the heart of the necessary reform.

Specific proposals included the development of an NHS constitution, the piloting of personal health budgets for patients with chronic disease, payments to reward health organisations that delivered higher-quality care, eschewing any growth in national targets and enhancing professionalism.

It is too early to judge the overall success of this programme to reform the National Health Service and make it fit for the twenty-first century. It is fair to say that while the service always attracts criticism and controversy from within the country, many other countries strive to provide health care within a realistic budget and the National Health Service principle of equity is still greatly admired internationally.

The next sections of the chapter set out in more detail the main structural and managerial elements through which the health service is organised.

THE DEPARTMENT OF HEALTH

The secretary of state for health is accountable to parliament for the National Health Service in England. He or she is based in the central government Department of Health. The Department of Health has a number of major functions, including accountability for the National Health Service, social care, the promotion of health and the protection of the public health.

Most of the responsibilities of the secretary of state for health in relation to the NHS

are devolved to strategic health authorities and primary care trusts. This is different, for example, to local authorities, whose powers are given directly from parliament.

Although ultimate accountability for the NHS at national level rests with the secretary of state for health, he or she is assisted by other ministerial colleagues. The secretary of state for health determines policy for the NHS, as well as on health matters more generally, but he or she receives advice from a range of sources, including senior civil servants, health service managers, health professionals, special advisers, external advisers and expert committees. A parliamentary Select Committee on Health also scrutinises and comments on the work of the NHS and addresses other contemporary themes in health and health care. Different arrangements exist for health services in other United Kingdom countries (see later).

The broad aim of the Department of Health is to improve health and well-being, through the following aims:

➤ to secure, through the National Health Service and within available resources, significant improvements in the health of the population through the delivery of services providing health promotion, prevention and diagnosis of illness, and high-quality cure, care and rehabilitation

➤ to ensure that these services are provided effectively, efficiently and economically, in response to identified needs of the population and with regard to the wishes of the patients

➤ to establish that the National Health Service is able to provide the structure and support for its staff to carry out

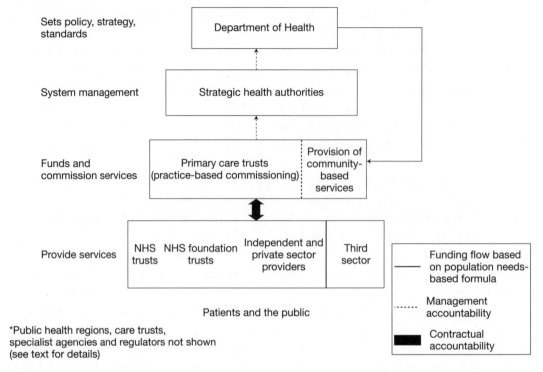

Figure 4.2 Organisational relationships in the NHS

their jobs satisfactorily and develop their careers

➤ to improve the health of the population, reduce health inequalities and protect the public health

➤ to ensure that local authorities with social care responsibilities promote independence through the provision of services, improve the life chances of children and improve protection for children and vulnerable adults

➤ to provide a legislative framework and ensure accountability to the public and parliament.

The day-to-day work of the Department of Health is led by a team of senior officials. There are three permanent secretaries: an

administrative head of department, a chief medical officer and a chief executive of the NHS. There are senior professional staff (such as the chief nursing officer, the director of research and development and the director of finance) as well as a cadre of other senior officials covering roles in the NHS or other areas of the Department's work.

The Department of Health is staffed by senior and junior career civil servants, professional, scientific and technical staff and health service managers. Traditionally, civil servants have been skilled in the areas of policy analysis and development and in preparing legislation but less experienced in implementation. However, by the beginning of the twenty-first century this had begun to change. The modern civil servant in a central government department such as the Department of Health is expected to be able to formulate policy and also to lead and facilitate change and improvement in public services. Reforming the traditional culture of public services such as health and education is important in order to make them more outward looking, more consumer-focused and more change-orientated.

The challenge is to ensure that the 'centre' does not interfere in the day-to-day delivery of services, does not place excessive demands on local service providers to supply monitoring information and is not unduly prescriptive about how things should be done (as distinct from being clear about what needs to be delivered); in short, the challenge is to ensure that goals are achieved with a 'hands-off' management style.

The Department of Health staff will often be in contact with staff at operational level (whether managers, doctors, nurses or other professional staff) through site visits to see at first hand and to learn about service developments and problems. The management of the health service at national level is also characterised by a great deal of teamwork involving staff of all disciplines. On any one day, government buildings will host a substantial number of meetings involving managers from national or local level as well as doctors, nurses and other professional staff. Such meetings will vary in their purpose, format and content but will range from single ad hoc events to discuss a particular issue, through working parties considering service programmes, to more permanent advisory committees.

This is an important and consultative part of the management of the service. It aims to ensure that there is commitment to national policies and programmes by those working in the field and that action initiated by the secretary of state for health and his or her department is informed by the knowledge and expertise of those closer to the operational service level.

STRATEGIC HEALTH AUTHORITIES

Below the Department of Health, the next organisational and managerial level of the health service consists of 10 strategic health authorities, which came into being on 1 July 2006. Each one on average covers a population of around 5.5 million.

The broad functions of a strategic health authority are:

➢ providing strategic leadership for health and health care in their region through developing commissioning and ensuring that local populations have access to a choice of services that are of high quality

➢ ensuring that service response and other activities in their region effectively meet need and improve health status

➢ accounting to the secretary of state for health for the performance of the NHS in their region

➢ troubleshooting and resolving conflicts between local NHS bodies that threaten the delivery of objectives

➢ working with all NHS bodies, other health care providers and other local stakeholders to improve the health of the population, reduce health inequalities and build capacity for improvement into local services.

Strategic health authorities are staffed by a team of managerial and professional staff, each of whom is ultimately accountable to the authority's chief executive, who in turn is accountable to the authority's chairman and board of non-executive directors (or 'members' as they are often called) as well as to the chief executive of the NHS. Individual strategic health authorities have taken different approaches to the organisation of their core staffing structure.

In carrying out these functions, strategic health authorities maintain a close working partnership and joint working with local government authorities and the government offices for the regions. This is particularly important in improving the public health and in commissioning and providing services for people with long-term or complex care needs (e.g., the elderly and mentally ill).

PRIMARY CARE TRUSTS

All general practices, family health service practitioners and other primary health care staff working with them are part of primary care organisations called primary care trusts (PCTs). Currently, 152 primary care trusts cover the population of England. The population served ranges between 90 000 and 1.2 million. The main broad responsibilities of primary care trusts are:

➤ improving the health of the community by addressing health needs
➤ commissioning high-quality services

in primary, secondary and tertiary care to meet health needs
➤ integrating health and social care locally (working with local authorities)
➤ reducing health inequalities.

Primary care trusts are also responsible for contracting with general medical practitioners, general dental practitioners, ophthalmic opticians and community pharmacists. These various primary care practitioners mainly work on a so-called *independent contractor* basis. Primary care trusts must maintain lists of these contractors and take responsibility for their remuneration. Other administrative functions relating to primary care are also the responsibility of primary care trusts, for example, appraisal of doctors' surgery premises, arranging for improvements to premises, reimbursing doctors for the employment of practice staff and the investigation of complaints.

Although the majority of practitioners are remunerated on this independent contractor basis, legislation also allows for different arrangements for delivering primary medical services. Essentially, there are four contractual mechanisms for securing primary medical services within an area:

1 *General Medical Services (GMS)* – general medical practitioners operate under a national contract, although there is some local flexibility
2 *Personal Medical Services (PMS)* – a locally negotiated alternative to the general medical services contract that allows greater flexibility on what services are provided and at what price
3 *Alternative Provider Medical Services (APMS)* – allows competent providers

1   NHS North East
2   NHS North West
3   Yorkshire and the Humber
4   East Midlands
5   West Midlands
6   South West
7   South Central
8   South East Coast
9   London
10 East of England

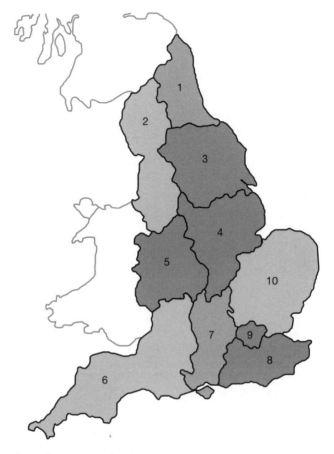

Figure 4.3 Strategic health authority boundaries in England

from any sector (public, commercial, not-for-profit) to provide primary care services and introduces an element of competition

4   *Primary Care Trust Medical Services (PCTMS)* – primary care services provided directly by the primary care trust.

General medical practitioners who are paid under the General Medical Services contract receive payment in a number of strands: a global sum linked to list size and workload, payment for meeting quality indicators or targets (the Quality and Outcomes Framework), payment for extra services provided and administrative payments.

Primary care trusts devolve part of their commissioning function to individual general practices. Under this practice-based commissioning scheme, practices are allocated resources and supported in developing their own commissioning arrangements, including hospital services. Often practices will cluster together for this purpose, thus serving populations of over 100 000 people. They may retain savings generated through this process.

Every primary care trust board has its own director of public health with statutory responsibilities for improving the health of the primary care trust's population, protecting the public health and ensuring that screening, infectious disease control and emergency planning services are provided (see later for a detailed description of the public health function).

CARE TRUSTS

Care trusts are statutory NHS bodies redesignated as care trusts under Section 45 of the Health and Social Care Act 2001. They build on primary care trusts, NHS trusts and Health Act flexibilities. They deliver integrated (whole systems) services in a single organisation. NHS and local authority health-related functions are delegated to them, not transferred. They are able to commission and/or provide. They are voluntary – partners can withdraw.

Care trusts are established on a voluntary basis and in partnership where there is a joint agreement at a local level that this model will offer the best way to deliver better health and social care services.

Care trusts commission (if they are a primary-care-based care trust) health care as well as local authority health-related functions. They also deliver those services that the NHS organisation would normally provide and local authority functions, most typically adult social care. Functions are delivered under delegated authority from local authorities.

Care trusts deliver integrated health and social care, offering the following advantages:

➤ improvements in service provision and an integrated approach
➤ a system that is designed around patient and user needs
➤ better and clearer working arrangements for staff, with more and varied career opportunities
➤ a single management structure, multidisciplinary teams managed from one point, co-location of staff and single or streamlined cross-disciplinary assessments
➤ financial flexibility and efficiency resulting from integration of functions
➤ a single strategic approach for health and social care, with a single set of aims and targets
➤ a stable organisational framework designed to improve quality of service provision through a single agency.

NHS TRUSTS

NHS trusts are a service entity created by legislation in 1990. Originally, the purpose of the trust concept was to establish considerable managerial freedom for hospitals, community units and other providers of care or services (for example, ambulance services) while retaining them under the overall organisational umbrella of the National Health Service.

The managerial team of an NHS trust is headed by a chief executive, with a board that comprises a non-executive chairman and non-executive directors (appointed by an independent appointments commission after open competition), together with executive directors (which must include a medical director, finance director and nurse director).

NHS trust hospitals participate in local service planning. They enter into service agreements with primary care trusts to provide defined services in return for funding.

NHS trusts have a responsibility to maintain a balance of services for patients (depending on the type of trust) and to ensure that major investment decisions, such as new buildings, equipment or employing new specialist doctors, are consistent with local priorities.

NHS FOUNDATION TRUSTS

NHS trusts that perform to a high standard can apply for foundation status. This new form of NHS provider was created by legislation introduced in 2003. NHS foundation trusts are independent 'public benefit organisations' but remain part of the NHS, subject to its standards and inspection regimes. They are not accountable to the secretary of state for health through the strategic health authorities, but their services and financial performance are independently regulated.

Local people, patients, carers and staff are eligible to become members of an NHS foundation trust; the members elect a board of governors, who are responsible for appointing the chair and non-executives to the board of directors and for informing and influencing how the organisation is run. NHS foundation trusts have additional freedoms beyond those of other NHS organisations. They:

➤ are not subject to direction by the secretary of state for health

➤ can borrow and invest subject to approval by the regulator (Monitor)
➤ have greater operational freedom in meeting national standards.

The NHS foundation trust regulator, Monitor, can authorise foundation status and has powers to intervene if the terms of the authorisation are breached.

NHS WALK-IN CENTRES

Walk-in centres were established in the mid-2000s to provide greater access for people with minor illness or injuries without the need for them to make general practitioner appointments. They are particularly convenient for people whose workplace is not near their home. There are about 100 such centres around the country.

PRIVATE AND INDEPENDENT HOSPITALS

The majority of hospitals and other providers of services in the British health service are operated by National Health Service organisations, but a proportion of care and services is provided by hospitals managed by the independent sector (either for-profit or not-for-profit organisations). Primary care trusts may purchase care, through agreements, from independent-sector providers, although a proportion of purchasers of private health care are generally still the patients themselves, either paying directly or through medical insurance plans.

A particular strand of independent provision is the group of independent-sector treatment centres that were centrally procured by the Department of Health to inject additional capacity for diagnostic facilities or surgical treatment. They were also intended to create competition for local NHS services. In the early stages of this programme, primary care trusts were expected to commission a proportion of services from independent sector treatment centres.

NHS DIRECT

NHS Direct was introduced in the late 1990s as an alternative way of accessing NHS services. It is a nurse-led telephone helpline service that exists to respond to public enquiries on a variety of health matters and acts as a gateway into all local health services. The service provides professional advice 24 hours a day, 365 days a year. It takes about 20 million calls a year. NHS Direct is available throughout England and provides a range of health information and services to help people maintain their health and know how to deal with common ailments. It provides advice on how to act on symptoms and signs and on how to access services.

NHS Direct Online (www.nhsdirect.nhs.uk) provides high-quality health advice and information on the Internet. It contains a comprehensive health encyclopaedia of illnesses and conditions, an easy-to-use 'self-help guide' to treating common health problems at home and a searchable database of local health services. An online enquiry service allows users to submit requests for health information to the website and receive an individual response.

THE PUBLIC HEALTH FUNCTION

Public health policies and action programmes are led at national level by the central government Department of Health and, within it, the chief medical officer. Increasingly, improving the population's health and reducing health inequalities is seen as a cross-government task. At national level, the Department of Health works closely with other relevant government departments such as the Department for Children, Schools and Families on healthy schools, the Department for Work and Pensions on workplace health and the Home Office and Ministry of Justice on drug misuse and prison health.

The public health function is an integral part of the National Health Service. In England, each primary care trust has a director of public health and his or her team. Most director of public health posts are joint appointments with local authorities. The role of public health in primary care is to ensure that attention and action is focused on improving the health of local communities and reducing health inequalities. In this task, the director of public health and his or her team ensure that the primary care trust forges strong partnerships with other local agencies that are in a position to contribute to health improvement. An essential partner is the local authority, but the role of other statutory and non-governmental organisations is particularly important. Tackling deep-seated problems like drug and alcohol misuse, teenage pregnancy and high levels of premature mortality from cancer and heart disease can only be effective through multi-agency action. It is essential also to engage local communities themselves in such programmes.

Directors of public health in primary care trusts play a pivotal role in leading, influencing and mobilising expertise to create effective multi-agency public health programmes, particularly in the most disadvantaged communities. They also have responsibility for ensuring that those preventive services that are provided in primary care by general practitioners, health visitors and other professional staff are delivered effectively. Thus they ensure, for example, that immunisation and vaccination uptake levels are high, that cervical cancer screening coverage is good, that people with hypertension are identified and their blood pressure is controlled and that smoking cessation clinics are working well.

Today's directors of public health have been recruited from a number of professional backgrounds, not just medical, creating a dynamic multidisciplinary workforce, which focuses on participation and delivery of public health services as well as on providing public health information.

A director of public health is on the board of every strategic health authority. He or she is also a director of public health in the relevant government office for the region. These dual post holders are called regional directors of public health. The strategic health authority is responsible for oversight and performance management of local health services, including those provided by primary care trusts. The regional director of public health thus has responsibilities to ensure that the public health function provided at primary care level is delivered to a good standard and that targets and objectives are being met. He or she also has an essential role in ensuring that networks of clinical services covering, for example, cancer and heart disease are well organised and perform effectively and that sound clinical governance arrangements are in place in every health organisation within the strategic health authority area. From early 2009, some of these health care responsibilities have been taken on by separate medical directors, an initiative in the NHS Next Stage Review.

A regional public health team is located in each of the nine government offices for the regions. Regional directors of public health have an important leadership and coordinating role. The regional director of public health is a member of the Department of Health's senior staff and is part of the chief medical officer's national team, and he or she also operates as part of the government office of the regional team, alongside staff from other central government departments covering areas such as economic development, the environment, transport and drug misuse. Representation at this level creates an important basis for health to be an integral part of regional regeneration programmes, addressing some of the wider determinants of poor health and health inequalities.

The regional director of public health integrates the NHS and the wider aspects of public health through this dual role. He or she also is responsible for the public health function in the region in relation to health protection and emergency planning measures. He or she also becomes involved in troubleshooting and intervention where services are failing to match standards of care.

Regional directors of public health have a role in developing and mentoring the public health function in their regions. In particular, they are responsible for ensuring that appropriate public health networks are established, involving public health staff from a wide range of organisations to provide specialist expertise, share good practice and progress professional development.

A public health observatory supports the work of each of the public health regions. Its key tasks are described in Chapter 1.

The health protection function (infectious disease prevention and control and protection of the public against hazards from chemical and radiation sources) is a vital and integral part of the local and regional public health function. This element of public health is supported by a national agency – the Health Protection Agency (*see* Chapter 9).

The detailed public health function described in this section applies to England, but public health is an essential part of the NHS structures of the other three United Kingdom countries, though precise structural arrangements differ.

The scope of a modern public health service encompasses a wide range of functions (Table 4.1), delivered through the structures described above.

THE UNITED KINGDOM DEVOLVED ADMINISTRATIONS

Most health and social care responsibilities are devolved matters under the Devolution Acts for Scotland, Wales and Northern Ireland. While the organisation of these functions in each of the four countries differs quite markedly, fundamental values are unaltered.

A common purpose of remaining true to its original ideals while modernising and becoming more health-focused, developing primary care and ensuring that evidence transfers more rapidly into practice are key features of the NHS in all parts of the United Kingdom. The interpretation of modernisation may be different, as it is, for example, between the Scottish Intercollegiate Guidelines Network (SIGN) in Scotland and the National Institute for Health and Clinical Excellence (NICE) in England and Wales, but these are variations on a theme, not a different tune.

Devolution means that there are four centres of political decision-making in the United Kingdom. The implications of devolution for the NHS and health care are still emerging. However, even where different policy priorities may pose a challenge, they also provide an opportunity to learn and to broaden the evidence base and experience of what works.

Devolution, at its simplest, means the delegation, from Westminster to either Scotland or Northern Ireland, of powers to pass primary legislation in devolved subject areas. The Scottish Parliament and the Northern Ireland Assembly can make primary legislation on any matters not reserved for the United Kingdom Parliament. The Government of Wales Act 2006 enables the National Assembly for Wales to ask the United Kingdom Parliament for legislative competence, and responses are made. In practice, most health and social care matters now rest with Welsh ministers.

Certain population protection functions

that are more effectively and beneficially conducted on a UK-wide basis are not devolved and remain powers reserved to Westminster. In health, these broadly include functions controlling and regulating medicines, medical devices, the registered health professions, abortion, human genetics, surrogacy, xenotransplantation and the regulation of prices charged for medicinal products and medical supplies.

PRESSURES ON HEALTH SERVICES

Modern health services face increasing calls on their limited resources. In industrialised nations of the world, the sources of this growth in demand include demographic change (particularly the ageing of populations), advances in medical science and technology, greater patient expectation of what health care can do for them and innovations in service delivery (Figure 4.4).

For any individual health care organisation, such as a hospital, the consequences of rapid growth in demand are enormous. It results in pressure to balance three conflicting imperatives: managing within a financial budget, meeting the needs of patients who present as emergencies and maintaining high standards of care for all patients – in particular, keeping response times short (Figure 4.5).

If the three are not met, one element of the triad will be sacrificed (in Figure 4.5, one side of the triangle will burst open). For example, a massive surge of emergency admissions during the winter months as large numbers of people are admitted with severe respiratory illnesses can mean planned admissions being cancelled. Meeting the needs of emergency admissions and continuing to keep waiting times short for patients requiring planned surgery means ensuring that the budget will not be over-spent through loss of financial discipline.

Table 4.1 Key elements of the public health function

● Health surveillance, monitoring and analysis
● Investigation of disease outbreaks, epidemics and risks to health
● Establishing, designing and managing health promotion and disease prevention programmes
● Enabling and empowering communities and citizens to promote health and reduce inequalities
● Creating and sustaining cross-governmental and intersectoral partnerships to improve health and reduce inequalities
● Ensuring compliance with regulations and laws to protect and promote health
● Developing and maintaining a well-educated and trained multidisciplinary public health workforce
● Ensuring the effective performance of NHS services to meet goals in improving health, preventing disease and reducing inequalities
● Research, development, evaluation and innovation
● Quality-assuring the public health function

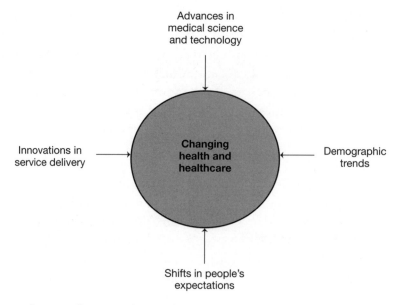

Figure 4.4 Key factors influencing change

These issues can be viewed positively as well as negatively. To some extent, the increased demand for health services is a reflection of success. Some diseases can be treated more effectively if diagnosed earlier, a new service innovation immediately generates its own demand (patients are able to be treated who could not be before) and patients expect more from the service.

KEY FUNCTIONAL PROCESSES OF HEALTH SERVICE DELIVERY

The overall purpose of health services in Britain is to improve the health of the population; to provide advice, assessment and treatment for patients; and to enhance the quality of life for those with special and long-term care needs (for example, the elderly, the mentally ill, the disabled and those with chronic diseases). There is also a responsibility to deliver services efficiently and,

where appropriate, to address problems of inequity (Figure 4.6).

The process begins with the formulation of strategic goals, aims and standards at national and local level and ends with a process through which health organisations in an area come together with local authority and other agencies to implement changes agreed in these strategies.

SETTING POLICY AND STRATEGY

The direction for the improvement of health and development of health care through the activities of the health service is set at a number of levels. National policy is formulated by ministers and the Department of Health, drawing widely on expert advice and information.

In the health service, the flow of new ideas, information, policy guidance, standards and new initiatives is constant, and one

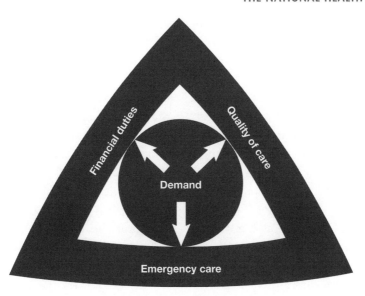

Figure 4.5 The bulging triangle: implications for a hospital of increasing demand

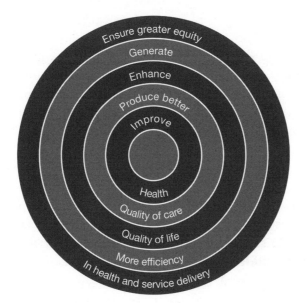

Figure 4.6 Functions of a health service

of the major challenges is to channel this stream into manageable courses to inform and stimulate health care development. It is important to be clear about priorities and not to overload local services with multiple targets and objectives.

The range of potential inputs to this planning process is very diverse and encompasses information arising from health needs assessment, learning and innovation, and policy and strategy, as well as wider influences such as the availability of resources and demographic and social change (Figure 4.7). There is a need to evaluate information, some of which is quite technical. It is important, for example, to draw in the research and development perspective to ensure that a proper evaluation is undertaken of new technologies and interventions that are claimed to be beneficial to patients or to the population. Policy and strategy set at national level are developed and extended through guidance to commissioners of services (*see* p. 218) and through formal planning mechanisms such as joint strategic needs assessments and local area agreements (*see* p. 219).

BUSINESS PLANNING

Business planning is a management process common to all organisations within the health service. It is often the process through which strategy is turned into action; it is the bridge between setting strategy and negotiating and forming service agreements. It is a continuous process rather than a discrete exercise.

The boards of strategic health authorities, primary care trusts, NHS trusts and NHS foundation trusts set vision, strategy, objectives and goals for the organisation. They identify likely available resources and assess the risks to successful delivery, identifying mitigating plans where necessary.

Contributions to the business planning process also come from the operational level of service. These involve identifying options for change in management and operational practices and in investment requirements. They also involve evaluating current service

levels, comparing the performance of other organisations ('benchmarking') and expressing the aspirations and requirements of the different functions within the organisation. In the case of hospitals, these will be the clinical services and the operational support services such as catering and portering, as well as the general management functions.

The National Health Service is no different from any commercial business environment, in that it is not possible to plan accurately for exactly what will happen in the year ahead. The business plan must therefore consider the implications of all likely situations that may arise during the course of the year. Financial planning is a key element of the business plan. The costs of action plans and programmes can usually be forecast with a reasonable degree of accuracy, but the organisation also needs to make provision for potential financial pressures that cannot be foreseen. This is called contingency planning.

The business plan document is a series of objectives and goals supported by specific programmes or action plans as the means to achieve them. The programmes and plans are prioritised and matched to likely available resources. Precise timescales are set for implementation. The plan will also identify the lead person in the organisation responsible for the implementation of each action.

Producing the business plan document is not the end of the business-planning process. The document provides the benchmark against which the organisation's performance is measured and evaluated, and this review must be continuous if the business-planning process is to be effective.

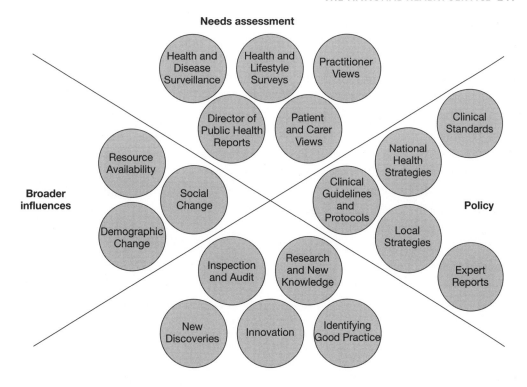

Figure 4.7 Inputs in the planning process

SERVICE AGREEMENTS AND CONTRACTS

The service agreement, or NHS contract, is the means through which a commissioner of NHS care (such as a primary care trust) secures a particular level and quality of services from NHS trusts that operate hospitals or that provide other services or health care. Service agreements may cover a longer period than annual contracts. They are not legally binding so cannot be challenged in a court of law should a dispute arise. Any disputes are settled by resolution under the secretary of state's authority. When the provider is not subject to direction by the secretary of state, however, as is the case

for foundation trusts or independent sector providers, contracts become legally binding and can be challenged in a court of law.

Patients who present to hospital as emergencies, either through referral by their general practitioner, by attending an accident and emergency department, after calling an ambulance or by telephoning NHS Direct, may require any element of the possible range of help that hospital-based specialist services are capable of providing. This may include specialist opinion, investigation, therapy with drugs or other measures, including operative intervention.

The majority of the non-emergency demand will arise from clinical workload generated by general practitioners referring patients following consultations. Thus, depending on the clinical specialty concerned, a relatively large proportion of the planned work of the hospital service will involve providing specialist assessment or an opinion (usually on an outpatient basis) to patients referred by a general practitioner. Such patients may require further investigation or treatment by hospital-based specialist services, but many will be referred back to their general practitioner with advice on further management of their problem.

In addition to baseline investigation, a group of patients will require more complex or advanced forms of investigation before their problem is defined. They may require further specialist intervention to resolve or alleviate their problem (provided either on an inpatient or outpatient basis), or they may again be referred back to the care of their general practitioner with advice only on treatment.

A further group of patients at any one time will have their problem defined as a need for intervention by specialist services, either in the form of an operation, another type of procedure or some kind of non-operative treatment. Some will have the condition or treatment monitored, and others will have further specialist interventions, either in response to changes in their health or at predetermined times as part of their overall clinical management plan.

It is not possible within this diversity of patients' clinical problems (and the consequent variation in care requirements and resource consumption) to accurately predict the numbers who will require particular programmes of care. Service agreements are therefore concerned with covering eventualities, and they can be framed to do so in a number of ways, ranging from a broad catch-all approach to a more specific basis for some groups of patients or some treatments. Service agreements are set following discussion and negotiation between the commissioner of services and the hospital or other provider and should be seen as part of continuing contact between the two.

COMMISSIONING

The Department of Health is no longer prescriptive in specifying the format for service planning and commissioning, preferring to delegate authority to local organisations – primary care trusts, trusts and other providers – to operate flexibly according to local needs and circumstances. Each year the NHS chief executive issues an operating framework, a short document that sets out guidance on priorities and 'deliverables' for the NHS in the year ahead. The guidance that outlines this process sets out the broad approach and specifies a small number of fixed requirements.

The commissioning function has become a key component of the way in which the reformed NHS operates at the end of the first decade of the twenty-first century. The term is mostly used quite loosely to describe the way in which the local budgets of the NHS are used not only to purchase services for patients but also to plan, shape and develop existing services and acquire new ones. A formal definition is set out in Box 4.1.

There are five main organisational entities that commission care:

1 primary care trusts
2 practice-based commissioners (many organised as a consortium of general practices) with delegated responsibility from the primary care trusts
3 specialised commissioning groups that commission specialist services on behalf of a number of primary care trusts that have pooled their budgets (on a regional or sub-regional basis)
4 National Commissioning Group for highly specialised services
5 local authorities.

Inevitably, the pressure on the commissioning process is to settle contracts for services with the major local and regional providers of care. Increasingly, though, the expectations of commissioners and the commissioning process have become much higher. The shaping and development of services is a much more difficult task, and this has led to the concept of world-class commissioning that aims to be strategic, long-term, outcome driven, evidence-based, partnership focused, clinically led and highly professional.

Another key element of commissioning is ensuring that patients have as much choice as possible. Policy evolved during the early 2000s to a point at the end of the first decade of the twenty-first century where patients being referred by their general practitioner for hospital or diagnostic services are entitled to a wide range of choice of provider (linked in some cases to maximum waiting times).

Commissioners in each locality are required to carry out a joint strategic needs assessment. In this way, primary care trusts, practice-based commissioners and local authorities come together to decide what needs to be done for their local populations. This joint assessment is a statutory requirement to support medium- and long-term planning.

LOCAL STRATEGIC PARTNERSHIPS AND LOCAL AREA AGREEMENTS

In 2000 the government published a neighbourhood renewal strategy, which placed local partnership working as a key element in leading local regeneration initiatives. Local strategic partnerships are non-statutory partnerships that bring together different public sector agencies as well as voluntary organisations, businesses, community organisations and local people. They are aligned with local authority boundaries. They operate at a level that allows strategy to be formulated but keep close to neighbourhoods and local communities so that action programmes are sensitive to their needs.

BOX 4.1 DEFINITION OF COMMISSIONING

'Commissioning is the process of specifying, securing and monitoring services to meet people's needs at a strategic level. This applies to all services, whether they are provided by the local authority, NHS or other public agencies or by the private and voluntary sectors.'

— *Source:* Audit Commission.

Local strategic partnerships essentially are charged with developing and implementing neighbourhood renewal strategies to deliver higher levels of employment, better education, lower levels of crime, improved health and better housing. In the 86 most deprived local authority areas, they have additional resources in the form of the Neighbourhood Renewal Fund. In these areas, their core purpose is tackling serious deprivation and addressing intractable and long-standing problems in disadvantaged communities.

Local strategic partnerships operate through local area agreements, binding partners to a programme to improve services, narrow gaps between deprived communities and the rest and achieve sustainable development. Through their participation in local strategic partnerships and involvement in local area agreements, primary care trusts ensure that health is an important consideration in this approach.

EVALUATION AND MONITORING

The process of evaluation and monitoring of health services is a continuous one. The basis for it is agreed before implementing service level agreements or health programmes. The lessons learned from the evaluation process can be used to inform the next year's commissioning decisions about service development and investment of resources.

QUALITY OF HEALTH CARE

In a modern, consumer-orientated society, one of the cornerstones of the process of supplying goods and services is an emphasis on quality. In turn, one of the principal stimuli in a market economy for improving quality and raising standards is competition amongst suppliers and providers to produce a better product or service as economically as possible and to produce one that meets the expressed needs or wishes of the purchaser. The question of quality and its improvement within a publicly funded health care system cannot be viewed quite in this way.

In the early years of the NHS, there was no formal and comprehensive approach to quality assurance and improvement. Much faith was placed in the belief that if standards of professional training and practice were high then they would ensure that the practitioner delivering the service would do so at a uniformly high quality. Over time, it has become recognised that the complexity of defining and measuring quality in the health care field is much greater than in many other sectors (industry, for example). This has been an impediment to developing a formal quality framework in health service provision.

During the 1980s and 1990s, certain local NHS services experienced serious failures in the standards of care they provided. These events quickly went beyond purely local media interest to become national news, often for weeks or months at a time. These incidents ranged from the high levels of postoperative mortality amongst children treated by the heart surgery service at the Bristol Royal Infirmary to problems with the conduct or performance of individual doctors at other services in the country.

Although almost certainly uncommon

in relation to the high standard of care provided by the NHS generally over this period of time, these service failures caused a great deal of public concern. They provided the opportunity for sustained negative media coverage of the NHS, damaging its caring image. They caused people to wonder whether such problems could be present in their own local hospital. The failures began to have a ring of familiarity, giving the impression, however unfairly, that the NHS could not stop history from repeating itself.

Two much more sinister cases also occurred during this period. Beverley Allitt, a hospital nurse in Grantham, Lincolnshire, was convicted of murdering some of her patients, while Harold Shipman, a general practitioner in Hyde, Greater Manchester, was found to have murdered elderly patients in his practice by deliberately overdosing them with opiates. There was a general acceptance that individuals with such criminal intent are encountered very rarely indeed in the health professions. Nevertheless, these depressing cases added to the perception of an NHS in the last two decades of the twentieth century that was beset by 'medical scandals' and an inability to recognise and act quickly on suspicion of serious criminal behaviour.

While the precise circumstances of these service failures differed, some common features began to emerge. Firstly, although problems in the services concerned often came to light through a serious incident or complaint, subsequent investigation would show that concerns had existed over a much longer period of time but had not been acted upon. Secondly, the culture of the hospitals in which serious problems occurred was often dysfunctional, with cliques and factions creating divisions between different groups of staff and between management and clinical staff. Thirdly, when confronted with serious problems in a service, managers and senior clinicians were sometimes unsure what to do about them or how to resolve the difficulties.

By the late 1990s the climate had changed. There was a widespread acceptance that quality and its improvement should be a central component of all health services and that major attention should be given to protecting patients against poor standards of care, whether arising from dysfunctional services or poor practitioner performance. There was a much greater willingness on the part of the NHS and major health professional bodies to accept that the traditional culture of the NHS needed to change. It was acknowledged that the NHS did not have good systems for the early detection of lapses in standards of care, and it did not have effective and well-understood mechanisms for intervening to resolve such problems. It had not always been clear in the past that the protection of patients should always be a priority over other considerations such as loyalty towards colleagues.

The Report of the Public Inquiry into Children's Heart Surgery at the Bristol Royal Infirmary (the Kennedy Inquiry) undertook a searching analysis of these issues and identified the need for a new patient-centred culture in medicine and in the NHS (Table 4.2).

The NHS Next Stage Review (*see* p. 202) set out an agenda for making quality and quality improvement a core objective for the NHS from 2009 onwards.

This section of the chapter describes some of the key themes underlying the approach to quality in health care and gives an account of the main mechanisms through which quality of care can be influenced.

CONCEPTS AND DEFINITIONS OF QUALITY

There are a large number of formal definitions of quality in health care. One of the most widely used is shown in Box 4.2.

The development of conceptual frameworks to define quality of health care has spawned a major literature on the subject in biomedical and health services journals, particularly since the 1970s.

Structure, Process, Outcome

One of the most important and widely respected classifications of quality in health care is that originally propounded by the North American Avedis Donabedian,[3] in which there are three aspects.

Structure

One aspect of assessing the quality of health care is examining the amount and nature of facilities and staff available. Examples of such structural measures would be hospital beds per thousand population and the number of senior doctors per thousand population. The structural aspects of quality in health care are often used in making comparisons between health services in different parts of a country or in international comparisons. Thus variation may be found between services in the number of surgeons per head of population or in the number of ophthalmology outpatient clinics available to different populations.

Such differences in the structural aspects of health care quality can be useful in initiating discussions about the adequacy of health care facilities available to different populations. They can also be valuable in stimulating change or improvement where, for example, levels of staff or facilities are very low compared to those that are agreed as being required to operate an effective service.

The main problem with relying on structural measures to assess how 'good' or 'bad' a health service is, is the fact that there is seldom adequate evidence to demonstrate what levels of facilities or staff are required to produce good results for particular types of patient care. It by no means follows, for example, that one service with a higher number of surgeons per head of population than a neighbouring service will yield better results for hernia repair operations (low in-hospital complication rates and low long-term recurrence rates).

Thus, while structural measures are still an important aspect of assessing the quality of health care, they are of limited value when taken alone and are best regarded as only one part of an overall concept that also embraces process and outcome measures.

Process

A second attribute of quality is concerned with what is done for and to a patient or group of patients and how well it is done. Assessment of the quality of care based on the process approach can be wide-ranging.

Table 4.2 Key findings of the Kennedy Inquiry into children's heart surgery services in Bristol

• Poor organisation
• Failure of communication
• Lack of leadership
• Paternalism and a 'club' culture
• A failure to put patients at the centre of care

Source: Kennedy I. *Learning from Bristol: the report of the public inquiry into children's heart surgery at the Bristol Royal Infirmary 1984–1995.* London: The Stationery Office; 2001 (Cm 5207).

BOX 4.2 A WIDELY USED DEFINITION OF HEALTH CARE QUALITY

'Quality of care is the degree to which health services for individuals and populations increase the likelihood of desired health outcomes and are consistent with current professional knowledge.'

— *Source:* Lohr KN, editor. *Medicare: a strategy for quality assurance.* Washington, DC: National Academy Press; 1990.

For example, the evaluation of a programme for control of high blood pressure (hypertension) might involve establishing how adequately the population at risk of developing hypertension had been identified; how thoroughly diagnostic criteria had been determined; how valid and accurate were the blood pressure readings that were taken; how other associated medical conditions were detected and managed; whether agreed treatment protocols were being followed; whether patients were complying with treatment regimes; what proportion of patients who had been diagnosed as hypertensive had their blood pressure stabilised at agreed levels; how often patients were followed up; and how adequate were their subsequent clinical assessments.

All of these are examples of processes of care that can be used as a basis for assessing aspects of the quality of clinical services given to hypertensive patients. In practice,

assessing quality in this way requires establishing agreed standards of good practice in the process of care concerned against which the actual service can be compared and hence assessed.

While the process approach adds much greater depth to the assessment of quality than does the structural approach, it cannot be viewed in isolation from it nor from the third attribute, outcome measurement. Indeed, there is no point in assessing the extent to which a process of care is in place unless the process is one that has a proven effect on an outcome of care.

Outcome

The final attribute of quality in the Donabedian triad is the outcome of the health care episode for the patient. Does he or she get better? Are there any clinical complications? Is he or she satisfied with the care delivered? Does he or she survive the illness or disease occurrence? Outcome is the final arbiter of the quality of care provided. There are numerous possible approaches to defining outcomes of health care or of a health service's activity.

One approach that is often quoted and easily remembered is based on the five D's: death, disease, disability, discomfort and dissatisfaction. Thus, for example, assessment of the outcome of care for a man admitted to hospital as an emergency for treatment of a ruptured aortic aneurysm might take account of whether he survived (death); whether the aneurysm was technically well-corrected surgically (disease): whether he returned to 'normal' physical, psychological and social functioning after discharge from hospital (disability); whether he remained free of residual pain (discomfort); and whether the interpersonal as well as the technical aspects of the nursing and medical care and the environment in which it was provided were pleasing to him (dissatisfaction).

This and similar classifications of outcomes are probably best used for illustrative purposes, because most are either too simplistic or too detailed to be operationally applicable. A great deal of work has been undertaken to define appropriate outcomes for use in clinical trials or service evaluations of particular health problems or therapies.

An important issue in considering outcome as an aspect of health care quality is to remember that there is a population and a patient care dimension. A conceptualisation of health care quality in the mid-1980s by Maxwell captures this wider scope and incorporates the population

dimension (Table 4.3). Like the Donabedian formulation, its principal use has been in shaping debate and improving strategies rather than in routine management and evaluation of services.

The practical application of outcome assessment to day-to-day health service management, whether at the population or at individual patient care level, is still in its infancy. This is partly because of the virtual absence of routinely available data through which outcome can be assessed. This situation is rapidly changing as greater emphasis is being placed on the importance of the outcome dimension in assessing the quality of care and on finding ways of using more widely the specific outcome measures that have been developed.

The Donabedian classification has been dealt with at length because it remains the most enduring and widely respected conceptual approach through which the quality of health care can be defined and assessed. It is important, however, to remember that these concepts are closely interrelated as well as dynamic. Determining the way in which health facilities (structural) are used (processes) to produce the end result of care for the patient (outcome) is the real route to improving the quality of care.

Technical, Interpersonal, Amenities

Donabedian has also pointed out that health care has different attributes upon which judgements about quality can be made. The health professional's definition of high-quality care would probably rely heavily on technical considerations (for example, how well the therapeutic or investigational aspects of the care were delivered). On the other hand, many patients would place a high or low value on the care they receive based on the interpersonal or amenity attributes of their care (for example, kindness, dignity, respect, explanation, information-giving and standards of lighting, heating, food, toilet and washing facilities).

All are important quality considerations, and it cannot be assumed that high quality in one attribute automatically means high quality in the others. For example, a surgeon may be excellent in the domains of communication and empathy with his patients but obtain less satisfactory surgical results than a colleague who is a masterly technical surgeon but treats his patients in an impersonal manner.

Effectiveness, Overuse, Underuse, Misuse

Another way in which quality can be viewed is the extent to which the health care interventions of known effectiveness are properly applied in the case of individual patients. The main concepts involved here are efficacy, appropriateness and effectiveness (Table 4.4).

It is important to distinguish efficacy from effectiveness, because the two terms are often confused or misused. Efficacy is whether the intervention (e.g., the drug or operation) delivers a particular outcome (e.g., restoration of lost function, relief of pain, five-year survival) under ideal conditions. For example, what was the efficacy of the intervention when it was first subjected to research evaluation in a randomised controlled trial? Effectiveness, on the other hand, assesses how well the intervention yields the desired outcome under everyday circumstances – such as a busy hospital service.

Appropriateness is whether the intervention that has been applied to a particular clinical situation is the right one. It brings in three important dimensions of quality: overuse, underuse and misuse. Extensive study around the world has shown that health care systems regularly have patients not receiving a treatment when they would have benefited from it, while others are receiving treatments when they will not derive improved outcome from them.

The misuse of diagnostic or treatment technologies that increase risks to patients highlights the concept of patient safety, which is discussed more fully later in the chapter. One of the main strategies for reducing inappropriate care is the creation

Table 4.3 Maxwell's dimensions of quality

- Access to services
- Relevance to need (for the whole community)
- Effectiveness (for individual patient)
- Equity (fairness)
- Social acceptability
- Efficiency and economy

Source: Maxwell RJ. Quality assessment in health. *BMJ.* 1984; **288**: 1471-2.

Table 4.4 Aspects of quality of a clinical intervention

Aspect	Meaning	In other words
Efficacy	The ability of an intervention to produce the desired outcome under ideal conditions (i.e., in the environment of a clinical trial)	What is the right thing to do?
Appropriateness	The application of the most effective intervention from the range of alternatives available to the particular patient's circumstances	Is the right thing being done to the right people at the right time?
Effectiveness	The performance of an intervention in producing the desired outcome in an ordinary service setting	Is the right thing being done right?

of clinical standards and guidelines that promote adherence to good practice based on the best research evidence.

The Philosophy of Continuous Quality Improvement

The experience of the commercial sector, both industrial and service, can inform strategies for quality improvement and quality management in health care. This wider quality debate is most clearly apparent in the recent history of the North American and Japanese manufacturing industries. It is not so long since the Japanese were renowned for producing cheap, poor-quality merchandise, and American industry predominated in such areas as camera production, stereo and hi-fi equipment manufacture. Today, the Japanese have gained a major share of the North American and, indeed, world markets in consumer goods. They now produce and export merchandise that competes with alternatives on quality – not simply on price.

The reason for this dramatic turnaround in the competitiveness and market position of Japanese industry is widely recognised as being grounded in the adoption of relatively simple theories of quality improvement. Ironically, the theorists who have been credited with stimulating this process in Japan are American – particularly W Edwards Deming[4] and Joseph M Juran.[5]

In the industrial field and in the service industries, this approach is based on the philosophy that by continually improving the processes of production (or the delivery of service), expensive consequences such as scrapping defective products, expenditure on warranty agreements and remanufacturing will be avoided. By concentrating on quality, productivity will improve. It is called total quality management (TQM) or continuous quality improvement (CQI).

The traditional approach to quality control in industry was initially based upon the concept of inspection to detect defects. This has a number of disadvantages.

Firstly, and most importantly, it does not gain commitment of the whole workforce to improving quality. Instead the issue is seen as the concern of a separate quality department or inspector. This instils in the workforce a feeling that they are not being trusted and, even worse, creates the situation in which they will only achieve a high standard of work when being watched or inspected. Secondly, when the process of manufacture is not properly designed and the raw material is inadequate, no amount of inspection will remedy the problem. This approach inspects out poor quality rather than building in good quality to the systems of management and production.

The CQI approach seeks to reduce the importance of inspection as a quality tool and instead to involve the whole workforce using fully their knowledge and expertise of the process of manufacture to constantly improve it so that the defects, errors and poor products are eliminated. The overall benefit for a company that is engaged effectively in CQI is success of its business. Reduction in errors and defects not only increases quality, it reduces costs (from remanufacture, replacement goods and inspection), improves profit ability and, by satisfying customers, attracts more of the market share.

While a key element of CQI is reducing unnecessary variation in the production process, another is the emphasis on the customer and his or her wishes and expectations. This customer ethos extends not just to the external customer but also to internal customers within the organisation. Indeed, in CQI terms, the very definition of quality of the product or service relies heavily on the customer's views of what constitutes good or bad quality.

The potential applications of CQI to the health care field are not yet fully apparent, so large numbers of practical examples cannot be cited. However, perhaps one example illustrates the potential benefits of quality improvement to a health service. A complication of hospital care, particularly in the elderly, is pressure (or 'bed') sores. In this example, good-quality care is a hospital inpatient stay for an elderly person in which he or she was free of pressure sores. An approach in which all nurses on the ward discussed, planned and reviewed the process of nursing care so that pressure sores were eliminated would have advantages over an approach in which a matronly figure inspected patients for evidence of pressure sores and then blamed individual nurses for failing in their duty if some were found. The former, TQM-based approach would reduce or eliminate pressure sores (improve quality of care), reduce costs (length of stay reduced, no need for skin grafts or other treatment), increase productivity (by enabling other patients to be admitted and treated) and improve market share (primary care trusts would be more likely to commission services from a hospital with a reputation for a low incidence of pressure sores).

Thus there are parallels between CQI in the business sector and in health care. In this example, the health service's aim of eliminating pressure sores could be seen as analogous to a Japanese electronics company in which concentration on improving the processes of production of television sets led to products in line with customer requirements (improved quality);

reduced costs (fewer defects resulting in rework, scrapping or payment of warranty agreements), increased productivity (less workforce time devoted to remanufacture or correcting defects) and increased market share (more satisfied customers).

The introduction of CQI is not simply a matter of exposing and adopting the techniques; it requires major organisation-wide change of the culture and orientation. It places responsibilities on senior management to create the kind of participative environment in which all members of the organisation are valued and their skills and efforts are rewarded. This is an environment which recognises that employees generally want to do their best and should be comprehensively and actively involved in the process of quality improvement.

One of the organisational approaches borrowed from private-sector experience, business-school teaching and the many management gurus who have written inspirational texts is that of restructuring. The concept of making an organisation 'fit for purpose' (including delivering quality strategies) has led to 're-engineering', 'downsizing', 'right-sizing' and a variety of other methods of reshaping organisations.

While these restructurings have often been adopted enthusiastically by the senior management of health care organisations, they have also been less popular with staff. Many health professionals are organised in fairly traditional hierarchies, and practitioners enjoy considerable autonomy in the delivery of their role. Sudden and dramatic reorganisations threaten job security and require entirely new models of working. They are sometimes less successful in developing health care organisation than more subtle and low key ways in which health care professionals are drawn into the management process.

Many different approaches have been advocated to create a quality organisation. They have important common features that have been shown to be successful (Table 4.5), including that the organisation should be well-led, have good systems in place, listen to and be supportive to staff and create a positive culture for quality improvement.

QUALITY ASSURANCE AND IMPROVEMENT: PROGRAMMES AND PRACTICE

Any health care system must have in place robust mechanisms for assuring the quality and safety of services provided to the patients it serves and also a way of ensuring that opportunities for quality improvement are recognised and acted upon.

As a result of changes introduced into the NHS in the late 1990s, a comprehensive framework for health care quality is in place. It consists of clear national standards; a programme of implementing quality assurance, patient safety and quality improvement in every local hospital and primary care service (this is called 'clinical governance'); and a set of mechanisms for inspecting and auditing performance to ensure that standards are being met and that quality assurance and improvement is indeed taking place at local service level.

Programmes have also been developed to ensure that patients are protected from harm during the process of care. This has led to the introduction of policies to ensure

Table 4.5 Quality management: an organisational philosophy

Leadership from the top
Empowerment of staff
Teamwork
Prevention (rather than correction) of adverse outcomes
Analysing, simplifying and improving processes
Strong customer focus

that poor practitioner performance is recognised early and acted upon and that the wider causes of risks to patients are identified and reduced.

From 2008 onwards, the goal of the *NHS Next Stage Review* that quality should be the 'organising principle' of the NHS, led to a renewed emphasis on quality of care. Technical measures (e.g., quality accounts, quality indicators and clinical dashboards) were developed to support this core purpose.

Setting Standards Based on Evidence

Every day, throughout each health service in the world, hundreds of thousands of decisions are taken by doctors, nurses and other health professionals during the diagnosis and treatment of illness. No systematic approach to improving quality of health care can afford to overlook the importance of clinical decision-making.

For many years, it has been recognised that there is wide variation in such decision-making. Between different health services internationally, thresholds for surgical intervention in patients with broadly similar clinical problems have been observed to vary greatly. Such variation can also occur between different parts of the same country and even different members of the same clinical team. In the example shown in Table 4.6, the Caesarean section rate varies greatly.

It has also long been acknowledged that the science and the practice of medicine do not go hand in hand in the way that they should. The failure to translate the results of research into practice quickly and effectively has meant that too few patients benefit in the way that they should from medical advances. It is also one of the reasons why there is wide variation in medical practice in many fields of care. This point can be reinforced by an example from obstetrics.

In the early 1970s, research carried out in New Zealand[6] focused on the babies of women who went into premature labour. Such babies are prone to respiratory problems partly caused by immature lungs. Treatment after delivery with agents called surfactants helps their lung function, but they will often also need a period of intensive care. Some will not survive, some will spend a long time in intensive care and some will have permanent disability. The New Zealand study showed that if selected women in premature labour were given an injection of corticosteroid before delivery,

Table 4.6 Caesarean section rates (per 100 live births) in selected countries

Country	Rate per 100 live births
Mexico	37.9
Italy	37.5
Korea	35.2
United States of America	29.1
Austria	23.6
United Kingdom	22.4
Iceland	16.4
Netherlands	13.6
OECD average (26 countries)	23.6

Source: Organisation for Economic Cooperation and Development (OECD), 2007; data relate to 2004.

these problems were significantly reduced. The benefits of this therapy were clear. It could save lives, reduce disability and produce major savings in the use of intensive care resources and drugs (corticosteroids are very cheap compared to surfactants).

The study appeared in a major medical journal at the time, and later studies confirmed the finding. The issue would have been widely read and talked about by obstetricians and in professional circles. It did not, however, impact in a major way on practice. The pattern of corticosteroid usage in premature labour 10 years later in one part of Britain is shown in Figure 4.8, and it is likely to have been similar in most parts of the country. The practice had only been adopted in a minority of eligible cases. The level of usage was higher in the regional teaching centre but even there was greatly suboptimal. Improvements in the region studied then took place. Since then substantial national improvements have taken place.[7]

Evidence-based Health Care

The example above and many other examples that could be chosen from other fields of medicine led health services during the 1990s to look critically at how clinical practice could be made more effective. Particularly influential was work from McMaster University in Ontario, Canada, which formulated the concept of 'evidence-based medicine'. It rapidly became an international movement. The original proponents of evidence-based medicine saw it as a paradigm shift in medical practice rather than merely a change in emphasis. Clinical decisions in the past relied upon intuition, impression and experience. The evidence-based medicine movement saw a future in which many more clinical decisions were based on the findings of valid research relevant to the particular patient's condition (Table 4.7). It was felt that evidence should be summarised from all published and unpublished research in whatever language and should be regularly updated.

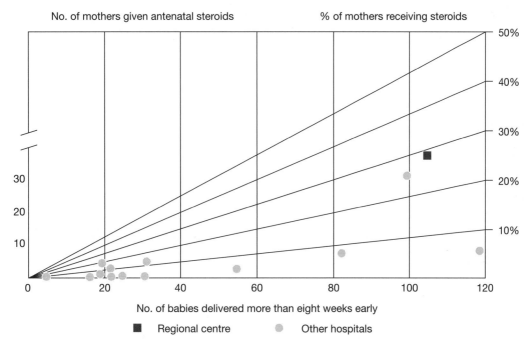

Figure 4.8 Use of steroids to prevent deaths and complications in premature babies: variations amongst maternity units

Evidence-based practice has not been free of controversy. Generally, health policy-makers and managers have welcomed it enthusiastically as a route to improving quality and reducing clinical variation. Within the health professions it has been embraced – but not in all quarters. Some have seen it as implying the end of clinical judgement based upon experience and the dawn of a mechanistic approach to patients. This is not the aim of evidence-based practice. There is an important place for traditional skills (the art of medicine) but clinical judgements should have a strong scientific basis as well as an experiential one.

The introduction of an evidence basis to professional practice, and to health care more generally, is a complex task involving a number of important steps (Figure 4.9).

There is a need to ensure that where there is a lack of research evidence in relation to a particular disease problem and its diagnosis and clinical management, research is commissioned to fill in the gaps.

Using the results of research studies to aid a clinical decision is not straightforward either. For example, a women patient aged 65 years who has suffered a number of transient cerebral ischaemic attacks may or may not benefit from an invasive carotid endarterectomy. How many studies are necessary before the correct use of the intervention is proven? How good are the studies on which current evidence is based? Does the evidence apply to all patients with transient ischaemic attacks or were the original studies limited to selected groups of patients? These are just some of the questions that are raised

Table 4.7 Evidence-based medicine

A process of life-long, self-directed learning in which caring for one's own patients creates the need for clinically important information about diagnosis, prognosis, therapy, and other clinical and health care issues, and in which clinicians:

- Convert these information needs into answerable questions.

- Track down, with maximum efficiency, the best evidence with which to answer them (whether from clinical examination, the diagnostic laboratory, the published literature, or other sources).

- Critically appraise that evidence for its validity (closeness to the truth) and usefulness (clinical applicability).

- Apply the results of this appraisal in their clinical practice.

- Evaluate their own performance.

Source: Sackett DL, Straus SE, Richardson WS, *et al. Evidence-Based Medicine: how to practise and teach EBM.* 2nd ed. Edinburgh: Harcourt Brace; 2000.

when the use of information from published research studies is considered. The importance of evaluating the quality of the research evidence is now appreciated. Thus, for example, one clinical trial on the use of therapy may not be enough if it was not big enough to yield a benefit in the treatment compared to the control group (if such a benefit was present). Five clinical trials may not be enough to constitute good evidence if they were all flawed in their methodological design.

Different levels of evidence may be available, depending on the state of research in the particular field, and it is important to be clear what quality of evidence is being relied upon to formulate a clinical policy (Table 4.8). Part of the task of developing evidence-based practice involves ensuring that health professionals are trained in the evaluation of research evidence. Techniques and training programmes have been devised to enable health professionals to acquire so-called critical appraisal skills.

It has also been recognised that clinical staff cannot be expected to undertake this evaluation themselves from scratch prior to taking clinical decisions across a busy service. Increasingly, databases and information systems have been developed to provide topic-based summaries of research evidence that can be made available to health professionals. One of the best established is the Cochrane Collaboration, which was started in Oxford, England and is now an international network. The Cochrane Collaboration prepares, maintains and disseminates systematic reviews of research (usually randomised controlled trials). This process yields summaries of the effectiveness of treatments and other interventions in particular fields of care. In this way clinicians can obtain information.

A systematic review is a type of secondary research that takes the findings of the original (primary) research and carefully assesses them using a strict set of criteria. Often this will mean pooling data

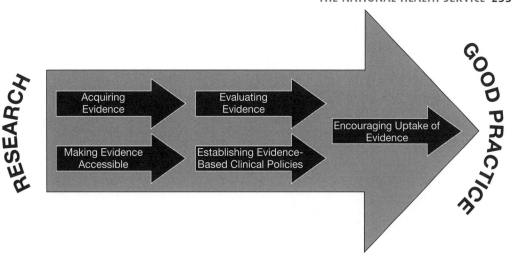

Figure 4.9 Evidence-based practice: key steps and activities

Table 4.8 Categories of evidence

Ia	–	Evidence from meta-analysis of randomised controlled trials
Ib	–	Evidence from at least one randomised controlled trial
IIa	–	Evidence from at least one controlled study without randomisation
IIb	–	Evidence from at least one other type of quasi-experimental study
III	–	Evidence from descriptive studies, such as comparative studies, correlation studies and case-control studies
IV	–	Evidence from expert committee reports or opinions or clinical experience of respected authorities, or both

Source: Eccles M, Freemantle N, Mason J. North of England evidence-based guidelines development project: methods of developing guidelines for efficient drug use in primary care. *BMJ.* 1998; **316**: 1232–5.

from the original studies and reanalysing them, a technique called meta-analysis. It is important to recognise that this form of secondary research is itself open to bias if the methods are wrongly applied or if it is undertaken superficially. Just as there can be bad randomised controlled trials, there can also be bad systematic reviews and bad meta-analyses.

Systems such as the Cochrane Collaboration, which is well established, rigorous in its methods and well respected scientifically, are very important in the development of evidence-based practice.

Aside from specialist evidence databases, there are many initiatives that circulate in short easy-to-assimilate form – summaries and advice given in a way that is of help to clinical decision-makers. They take the form of specialist journals dealing with evidence-based health care, clinical effectiveness bulletins and newsletters.

Making this clinical information available, particularly in specialist databases like the Cochrane Collaboration and also in good summaries on effective care, has been made much easier by the Internet. Nevertheless, individual practitioners must have the ability to gain access to these electronic media easily. Hospitals and other health care organisations have an important role in providing knowledge and evidence by ensuring that there is a proper infrastructure of information technology.

National Institute for Health and Clinical Excellence

One of the main ways in which new clinical policies are formulated is through clinical practice guidelines. Many clinical practice guidelines setting out the best way to manage a particular health problem are written by national or international bodies, drawing on the best evidence and expert opinion. Increasingly in England, statements about what represents good practice in particular fields are made by the National Institute for Health and Clinical Excellence (NICE).

The role of NICE is to provide guidance to the NHS, based upon clinical and cost-effectiveness. NICE guidance is used by NHS clinicians, those commissioning NHS services (including primary care trusts) and patients and their carers (Table 4.9).

NICE produces four main types of guidance – technology appraisals, interventional procedures, clinical guidelines and public health guidance. NICE technology appraisals and interventional procedures look at the clinical and cost-effectiveness of a new or existing treatment, either a drug, a device or a discrete procedure such as a surgical operation. The process of producing an appraisal has typically taken around a year, but a new fast-track appraisal system is now in place for particularly urgent critical issues, such as potentially life-saving cancer drugs, where there is often major public concern about apparently unnecessary delays. Appraisal involves the gathering and assessment of evidence, consultation with stakeholders, publication of a draft version of the appraisal on the NICE website and a chance for consultees to appeal against the final appraisal.

NICE clinical guidelines take longer to produce – usually at least 18 months – since they cover all aspects of the management of a condition, from self-care through to care by primary care, hospital and specialist services.

Some of the NICE appraisals cover drugs for the treatment of particular conditions. In some instances this will involve guidance on whether a new (and perhaps expensive) drug should be used in, and funded by, the NHS. Other NICE appraisals cover medical devices, diagnostics, surgical procedures and health promotion.

It cannot be assumed that merely disseminating guidelines will result in uniformly effective practice. Changing professional behaviour to conform with evidence of best practice is a complex process.

Research into the factors that influence change in professional behaviour has shown that no single measure will be effective; it is multifaceted strategies that are important. The factors that have been shown to contribute to such change are shown in Table 4.10.

Table 4.9 Appraisals and guidance issued by the National Institute for Health and Clinical Excellence (NICE): some examples

Guidance	Type
Coronary artery disease: drug-eluting stents	Technology appraisal
Induction of labour	Clinical guidelines
Laparoscopic gastrectomy for cancer	Interventional procedures
Promoting physical activity in the workplace	Public health intervention guidelines

National Service Frameworks

National service frameworks are national service plans that aim to improve service quality and reduce variation in outcome of care by setting out clear standards for particular services or care groups.

National service frameworks set national standards and define service models for a service or care group, putting in place strategies to support implementation and establishing performance measures against which progress can be measured within an agreed timescale. A programme of production of national service frameworks was launched in the late 1990s and covers mental health, coronary heart disease, older people, diabetes mellitus, renal services, services for children and young people and services for people with long-term medical conditions.

Delivering Better Quality: Clinical Governance

In the 1980s and early 1990s, issues such as achieving financial balance and meeting workload targets had started to dominate the agendas of many health care organisations in the NHS. Today all NHS organisations have a statutory duty for quality placed on them through legislation. This is implemented through programmes of clinical governance.

The concept of clinical governance (Box 4.3) was formulated in the late 1990s to provide a unified approach to quality assurance and quality improvement at the level of the local NHS provider.[8,9]

The organisations that make up any health service will vary in their performance against quality criteria. A hypothetical quality curve is shown in Figure 4.10. Health care organisations at the left-hand tail of the curve will be those that have demonstrated failures in standards of care, whether detected through complaints, inspection, audit, untoward incidents or routine surveillance. The challenge here is to learn lessons that can be built into future service delivery. Similarly, looking at the innovative organisations at the right-hand tail of the distribution, good practice must be recognised, the scope for more general applicability must be identified and methods must be found to transfer it both locally and nationally.

This process of learning lessons – both from exemplar and problem services – was never tackled systematically before, and it was an important part of the clinical governance programmes introduced at the beginning of the twenty-first century. In

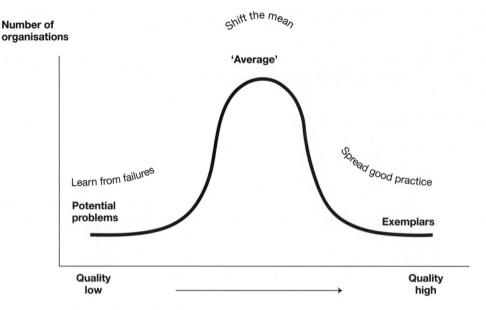

Figure 4.10 Variation in the quality of organisations
Source: Scally G, Donaldson LJ. Clinical governance and the drive for quality improvement in the new NHS in England. *BMJ.* 1998; **317**: 61–5.

Table 4.10 List of measures that may achieve professional behaviour change that have been subject to evaluation by trials

Intervention	No. of studies
Educational material	12
Conference	17
Outreach visit	8
Use of local opinion leader	5
Patient-mediated intervention	10
Audit and feedback	31
Reminder system	52
Marketing	3
Multifaceted intervention	15
Local consensus process	8

Source: Oxman AD, Thornson MA, Davis DA, *et al.* No magic bullets: a systematic review of 102 trials of interventions to improve professional practice. *Can Med Assoc J.* 1995; **153**: 1423–31.

BOX 4.3 DEFINITION OF CLINICAL GOVERNANCE

'Clinical governance is a framework through which NHS organisations are accountable for continuously improving the quality of their services and safeguarding high standards of care by creating an environment in which excellence in clinical care will flourish.'

— *Source:* Department of Health. *A First Class Service: quality in the new NHS.* London: DoH; 1998.

---

addition to addressing these tails of the quality curve, a major movement of any curve of this kind towards improved quality requires that health organisations in the middle range are engaged ('shifting the mean').

Most organisations lie relatively close to the 'mean', so the thrust of clinical governance is to improve quality in every organisation, not simply to concentrate on the best and the worst. The task is largely a developmental one – of organisations and staff. Clinical and management systems, quality-improvement mechanisms and the work of teams and individuals all need to be aligned to produce a new kind of health organisation.

When considering different hospitals and primary care services, the feature that distinguishes the best from the others most clearly is probably their culture. In an organisation where the culture is underpinned with an understanding of clinical governance, high standards tend to become a prevailing purpose rather than a desirable accessory. Patients measure a clinician's performance on what they understand and value. Clinicians communicate their attitude and culture in their daily behaviour when interacting with other members of their team and with patients and their families. An organisation that creates a working environment that is open, participative and team-based, where ideas and good practice are shared, where education and research are valued and where blame is used exceptionally is likely to be one in which clinical governance is prospering.

Clinical governance involves the integration of many aspects of quality (including those discussed in this chapter) that had previously been dealt with in a rather fragmented way (Figure 4.11). The introduction of the clinical governance framework seeks to modernise systems for quality control, incorporating established clinical standards, evidence-based practice and learning from the lessons of poor performance. Clinical governance includes all activity and information that allows an NHS organisation and those who work within it to assure and improve the quality of services locally. This will include work to identify and build on good practice, assess and minimise the risk of untoward events, develop a reporting and learning culture, investigate problems as they arise and ensure lessons are learned. Successful clinical governance relies on proper arrangements for accountability that are seen to be effective by the public.

These objectives can only be achieved if there is top-level commitment within the organisation. Clinical governance places accountable-officer status on the chief executive of the health care organisation, with regular reports to board meetings (of equal importance to monthly financial reports), and it places day-to-day responsibility in the hands of a senior clinician. It is for each organisation to work out these accountability arrangements in detail and ensure that they are communicated throughout the organisation.

Clinical governance activity involves individual teams spending time examining their services from the patient's perspective and seeking ways of improving them. This may involve examining data, looking at feedback from patient surveys, taking account of best practice or innovation elsewhere in the health service or other sectors, or pooling ideas and experience of how the service runs.

A traditional way in which the performance of a service is reviewed by a clinical team is through clinical audit. Clinical audit is the approach through which health professionals critically examine their own and one another's practice so that the lessons learned

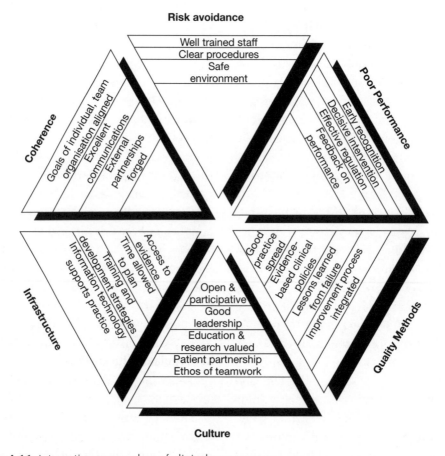

Figure 4.11 Integrating approaches of clinical governance
Source: Scally G, Donaldson LJ. Clinical governance and the drive for quality improvement in the new NHS in England. *BMJ*, 1998; **317**: 61–5.

from such a scrutiny can be used to make improvements in professional practice.

The process through which effective clinical audit is conducted is progress around the audit cycle (Figure 4.12). A key component of the cycle is the setting of standards based upon evidence comparing current practice against these standards. The setting of standards is something for all members of the clinical team to agree upon, but it should be undertaken using the best available medical evidence and knowledge drawn from reports by the National Institute of Health and Clinical Excellence, from specialist research databases (such as the Cochrane Collaboration) and from appraisal of the research undertaken by members of the clinical team themselves.

An equally important component of the audit cycle is the implementation of the agreed standard. There is only a loose and imperfect relationship between knowing what to do and the ability to act on that knowledge. Experience teaches that although clinicians understand the importance of standard-setting, they do not always do the things they know they should. The duty of quality imposed by clinical governance recognises the common failure to close the audit cycle loop and prompts a whole organisational responsibility for patient-centred, accountable care.

REGULATING AND INSPECTING FOR QUALITY

An important part of a system to assure the quality and safety of health care and to promote continuous quality improvement is the role of bodies that are external to local services. These can take various forms, but they essentially can give objective assessments of progress, identify problems and point to action necessary to bring about improvement. The majority operate on a national basis.

Care Quality Commission

The Care Quality Commission was established by legislation passed in 2008, and in April 2009 it became the regulator for quality of health and adult social care. It subsumed its predecessor bodies: the Healthcare Commission, the Commission for Social Care Inspection and the Mental Health Act Commission.

The Care Quality Commission regulates the health and social care system to ensure that essential standards for the quality and safety of care are met, that quality improvement is promoted and that poor care is rooted out. It also has responsibility for monitoring the Mental Health Act, particularly with respect to the treatment of compulsorily detained patients.

The Care Quality Commission has specific powers in relation to health-care-associated infection, including inspections, imposing fines and, if necessary, closing down wards with poor hygiene standards.

The Care Quality Commission has four key regulatory functions:

➤ *safety and quality assurance* – this involves registering providers of health and adult social care, assessing providers against a set of registration standards, investigating serious service failures and intervening with sanctions, conducting follow-up

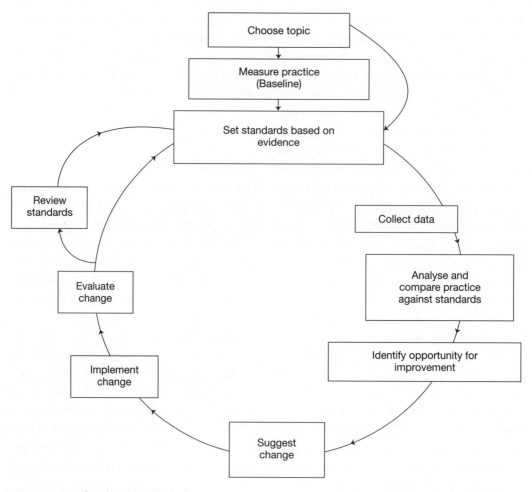

Figure 4.12 The clinical audit cycle

investigations and publishing information and reports

➤ *safeguarding patients' rights* – this is a power of the former Mental Health Act Commission and it involves monitoring the use of the Act and also the Mental Health Incapacity Act 2005

➤ *commissioner assurance and provider assessment* – this involves ensuring the availability of high-quality information to support patient and user choice, publishing an independent assessment of both provider and commissioner performance and carrying out and publishing service and thematic reviews

➤ *minimising the burden of regulation* – this involves adhering to the principles of good regulation and avoiding it becoming burdensome and bureaucratic, as well as coordinating the role of other inspectorates to avoid duplication.

Monitor

Monitor is the independent regulator of NHS foundation trusts. It assesses NHS trusts for foundation status and regulates existing foundation trusts to ensure that they are properly managed and delivering good financial performance; it has legal powers of intervention when they are not. Foundation trusts have a specific set of operating conditions ('authorisations') that they must meet. The regulator ensures that they are adhered to and also that there is no central government interference in areas where foundation trusts have been granted freedoms.

The Audit Commission

The Audit Commission is a body that has overall responsibility for the external financial audit of all local authorities as well as the National Health Service in England and Wales. The Commission audits the governance, the internal controls and the quality of financial systems in NHS trusts, primary care trusts and strategic health authorities.

Part of its role involves assessing how well the public funds that are allocated to the authorities concerned have been used. In addition to examining the way in which funds are used within individual authorities, the Audit Commission also undertakes regular reviews of specific subjects and makes recommendations that particularly focus on value-for-money issues. The usual method of conducting these reviews is for the Commission's staff to study services in a number of parts of the country and draw up a report based on its findings. Organisations are then encouraged to examine the implications for their local services in the light of the Audit Commission's report and implement changes as necessary. The Commission's overall aim is to improve efficiency, effectiveness and outcomes in local public services.

The National Audit Office

The National Audit Office (NAO) scrutinises public spending on behalf of parliament. It is independent of government. It audits the accounts of all government departments and agencies as well as a wide range of other public bodies and reports to parliament on the economy, efficiency and effectiveness with which government bodies have used public money. In this respect, it has the power to audit the work of the Department of Health as the central government department responsible for the NHS. Its work saves the taxpayer millions of pounds every year. Its aim is to promote the highest standards in financial management and reporting, the proper conduct of public business and beneficial change in the provision of public services.

National Clinical Audits of Services

Although the majority of clinical audit activity is carried out as an integral part of clinical governance at local level, there are examples of clinical audit initiatives on a regional or a national scale.

There are three major national inquiries of this kind. The National Confidential Enquiry into Suicide and Homicide by People with Mental Illness (*see also* Chapter 7) analyses cases and seeks to identify key causal and avoidable factors. The Confidential Enquiry into Maternal and Child Health (CEMACH) (*see also* Chapter 6) collects a standard data set of all maternal and perinatal deaths and reports each year on trends. Every three years it produces a themed report identifying causes and risks and making recommendations. This inquiry has a long tradition evolving from separate inquiries into maternal mortality and infant deaths. The National Confidential Enquiry into Patient Outcome and Death has evolved from the earlier Confidential Enquiry into Perioperative Deaths (CEPOD). The current inquiry has moved from examining a specific data set of deaths from surgery to examining deaths in hospital (or other health care facilities) on a thematic basis. For example, reports in 2008 looked at deaths following coronary artery bypass surgery and deaths in sickle cell anaemia patients. Reports in 2009 examined acute kidney injury and death in acute hospital settings.

Many individual medical royal colleges, professional societies or clinical networks organise and carry out their own national audits periodically or on an ongoing basis. For example, the Association of Coloproctology of Great Britain and Ireland has led a three-year national audit of standards of care in the prevention, diagnosis and treatment of bowel cancer, while the British Cardiovascular Society, other professional groups and interests lead an audit of the quality of clinical care in people who have had myocardial infarctions (MINAP).

In addition, the National Clinical Audit Support Programme is a clinical audit and information programme to support national service frameworks and clinical governance.

ASSURING THE QUALITY OF INDIVIDUAL PRACTICE

The delivery of high-quality health care does not depend only on creating health organisations with the leadership, culture and systems to assure and improve the standard of services they provide. It also requires a focus on the individual health practitioner to ensure that mechanisms are in place to assure the quality of his or her practice.

The first important set of activities that underpin the quality of individual practice is the provision of education and training programmes. These should be career-long, with continuing professional development reinforcing and extending the knowledge, skills and values acquired by health care professionals after graduation and completion of their foundation and specialist training programmes.

The second is the need for regular assessment of the individual, which is part of a reform of medical regulation set out in the Health and Social Care Act 2008. The system, called 'revalidation', is overseen by the General Medical Council, with the involvement of NHS and private-sector employers, the medical royal colleges and patient representative groups. It involves two separate processes: 'relicensing' (confirming that a doctor's practice is in line with the General Medical Council's generic standards) and 'recertification' (confirming that doctors on the specialist and general practice registers conform with standards appropriate to their specialty of medicine). Doctors will have to 'pass' these checks periodically if they are to remain on the medical register. The new system is a major revolution in medical regulation and gives the medical profession and the public more objective assurance than in the past that a doctor is up-to-date and practising safely and to acceptable standards.

The third mechanism needed to ensure the quality of individual practice involves addressing situations in which an NHS doctor's performance is so poor as to give rise to concerns about patient safety or the effective functioning of a clinical team or service. A doctor's employer can seek advice from a specialist national agency, the National Clinical Assessment Service (NCAS), a division of the National Patient Safety Agency. The Service does not take over the role of an employer, nor is it a regulator. It does, however, help the employer by giving advice in resolving performance issues locally and carrying out objective assessment. Following assessment, the Service will advise the referring organisation on appropriate courses of action, which could include recommendations for remedial training. In serious cases, the General Medical Council will also become involved and will consider whether issues with a doctor's professional conduct, performance or health are serious enough to affect their licence to practice.

The National Clinical Assessment Service now includes dentists and (from 2009) pharmacists. Poor performance involving a nurse or a physiotherapist would be a matter for the NHS employer alone (taking ad hoc professional or specialist advice as appropriate). However, in serious cases

there are national professional regulatory bodies broadly equivalent to the General Medical Council. Including the General Medical Council, there are nine councils that regulate health professions. Three of these are the Nursing and Midwifery Council, the General Optical Council and the Health Professions Council (which covers a wide range of professions allied to medicine).

The Council for Healthcare Regulatory Excellence (CHRE) is an independent body (accountable to parliament) that has an oversight function for the individual health professional regulators. The Council has a number of discrete statutory functions, such as promoting the interests of the public and patients, reviewing fitness to practice systems of individual regulators and identifying learning points. It also seeks to promote good practice and harmonise functions across the regulators.

PATIENT SAFETY

One important strand of quality programmes in health care is to ensure that the services provided to patients are as safe as possible. Until recently, safety as a concept in health care has been much less developed than in some other sectors. A careful, conscientious approach to clinical practice has always been part of the training and ethos of health professions. Similarly, reducing risks and maximising benefits has been essential when introducing new medicines and equipment into the health care arena. Yet it is now realised that the scale of the problem of harm to patients as a consequence of them experiencing health care is substantial.

The epidemiology of medical error and patient safety more generally is still an under-researched field. Data suggest that medical error is a large and previously unrecognised cause of avoidable mortality and morbidity. Studies in the United States, Australia and the United Kingdom have suggested a level of adverse events amongst hospital inpatient admissions varying from 3.7% to 16.6% – broadly equivalent (in the United Kingdom figure) to 850 000 hospital admissions per year (Table 4.11). Worldwide it is estimated that around a quarter of all adverse events are due to medication error alone (although this figure requires careful interpretation of the definition of a 'mistake', which may range from the serious to the inconsequential).

The issue of safety in health care has many similarities with safety in other sectors. In the airline industry, for example, it has long been recognised that improving safety means understanding what makes an aircraft, its crew and its passengers more likely to experience an accident or serious incident. The change necessary to improve safety in the airline industry has been profound and has included transforming organisational culture, staff training, information gathering and analysis and senior management commitment.

The perspective necessary to address safety in health care is best understood by considering an example of a serious 'accident' during the treatment of a patient. The death of a teenager in a hospital in the East Midlands area of England (Table 4.12) in 2001 occurred because he was given a drug by injection intrathecally (into his spine) when it should only ever have been given intravenously.

For treatment of his cancer, he in fact needed two different drugs, one to be given intravenously and one to be given intra-thecally. The two syringes looked very similar (Figure 4.13). In the event, he was given the wrong drug by the wrong route, so a treatment that was intended to play a part in saving his life was responsible for his death. In short, there was a 'mix-up' – one that was to prove catastrophic for the teenage patient. More than 50 similar incidents have been reported world-wide and others may have gone unreported.

On the surface, serious medication errors seem to be tragedies caused by human error: doctors making fatal mistakes. Investigation of such incidents shows that far from being a simple human error, the true cause of the catastrophe is often human error in a weak system: a weak safety culture, weak operational practices, weaknesses in the presence of protocols and training, weaknesses in communication and serious weaknesses in the packaging and design of drugs and equipment. In short, the cause is comprehensive systems weaknesses.

Accidents in which people are killed or seriously injured happen in many service industries (particularly transport), not just in health care. Research and experience outside health care has shown that safety comes down to appreciating that big improvements are not made by telling people to take care but by understanding the conditions that provoke error. There is usually no simple explanatory cause for a catastrophic event. Instead there is a complex interaction between a varied set of factors, including human behaviour, technological factors, socio-cultural factors and a range of organisational and management

Table 4.11 Research into adverse events in hospitals

- In the USA, 3.7% of inpatient episodes lead to unintended harm (The Harvard Medical Practice Study, 1991).[10]

- In Australia, 16.6% of inpatient episodes lead to unintended harm – around half are preventable (The Quality in Australian Health Care Study, 1995).[11]

- In the UK, 10% of inpatient episodes lead to unintended harm – around half are preventable (Vincent C, Neale G, Woloshynowych M, 2001).[12]

Table 4.12 Death of a patient due to maladministration of an anti-cancer drug

A teenager who was a day-case patient attended the ward of a large teaching hospital for an intrathecal (spinal) administration of chemotherapy as part of his medical maintenance therapy following successful treatment of leukaemia. Two junior doctors carried out the procedure. One gave the injection and the other assisted. A drug that should only ever be administered by the intravenous route (into a vein) was given intrathecally by mistake. Despite emergency treatment to try to rectify the error, the patient died. The investigation carried out into this catastrophic event concluded that while human error occurred, it was at the end of a chain of events in which some 40 systems failures occurred, for example:

- staff untrained in cytotoxic drugs were allowed to dispense chemotherapy from the pharmacy

- there were no explicit protocols for staff to follow in undertaking this high-risk procedure

- there was no formal induction programme for junior doctors starting in the service

- the design, packaging and labelling of the drugs intended for intravenous and intrathecal use was potentially confusing.

Although this was a rare, catastrophic event, it was not unique. It had occurred previously in other hospitals, often in very similar circumstances. General guidance and warnings to the NHS to be more careful had not been effective. Action taken following this tragedy included a standardised procedure for the administration of cytotoxic drugs for the whole of the NHS, together with work to identify a 'design' solution so that it is impossible to connect a syringe containing a drug intended for intravenous administration to a spinal route of administration.

weaknesses. This is the 'cause' of many medication-associated deaths and major accidents, such as the Kegworth air crash (Table 4.13).

This view of accident causation compares the risks of something going wrong to the holes in slices of a Swiss cheese (Figure 4.14). The solid parts of the slices of cheese are the systems defences, and the holes are the vulnerabilities. Unlike the holes in a real Swiss cheese, the holes in the imaginary slices of cheese – the organisation's system – are constantly opening, closing and shifting position. Danger arises when a set of holes line up. Some of the holes – the risks – are caused by unsafe actions committed by individuals. These are slips, lapses, mistakes or violations of procedures. However, many more are due to so-called latent conditions. These are factors in the system – lack of training, poor equipment, absence of procedures – that create preconditions for

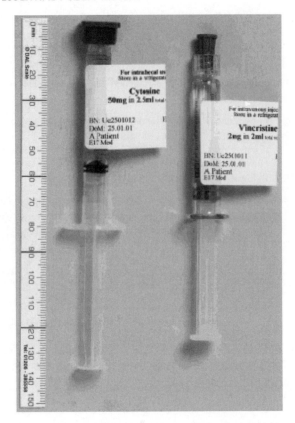

Figure 4.13 Two syringes looking similar

failure. When human error occurs in the presence of these latent conditions, a serious incident can happen. The importance of the Swiss cheese analogy is that it helps to encourage systems thinking and a preventive approach based on anticipating risks and trying to reduce them.

The National Patient Safety Agency (NPSA) is an arms-length body of the Department of Health configured as a special health authority. It houses a number of specialist functions: the National Clinical Assessment Service (*see* p. 243), three national confidential inquiries (*see* p. 241) and a UK-wide national research ethics

service. This agency was established by a comprehensive report on patient safety published in 2000 (*An Organisation with a Memory*).[13] Its role and the patient safety programme in the NHS more generally were strengthened by a report in 2007, *Safety First*.[14]

The National Patient Safety Agency gathers reports from the NHS of all adverse events, incidents and 'near misses'. By the end of 2008, it had a cumulative database of 2.8 million incidents and had produced regular analyses of the key problems. The Agency produces regular patient safety alerts; for example, it identified the risk

Table 4.13 The Kegworth air crash

In 1989, 47 people died when a British Midland Boeing 737 travelling from Heathrow to Belfast crashed onto the M1 motorway. In the media, human error was blamed for the catastrophe. In fact, the accident at Kegworth illustrated how systems failure can occur at a number of levels:

- *technical failure* – fracture of engine blade not identified by aircraft's warning system

- *failure in decision-making process* – leading to incorrect diagnosis of source of engine failure and then to closing down of wrong engine

- *communications failures* – pilots distracted by air traffic control, and cabin staff and passengers failed to communicate their observations on smoke and flames from left-hand engine

- *organisational and environmental factors* – design of cockpit and its instrumentation, new and insufficient training for pilots converting to new types of aircraft.

Source: Adapted from Reason J. *Managing the Risks of Organisational Accidents.* Farnham: Ashgate Publishing, 1997.

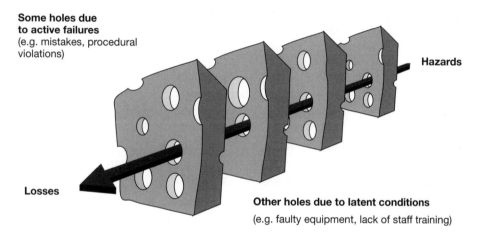

Figure 4.14 The Swiss cheese model of accident causation
Source: Adapted from Reason J. *Managing the Risks of Organisational Accidents.* Farnham: Ashgate Publishing, 1997.

that strong potassium chloride solutions, if given inadvertently without proper dilution, could kill or harm patients. As a result, all hospitals were given detailed guidance on how to avoid this source of error, including removal of concentrated solutions of potassium chloride from day-to-day clinical areas and making available prediluted alternatives.

The National Patient Safety Agency also organises and runs nationwide campaigns (including the *Clean Your Hands* campaign), promotes good practice in patient safety and networks with similar bodies internationally.

Worldwide, the World Health Organization's World Alliance for Patient Safety plays a major leadership role through its programmes and 'global patient safety challenges'.

In the past, the NHS had no way of learning systematically from its mistakes, so the bad experience of one patient was not used to make the care of a future patient safer (Table 4.14). The promotion of the concept of patient safety does not end with the creation of a system of reporting, analysis and learning from adverse events. It also entails creating a culture where health care professionals are willing to report mistakes without fear of blame or retribution. Moving towards an organisational culture that is free from blame within health care is not easy, but experience in other sectors shows that if there is fear of reporting, errors will not be admitted. No learning can then take place, and the opportunity to reduce risk is lost. This does not mean that no one can ever be held to account for his or her actions. Wilful misconduct or neglectful behaviour is not acceptable. Instead it means that the balance has been too much towards blaming an individual when something goes wrong rather than recognising that the root cause is most likely to be systemic.

PATIENT PARTNERSHIP

In the past, concern with quality has largely focused on improving standards of diagnostic and treatment techniques delivered by doctors and other health care professionals. This perspective on quality improvement is still very important, but attention is increasingly being given to seeking and acting upon the views and expectations of users and potential users of health services.

In a message to the United States Congress in 1962, President John F Kennedy identified four basic rights of consumers (Table 4.15). These rights embody fundamental principles that if applied to health services would constitute a powerful commitment to users of services.

In the United Kingdom there has been a trend in the health service and other public services to formulate charters and entitlements for patients as consumers of services. Such an approach is aimed at raising standards and ensuring greater accountability in the delivery of public services. This approach deliberately encourages patients to have high expectations of services and uses the criteria set out (such as response

Table 4.14 What a service working well should expect

- Serious failures of standards of care are uncommon.
- Serious failures of a similar kind do not recur on a future occasion.
- Incidents where services have failed in one part of the country are not repeated elsewhere.
- Systems are in place that reduce to a minimum the likelihood of serious failure in standards of care happening.
- Attention is also paid to monitoring and reducing levels of less serious incidents and near misses.
- The culture in health organisations encourages openness in reporting and values learning from error rather than retribution.

times) as one of the levers for improving quality.

Genuine empowerment of patients as consumers of health care requires a cultural shift in the way in which services are traditionally delivered. It involves not only listening and talking to patients about the care that they receive but also genuinely taking their views and opinions into account when designing services. It is about being open and accessible and inviting feedback on their experiences as a whole, not just their care. It also means enabling them to make informed choices and become partners with health professionals in the care provided.

True patient-centredness in health care has been historically limited by a range of factors. Infrastructure within local services has often been lacking. Health care professionals do not always have the training or skills to enable patients to participate effectively in their own care. Particular groups of patients, such as those who are in ethnic minority populations or who are disabled, can experience even greater barriers. Strategies must be actively pursued if patient-centred care is to become a major part of high-quality health care.

A first step involves creating an infrastructure that supports active engagement of patients, both as individuals and partners in their own care and collectively in planning and shaping health services. The public have told government that they want a greater say over how their money is spent on care services.[15] Services deliver better care if they listen to the people who use them. In the late 2000s, the government put in place a series of initiatives to make services more accountable and responsive and to give citizens more opportunities to influence the care they receive.

In 2006, the Department of Health published *A Stronger Local Voice: a framework for creating a stronger local voice in the development of health and social care services.*[16] The document set out plans that were introduced via the Local Government and Public Involvement in Health Act 2007.

In 2008, the Commission for Patient and

BOX 4.4 THE CAUSE OF MISTAKES

'Human beings make mistakes because the systems, tasks and processes they work in are poorly designed.'

— Lucian Leape. Testimony before the President's Advisory Commission on Consumer Protection and Quality in the Health Care Industry, 19 November 1997.

Table 4.15 Basic rights of consumers

- The right to be informed
- The right to be heard
- The right to choose
- The right to safety

Source: President John F. Kennedy. Message to the United States Congress, 1962.

Public Involvement in Health was abolished, along with the system of patients' forums. These were replaced by local involvement networks (LINks). As an independently run network of local individuals and groups, a LINks' role is to find out what people want from services, to monitor local delivery and to use its powers to hold health and social care services to account. LINks make it easier for more citizens to get involved in shaping services and also make dialogue between communities and services easier.

By the end of the last decade of the twenty-first century, the voice of patients was seen as lying at the heart of the commissioning process. Under the Local Government and Public Involvement in Health Act 2007, the NHS duty to involve citizens was strengthened and a new duty of reporting on consultation was established. The duty of involvement obliges all NHS bodies to involve patients and the public in planning, service development and decision-making. The new duty of reporting on consultation requires strategic health authorities and primary care trusts to report back to their communities on how they have involved users and how such involvement has impacted on their commissioning decisions.

A further step involves gathering regular feedback. An annual national survey of user and patient experience was begun in the late 1990s. This was reinforced by the introduction of the National Patient Survey Programme. This programme, conducted by the Healthcare Commission (now the Care Quality Commission), is one of the largest and most extensive regular patient survey programmes in the world. Since its inception, over 20 surveys have been conducted, with well over a million patients taking part. These surveys have covered seven different health care settings – acute inpatients, acute outpatients, emergency departments, maternity services, users of mental health services, local primary care services and ambulance services.

The National Patient Survey Programme collects structured and systematic feedback on the quality of service delivery from the patient/service users' point of view. In this way, it provides highly robust measures of NHS performance – at organisation level, but also both regionally and nationally. The National Patient Survey Programme is a well-established feature of health care regulation in England – and patients' views count in the assessment of trusts more than ever before.

Survey results are used by a number of organisations in a variety of ways to meet different requirements. Some examples follow.

➤ *NHS trusts and primary care trusts* – results are used to track their own performance over time, benchmark their results against similar organisations, inform local improvement activities (including local delivery plans) and monitor the impact of these activities on the patient experience.

➤ *Strategic health authorities* – results are used to monitor performance of trusts within their geographical area.

➤ *The Care Quality Commission* – results feed into the Annual Health Check for NHS organisations via national targets and standards-based assessments. Results are also widely used in relevant service reviews and investigations.

➤ *Department of Health* – results provide feedback on policy delivery and implementation and provide the metrics for measuring progress against the national 'improving patient experience' target.

In addition to the National Patient Survey Programme, a number of other initiatives are operated locally to obtain patient feedback. These include patient experience trackers, comments cards and feedback websites.

The Expert Patients' Programme

In 2002, a new NHS programme was established to support patients with chronic disease to manage their own conditions.[17] The programme was based on work at Stanford University that demonstrated that teaching people to manage the consequences of their chronic disease improved outcomes of treatment, reduced dependence on health services and increased people's sense of empowerment and well-being.[18] It relied on a lay (i.e., patient-led) training programme. The Expert Patients' Programme in the NHS is now organised as a community interest company, an innovative governance model that is a not-for-profit social enterprise.

By the end of the last decade of the twenty-first century, 30 000 people had attended the programme in England. Evaluation has shown improvements, including reduced use of health services, improved confidence of patients in managing their own disease,

higher energy levels and better quality of life.

COMPLAINTS AND REDRESS

While the majority of patients are satisfied with their care, evidence from recent surveys of service users and from complaints data suggests that sometimes people who wish to complain do not do so. The main reasons for this are lack of awareness of the complaints system; concerns about the effect complaining might have on their ongoing treatment or care; or feeling daunted by the formality of the process.

Complaints and other sources of feedback from patients in the form of compliments, comments and concerns represent an important opportunity to learn lessons about possible service failures, which can then be translated into improvements in service quality. An important factor in judging the quality of a health service should be how quickly and effectively complaints are resolved and how the lessons learned are embedded into service improvement. Patients want to see their concerns taken seriously and their complaints investigated speedily, fairly and using appropriate mechanisms, such as mediation or independent investigation, with an apology, a clear explanation given and follow-up action taken.

Services are expected to respond to complaints in the most suitable, sensitive and appropriate way for the individual and the circumstances. There is a strong focus on local resolution and outcome, with recourse to the Health Ombudsman if the complainant is still dissatisfied.

The NHS objectives on patient-centred responsiveness to complaints were enshrined in the NHS constitution, developed as part of the NHS Next Stage Review (the Darzi Report). The following rights and pledges were set out:

➤ you have the right to make a complaint about your NHS services; to have your complaint dealt with efficiently and investigated appropriately; to know the outcome; and to compensation when harmed by negligent treatment

➤ you have the right to take your complaint to the health service ombudsman, or to make a claim for judicial review, if you have exhausted other rights of appeal

➤ the NHS will strive to ensure that if you make a complaint, you are treated with respect and courtesy, you receive a timely and appropriate response, any harm that you suffered is corrected and any necessary changes are put in place.

Patient Advocacy and Liaison Service (PALS)

The patient advice and liaison service known as PALS was introduced to the NHS in 2002 to make sure that trusts have dedicated staff who can provide information to patients and their families and carers and who try to resolve any concerns as quickly as possible. PALS main functions are to:

➤ provide on-the-spot help – they have the power to negotiate immediate solutions or speedy resolutions of problems

➤ act as a gateway to appropriate advice and advocacy support from local and national sources

➤ provide accurate information to patients, carers and families about the trust's services and other health-related matters

➤ act as a catalyst for change and improvement by providing the trust with information and feedback on the problems arising and on gaps in services

➤ operate within a local network with other PALS in their area and work across organisational boundaries

➤ support staff at all levels within the trust to develop a responsive culture.

The Health Service Commissioner (Ombudsman)

The health service ombudsman can carry out independent investigations into complaints about poor treatment or service provided through the NHS in England. If someone has suffered because they have received poor service or treatment or were not treated properly or fairly – and the organisation or practitioner has not put things right where they could have – the health service ombudsman may be able to help.

Investigations look into complaints against NHS services provided by hospitals, health authorities, trusts, general practitioners dentists, pharmacists, opticians and other health care practitioners. The ombudsman can also investigate complaints against private health providers if the treatment is funded by the NHS.

Courts

A patient has recourse to the courts of law, where he or she may allege clinical negligence. Settlements are usually made out of court, and this is the main route of complaint through which people can obtain financial redress. This is an increasingly common route for complainants in Britain and is a major feature of medical practice in the United States, where patients are much more litigation-minded and doctors are inclined to plan their clinical management in a way that is least likely to lead to litigation, even if it may not be the best approach to a particular clinical problem (so-called 'defensive medicine').

The National Health Service Litigation Authority (NHSLA) is a special health authority that handles negligence claims against the NHS bodies in England. In total, almost £600 million is paid out in response to clinical negligence claims (damages to patients and NHS legal costs). Around 96% of all claims are settled out of court.

REGULATION OF MEDICINES, MEDICAL DEVICES AND BLOOD

The Medicines and Healthcare products Regulatory Agency (MHRA) is a central government agency that accounts to the Department of Health and is responsible for ensuring that medicines and medical devices work and meet an acceptable standard of safety. The field that is regulated by this agency is very wide; as well as medicines and medical devices, it includes blood and blood components for transfusion and therapeutic products derived from tissue engineering.

The legal basis for control and monitoring of medicines in the United Kingdom is the Medicines Act 1968, but European Union medicines legislation takes precedence over domestic legislation in many circumstances. The criteria on which legislation to control medicines are based are safety, quality and efficacy. Experts and committees advise the agency in its task of assessing all new medicines to ensure that they meet the necessary standards and on ongoing systems of inspection, testing and safety monitoring. Increasingly, new medicines are being licensed via a centralised European procedure operated by the European Medicines Agency (EMEA). The MHRA works closely with Europe in the assessment of these innovative products.

The legislation and approach to medical devices is different to that for medicines. There is no United Kingdom 'Medical Devices Act' that is comparable to the Medicines Act 1968. Instead, legal regulations implement the European Commission devices directives into United Kingdom law. They place requirements on medical device manufacturers to ensure that their products are safe and fit for purpose before they are CE marked and used in any European Union member state.

The Medicines and Healthcare products Regulatory Agency functions can be summarised as follows:

> on behalf of the government, to ensure that medicines are sufficiently efficacious and acceptably safe and that they meet appropriate quality standards

> to ensure that medical devices (which includes in-vitro diagnostic products) and equipment meet appropriate

standards of safety, quality and performance and that they comply with relevant directives of the European Union

➤ to provide regulatory approval for clinical trials of medicinal products and clinical investigations of medical devices

➤ to operate an effective system for the reporting of serious adverse events and reactions to blood transfusion and ensure that blood banks and blood establishments operate to required standards

➤ to inspect manufacturers and distributors to ensure compliance of procedures with the product licence and good manufacturing or distribution practices

➤ to inspect laboratories that conduct safety studies on chemicals, including those used in medicines, for compliance with good laboratory practice

➤ to monitor suspected adverse reactions to medicinal products (together with the Commission on Human Medicines) and take steps to optimise safe usage

➤ to monitor reports of suspected quality defects in medicinal products and medical devices and liaise with manufacturers with a view to a possible recall

➤ to take enforcement action in relation to breaches of legislation and regulations

➤ to provide information on risk/benefit to health professionals and patients and ensure advertising is not misleading

➤ to maintain international collaborations with other regulatory bodies, particularly through the European Union and the World Health Organization.

The strategic direction and governance of the MHRA are overseen by a non-executive agency board whose members bring wide external experience. The decisions taken by the Agency's own staff (medical, scientific, technical and managerial) in their day-to-day work are supported by reference to advisory committees of independent experts and lay members – in particular the Commission on Human Medicines and the Committee on the Safety of Devices. Using all available scientific and practical evidence, these play a crucial role in providing advice on whether medicines and devices work and are acceptably safe. Legally, the Agency's powers are vested in the secretary of state for health.

A particularly important role of the Agency is the process of detecting untoward reactions from drugs and adverse incidents involving medical devices. For medicines, a long-standing mechanism for doing this is the Yellow Card Scheme. The Scheme receives reports from health professionals, patients, carers and parents on suspected adverse reactions to medicines (whether prescription drugs, over-the-counter medicines or herbal products). Such reports are then evaluated, both individually and by the application of data-mining techniques to the whole database of over half a million reports. The Yellow Card Scheme is only one part of the wider process of pharmacovigilance by which the risk/benefit of medicines is continually monitored in population use.

In addition to the mandatory adverse incident reporting by medical devices manufacturers under the European Union 'Vigilance' post-marketing surveillance system, the MHRA also receives reports from health care professionals and members of the public. Over 50% of these reports are now submitted via the MHRA's online systems, including the innovative MORE (Manufacturers' Online Reporting Environment).

DRUG SAFETY

Before a drug receives a marketing authorisation (product license), the Licensing Authority must be satisfied that it is safe in relation to its intended use. This is a relative judgement, termed the risk/benefit analysis. For example, a new anti-cancer drug or an antiviral agent for use in AIDS would be permitted to exhibit more frequent or serious toxicities than a new agent for a less serious indication.

Information on safety of new drugs is initially generated through a range of pre-clinical studies, including carcinogenicity, mutagenicity and reproductive toxicity in several species. Appropriate standards of chemical and pharmaceutical quality must also be achieved. After appropriate animal testing, new drugs are introduced into clinical use through a continuous process of clinical development that is conventionally divided into four phases, the first three of which would normally be complete before marketing approval.

➤ Phase 1 studies constitute first use in humans, where the clinical pharmacology of the drug is investigated in small numbers of healthy volunteers or patients.

➤ Phase 2 studies comprise clinical investigation for efficacy and safety in larger numbers of patients, typically 200–300.

➤ Phase 3 studies are randomised clinical trials on a substantive scale, often more than 1000 patients to confirm safety and efficacy identified in phase 2 studies.

➤ Phase 4 studies, also known as post-licensing studies or post-marketing surveillance, consist of further surveillance, particularly for safety, in large populations after the drug has been launched.

Adverse reactions to drugs can be broadly subdivided into two groups. Type A (augmented) reactions are exaggerated responses to the drug's normal pharmacological action – for example, bradycardia with beta-blocking drugs. They are common, predictable, usually dose-related and rarely fatal. Type B (bizarre) reactions are unrelated to the drug's normal pharmacological actions, uncommon and usually not dose-related. However, they are often serious and may carry a high mortality – for example, agranulocytosis with the atypical antipsychotic clozapine or Stevens-Johnson syndrome with carbamazepine. Much effort in adverse-reactions monitoring and post-marketing surveillance is therefore directed at identifying and minimising the risk of Type B reactions. Specific risk-management strategies may be possible. For clozapine, this consists of close blood-count monitoring during treatment. For carbamazepine, pre-treatment genetic testing for the HLA-B*1502 allele in some Asian ethnic groups (Han Chinese, Hong Kong Chinese and Thai) will identify individuals at greatly increased risk of skin toxicity for whom an alternative drug should be used if possible.

MEDICAL DEVICES SAFETY

The Medicines and Healthcare products Regulatory Agency receives over 8000 adverse incident reports each year. After risk assessment, it directly investigates over 20%, and a further 30% are investigated by the manufacturer in collaboration with the Agency.

As a result of information gained from reports and investigations, the Agency issues medical device alerts within the UK and shares information on a range of safety issues with other competent authorities in Europe and elsewhere around the world. Additional safety guidance of a more general nature is published in MHRA Device Bulletins.

BLOOD SAFETY AND QUALITY

Following new regulatory requirements, the SABRE (Serious Adverse Blood Reactions and Events) system was implemented to capture individual incident reports submitted by transfusion and blood service staff. Annual summary reports are collated across the European Union.

Blood establishments are subject to Medicines and Healthcare products Regulatory Agency inspection, as are blood banks where indicated by the audit of annual compliance reports. The Agency increasingly uses risk-assessment methodology to maximise public health gain while minimising regulatory burden.

RESOURCES FOR THE HEALTH SERVICE

The health service in the United Kingdom represents a major area of government expenditure. This section of the chapter describes how the resources of the health service are determined and deployed. In addition to financial resources, there are three other major elements of health service resources: staff, estate and information. These first three elements are explored further here, and the fourth element of the health services resources, information, is considered in Chapter 1.

The National Health Service is mainly funded from public finances. In its first full year of operation, the NHS cost approximately £10 per head of population, but by 2008 this had increased to around £1800 per head. The NHS accounts for a high proportion of overall public expenditure: 16% in the financial year 2007/08.

Total NHS expenditure increased from £33 billion in 1996/97 to £49.7 billion in 2001/02 and £92.64 billion in 2008/09, real terms growth of 6.1% annually over the period. This compares with an annual average over the preceding 35 years of 3.1%. Spending on health care and the proportion funded by public expenditure varies greatly across countries of the world (Figure 4.15).

Resources committed to the NHS fall into two broad categories:

1 *revenue* – money spent on day-to-day running costs, such as staff, drugs and consumables

2 *capital* – money spent on buildings or equipment.

More than 80% of the NHS revenue budget is allocated directly to primary care trusts, with the remainder being used for central budgets in programmes such as research and development, training and information technology.

The exact allocation of funds to each of the 152 primary care trusts in the country is determined by a formula that is intended to give equal level of services for people with equal need and also to tackle health inequalities. The allocation is made on the basis of the number of people resident in the primary care trust area, adjusted by three factors:

1 *age* – areas with more elderly or very young people receive a larger allocation

2 *need* – areas with higher levels of particular diseases and deprived populations receive a larger allocation

3 *higher cost of provision* – areas with higher costs (e.g., labour costs), predominantly in London and the South East, receive a larger allocation designed to cover unavoidable costs.

The resulting 'weighted capitation formula' gives each primary care trust a target allocation. Their actual allocation depends on how quickly ministers in the Department of Health choose to move them towards their target allocation.

The system results in a wide range in allocations between primary care trust populations. For example, in 2007/08 Islington Primary Care Trust received an allocation of £1956 per head of population, the highest in the country. In contrast, the lowest per capita allocation in the country went to Leicestershire County and Rutland Primary Care Trust. It received £1140 per head of population. Unsurprisingly, the operation of the funding allocation formula proves controversial and is subject to regular review.

The Treasury undertakes a Comprehensive Spending Review (CSR) usually every three years. These involve ministers of the various departments of state submitting bids to the chief secretary to the Treasury, who then makes proposals to the Cabinet on public expenditure levels. These are accompanied by an economic assessment by the chancellor of the exchequer. Each department is then given a three-year departmental expenditure limit and a set of outcomes agreed with the Treasury on which the department is held accountable. The funding of the NHS is part of the allocation to the Department of Health under this system.

Typically, a private sector finance consortium will consist of a large construction company (to build the scheme), a design team (to design the facility) and one or more facilities management companies (to provide, for example, estates, security, portering and cleaning services). The hospital facility is managed by the consortium, with a trust paying regular revenue payment for the use of the hospital.

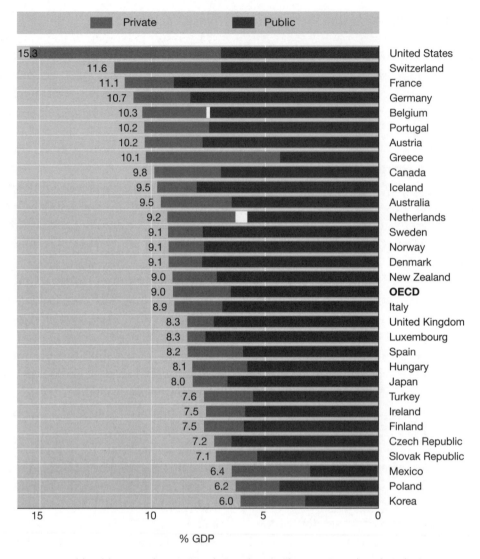

Figure 4.15 Total health expenditure as a share of gross domestic product (GDP), 2005
Source: Organisation for Economic Co-operation and Development (OECD). *Health at a Glance.* Paris: OECD; 2007.

HUMAN RESOURCES

The most important asset of a service industry like the health service is the people it employs (Table 4.16). Either directly or indirectly, they are the means through which the patients or consumers of health services receive the help they need. The health service has traditionally employed a wide range of professional staff; doctors, nurses, physiotherapists, clinical psychologists and occupational therapists are examples, but there are many others. In addition, there are many groups of staff that perform specialist technical jobs – for example, medical physicists and information technologists. During the 1980s and early 1990s, there was a growth in general management posts covering specialist management functions such as finance and personnel. Finally, a further group of staff essential to the efficient and effective running of the service is the very wide range of personnel providing an infrastructure of key support to the service – for example, drivers, porters, catering staff, ward clerks, records officers, medical secretaries, engineers, laboratory technicians and public relations officers.

The beginning of the twenty-first century saw a much greater awareness on the part of the NHS of the need to identify and address the workforce implications of its policies and the need for developing staff who were equipped for the new health policies that were being put in place.

Major changes have taken place in the professions. For example, the traditional role of nurses has been greatly extended into areas such as prescribing, clinical assessment of patients, dealing with minor injuries and providing community care and health promotion services. These areas would in the past have been the sole province of doctors, but today nurses have a much greater degree of autonomy. Other professions have extended their roles similarly, while all health care professionals, including doctors, have had to further develop their skills in areas such as primary care, health promotion, information technology, evidence-based practice and counselling and advising patients.

All this was recognised as part of the NHS Next Stage Review (*see* p. 202). A report on the future of the health workforce, *High Quality Workforce: NHS Next Stage Review*,[19] set out proposals on roles, education and career pathways, seeking to embed a clear set of principles in all three: a focus on quality, patient centredness, being clinically

Table 4.16 NHS staff in England, 2007

Staff group	Numbers
Doctors	127 645
Qualified nurses	399 597
Qualified scientists, therapeutic and technical staff	136 976
Qualified ambulance staff	17 028
Support to clinical staff	346 596
Infrastructure support staff	207 778
Managers and senior managers	36 499
Other	94 924
Total*	1 330 544

*Some exclusions not shown in table
Source: Information Centre for Health and Social Care.

driven, flexibility, valuing people and life-long learning. These wide-ranging changes are a long-term project. Work commenced to implement them in 2009.

THE ESTATE

A major element of the resources of the health service is its estate: the buildings, land, plant and equipment from which services are delivered. The management of the resources that make up the estate is a complex and wide-ranging process. It involves the deployment of existing capital assets to meet service needs and strategic decisions about new investments. The planning and building of new hospitals is itself a complex process that includes the establishment of an initial business case, detailed planning and design, acquiring land, procurement, construction and commissioning (*see also* the preceding information on capital funding allocations).

Management of the estate also involves maintenance and renewal of buildings machinery and equipment. It involves ensuring that rigorous safety standards are met and, increasingly, it involves addressing environmental issues (such as energy consumption and waste management).

SOCIAL CARE

Social care has been defined as 'the wide range of services designed to support people to maintain their independence, enable them to play a fuller part in society, protect them in vulnerable situations and manage complex relationships'. Care is indeed provided to a wide range of adults and children.

The provision of services to children, older people, those with mental health problems and people with disabilities are described in other chapters.

In England alone, some 1.26 million people receive social care funded by local authorities. About 259 000 of these people are in residential care. The largest group of users of social care services are older people: approximately two-thirds of service users are over 65 years of age. The provision of social care services for adults is a local government responsibility, and it rests with the upper tier or unitary local authority in England, rather than with districts where they exist, and with local authorities in Wales and Scotland. In Northern Ireland, there is an integrated health and personal social services structure. The professional leadership role in local authorities is held by a director of adult social services. In a small number of instances in England, the roles of director of adult social services and chief executive of the primary care trust are combined.

There are many different disciplines within the social care workforce, ranging from qualified social workers to residential workers to unqualified care workers. Social care services themselves are again wide-ranging, encompassing residential care, foster care, child protection services, home helps, meals-on-wheels, day care and counselling services.

The number of adults needing social care continues to grow as the population of the United Kingdom and many other developed countries ages. In addition, medical advances mean that people with serious conditions resulting in substantial disability can survive for many more years. There has also been a substantial shift towards care in the community. This gives vulnerable adults much more independence, control and choice over how they live their lives. It may, however, place additional burdens on families and carers. The programme for transforming social care to cope with these challenges was laid out in England in a policy document, *Putting People First*, published in 2007.

CONCLUSIONS

The basic principles of the National Health Service have remained intact since it was introduced after World War II. This is despite a number of major reorganisations that have changed its structure and management. When viewed internationally, it is generally acknowledged as a relatively efficient system of delivering health care to the population.

Changes that will occur in the first few decades of the twentieth century and beyond are likely to include a further growth in diagnostic and treatment technology, further ageing of the population, a greater emphasis on the promotion of health, a change in the role that the hospital will play in the health care system and rising consumer expectations (Table 4.17). It will be important for the National Health Service to adapt to and meet these challenges as they occur.

REFERENCES

1 Wanless D. *Securing Our Future Health: taking a long-term view. Final report*. London: HM Treasury; 2002.
2 Wanless D. *Securing Good Health for the Whole Population*. London: HM Treasury; 2004.
3 Donabedian A. Evaluating the quality of medical care. *Milbank Mem Fund Q*. 1966; **4**: 166–206.
4 Deming WE. *Out of the Crisis*. Cambridge: Cambridge University Press; 1986.
5 Duran JM. *Managerial Breakthrough*. New York: McGraw-Hill; 1964.
6 Liggins GC, Howie RM. A controlled trial of antepartum glucocorticoid treatment for prevention of the respiratory distress syndrome in premature infants. *Paediatrics*. 1972; **50**: 515–25.
7 Wilson B, Thornton JG, Hewison J, *et al*. The Leeds University maternity audit project. *Int J Qual Healthcare*. 2002; **14**: 175–81.
8 Scally G, Donaldson LJ. Clinical

Table 4.17 The changing philosophy of the NHS

Earlier decades	Twenty-first century
Treatment emphasis	Public health emphasis
Demand-led priorities	Needs-driven priorities
Hospital care centred	Primary care centred
Provider dominated	Consumer empowered
Professional opinion and therapeutic fashions	Evidence-based standards

governance and the drive for quality improvement in the new NHS in England. *BMJ*. 1998; **317**: 61–5.

9 Halligan A, Donaldson LJ. Implementing clinical governance: turning vision into reality. *BMJ*. 2001; **322**: 1413–17.

10 Brennan TA, Leape LL, Laird NM. Incidents of adverse events and negligence in hospitalised patients. *N Engl J Med*. 1991; **324**: 370–6.

11 Wilson RM, Runciman WB, Gibberd RW, *et al*. The Quality in Australian Health Care Study. *Med J Aust*. 1995; **163**: 458–71.

12 Vincent C, Neale G, Woloshynowych M. Adverse events in British hospitals: preliminary retrospective record review. *BMJ*. 2001; **322**: 517–19.

13 Chief Medical Officer. *An Organisation with a Memory*. London: The Stationery Office; 2000.

14 Department of Health. *Safety First*. London: Department of Health; 2007.

15 Department of Health. *Your Health, Your Care, Your Say*. London: Department of Health; 2006.

16 Department of Health. *A Stronger Local Voice: a framework for creating a stronger local voice in the development of health and social care services*. London: Department of Health; 2006.

17 Department of Health. *The Expert Patient: a new approach to chronic disease management for the 21st century*. London: Department of Health; 2001.

18 Lorig KR, Mazonson PD, Holman HR. Evidence suggesting that health education for self-management in patients with chronic arthritis has sustained health benefits while reducing health care costs. *Arthritis and Rheum*. 1993; **36**(4): 439–6.

19 Department of Health. *A High Quality Workforce: NHS Next Stage Review*. London: Department of Health; 2008.

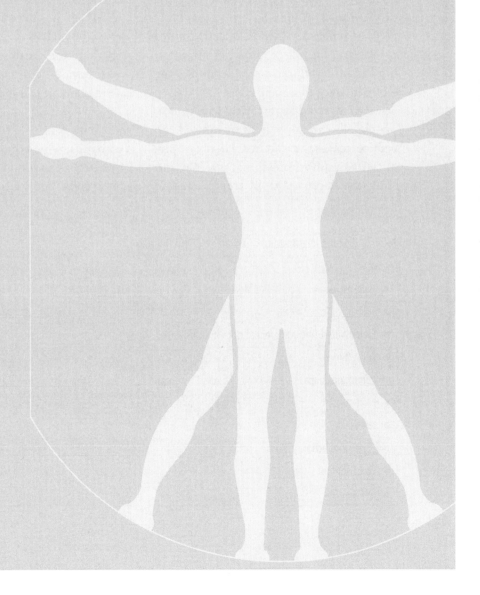

CHAPTER 5
Physical Disability

INTRODUCTION

Many disease processes are wide-ranging in their impact. In some, the result is disability: a state in which the individual may experience loss or limitation of physical function, reduced opportunities in social functioning, economic hardship or disadvantage, negative attitudes and prejudice. Aside from disease, disability can arise through other causes, such as foetal abnormalities and accidents.

Disability is an important public health issue for a number of reasons. Firstly, the proportion of people who develop disability could be reduced with more effective health promotion measures aimed at eliminating the underlying causes. Secondly, the effective use of treatment and rehabilitation services directed at restoring function in people who are already ill or injured can reduce residual disability. For example, an active multi-professional approach to the clinical recognition, treatment and rehabilitation of people with stroke helps to prevent long-term major disability in some of those affected. Thirdly, disabled people have additional needs. It is a responsibility of those planning and providing services to ensure that the needs of disabled people are clearly identified and that an appropriate and personalised response is made to them. To undertake this task properly poses enormous challenges. It is not simply a question of making adjustments in the delivery of health and social care services. The needs of disabled people are very wide-ranging, and addressing them requires a variety of approaches across many areas (Table 5.1).

Perhaps the greatest challenge is to create an infrastructure of help, support and care that enables disabled people to be fully integrated within, and make a meaningful contribution to, society, as well as creating a climate in which they are recognised and respected as individuals, with commensurate rights and entitlements. Disabled

Table 5.1 Some key areas of need for disabled people

- Medical care
- Building and environmental design
- Transport
- Employment (including equal opportunities)
- Education
- Communications
- Leisure
- Financial
- Social interaction
- Carer support
- Information

people must never be regarded as passive recipients of care. This chapter deals with the nature and causes of physical disability as well as the needs of people who are so affected and the range of responses that can support them.

THE MEANING OF DISABILITY

The language that is used in the area of disability is complicated and is sometimes disputed. The societal view of disability continues to shift from an approach that in the past has sought to define disability in terms of the features of an individual that are directly caused by disease or trauma and require medical treatment of some form. The move is from this 'medical model' towards a 'social model' that sees disability not in terms of the individual but in terms of a society that must find ways of accommodating a wide range of individuals with problems that result from the attitudes of society and the inadequacies of the built environment. Neither model is adequate on its own, and a synthesis of the two approaches, sometimes described as the 'biopsychosocial model', is probably the most effective approach.

In an attempt to provide a tool to describe and analyse disability and to move beyond the purely medical approach represented by the International Classification of Diseases, the World Health Organization has developed a classification system know as the International Classification of Functioning, Disability and Health (or ICF for short). The name of the classification reflects its concentration on functioning and health as well as on disability. The ICF is designed to be used for a wide range of functions, including assessment of individuals, institutional management, research and service planning. The definitions that form the basis of the ICF are shown in Table 5.2.

In addition to the ICF, the World Health Organization has developed an interviewer-administered assessment instrument, the WHO Disability Assessment Schedule II (WHO DAS II), which is designed to be used

Table 5.2 Definitions of the components of disability

- Body functions are physiological functions of body systems (including psychological functions).
- Body structures are anatomical parts of the body, such as organs, limbs and their components.
- Impairments are problems in body function or structure, such as a significant deviation or loss.
- Activity is the execution of a task or action by an individual.
- Participation is involvement in a life situation.
- Activity limitations are difficulties an individual may have in executing activities.
- Participation restrictions are problems an individual may experience in involvement in life situations.
- Environmental factors make up the physical, social and attitudinal environment in which people live and conduct their lives.

Source: Towards a Common Language for Functioning, Disability and Health: The International Classification of Functioning, Disability and Health. World Health Organization; 2002.

with individuals to provide an indication of both functioning and disability that is reliable and comparable internationally.

The United Kingdom has a strong statutory basis for ensuring that people with disabilities do not suffer discrimination and that all public bodies have an obligation to reduce the impediments that prevent people with disabilities leading as normal a life as is possible. This is sometimes referred to as the 'Disability Equality Duty'. Under the key legislation, the Disability Discrimination Acts of 1995 and 2005, a person has a disability if they have a physical or mental impairment that has a substantial and long-term adverse effect on their ability to carry out normal day-to-day activities. Taken together with the Equality Act of 2006, the disability discrimination legislation seeks to ensure the unimpeded participation of people with disabilities in society.

PRACTICAL IMPLICATIONS OF DISABILITY

The applicability of the definitions in Table 5.2 depends very much on the underlying cause of the disability, the characteristics of the individual and the characteristics of the community or society in which they live. Even for particular causes of disability, people can vary greatly in the impact that the disease process has upon them. For example, a person with diabetes mellitus is impaired by definition, since there is a disturbance to normal functioning of one organ of the body. For many diabetic people, careful self-regulation of their disease through urine glucose monitoring, diet, exercise and insulin injection will mean

that they are not disabled: there is no loss or restriction of functional ability or activity because of their impairment. On the other hand, a diabetic person whose disease has progressed or been badly controlled may have complications of the illness (for example, blindness, poor circulation to the limbs) that will seriously interfere with his or her ability to function.

Of even greater importance when considering the needs of disabled people are the ways in which disability is perceived by society and its individual members, the ways in which disabled people themselves are affected by these attitudes and the extent to which they cope with them. As a result of the way in which disabled people may be treated by other members of society, they may develop feelings of frustration, resentment and serious loss of self-esteem. It is particularly important that health and social care professionals supporting disabled people (and their carers) are sensitive to their perceptions and have the training to deal with complex issues (Table 5.3).

THE ASSESSMENT OF NEED

There are no comprehensive data available to describe how many people are disabled and the nature of their disabilities at local population level. This is for a number of reasons. Firstly, most information systems are derived from contact with hospital services, but many disabled people will be living in the community and will not necessarily be receiving care from hospital-based services. Secondly, the needs of disabled people have not, in the past, been a high priority for service providers. Therefore, building up

Table 5.3 Perceptions of quality care by disabled people and their carers: some wants

To be respected and understood by professionals providing services
To be given an accurate diagnosis and prognosis sensitively
To be involved in the planning and decision-making about their care and services

Source: Seminar report: be prepared for action. Disability and Rehabilitation Open Learning Project; 1998.

accurate information on the numbers of those disabled people and on their needs has not been a concern. Thirdly, for information on disability to be of any value, it must encompass some of the definitional issues that were discussed in the previous sections. Gathering valid data on this basis is extremely complex in practice given that, for example, many elderly people with severe mobility problems do not consider themselves to be 'disabled'. It is estimated that in the United Kingdom, using a wide survey definition of disability, that there are approximately 11 million disabled adults and 770 000 disabled children.

CAUSES OF DISABILITY

The major underlying causes of disability worldwide (Figure 5.1) are consistent across a number of surveys. In examining population need locally, some insights into the number of people with disabilities can be derived by estimating the number of people with conditions such as stroke. This disease-based approach does not provide information on the full range of disability, nor does it yield data on levels of incapacity amongst disabled people, the most important issue when assessing need and planning service responses. Some information is available from the National Sample Survey, the Integrated Household Survey and

its predecessor, the General Household Survey, which ask questions about long-term incapacity.

PATTERNS IN THE POPULATION

The most comprehensive information on the numbers of disabled people and the nature of their impairments comes from a series of national surveys undertaken during the 1980s. Originally commissioned by the government in 1984, the Office of Population Censuses and Surveys (OPCS) carried out four separate surveys between 1985 and 1988. In 1995 and again in 2001, the Health Survey for England repeated major parts of the 1985 disability survey series using an adapted form of the World Health Organization's questions for determining levels of disability.

The Health Survey covered private households in England and found that 17% of men and 18% of women aged 16 years and older had at least one type of disability out of the five covered. Overall, 4% of men and 5% of women were judged to have a serious disability. The prevalence of disability increased with age for both men and women, with almost three-quarters of men and women aged over 85 years having at least one disability (Figure 5.2).

The most commonly reported cause of disability was disease of the musculoskeletal

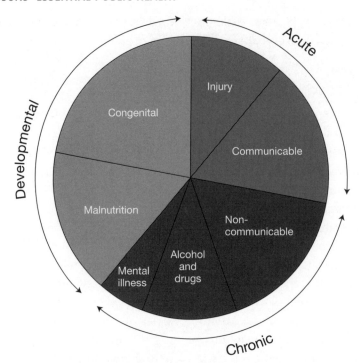

Figure 5.1 Classes of disorder giving rise to disability in the world
Source: Wood P, Bradley E. The epidemiology of disablement. In: Goodwill CJ, Chamberlain MA (eds).
Rehabilitation of the Physically Disabled Adult. London: Croom Helm; 1988.

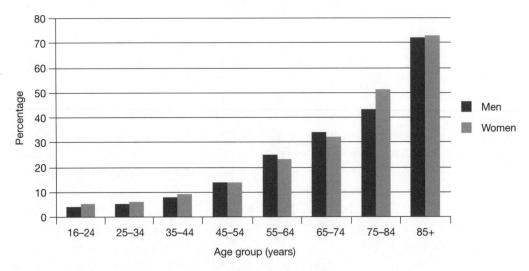

Figure 5.2 Percentage of adults with one or more disabilities, by age and sex
Source: Health Survey for England 2001. London: The Stationery Office; 2003.

system (in particular, arthritis) – see Table 5.4. There was a strong relationship between disability and social class (Figure 5.3). For men of working age who had a disability, 46% of those with any disability were permanently unable to work. The comparable figures for women were slightly lower at 34% (Figure 5.4). Overall, 5% of children (boys and girls aged 10–15 years) had at least one disability and 1% had a serious disability.

These major national surveys were very important in describing the proportion of

disabled people in the population and the nature of their impairments. Increasingly, it will be necessary to gather similar data at a more local population level if the needs of disabled people are to be properly assessed and then addressed by those planning and providing services.

SENSORY IMPAIRMENT

People with sensory impairments are individuals with additional needs within the

Table 5.4 Reported causes of disability among adults

Health complaint	Percentage*
Diseases of the musculoskeletal system and connective tissue	40
Arthritis	21
Others	19
Diseases of the circulatory system	13
Injury and poisoning	9
Congenital abnormalities	8
Diseases of the nervous system (other than eye or ear)	8
Diseases of the ear and mastoid processes	7
Diseases of the respiratory system	7
Mental disorders	6
Eye disorders	5
Endocrine, nutritional and metabolic diseases and immunity disorders	3
Infectious and parasitic diseases	1
Neoplasms	1
Diseases of the digestive system	1
Diseases of the genitourinary system	1
Diseases of the skin and subcutaneous system	1
Old age and problems not included in other categories	8

* Percentage add to more than 100 because some informants had more than one complaint.
Source: Health Survey for England 2001. London: The Stationery Office; 2003.

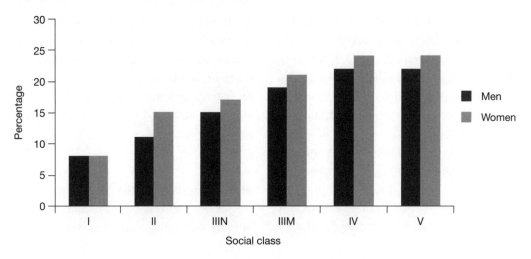

Figure 5.3 Prevalence of disability by sex and social class (age-standardised)
Source: Health Survey for England 2001. London: The Stationery Office; 2003.

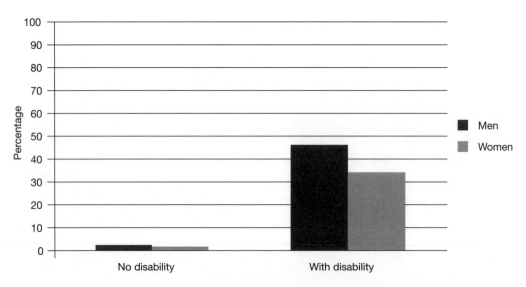

Figure 5.4 Percentage of adults of working age who are permanently unable to work
Source: Health Survey for England 2001. London: The Stationery Office; 2003.

disabled population. The three principal categories are people with blindness, those with deafness and those who are both deaf and blind.

There are various definitions of blindness and deafness in use, depending on the context. The National Assistance Act 1948 defines blindness as 'that a person should be so blind as to be unable to perform any work for which eyesight is essential'. There is no statutory definition of partial sight. However, in practice this category refers to those who, although not blind within the meaning of the Act, are substantially and permanently disabled by defective vision caused by congenital defect, illness or injury.

Social services authorities are required to maintain registers of people in their areas who are blind or partially sighted. Individuals are not obliged to register in order to access social services, although some concessions provided by other agencies and not related to social services are available only to people who are registered. The concessions available for blind people (e.g., the blind person's income tax allowance) are generally more significant than those available to partially sighted people, so there is a stronger incentive for blind people than for partially sighted people to register. Even so, it is estimated that registers significantly under-record the prevalence of blindness.

Social services authorities are advised to register people as blind or partially sighted only when they have been certified as such by a medical practitioner with experience in ophthalmology (usually a consultant ophthalmologist). Absolute standards are not laid down, but the advice is that most people with visual acuity below 3/60 Snellen can be certified blind, as can people with greater visual acuity but a very contracted field of vision. People with visual acuity between 3/60 and 6/60 with full field, or with greater acuity but a contracted field, may be certified partially sighted.

Social services authorities are also required to maintain registers of people who are deaf or hard of hearing. As with visual impairment, there is no requirement

for individuals to register to access social services, although some unrelated concessions provided by other agencies may be available to those who do. There is no requirement for a person to be medically certified as deaf or hard of hearing before he or she is registered. Some deaf people do not regard themselves as being disabled but rather that they simply use different forms of communication.

Different agencies use different terminology, but in helping users to access services it is often useful to distinguish between those who are:

➤ 'deaf' (often written with a capital D): people who are born deaf or who become profoundly deaf in childhood and whose preferred language is British Sign Language (BSL)

➤ 'deafened': those who become profoundly deaf after acquiring spoken language in the usual way and who identify mainly with hearing people

➤ 'hard of hearing' or 'partially hearing': those who are hard of hearing but not profoundly deaf (mainly older people)

➤ 'Deafblind': those who have a severe degree of both visual and hearing impairment. It is not precisely defined, but does not necessarily imply that a person is completely blind or completely deaf. It has been estimated that 40 people in every 100 000 are deafblind. People aged over 65 are thought to account for more than 50% of those who are deafblind, and the incidence of deafblindness increases sharply after the age of 75. Causes of deafblindness vary, as does the point in life when a person becomes deafblind.

Until recently, the most common cause of dual sensory impairment among newborn babies was rubella contracted by the mother during pregnancy. Vaccination has reduced the incidence of rubella, but congenital deafblindness can also result from premature birth and birth trauma. Many of those who are deafblind from birth also have other disabilities (e.g., learning disability).

Some genetic conditions mean that people will become deafblind by the time they are young adults. For example, Usher's syndrome results in deafness from birth and gradual loss of sight in late childhood.

As the population ages, the number of people who are deafblind because of age-related visual and hearing impairment is growing.

It is important to take account of the particular needs of deafblind people in planning services. Mainstream services for people who are either visually or hearing impaired may not be appropriate, as they are likely to assume, for example, that a visually-impaired person has unimpaired hearing, which a deafblind person, by definition, does not. Social services authorities may be able to provide some figures on the number of people in the area whom they know to be deafblind, but it is important to recognise that, because of their disabilities, deafblind people may be less likely to access services on their own initiative. It is therefore all the more important for service providers to take active steps to identify the level of need.

The prevalence of hearing loss in the adult population of Britain is not available from routine data sources but can be derived from well-designed surveys (Figure 5.5).

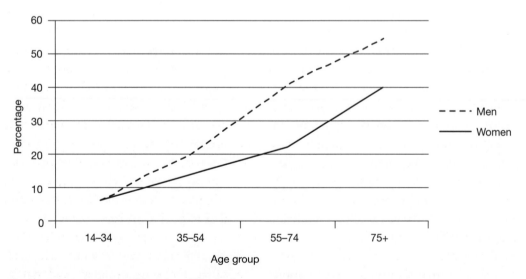

Figure 5.5 Prevalence of hearing difficulty by age and sex
Source: Davis A, Smith P, Ferguson M, *et al.* Acceptability, benefit and costs of early screening for hearing disability: a study of potential screening tests and models. *Health Technol Assess.* 2007; **11**(42): 1–294.

SERVICES FOR DISABLED PEOPLE

During World War I, rehabilitation regimes, including physiotherapy, hydrotherapy, remedial exercises and occupational therapy, were organised for orthopaedic cases. Meanwhile, the work of St Dunstan's Hospital for blinded soldiers and sailors showed how experts with a medical approach could train disabled people to acquire self-reliance and compensatory skills.

The large number of military and civilian casualties sustained during World War II brought about rapid innovations in rehabilitation methods and special schemes for disabled people. Under the Emergency Medical Service, a large number of hospitals were taken over by the Ministry of Health for the care of war casualties and evacuated civilian patients. The improved resources together with a commitment towards treating war casualties stimulated a progressive attitude. The range of occupations for which disabled men were trained greatly widened to include, for example, skilled engineering work. Rehabilitation methods similar in principle to those used in orthopaedic practice were applied to other categories of sick and injured people. Furthermore, an increasing emphasis was placed on the involvement of patients in their own treatment through techniques such as group exercise and remedial games.

The development of services for the rehabilitation of people with spinal injuries, although a specialised field, has also done much to stimulate improvements in rehabilitation services generally.

As with other groups with special needs, the emphasis in providing help, support and care for people with physical disability must lie in comprehensive needs assessment by all relevant agencies working together. Meeting the large range of health, social and other needs of people with a disability requires well-coordinated and managed services and a personalised approach in organising the care and support required. The Health Service is only one of the agencies involved in providing such care. Social services departments have the lead role in community care. Increasingly, the role of statutory health and social care bodies is to commission services that are provided by the 'third sector', which includes social enterprises and voluntary organisations.

MEDICAL AND REHABILITATION SERVICES

A cornerstone of the health services' response to disability is the provision of high-quality rehabilitation services. In the past, such services have grown up around wartime medicine, notably that of World War II and the Vietnam War. Survivors of serious injury often had considerable residual disability, and their function was often greatly improved by targeted intensive rehabilitation programmes. This whole issue is still very pertinent with the revival of interest in military medicine (and with it, rehabilitation techniques) as a result of the 21st century wars in Iraq and Afghanistan.

In Britain, although there have been some centres of excellence for rehabilitation medicine, the majority of local services have had to make do with general, rather than special, expertise. This is changing rapidly. It is now recognised that an organised, team-based approach to rehabilitation is an essential feature of local services for people with disability. Not only has there been a growth in rehabilitation as a specialty of medical practice, there has also been increased recognition of the value of therapy services. The continuing growth of voluntary and charitable organisations and of the disabled persons movement have also been important forces for change. It was the advent of the disabled persons independent living movement in the United States that was a major force in the development of rehabilitation and disability services in that country.

Rehabilitation services have a number of functions. Firstly, they must undertake a full assessment of the disabled person, ideally in their home or other place of residence. This will enable functional capacity to be assessed and the scope for restoration of lost functions and acquisition of new skills to be identified. It will also identify the need for equipment to be supplied or for adaptation to the person's home environment. Secondly, rehabilitation services will set out to establish a clear care plan, agreed with the person concerned and their carers (if any). Thirdly, the service will set in hand measures and services to deliver the care plan. The circumstances vary greatly. In some cases, rehabilitation will begin following an acute hospital admission – for example, because of stroke or traumatic injury. In other cases, rehabilitation services may be offered to someone who has had a long-standing condition, such as multiple sclerosis, but has never previously had help of this sort.

It is important to recognise that disabled people often have long-term care needs that will continue to benefit from rehabilitation services, and the notion of rehabilitation

as a single course of therapy is increasingly outmoded. This means that rehabilitation services will not be exclusively provided on a hospital site, but will be delivered on a community basis. Local rehabilitation teams are multi-professional, using skills such as physiotherapy, occupational therapy and speech and language therapy in addition to those of medicine and nursing.

Within the National Health Service, there are increasing numbers of consultant posts in rehabilitation medicine that are filled by people with specialist training. In addition to being core members of local rehabilitation teams, such consultants perform a liaison and specialist advisory role with consultants in other disciplines (for example, neurology, geriatric medicine, orthopaedics, rheumatology) where conditions giving rise to disability are commonly seen amongst their patient population.

While many hospitalised patients will be able to receive help from the rehabilitation team and still remain within the service that is treating their underlying condition, some designated hospital inpatient facilities are required specifically for the treatment of disabled people. During the latter part of the 1990s, there was a clear trend to establish a three-tier system of rehabilitation services. Local general hospitals have specialist inpatient units (stroke units are common, but more widely orientated disability units are also developing). Community teams then provide a link to the hospital-based service. Some of these community teams cover the full range of rehabilitation services and deal with all conditions. Others are more specialised (e.g., community multiple sclerosis teams, stroke early discharge teams).

Specialist facilities are also required for the rehabilitation of people with acute traumatic injury of the spinal cord and people who have sustained head injuries. The physical, psychological, social and financial consequences of both of these types of disability are profound and justify the specific attention of services to ensure high standards of care for the groups of patients concerned.

It is also important to ensure that services specifically address the needs of young people so that the transition from childhood to adulthood and from children's services to adult services is as smooth as possible. In many areas, advisory services for the disabled young school-leaver have been developed.

INDEPENDENT LIVING CENTRES AND CENTRES FOR INDEPENDENT LIVING

A major focus of local services for disabled people are the 'independent living centres' and 'centres for independent living' (two different types of body, despite their similar title). Independent living centres are still infrequent in the United Kingdom, but where they exist they act as a valuable resource and information facility and provide a wide range of aids, appliances and equipment for disabled people. Centres will undertake assessment to help people decide what sort of aids and equipment are most appropriate to their needs and will also provide advice and training on their use in the home environment. In some cases, this will involve home visiting by the centre's staff.

Most centres for independent living provide many additional services. Typically, they will give information and advice to disabled people and their families on issues such as health and social services, employment, benefits and entitlements. Their advisory function in relation to benefits may extend to an advocacy role and to representing disabled people at tribunals and hearings. They will also often serve as an educational resource to pass on expertise about caring for disabled people. Many centres are funded from charitable sources, but additional funding is usually also provided by health and local authorities. A local centre for independent living can provide continuity of support, advice and information to empower and enable disabled people to have access to the complex range of services that are available. Increasingly, organisations working with disabled people are user-led, and the 2005 government report *Improving Life Chances* recommended that by 2010 every local authority area should have a user-led organisation modelled on the existing centres for independent living.

SOME SPECIALIST SERVICES

While services such as those provided by the independent living centres and centres for independent living are intended to be accessible to all disabled people in a particular locality, the nature of some people's disabilities will mean that they have needs that can only be met by more specialised services. The nature of such services has developed in different ways around the country, either in response to a particular need, because of local initiatives, or as a result of the enthusiasm and commitment of certain individuals or organisations. Nevertheless, there are some specialist services that are more generally available. These may be based at independent living centres or centres for independent living or delivered from other locations.

Continence Services

Many disabled people experience a degree of urinary incontinence. This subject is discussed more fully in the chapter on elderly people, but much of the core service is the same. Because the embarrassment and stigma of incontinence of urine or faeces is particularly great, an important function of continence services is to promote awareness of the problem, as well as to provide practical help and support. Continence services are usually run by a continence adviser, invariably with a nursing background, who assesses the extent of the person's problem and advises on the most appropriate continence treatment, including continence and toileting equipment.

Stoma Care Services

A stoma is an artificial opening to the outside of the body from one of the internal organs. The more common types of stoma are created after bowel surgery for diseases such as cancer of the bowel, ulcerative colitis and Crohn's disease. A stoma may also involve the urinary tract. People who have a stoma have special needs for advice, counselling and practical support. Although this may be provided by the hospital surgical service that created the stoma, increasingly, specialist services using trained stoma care nurses or therapists provide preoperative counselling, after-care and continuing support to patients.

Tissue Viability Services

Pressure sores are a particular hazard for disabled people. Their consequences can be serious and their treatment is potentially very costly. They are preventable. Many pressure sores develop amongst people who are hospitalised, particularly the elderly. The avoidance of pressure sores in this group relies upon high-quality nursing care. Similarly, for people who are confined to bed in their own homes, skilled nursing care in the community will reduce the occurrence of pressure sores. For disabled people who use wheelchairs or whose mobility is seriously restricted, it is important that they receive advice and counselling from expert staff on the measures they need to take (regular shifting of position, weight distribution cushions, special mattresses) to avoid developing a pressure sore.

Counselling Services

The psychological consequences of disability are, for most affected people, profound. Counselling and psychological intervention can provide, therefore, an important and much valued element of core services for disabled people. Therefore, it is very important that this domain of disability is not regarded as a need to which services respond as an afterthought. There are very strong arguments for a counsellor being a core member of the professional team of every local disability service.

Driving Assessment Services

The dominant feature of many disabilities is restriction of physical mobility, with its potential to limit social contacts and produce difficulty in coping with aspects of independent living such as shopping, leisure or visiting places of entertainment. For many disabled people, a car or other means of personal transport will be one of the most important features of their lives. Disability arising from a wide range of causes will affect people's ability to drive (for example, stroke, epilepsy, muscular dystrophy, amputation, rheumatoid arthritis). A person's fitness to drive must be taken into account by the Driving and Vehicle Licensing Agency (DVLA), based in Swansea, whose staff (making use of medical advisers) will decide whether the disability could constitute a danger when driving. Medical reports and assessments will usually be required from the person's local doctor.

A disabled driver has three main needs: firstly, to be fully assessed; secondly, to be advised on the type of car most suited to his or her needs (with adaptations and modifications where appropriate); and thirdly, to receive advice on how to finance the purchase.

There are a number of assessment centres for disabled drivers around the country that provide these services, including the opportunities to try out particular vehicles and adaptations. Some also offer advice on wheelchairs and pavement vehicles. It is important that local disability services have good links with these centres so that they can ensure disabled people have access to them even though they may live some distance away.

Prosthetics and Orthotics

A prosthesis is a device that replaces a missing part – for example, the fitting of an artificial limb to a person who has lost all or part of their limb due to amputation because of trauma, vascular disease or cancer. There are many other types of prostheses, and they are becoming increasingly sophisticated as a result of advances in modern science and technology, as well as higher expectations of people themselves.

The fitting of prostheses is highly specialised and, in common with other services for disabled people, requires a service based upon an ethos of high-quality and patient-centred care. In the case of an artificial limb, the scope of the service should involve pre-operative counselling, the operation itself, the assessment and fitting of the prosthesis, gait or dexterity training, after-care and support. Such an approach requires general practitioners, surgeons, physiotherapists, occupational therapists, other members of the rehabilitation team, prosthetic fitters, engineers and suppliers working closely together. Increasingly, for example, it is recognised that the quality of a surgical amputation is a vital determining feature of a successful prosthesis for the patient. It is a growing practice for amputations to be performed by senior surgeons who undertake larger numbers of such operations and who work closely with the prosthetic and rehabilitation teams.

An orthosis is an appliance or piece of equipment that is attached to the body to enhance function. Orthoses can range from splints or collars applied to support an arthritic joint, through calliper-type devices used to assist movement where muscles are weak or paralysed, to devices that support or redistribute weight (for example, special footwear). The orthosis is usually arranged following a prescription by a consultant or physiotherapist. Orthotics is a well-established service for disabled people, but it could be better integrated into rehabilitation services. Many orthoses are supplied by private firms whose orthotist also does the assessment. This can lead to a conflict of interest. However, the NHS Purchasing and Supply Agency is well qualified to offer advice on contracting, quality and value for money.

Wheelchair and Special Seating Services

Wheelchairs are an important aid to mobility for disabled people. The majority are prescribed and supplied at local level by a therapist. Some disabled people will require a more specialised chair, and, in such cases, assessment and supply may have to be arranged at a centre serving a wider population. A wide range of wheelchairs (non-powered and powered) are available, both for indoor and outdoor use. The wheelchair service is also responsible for assessing and providing special seating for disabled people with major postural problems.

Communication Devices

Difficulties with speech and communication are an important consequence of some causes of disability. For this reason, a speech and language therapist should also be a member of the team providing core rehabilitation services for disabled people at local level.

In addition to speech and language therapy services, some people can greatly benefit from an electronic device for communication. Each person should receive careful individual assessment to determine which of the many communication devices is best suited to his or her needs. Communication devices are normally provided through a network of communication aids centres. Equipment ranges from simple voice amplifiers to devices controlled by non-affected parts of the body (for example, eyeball, finger, chin, and toe) that will link up to electronic typewriters, computers, or to the more complex communication and environmental controls systems.

The most fundamental development for those who otherwise would be profoundly deaf has been the cochlear implant programme which operates through a network of centres across the United Kingdom serving both children and adults. Implants work through stimulation of the auditory nerve by means of an internally implanted electrode assembly. The level and quality of the follow-up following implantation is crucial to achieving maximum benefit.

Equipment for Sensory Impairment

It is important to ensure that people with sight or hearing impairments have had a proper clinical assessment. They must also have access to medical and surgical treatment where they can potentially benefit from it. Having said this, a proportion of people with sight or hearing impairments will have a condition that is not amenable to specific intervention. The approach is then to ensure that they receive equipment to minimise the degree of disability caused by their condition. For deaf people, this can mean the fitting of a hearing aid or other devices to assist amplification of sound, provision of equipment for the home (such as lights on telephones and door bells) and provision of vibration devices for the profoundly deaf.

Similarly, the range of equipment available for blind people is now quite large. Longer-term measures used in the rehabilitation of blind people include teaching them to read Braille and Moon and to touch-type. Some of these services are more appropriate for the younger blind rather than they are for very elderly people. The British Wireless for the Blind Fund can arrange for any registered blind person in need of a radio to have one. Free membership is available to blind people for the National Library for the Blind and for the Royal National Institute for Blind People, which also has a large talking-book library.

Braille dials can be fitted to most gas and electric cookers. Clocks and watches are available with special markings, and embossed playing cards, chess, dominoes, draughts and other games are obtainable.

Telecare

The ability to use remote monitoring to support people with disability to live independently has led to a substantial growth in the field of telecare. It is estimated that there are 1.5 million telecare installations in England alone. The services provided using telecare can range from simple pendent alarms to more complex telehealth systems that can remotely monitor cardiac and respiratory conditions. The potential benefits from the development of telecare include reduction in the frequency of admissions to hospital or residential care and the reassurance provided to users and their relatives and carers.

PRIMARY CARE AND COMMUNITY SERVICES

Many of the services for disabled people already described in this section are delivered to people living in the community. Most disabled people will be registered with a general practitioner. Through this, they will have access to the services provided by or commissioned by a primary care trust, including home nursing, dietetic services and chiropody services, as well as general medical care. However, many disabled people may not be in regular contact with their general practitioner. Thus, while general practitioners provide a logical point of contact for disabled people, the numbers and requirements of disabled people in the practice population may not be clearly identified. Community social care services such as meals at home, home care help and care assistants that are most often provided for older people (as described in Chapter 8) can also be provided to younger disabled people.

DAY CARE

Day care should be an important component in the network of services for disabled people. It is mainly provided by either social services departments or by certain voluntary organisations, although specialist hospital facilities may develop a day care service alongside acute work.

Regular attendance at a day care centre can facilitate important social contact and access to other specialist services. On a more practical level, meals are usually provided in the day care setting. Such measures also provide a safe and comfortable environment. Some day care, particularly that provided by voluntary organisations, has social integration as its main aim. It focuses on providing social activities for both able-bodied and disabled people. Such organisations tend to operate on an informal, drop-in basis.

SUPPORT FOR CARERS

Adequate support for those providing informal care for disabled people is an increasingly important aim of statutory services. It is a key feature of the formal arrangements for community care described at various points in this book in relation to other care groups. Carers must be fully involved in the assessment process, not only as partners with statutory agencies in providing care for disabled people, but also as individuals who have their own needs.

The support that carers need has two dimensions. The first is aimed at providing the carer with a break. Services such as sitting services, respite care services, emergency cover and holiday care are all examples of what is required to enable the carer to be relieved of the task of caring for a short time. It is particularly important that respite services are available when carers want them and that there is continuity of care among respite personnel.

The second type of support for carers is aimed at helping the carer directly in the caring role. Examples would be education about lifting the disabled person and preventing pressure sores or about managing incontinence. Opportunities to form and participate in carers' support groups are also useful. Here, as is the case with all disability services, it is extremely important that health and social services agencies work together so that the full spectrum of carers' needs can be addressed.

RESIDENTIAL CARE

Different agencies are involved in providing residential accommodation: local authorities, voluntary organisations and the private sector. The NHS has responsibility for those with continuing health care needs. The type of residential accommodation needed by disabled people depends on individual requirements.

EMPLOYMENT AND TRAINING

Work, although a means of financing household necessities and leisure pursuits, also provides status and self-esteem for the individual and is the basis of many social contacts. Indeed, for some it represents the main focus of their lives. The work orientation of many modern societies is a source of additional pressure for disabled people. Even those who are more severely disabled will perceive work as a means of drawing closer to other members of society.

Careers guidance is important to help people, particularly young people, decide which option is best for them to fulfil their potential. The Careers Service, as part of its ongoing work, will focus its help on those who need it most, including those with learning disabilities.

There are a number of measures in place to help disabled adults and young people access and remain in employment. Work-based provision for young people is important and includes Modern Apprenticeships, National Traineeships and other specific training provisions.

The majority of disabled adults will be helped through the mainstream employment and training measures delivered by the Jobcentre Plus, an agency of the Department for Work and Pensions. Advice is available from the local Jobcentre. This provision includes Programme Centres, which modularise training to meet individual needs, Work Trials and work-based learning for adults.

In addition, there is a range of specialist disability measures. Disabled people have access to the specialist disability employment advisers in the local Jobcentres or Jobcentre Plus offices. As well as providing general advice to individuals and employers, they will be able to give details of the specialist disability measures. These include Access to Work, which provides help in the form of funding for equipment, adaptations, fares to work and communicator/interpreter support. The Job Introduction Scheme provides a subsidy to employers for an agreed number of weeks to assist employers to introduce an individual into a particular job.

The supported employment programme known as WORKSTEP assists in providing employment for people whose disabilities are more severe. The actual employment is provided by organisations such as Remploy and voluntary bodies and local authorities, and it can be supported placements with employers or in sheltered workshops or factories. Remploy was founded in 1944 and was created to assist ex-service people. It provides both direct employment opportunities and recruitment services to help people with disabilities gain mainstream employment.

Courses under the title Work Preparation are available to help individuals to return to work following a long period of illness. The courses are short-term and help individuals by addressing the specific employment-related needs that result from their disability and prevent them from taking up work or vocational training of a type that would otherwise be suitable for them.

In addition to work-based learning for adults, mentioned earlier, there is specialist residential training provision for adults at 10 colleges throughout England, and the courses can also be accessed by Scottish and Welsh residents, as there is no provision in those countries. These courses are accessed by disabled people in collaboration with their local disability employment adviser in the first place.

BENEFITS AND ALLOWANCES

Many disabled people have a lower earning capacity than other members of society and are over-represented in the lower socio-economic groups. By the nature of their disability as well as on the basis of their level of income, disabled people are entitled to a wide range of benefits, special payments and income support. Informal carers for disabled people also have certain entitlements.

The whole system of financial support is quite complex and changes rapidly but the broad range of benefits available covers a wide range of areas of need (Table 5.5). An important component of services for disabled people and their carers is a mechanism to ensure that they are receiving their full entitlements. In practice, this means the provision of leaflets and other printed information in an easily readable form coupled with access to people who are skilled in the interpretation of the regulations and who can give specific advice and help. It is not surprising that specialist advisory staff are often in great demand where they are part of a Centre for Independent Living.

DISABLED RIGHTS

The Disability Discrimination Acts of 1995 and 2005 have substantially increased the rights of people with disabilities. Not only is it illegal to discriminate against disabled people, but the legislation gives rights to disabled people in the areas of housing, transport, education and in access to everyday services and locations. As well as rights in service provision, the legislation also places duties on health service providers to make information available in accessible formats where it is reasonable to do so.

In 2007, the Equality and Human Rights Commission came into being, thus replacing separate bodies covering the fields of racial, gender and disability rights. The Commission also took on new equality roles in the areas of age, sexual orientation and religious belief. The Commission has extensive powers to enforce the equality duties that rest with health services and other public bodies.

CONCLUSIONS

The value attached to disabled people and the extent to which they are regarded and treated as full members of the population is an important indicator of how caring a society is. Identifying the number of people in the population who are disabled and describing the nature of their disability and the needs that result from it has not been accorded a high priority in the past. Assessing need at both individual and population level is a key prerequisite to the provision of appropriate services and requires attention being given to gathering and maintaining high-quality information. Services for disabled people will be most effective when they are based on such needs assessment and when they are founded on teamwork – both at the organisational (health, local authority and voluntary agency) and at the individual level (doctors, nurses, therapists, social workers).

Table 5.5 Key components of the benefit system

Benefit/Allowance	Eligibility
Disability Living Allowance (DLA)	Available to both children and adults up to the age of 65. Two components: Care component Mobility component. Not means-tested.
Carer's Allowance (CA)	Available to a parent or person who regularly spends 35 hours or more caring for someone who is disabled. Not means-tested.
Incapacity Benefit	Available to adults who are unable to work because of sickness or disability and who do not qualify for statutory sick pay (SSP). Paid at three rates – short-term low, short-term high and long-term. A contribution record may be required in some cases.
Income Support (IS)	Available to all adults under the age of 60 and on a low income. If a disabled person qualifies for Income Support, they may be entitled to additional payments (known as premiums). Income Support is means-tested.
Housing/Council Tax Benefit	Available to those on a low income to assist with paying rent or council tax bills. Means-tested.
Community Care (Direct Payments) Act 1996	This gives authority for local social service departments, after assessing a person's need, to award a financial payment as an alternative to giving a service. This then enables an individual to purchase and administer their own care service.
Working Tax Credit	For disabled persons, this benefit incorporates Disabled Person's Tax Credit and Working Family Tax Credit. Available to people working more than 16 hours a week and whose disability puts them at a disadvantage in finding employment.
Motability/Blue Badge Scheme	Motability is a scheme to help people with disabilities and those that care for them buy or hire a car, wheelchair or scooter. The Blue Badge Scheme (formerly known as the Orange Badge Scheme) covers parking entitlements, such as free parking in metered areas.
Attendance Allowance	Available to anyone aged 65 and over who requires care and attention with their personal needs.
Independent Living Fund (ILF)	A weekly financial allowance to support disabled people to continue to live independently in the community. Available to those who are already in receipt of local authority services; a care plan is agreed between the local authority, ILF and claimant, to which the ILF make a financial contribution. Contributions are made as a direct payment.

CHAPTER 6
Mothers and Children

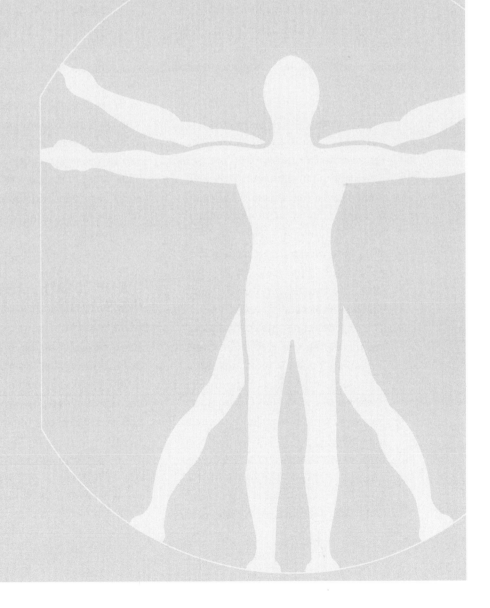

INTRODUCTION

Until about 70 years ago, childbirth was an event that threatened the life of both mother and baby. Deaths of women in labour were not uncommon, and children's funerals were a prominent feature of everyday life.

Throughout the ages, children have been subjected to harsh and inhuman treatment and, until the twentieth century, infanticide was a common occurrence in England. It is not always appreciated that the famous politician and Prime Minister of the last century Benjamin Disraeli (1804–81) was also a novelist. A quotation from *Sybil, or the Two Nations* is an eloquent commentary on life at that time for some mothers and children:

> About a fortnight after his mother had introduced him into the world, she returned to her factory and put her infant out to nurse: that is to say, paid three pence a week to an old woman, who takes charge of these newborn babies for the day and gives them back at night to their mothers as they hurriedly return from the scene of their labour to the dungeon or the den, which is still by courtesy called 'home'. The expense is not great: laudanum and treacle, administered in the shape of some popular elixir, affords these innocents a brief taste of the sweets of existence and, keeping them quiet, prepares them for the silence of their impending grave. Infanticide is practised as extensively and as legally in England as it is on the banks of the Ganges: a circumstance which apparently has not yet engaged the attention of the Society for the Propagation of the Gospel in Foreign Parts.

From the beginning of the last century up to modern times, there has been a steep decline both in maternal deaths and in mortality in the early years of life and later childhood. There is still considerable scope for improvement. In particular, many aspects of health inequalities are at their starkest amongst children.

This chapter deals with the health of children and the health of mothers around the time of childbirth. The main ways of assessing health and need in these sections of the population are described. The scope for the promotion of health in the early years of life is discussed in relation to the prevention of foetal loss and of foetal anomalies, as well as the measures required to improve health amongst women of childbearing age. The range of services that are provided for mothers and children are described and, where appropriate, set in their statutory framework.

BIRTHS, DEATHS AND FERTILITY
REGISTRATION OF BIRTHS AND STILLBIRTHS

Registration of births and stillbirths is a legal requirement. The information is collected by the local registrar of births, marriages and deaths and transmitted to the Office for National Statistics in England and Wales. Every birth must be registered:

➤ by a parent or other informant
➤ with the local registrar
➤ within 42 days of birth.

In Northern Ireland, comparable arrangements apply, while in Scotland they are slightly different (e.g., births must be registered within 21 days).

If a birth occurs anywhere in the world on a United Kingdom-registered aircraft, under the Civil Aviation Act 1982 the owner of the aircraft must notify the Civil Aviation Authority by completing a birth notification form. The Civil Aviation Authority will then send a copy of the entry from their register to the appropriate registrar's office.

Information collected on the public record of a birth registration covers date and place of birth; the baby's name and surname and its sex; the name, address and place of birth of parents (although father's details may be omitted if the mother is unmarried); the occupation of the father and, optionally, the mother (if both names appear on the certificate) or the mother (if only her name appears); the surnames by which the mother has been known (e.g., name at the time of the birth, other former names, maiden name at first marriage); and details of the informant. Confidential information is also collected (but not entered in the register) that includes:

- the father's date of birth, if his name is entered in the register
- the mother's date of birth in all cases
- If the child's parents were married to each other at the time of the birth
- the month and year of the parents' marriage
- whether the mother has been married more than once
- the number of the mother's previous children by her present husband and any former husband – those born alive (including any who have died since) and those stillborn.

Further information is also collected on a voluntary basis or obtained from the birth notification for statistical purposes (e.g., birth weight, additional details on multiple births, parent's employment status).

As with live births, the same legal obligation exists to ensure registration of stillbirths. The legal definition of a stillbirth as amended by the Stillbirth (Definition) Act 1992 is: 'A child which has issued forth from its mother after the 24th week of pregnancy and which did not at any time after, having been completely expelled from its mother, breathe or show any other signs of life.'

Stillbirths may only be registered within three months from the date of stillbirth. In addition to the information recorded at a live birth, information is obtained from the medical certificate of stillbirth (e.g., on cause of death, gestational age, post-mortem).

NOTIFICATION OF BIRTHS

In addition to birth registration, a parallel process of birth notification takes place. The midwife, doctor or other attendant at the birth is required to notify the primary care trust in England (or local health board in Wales) for the area where the birth took place (s.124(4) of the NHS Act 1977, as amended by Statutory Instrument 2002/2469) within 36 hours.

The Central Issuing System (CIS) now has responsibility for issuing blocks of NHS numbers under the NHS Numbers for Babies (NN4B) project. This system checks notifications and passes them to child health departments in primary care trusts. The information usually reported in this notification includes birth weight, length of gestation, parity and the presence of foetal anomaly.

It is important to understand that registration and notification of births serve different purposes. Registration is essentially intended to record the fact of birth, legal parentage and the name by which the child will be known and to issue a birth certificate. It also enables the collection of certain information for statistical purposes. Notification is intended to alert health services to the birth of the child so that the necessary care can be provided to support the mother and her new baby. Here there is a need for urgency in passing on the information about the birth of the child. There is also an exchange of information between the health service and the registrar of births and deaths. NHS trusts and primary care trusts pass on brief information on the notification of births to the registrar as they are received in order to assist in obtaining full registration. The only medical information that is transferred is birth weight, which is passed by registrars to the Office for National Statistics and is not a legal requirement. When added to the other data collected at birth registration, it allows statistics of live and stillbirths to include this important variable.

REGISTRATION OF DEATHS

As with births, deaths of babies must also be registered, in this case within five days of their occurrence. In the mid-1980s, new certificates were introduced in England and Wales to cover stillbirth and neonatal death (death of a baby born alive but dying in the first four weeks of life). Certification accords with World Health Organization standards. The certificate includes information on both maternal and foetal causal factors (Table 6.1). Deaths occurring after the neonatal period are certified by a doctor and are also then registered with the local registrar of births, marriages and deaths.

ASCERTAINMENT AND VALIDITY

Ascertainment of births through the registration process in Britain is high. The vast majority of births are registered by the parent or another proper informant. Any birth where there has been contact with a health care professional will, in addition, be picked up through the crosscheck of the notification system. There are a small number of births (for example, as a result of concealed pregnancy) where there may be further delay in registration. On the whole, in Britain the quality of information on birth certificates is very good, although there may be problems with variation in the names used by parents on certificates.

Ascertainment of death in infancy is also virtually complete. Only those deaths that are concealed following criminal violence may fail for a considerable period to be recognised. However, there is delay in the registration of those deaths where there has been a coroner's inquest. Information on cause of death as registered is not always reliable. It is most likely to be accurate if there has been a post-mortem examination.

Internationally, systems for birth and death registration vary and may be weak in some parts of the developing world. It is important to bear this in mind when comparing mortality rates in infancy and childhood internationally. In some parts of the developing world, particularly those where there is disruption due to natural disasters, war or famine, information on infant and perinatal mortality is available only from ad hoc surveys, usually conducted by international aid organisations.

INDICES OF FERTILITY
Crude Birth Rate

The number of live births, expressed as a rate per 1000 total population per annum, is the annual crude birth rate. Although often quoted, it is a poor indicator of fertility because included in the denominator are men, children and post-menopausal women (the limitations of crude rates are discussed in Chapter 1).

General Fertility Rate

A better denominator is used in the general fertility rate, which is calculated by expressing the number of live births per 1000 women in the population of childbearing age (by convention this is usually taken as those aged 15–44 years).

Age-specific Fertility Rates

Because there are differences in levels of fertility amongst women of different ages within the childbearing years, an even more precise measure of fertility is obtained by calculating the number of births to a specified age group per 1000 women of that same age group. For example, the fertility rate for women aged 20–24 is calculated by taking the number of live births occurring to mothers aged 20–24 and expressing them per 1000 women aged between 20 and 24 in the population.

Total Period Fertility Rate

The total period fertility rate is a convenient summary of all the age-specific rates. This rate is the sum of the age-specific fertility rates, in this case expressed as live births per woman of a single age, rather than per 1000 women. It measures the average number of live-born children per woman that would occur if the current age-specific fertility rates applied over the entire 30 years of the reproductive span. It therefore takes account of differential fertility within the different reproductive age groups, while providing a convenient summary measure in a single figure. It can be thought of as reflecting the average number of children that would be

Table 6.1 Cause-of-death categories in the certification of stillbirth and neonatal death

• Main diseases or conditions in the foetus or infant
• Other diseases or conditions in the foetus or infant
• Main maternal diseases or conditions affecting the foetus or infant
• Other maternal diseases or conditions affecting the foetus or infant
• Other relevant causes

born to women who experienced the age-specific fertility rates of the year in question throughout their reproductive lives. It enables comparisons to be made between countries and within the same country over time because it is not affected by the age distribution of women in the reproductive age groups.

Cohort Measures of Fertility

All indices of fertility so far described have referred to births at a specific period of time, most often a single year. However, births in any given year occur to a cross-section of women married at different ages and with differing numbers of previous children. Temporary fluctuations in 'period' indices may simply reflect the timing of births within a reproductive lifespan without any important change in the number of children women will have by the time they have come to the end of their reproductive years.

A cohort of women is a population of women who were born in a particular year (generation or birth cohort). Studies of fertility following such cohorts of women observe the occurrence and timing of births in their reproductive lifetime. The cohort fertility rate (which gives the completed family size for women born around the same time) provides a much more stable basis for commenting on trends and predicting future levels of fertility than do measures based on a specific period of time (Figure 6.1). The cohort fertility rate has the disadvantage that it cannot properly be calculated until the cohort concerned has completely passed out of the childbearing years.

TRENDS IN FERTILITY

A fall in fertility in Britain during the economic depression of the 1930s stimulated considerable national concern about the long-term growth of the population. An increase in the birth rate occurred after World War II, and since that time fertility has been dominated by two distinct trends. During the decade between the mid-1950s and the mid-1960s, the number of births, the crude birth rate, the general fertility rate and the total period fertility rate all rose, reaching a peak in the mid-1960s (the so-called 'baby boom' generation). The succeeding decade showed a sharp fall in the same indices of fertility. In 1977, the crude birth rate, the general fertility rate and the total period fertility rate all fell below their corresponding values in 1933 – the previous lowest level of this century.

By the beginning of the 1990s, fertility had increased well above its low point in 1977, but not to the high level of the 1960s. Changes in the fertility rates in the 1960s and 1970s have not been properly explained and were largely unpredicted. There has been a recovery from the low of the mid-1970s, and by 2007 the total period fertility rate had reached 1.91 – its highest level since 1973. This is, however, still below the natural population replacement level of 2.1. This has not stopped the population growing, because the number of deaths remained below births and inward migration. Trends in the key indices over the past decade are shown in Table 6.2.

The greatest numbers of births now occur in the 30–34 age group (Figure 6.2). Fertility rates amongst younger women declined from the late 1960s onwards. For example, in England and Wales in 1971 the birth rate amongst women aged 20–25 years was more than double that of women aged 30–34 years.

There has also been an increase in childlessness over successive cohorts of women. Amongst the 1945 cohort, 34% were childless at 25 years of age, compared with 61% for those born in 1969. There may be some catching up in the older years for this cohort, but not enough to reverse what seems to be the genuine option of childlessness for more couples.

Another trend during the final part of the twentieth century in the United Kingdom was the increase in the proportion of births that occurred outside marriage (from around 9% in 1976 to 44% in 2007). The change in the structure of society is also illustrated by the decline over time in the proportion of births outside marriage

where the birth registration contained the details of only one parent. This reduced from 55% in 1971 to only 15% in 2007.

Generally, levels of fertility have been higher for women born outside the United Kingdom. In England and Wales in 2007, the estimated total fertility rate for women born in the United Kingdom was 1.8, while the rate for women born outside the United Kingdom was 2.5.

FACTORS AFFECTING FERTILITY

In few societies do women produce the maximum number of children of which they are physiologically capable. Factors that determine sexual behaviour in society are wide-ranging and complex. They include the influence of society's norms and expectations, the family, the law, social and psychological factors, religion and lifestyle.

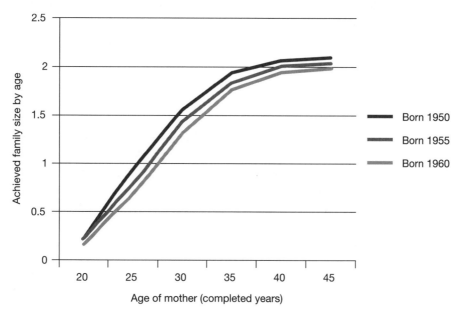

Figure 6.1 Cohort fertility of women born in the United Kingdom
Source: Government Actuary's Department.

Table 6.2 Changes in the key live-birth statistics for England and Wales, 1997–2007

Year	1997	1998	1999	2000	2001	2002	2003	2004	2005	2006	2007
General fertility rate	60.0	59.2	57.8	55.9	54.7	54.7	56.8	58.2	58.3	60.2	61.9
Total period fertility rate	1.73	1.72	1.70	1.65	1.63	1.65	1.73	1.78	1.79	1.86	1.91

Source: Office for National Statistics, 2008.

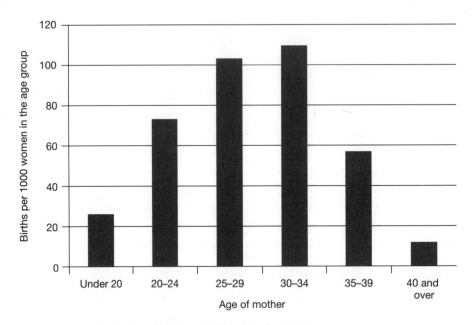

Figure 6.2 Age-specific fertility rates, England and Wales 2007
Source: Office for National Statistics, 2008.

Availability and use of contraception, levels of economic prosperity and patterns of marriage and cohabitation may also have independent effects on the number of children a woman may have.

A number of explanations have been put forward to account for the changes in fertility that have occurred during the twentieth century. Three common interpretations of the trends are as follows:

a   *Contraceptive availability*. This refers to the widespread availability of modern contraceptive methods, particularly the introduction of oral contraception in Britain in the early 1960s. However, fertility fell in a similar way in the 1930s, when contraceptive technology was primitive. Trends in fertility similar to those seen in Britain over the last 20 years occurred in other industrial societies in western Europe, North America and Australia and not all these countries had well-developed family planning services. It seems unlikely that the availability of the oral contraceptive pill is the entire story.

b *Level of affluence.* Levels of income and attitudes towards future prosperity are said to be influential. Hence a parallel is drawn between the economic depression of the 1930s, which is considered to have been largely responsible for the reduction in fertility at that time, and the downturn in fertility in the early 1970s, when an economic recession also prevailed. However, the decline in fertility had started well before the financial crisis brought about by the increase in oil prices in 1973; so, once again, this cannot be the whole explanation.

c *Working women.* More women of childbearing age now enter the labour force. It is believed that women restrict their family size in order to progress their career. However, the upward trend in the proportion of married women at work was just as steep during the rise in fertility in the early 1960s as it was during the decline in the 1970s.

It is probable that all three factors, as well as others, influence fertility in a complex manner that is not fully understood – which illustrates the difficulty in predicting trends in fertility, even in the relatively short-term.

FEMALE GENITAL MUTILATION

Female genital mutilation, a problem usually associated with developing countries, particularly in Africa, has serious short- and long-term consequences for the health of the girls and women on whom it is inflicted. It involves damaging the female genital tissue and it interferes with normal biological functioning.

It is estimated that across the world some 100 to 140 million girls and women have been subjected to this form of mutilation. There are reports of it being performed amongst some immigrant communities in Europe, and the consequences of the mutilation are seen in hospital settings in many countries, including the United Kingdom. As well as the immediate consequences of mutilation, which is often carried out under unsanitary conditions, there are long-term risks of maternal morbidity and higher rates of perinatal mortality amongst the babies of women who have been subject to the practice.

The campaign to end this barbaric practice is making slow progress, and a major concern is the evidence of increasing numbers of medical professionals being involved in carrying it out. The main thrust of the campaign to eliminate the practice is to enact legislation and to ensure enforcement of those laws. In addition, community education activities, amongst men as well as women, are seen as an important way of turning the tide against mutilation.

Successive United Kingdom governments have taken a strong position on the subject of female genital mutilation, and the practice was made illegal in the United Kingdom in 1985. Further legislation in 2003 (2005 in Scotland) made it illegal for United Kingdom nationals or permanent residents to have any role in the procedure, whether in the United Kingdom or abroad.

MORTALITY AMONGST MOTHERS AND BABIES

Internationally, comparison of maternal, infant and childhood mortality is a vital epidemiological tool, and these three measures are powerful indicators of the general health of the population. Traditionally they have been used as an indicator of a nation's health since they are closely related to standard of living, to inequalities in social and economic status within the country concerned and to the quality of medical care. In the developed world, differences still occur across populations in maternal, perinatal and infant mortality because of these underlying influences. However, as rates fell during the twentieth century, the number of deaths in developed countries has been relatively small. Measures of mortality are not, therefore, as useful – particularly when looking at smaller populations. It is also important to measure disease and disability and to concentrate on underlying factors in exploring unexplained deaths or foetal anomalies.

MATERNAL MORTALITY

Improvements in the general health of women, general medical advances (for example, the advent of antibiotics and blood transfusion), a reduction in the number of illegal abortions, together with improved standards of obstetric care and anaesthetic care, all contributed to a major decline in maternal mortality during the twentieth century. In 1847, the maternal mortality rate was around six per 1000 total births and fell to around four per 1000 births by 1937. A sharp fall in the rate occurred after 1937, probably due to the introduction of sulphonamides. The rate for the United Kingdom in 2003–05 was 14 per 100 000 maternities. The denominator for this rate, 'maternities', refers to pregnancies that result in a live birth or stillbirth. There is real concern that the rate has ceased to fall in recent years (Table 6.3).

A maternal death is defined by the World Health Organization as: '. . . the death of a woman while pregnant or within 42 days of termination of pregnancy, from any cause related to or aggravated by the pregnancy or its management, but not from accidental or incidental causes.'

Maternal deaths are subdivided into 'direct', 'indirect', 'fortuitous' and 'late'. Direct maternal deaths are those resulting from obstetric complications of pregnancy, labour and the puerperium. Indirect maternal deaths are those arising from an existing disease or from one that developed in pregnancy and whose effects were accelerated or altered by the pregnancy. Fortuitous maternal deaths are those resulting from causes not related to or influenced by pregnancy. The term 'fortuitous' is replaced by the term 'coincidental' in the United Kingdom because of the happy connotations of the former term. Late deaths are those that occur more than 42 days but less than one year after the end of the pregnancy, and these can be direct, indirect or fortuitous.

There are two measures of maternal mortality used in this country. The most accurate is based on the working of the Confidential Enquiry into Maternal and Child Health (CEMACH), as it is based on a proactive system of ascertainment. The rate used for the purpose of international

Table 6.3 Maternal mortality* in the United Kingdom, 1985–2005

Years	1985–87	1988–90	1991–93	1994–96	1997–99	2000–02	2003–05
Number	223	238	228	268	242	261	295
Rate**	9.83	10.08	9.85	12.19	11.40	13.07	13.95

* Direct and indirect deaths known to the Confidential Enquiry into Maternal and Child Health. ** Rate per 100 000 maternities.
Source: Lewis G, editor. Confidential Enquiry into Maternal and Child Health (CEMACH). *Saving Mothers' Lives: reviewing maternal deaths to make motherhood safer 2003–2005. The Seventh Report on Confidential Enquiries into Maternal Deaths in the United Kingdom.* London: CEMACH; 2007.

comparison is calculated by the Office for National Statistics (ONS) on the basis of death certificates that indicate a pregnancy-related cause. The former rate is significantly higher than the ONS-calculated rate.

The system of reviewing individual maternal deaths was established in England and Wales more than 50 years ago and has covered the whole of the United Kingdom since 1985. Because of the small numbers involved, the review reports every three years and is carried out on a confidential basis. The triennial report of the Confidential Enquiry into Maternal Deaths in the United Kingdom covering the years 2003–05, entitled *Saving Mothers' Lives*, was published in 2007.

The Enquiry has five regional offices in England and partner offices in Northern Ireland, Scotland and Wales. Using a standard enquiry form, information is collected from the various health staff concerned with the care of the woman. These may include general practitioners, midwives, health visitors, consultant obstetricians and anaesthetists. The completed form is forwarded to an obstetric and midwifery assessor (and, where appropriate, to an anaesthetic, pathology or midwifery assessor). The assessors add their comments and opinions regarding the cause of death. Each case is subject to a two-stage, regional and then central review and assessment process. Strict confidentiality is observed at all stages, and reports based on the analysis are published every three years. The reports draw general conclusions about causes of maternal deaths and changes over time, and they make recommendations for action based upon the lessons learned.

Since the 1970s, the two leading causes of direct maternal death have been pulmonary embolism and hypertension in pregnancy. However, the rate of death from genital-tract sepsis continues to rise, and in the most recent report the number of deaths from this cause equalled the number caused by hypertensive disorders. Suicide, which had been the single greatest cause (direct or indirect) of death in the previous period, showed a decline. Of those women who died from any cause, including those unrelated to pregnancy, a third were either single and unemployed or in a relationship where both partners were unemployed. A total of 14% were victims of domestic abuse and 11% had problems with substance abuse.

Despite the relatively low level of maternal deaths compared to the past, reports of the Confidential Enquiries into Maternal

Deaths continue to make recommendations that, if implemented, would bring about further improvements. The most recent triennial report contains a 'top ten' of recommendations that contain important public health messages concerning migrant women and other issues surrounding access to care. Past reports have highlighted issues such as diagnostic errors; inappropriate treatment; the need for better communication between doctors, midwives and other professional staff involved in caring for pregnant women; greater involvement of consultants during pregnancy and labour; and a failure to recognise and act upon potential problems when they develop.

REGIONAL INEQUALITIES IN MORTALITY

The nature of the causative factors for deaths around the time of birth and up to one year of age would suggest there might be a significant inequality in the mortality rates across the country because of the variation in social conditions. This is indeed borne out by the data. Such regional variation occurs across the various mortality rates in a fairly consistent pattern. For example, the infant mortality rates for 2007 show the highest level of infant mortality to occur in the West Midlands and the lowest in the South East (Figure 6.3).

To look comparatively at one year's figures for areas smaller than regions is difficult because of the small numbers involved. For example, in Wales in 2006 the lowest infant mortality rate was 1.7 in Ceredigion and the highest was 7.2 in Anglesey, but the number of deaths involved was only one in the former and five in the latter. It is for this reason that five-year rolling rates are frequently used, as this smoothes out the wide year-on-year variation that can occur if only one year's data is examined.

MORTALITY IN EARLY LIFE

Death rates in infancy are constructed differently from the mortality rates of later childhood and adult life. Births occurring during the same period as the deaths, not the population of a particular age group, is the denominator. 'Infancy' is taken as the first year of life, and thus the infant mortality rate in a given period of time (usually a year) is the number of deaths of children under the age of one year (numerator) per 1000 live births in the same period.

The infant mortality rate has long been regarded as an important measure of the health of a community. However, it is a rather crude indicator because deaths occurring during different periods of the first year of life usually reflect different groups of causal factors. It has become customary to consider deaths in infancy in a number of different time periods.

a   Perinatal deaths – deaths from the 24th week of gestation up to six completed days of life.

b   Early neonatal deaths – deaths between birth and six complete days of life.

c   Late neonatal deaths – deaths from seven to 27 completed days of life.

d   Neonatal deaths – deaths in the first 27 completed days of life.

e   Post-neonatal deaths – deaths at 28 days but under one year of life.

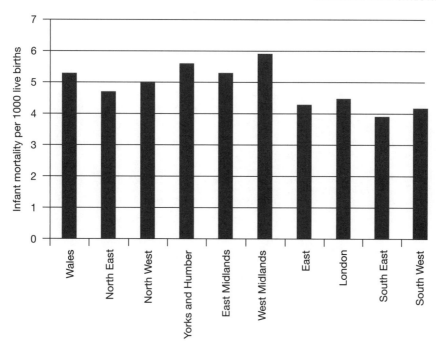

Figure 6.3 Infant mortality in Wales and the English regions, 2007
Source: Office for National Statistics.

The formal definitions of these rates are shown in Table 6.4. The various mortality rates are constructed around these different periods of infancy (Figure 6.4). The numerator is all deaths occurring within the period of infancy in question (usually during a calendar year), the denominator is the number of registered live births during that same calendar year. The exceptions to this general rule are stillbirths (babies born dead after 24 weeks of gestation) and perinatal deaths (stillbirths plus babies dying in the first week after birth), where the denominator in each case is total births (i.e., both live and stillbirths). In other words, when stillbirths are included in the numerator, then the denominator is total births, not live births alone. Records of infant deaths

are routinely linked nationally to their birth certificates. This enables such deaths to be analysed using data collected at birth registration (which is more extensive).

Perinatal deaths

Amongst the reasons for using this index, which groups together stillbirths and deaths in the first week of life, is that the factors responsible for these two types of death are often similar, being those operating before or around the time of birth. Another practical reason is that it overcomes some of the difficulties (particularly in making international comparisons) of variation between different localities as to which babies are regarded as stillborn and which as having

Table 6.4 Definitions of annual mortality rates of infancy

Stillbirth rate	Number of stillbirths per 1000 total births per annum
Perinatal mortality rate	Number of stillbirths together with deaths up to six completed days of life per 1000 total births per annum
Early neonatal mortality rate	Number of deaths up to six completed days of life per 1000 live births per annum
Late neonatal mortality rate	Number of deaths between the 7th and 27th completed days of life per 1000 live births per annum
Neonatal mortality rate	Number of deaths in the first 27 completed days of life per 1000 live births per annum
Post-neonatal mortality rate	Number of deaths at ages 28 days and over but before the end of the first year of life per 1000 live births per annum
Infant mortality rate	Number of deaths from the first day of life to the end of the first year of life per 1000 live births per annum

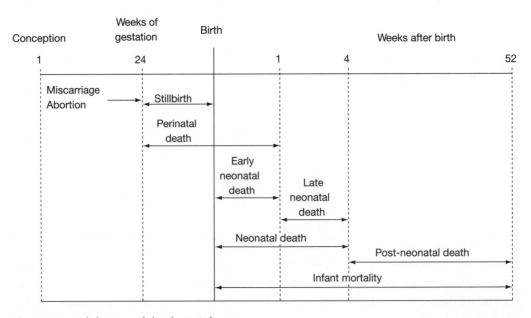

Figure 6.4 Subdivision of deaths in infancy

been born alive but died shortly after birth. Information on perinatal deaths is determined from national death certification and birth registration data. In addition, each region in England, together with Wales and Northern Ireland, is required to participate in the analysis of perinatal mortality by CEMACH. In this way, causes of death are established and potentially avoidable factors can be identified.

Just 60 years ago in Britain, one in every 20 babies was either born dead or died within the first week of life. By the late 1990s, these major risks of foetal life and of birth had receded to the extent that only one in 120 babies failed to survive the first week of life. While the perinatal mortality rate has fallen steadily (Figure 6.5), there is still considerable regional variation, as has already been noted with respect to infant mortality.

However, the perinatal mortality rate varies between localities and fluctuates from year to year. Conclusions based upon comparisons between places and within places over time must be very cautiously drawn because the variations observed may be arising from very small numbers. A statutory change to the definition of stillbirths (commencing from the 24th week of gestation, not the 28th as previously) introduced in October 1992 has implications for the interpretation of trends over time. Figure 6.6 summarises the factors contributing to perinatal death, together with ascertainment processes. This is useful to consider when making international comparisons or exploring or interpreting variation between localities.

Much of the reduction in perinatal mortality has been associated with an overall improvement in the health and nutrition of the population; also, far fewer women are having a large number of pregnancies. In addition, over the last several decades there have been major technological advances in the care of pregnant women and the newborn. Such treatments are now accepted as commonplace today, but at the time of their introduction may have appeared to be as unnatural as some of the techniques used in the care of women in labour or very tiny babies today. Natural childbirth arguments have led to the acknowledgement that high-technology care is not necessarily appropriate for every mother, but recent improvements in perinatal mortality would have been hard to achieve without it.

Low birth weight is the most important factor that is linked to perinatal death. Survival of babies with very low birth weight has improved over the last 40 years, although the most marked change did not occur until after 1980. This improvement is due in part to the wider availability of intensive care facilities for newborn babies, together with advances in technology in this field of care. The importance of low birth weight is apparent in the infant mortality rate, where difference in the death rate according to birth weight is of very large proportion (Figure 6.7).

It is important to understand the factors that contribute to, or are directly associated with, low birth weight or perinatal mortality and to identify those elements where there are clear associations and opportunities for improvement. If lethal congenital malformations are left to one side, the major factors associated with low birth weight are plural pregnancy, poor nutrition, low socio-economic status, teenage pregnancy and smoking and drinking in pregnancy. Many of the factors associated with low birth weight and perinatal mortality are interrelated. Their independent contribution is hard to assess.

The association between smoking and low birth weight was first reported in the mid-1950s, and there is now no doubt that

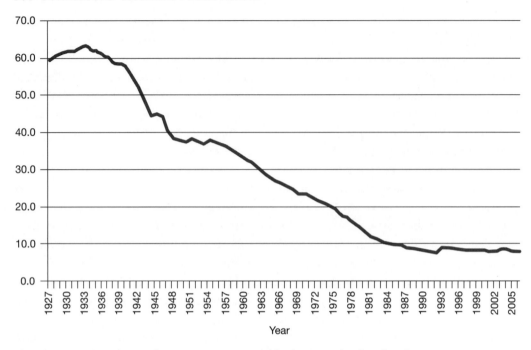

Figure 6.5 Perinatal mortality rate per 1000 total births in England and Wales
Source: Office for National Statistics.

smoking during pregnancy has an adverse effect on the unborn child. The more the mother smokes, the greater the risk to the baby. The average reduction in birth weight of a baby born to a smoker is of the order of 150 to 250 grams. Smoking is also associated with impairment of the child. The increased risk of perinatal mortality due to smoking has been estimated at 28%.

Drinking alcohol is also potentially damaging to the developing foetus. Heavy alcohol consumption, particularly in early pregnancy, can lead to a baby being born with foetal alcohol syndrome. This is characterised by retarded growth and anomalies of the face and nervous system, as well as abnormal behaviour of the baby in the period after birth.

Women from poorer social backgrounds are one and a half times more likely to produce a low-birth-weight baby or suffer a perinatal death than are those in the other social classes. Similarly, the youngest and the oldest women who are pregnant have much greater risks of poor outcomes of their pregnancies. For teenage pregnancies, the opportunities to effect change include better sex education, easier access to contraception and wider availability of counselling and support services, as well as enhanced antenatal care for young expectant mothers (this issue is discussed more fully later in the chapter).

Some parts of Britain have large ethnic minority populations. Some women within ethnic minority communities are at higher risk of perinatal loss than are pregnant women as a whole. The factors contributing

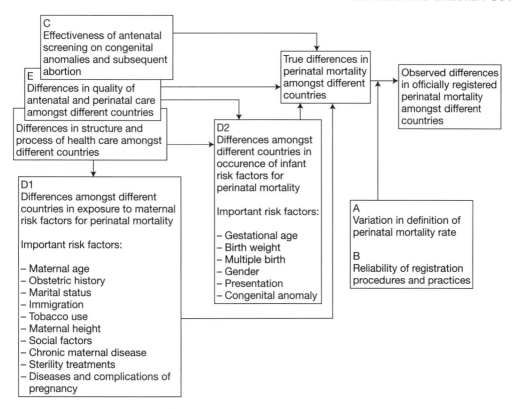

Figure 6.6 Conceptual model of the relationship between quality of antenatal and perinatal care, risk factors for perinatal mortality, and registration procedures and practices in the construction of the perinatal mortality rate

Source: Richardus JH, Graafmans WC, Verloove-Vanhorick S, *et al.* The perinatal mortality rate as an indicator of quality of care in international comparisons. *Med Care.* 1998; **36**(1): 54–66.

to such differences are not fully understood but include the presence of certain mother and baby illnesses, dietary practices and the availability, or otherwise, of services that are responsive to the special needs of women in ethnic minority groups – including interpreters, translations of written materials and familiarity of health care professionals with cultural and religious beliefs. Innovative approaches to this problem have already been taken in some parts of Britain – such as special link workers to ensure that the needs of ethnic minority mothers are

more comprehensively met. In areas where ethnic minority populations are present, the need for services to be appropriately targeted and designed to respond to these mothers and their families should be recognised and actively addressed.

Neonatal, Post-neonatal and Infant Deaths

At the end of the nineteenth century, about 150 children in every 1000 live births died during the first year of life. The decline in

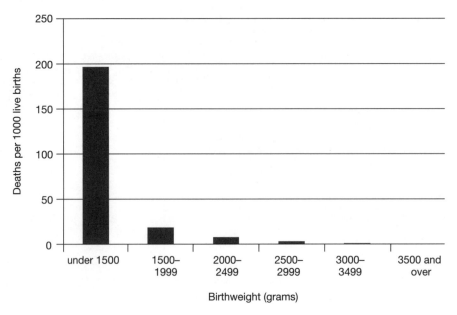

Figure 6.7 Infant mortality rate by birth weight, England and Wales, 2006
Source: Office for National Statistics.

this rate since then has been both consistent and dramatic. By 1936 it had fallen to 58.7, by the beginning of the 1960s it had halved again, and by 2006 it was five deaths per 1000 live births. The decline is unlikely to have been due to a single factor. Better nutritional standards, better education and improved environmental conditions of the large working-class population of late Victorian England, together with the emergence of the middle class, have all contributed. Improvements in medical care and the advent of comprehensive vaccination programmes have also played a part.

Deaths occurring in the first year of life are a fair reflection of the health of a population generally. For descriptive epidemiological purposes, infant deaths are usually divided into neonatal and post-neonatal deaths (definitions given earlier). The factors affecting neonatal deaths have many similarities with those that influence perinatal mortality.

Post-neonatal deaths are more strongly related to social and economic factors as reflected by place of residence, father's occupation and social class. Even since the mid-1970s, there have been further sharp declines in neonatal and post-neonatal mortality and in infant mortality as a whole (Table 6.5). The data are presented for each fifth year in order to more readily show the decline. In recent years, some of the rates have reached comparatively low levels, and decline has slowed.

Undertaking analyses using routinely available national data shows that infant mortality varies according to birth weight, maternal age and maternal ethnic origin. In 2006, the infant mortality rate for babies of normal weight (2500 grams or more) was 1.7 per 1000 live births, compared to a rate of 196 amongst very low-birth-weight babies (less than 1500 grams). Fifty percent of infant deaths occur amongst very low-birth-weight babies. The infant mortality rate was lowest amongst mothers aged 30 to 34 years, at 4.1 per 1000 live births. This compared to rates of 6.4 amongst teenage mothers and 5.9 for babies born to mothers aged 40 years or more.

As a result of rules for certification of stillbirth and neonatal death (introduced in 1986), causes of neonatal deaths are analysed by the main maternal and foetal conditions, but not by a single underlying cause. The conditions cited most often for neonatal deaths are immaturity, congenital malformations, intrapartum causes and infection.

For post-neonatal deaths, where certification rules are different, a single underlying cause can be analysed. The leading causes of death in this period are sudden infant death syndrome (SIDS), diseases of the respiratory system, and other infections and congenital malformations. Since the early 1970s, death certified with terms such as 'cot death', 'sudden unexpected death in infancy' or 'sudden infant death syndrome' have been separately

identified and analysed for epidemiological purposes. The category is defined as 'sudden death of an infant or young child, which is unexpected by history, and in which a thorough post-mortem examination fails to demonstrate an adequate cause of death'.

The whole issue of sudden unexpected deaths in apparently healthy babies is one that has caused a great deal of public concern. At the same time as interest in this syndrome rose, its frequency as a certified cause of death increased in the mid-1980s, while respiratory causes declined. This suggested a change in certification practice. The post-neonatal mortality rate as a whole is strongly influenced by changes in the occurrence of sudden infant death syndrome. A major fall in mortality attributed to SIDS occurred during the first half of the 1990s when the Department of Health issued advice that was widely publicised about babies' 'sleeping position'.

Research had shown that the 'prone' position increased risk, so parents were told to place babies on their backs. Advice also contained warnings about overheating of babies through placing too many covers on them and about keeping them in an environment free of cigarette smoke. The 'Back to Sleep'

Table 6.5 Trends in the components of infant mortality, England and Wales

Mortality Rate*	Year					
	1981	1986	1991	1996	2001	2006
Stillbirth	6.6	5.3	4.6	5.4	5.3	5.4
Neonatal	6.7	5.3	4.4	4.1	3.6	3.5
Post-neonatal	4.4	4.3	3.0	2.0	1.9	1.5

*See text for definitions.
Source: Office for National Statistics. *Mortality Statistics: childhood, infant and perinatal.* Series DH3, no. 39. London: ONS; 2008.

campaign is thought to be a major contributor to the fall in mortality due to sudden infant deaths but would not explain all of it. It is, however, one of the most successful public health campaigns ever.

Dramatic improvement in the infant mortality rate has occurred in most of the countries in western Europe. The scope for further improvement is evident from the lower rates of some other countries (Figure 6.8). Developing countries and eastern European countries have much less favourable rates, while Japan has one of the lowest infant mortality rates in the world.

FOETAL ANOMALIES

An important cause of foetal death, impairment, disability and handicap are the disorders that develop during intrauterine life. The decline in other causes of death over the last several decades has meant that congenital anomalies have accounted for an increasing proportion of infant deaths, some 29% of such deaths in 2006. Such anomalies also cause some of the deaths that occur in later childhood.

Information on the reported frequency of congenital malformations and other foetal anomalies in the population is available from the National Congenital Anomaly System (NCAS) (run by the Office for National Statistics), which was introduced in 1964 for England and Wales following the thalidomide tragedy. The system is voluntary and since 1995 takes account of anomalies detected at any age. It relies on information being supplied by doctors, nurses and midwives in NHS trusts and on primary care trusts extracting information on congenital malformations from birth notifications. Minor anomalies have been excluded from the reporting system since 1990.

Returns are subjected to statistical analysis

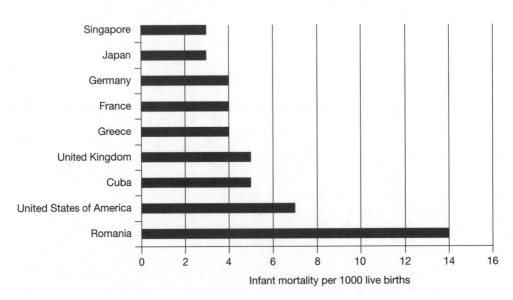

Figure 6.8 Infant mortality per 1000 live births, selected countries, 2006
Source: World Health Organization. *World Health Statistics 2008.* Geneva: WHO Press; 2008.

on a quarterly basis, and any significant increases are reported to the health authority concerned. The statistical approach used is the cumulative sum technique, and it seeks to detect any significant rise in notification in any of the nearly 100 anomaly groupings. The system is therefore primarily a method of surveillance to compare trends over time. An increase in notification may be the result of a change in local notification practice. It is of less value exploring variations in incidence between different localities, testing aetiological hypotheses and detecting overall prevalence.

It has been recognised that there is under-reporting in the National Congenital Anomaly System, and since 1998 a programme to improve the level of reporting has been undertaken by exchanging information with some of the local congenital anomaly registers that exist in various parts of England and Wales. Despite some limitations of the data, congenital malformation statistics from the national monitoring scheme yield much valuable information. The most accurate figures come from areas that have local anomaly registers that cooperate in data exchange with the National Congenital Anomaly System. Table 6.6 shows rates of congenital malformations for some selected causes.

Congenital anomalies often are not isolated occurrences, and just less than one in four of the notifications received by the National Congenital Anomaly System in 2006 from areas with good data capture were for babies with multiple anomalies. The incidence of anomalies is higher in male babies than in female babies and is also higher for multiple births. Unsurprisingly,

the incidence of anomaly is higher in stillborn infants, at 14%, compared with live-born infants, at less than 2%. The incidence of congenital anomalies also varies with maternal age, with the highest levels present under the age of 20 years and over the age of 40 years (Figure 6.9). This analysis of congenital anomaly and maternal age uses data from the areas of England and Wales where a local register allied to the National Congenital Anomaly System is in operation.

An important cause of foetal anomalies is a group of conditions called neural tube defects, which occur in differing forms, including that of spina bifida. Neural tube defects arise from a failure of normal development of the central nervous system during the first few weeks of embryonic life; specifically, from the failure of proper closure of the neural tube. A spectrum of disorders may result, depending on the site and severity of the defect:

- *anencephaly* – failure of development of the forebrain, its coverings and the skull. This defect is incompatible with life; most affected infants are stillborn, while the remainder usually die within hours of birth
- *spina bifida occulta* – failure of fusion of the vertebral arches with no protrusion of tissue and seldom any neurological impairment
- *spina bifida cystica* in two forms:
  - *meningocoele* – this less serious and less common form consists of a protrusion of meninges, but not the spinal cord, through a defect in the vertebral column. The sac consists of spinal

Table 6.6 Rates of notification of main groupings of congenital anomalies per 10 000 total births (areas covered by a register in England and Wales, 2006)

Condition	Rate
Central nervous system anomalies	9.3
Cleft lip and palate	10.8
Heart and circulatory	39.4
Alimentary	15.4
Genital organs	17.3
Urinary system	25.3
Musculoskeletal	45.7
Chromosomal anomalies	17.2

Source: Office for National Statistics. *Congenital Anomaly Statistics: notifications England and Wales 2006.* Series MB3, no. 21. London: ONS; 2008.

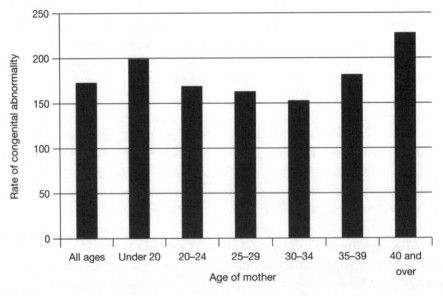

Figure 6.9 Rates of notification of congenital anomaly (in areas covered by a local register) by maternal age, England and Wales, 2006
Source: Office for National Statistics.

membranes and is covered by skin ('closed' neural tube defect). After surgical closure, prognosis is usually good, with minor residual impairment

— *myelomenigocoele* – this type is more serious and more common (accounting for 80–90% of all spina bifida cystica births). In this 'open' neural tube defect, the protruding sac contains spinal cord that is partly uncovered. This defect often results in severe handicap of the nervous, urinary and locomotor systems, even if surgical treatment is undertaken (although this depends on the spinal level at which the defect occurs). Hydrocephalus and learning disability may also be accompanying features.

Neural tube defects are a worldwide phenomenon. Their aetiology is not fully elucidated. They have declined sharply in England and Wales and a number of other countries. There is a strong social-class gradient for the prevalence of neural tube defects; they occur more frequently in social class IV and V than in I and II. In part, the fall has been due to a reduction in the natural incidence of the condition for reasons that are so far unexplained but that may be due to dietary and environmental factors. Support for this theory came from an important seven-year Medical Research Council study that showed the risk of conception of a second child with such a defect was greatly reduced if the mother took folic acid supplements prior to conception of the next child. In 2007 the Food Standards Agency recommended that mandatory fortification of flour should take place in the United Kingdom. Until such time as that policy is implemented, the advice is that all women planning a pregnancy should consume additional folic acid prior to conception and in the first 12 weeks of pregnancy in the form of folate-rich foods supplemented by an extra daily dietary supplement of folic acid.

Another factor that has contributed to the decline in births of babies with neural tube defects is the advent of techniques for detecting open neural tube defects during pregnancy. Prenatal diagnosis enables parents to be offered the option of terminating the pregnancy and so avoiding giving birth to a severely handicapped baby or one who may die in the perinatal period. About one-third of the reduction in the number of babies born with open neural tube defects in the last 10 years is estimated to be due to screening and termination.

Another important foetal anomaly is Down's syndrome, which is discussed more fully in Chapter 7. Screening for Down's syndrome and neural tube defects is discussed again later in this chapter.

HEALTH INEQUALITIES IN INFANCY

The effect of social and economic conditions is particularly powerful in infancy and is clearly seen in the very substantial variation in the outcomes as represented by perinatal and infant mortality rates (Figure 6.10). Information on the occupation of the father is coded for all stillborn babies and for all babies dying in the first year of life. It is also coded for a one in 10 sample of live births. Since 2001 the National Statistics Socio-economic Classification has been used to describe the socio-economic structure of society, and this is based upon the occupation of the father of the baby. The numbers in the last of the eight categories (never worked and long-term unemployed) are too small to provide meaningful statistics, but there is a distinct socio-economic gradient in perinatal and infant mortality rates across the other seven categories.

HEALTH AND DISEASE IN CHILDHOOD

Beyond the first year of life, mortality rates for the remainder of childhood (until the age of 15 years) are expressed in relation to the numbers in the population at risk. Deaths in childhood in England and Wales, like mortality in infancy, fell during the twentieth century and have fallen further in the twenty-first century (Figure 6.11). The main reason for this improvement was a substantial reduction in the importance of infectious diseases as a cause of death in this age group. In the 1930s the majority of childhood deaths were attributable to infectious

diseases, including pneumonia, tuberculosis, diphtheria, measles and whooping cough. By 2006 infectious diseases accounted for only 6% of deaths between one month and 15 years of age. The change was brought about by a combination of socio-environmental changes (such as improvements in standards of nutrition, housing and sanitation), preventive measures (immunisation) and therapeutic medical advances (antibiotics in particular). The decreased impact of infectious diseases means that the mortality rates within the different phases of childhood and after the first year of life are lower than at any other period of life.

While this overall improvement in childhood mortality has occurred, other conditions have assumed greater importance.

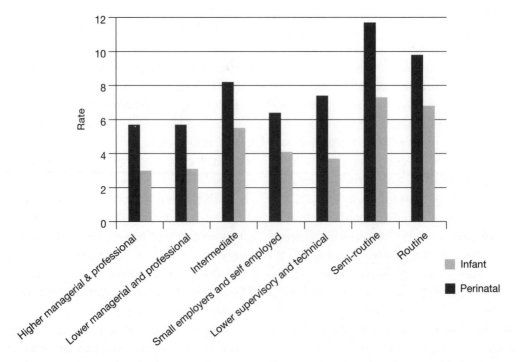

Figure 6.10 Perinatal and infant mortality rates and socio-economic classification of father, 2006
Source: Office for National Statistics.

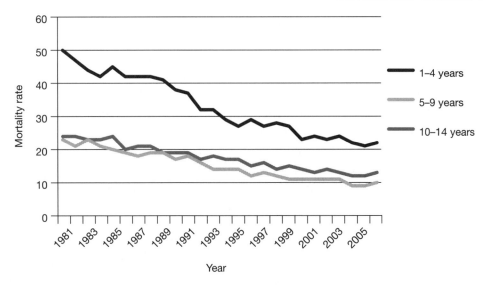

Figure 6.11 Childhood mortality rates per 100 000, England and Wales, 1981–2006
Source: Office for National Statistics.

For children aged 1–4 years, unintentional injury is the most common cause of death. Cancer represents 14% of deaths in this age group, and a further 14% are due to diseases of the nervous system. Between 5 and 14 years of age, injuries and cancer both represent about a quarter of deaths, and diseases of the nervous system represent 13% of deaths. The pattern shifts markedly in the 15–19 years group, with injury accounting for more than half of all deaths. The majority of these deaths are road traffic deaths, but 18% of the total are attributed to deliberate self-harm or have an undetermined cause. Mortality in all age groups shows a very direct relationship with deprivation. This is very markedly so in relation to deaths in fires.

There are various measures of morbidity available. None of these are as robust as the measures of mortality. The three main national sources are parents' perception of their children's health as reported by the General Household Survey, morbidity statistics from general practice relating to children and information from hospital episode statistics. The national study of morbidity statistics from general practice of 1991–92 gave information from a sample of practices about consultation patterns for children. Across childhood, a third of consultations are for diseases of the respiratory system. In contrast, injury and poisoning, which is the major cause of childhood death, accounted for only 13% and 19% of consultations of children aged 0–4 years and 5–15 years respectively. However, the survey has not been repeated since then, and the data must therefore be regarded with caution.

Hospital episode statistics (HES) are collated nationally on inpatient and day-care surgery episodes. For the majority of serious diseases of childhood (for example, asthma, epilepsy and diabetes), hospital episode statistics are of only limited value in describing overall morbidity. There are specific data-collection systems for some conditions. The British Paediatric Surveillance Unit receives notification from paediatricians on certain rare disorders (for example, AIDS, scleroderma, neonatal herpes and congenital adrenal hyperplasia) and produces information on incidence and prevalence. Cancer registries hold information on childhood cancers, often supplemented by detailed regional treatment and follow-up registers – for leukaemia in particular. Detailed national surveys of children's dental health were carried out each decade from the 1970s onwards.

Local information on specific conditions may exist as registers (for example, for paediatric renal disease, diabetes and specified tumours). These often start as treatment registers or for research purposes and may not necessarily have a population base to which the incidence of disease can be related.

PREVENTING UNWANTED PREGNANCY
CONTRACEPTIVE METHODS

Contraception has a long history stretching back thousands of years. The practice of coitus interruptus was perhaps the first method and is still used today. The use of various acidic or alkaline substances inserted into the vagina also has ancient roots. Spermicidal creams and pessaries are available today, and research is being undertaken into microbicides that might be effective against sexually transmitted diseases as well

as being contraceptives. Effective male and female barrier methods of contraception were introduced in the nineteenth century, and condoms in particular are still seen as an effective method of contraception and avoiding sexually transmitted disease. Since the 1960s, contraceptive methods have been dominated by the so-called 'high technolzogy' measures – the oral contraceptive pill, new hormonal delivery systems and, to a lesser extent, the intrauterine device (IUD).

In 2006/07, amongst women attending a community contraceptive clinic for the first time, 46% used the oral contraceptive pill, 28% used male condoms and 21% used long-acting reversible contraceptives such as IUDs and injectable contraceptives and implants.

The efficacy for the average user of the various methods of contraception varies substantially. Typically, the percentage of women experiencing an unintended pregnancy within the first year of use will be 8% for the contraceptive pill, 15% for the male condom, 0.05% for the long-acting implant and 0.5% for female sterilisation. It should be noted that some methods, such as sterilisation and implants, will have little variation between users, while other methods, such as condoms and the contraceptive pill, will have a lower failure rate with experienced users.

Emergency Contraception

If someone has unprotected sex or thinks their contraceptive method may have failed, emergency contraception is an option. There are two methods of emergency contraception: hormonal (levonorgestrel) treatment or the insertion of an intrauterine device. The hormonal method can be used up to 72 hours post-coitally and the intrauterine device method up to five days later. While the insertion of an intrauterine device requires professional involvement, the emergency contraceptive pill can be obtained from a wider range of places and can be purchased from most pharmacies by women aged 16 years or over. There has been controversy surrounding the wide availability of emergency contraception, with opponents arguing that it could encourage unprotected sex.

Safety of Contraceptive Methods

Most published data about mortality from the use of contraceptives concentrate on the risk from the method itself. Some investigators, however, deal with the wider aspect and calculate cumulative mortality. Thus not only inherent risk of death from the method is considered but also risk from pregnancy as a result of method failure. Additionally, in the case of the oral contraceptive, the potential beneficial effects of reducing the risk of ovarian and endometrial cancer are taken into account.

Precise risks are difficult to determine, and detailed information is limited to hormonal contraceptives, intrauterine devices, sterilisation and other hormonal delivery systems. Risk related to oral contraceptives has been most studied in this and other countries. The diseases that are more common among women while they are taking the combined pill include certain cancers, such as breast cancer, and also various disorders of the circulation – especially thrombosis and stroke. However, the benefits of the pill include a reduction in the risk of endometrial and ovarian cancer. Media scares about the safety of hormonal contraception have at times resulted in large numbers of women abandoning the method, and while they may have avoided a small risk of serious side effects, rises in the numbers of abortions in the years that followed have been attributed to the concerns. Women's health advocates argue that side effects such as emotional well-being, weight gain, menstrual bleeding and headaches are often ignored by researchers.

IUDs can be used by all women, providing they are not at risk of acquiring an infection. Sterilisation involves a one-time risk associated with surgery, unlike the sort of continuous exposure of the other two methods. However, sterilisation has a low ongoing failure rate.

PROVISION OF SERVICES

Family planning services in Britain are provided in three main ways: by general practitioners; in community family planning clinics and sexual health clinics; and in departments of obstetrics and gynaecology in local hospitals. Despite the move during the 1990s towards more family planning services being delivered by general practitioners, it has been national policy to maintain a choice of service, and hence the community family planning clinics have been preserved (albeit in smaller numbers than in the past). Women and men may prefer to visit such a clinic rather than their general practitioner for a number of reasons: they may prefer anonymity, it may be easier to see a woman doctor, there may be a fuller range of contraceptive methods and they will often regard the staff of the family planning clinic as 'specialists' with more detailed knowledge.

A number of principles underlie the provision of good family planning services (Table 6.7). These include ensuring that certain quality criteria are fulfilled, providing good access and enabling groups with traditionally low uptake (but who may be in particular need) to receive services. Of particular importance are the problems of sexual health amongst teenagers, where the risks of unwanted pregnancy are high. In addition, effective family planning services must give advice about reducing the risks of sexually transmitted diseases. Attendance for family planning advice also provides a chance for opportunistic health promotion, including offering cervical screening to women whose test is due or overdue. Many general practitioners now offer family planning in the context of a 'well women' service.

TEENAGE PREGNANCY

There has always been a proportion of women who become pregnant in their teens and for whom the pregnancy is both unplanned and unwanted. This proportion has varied over time as sexual and social mores have changed and women have both increased their participation in higher education and occupied an ever more prominent place in the workforce. It is recognised, however, that the United Kingdom has a rate of teenage pregnancy that is substantially higher than other countries in Western Europe and that this state of affairs is socially and economically undesirable.

The precise effects of teenage parenthood are difficult to study, as it is women who are already in disadvantaged groups that are the most likely to become teenage mothers. Research in the United Kingdom has shown that teenage mothers have significantly poorer mental health during the three years after the birth than older mothers or teenage non-mothers. Comparison of teenage mothers with teenagers who have had a miscarriage has shown that at age 30 there is little effect on a woman's qualifications, job prospects and income. There is, however, an effect in that if the teenage mother has a partner by the age of 30, he is more likely to have had no education beyond the age of 16 and to be unemployed. In contrast, the effects of being born to a teenage mother are more far-reaching and include lower educational attainment, higher levels of economic inactivity and, if female, a high risk of teenage parenthood.

Data on Teenage Conception

There are several difficulties in acquiring accurate, comprehensive and comparable data on teenage pregnancy. Firstly, some pregnancies end in spontaneous abortion and may not be recognised or recorded as such. The teenage pregnancy rate is therefore made up of two components: live or stillbirths and therapeutic abortions carried out under the Abortion Act 1967. Secondly, it is teenage conceptions that are of interest to policy-makers, so data is converted to an estimated date of conception. This

Table 6.7 Factors to be considered when organising family planning services

- Ensure the number, times and locations of clinics meet the needs of users.
- Provide a choice of male and female professional staff.
- Make available a wide choice of contraceptive methods.
- Provide accessible, objective, consistent information that is evidence-guided.
- Ensure the service is staffed by those with skill and knowledge of contraceptive methods and sexual health.
- Provide opportunities to discuss related subjects (for example, premenstrual tension, HIV).
- Offer an appointments system with flexibility to allow walk-in attendances (especially for emergencies).
- Provide facilities for children.

is done using the gestational data supplied as part of the notification of stillbirths and legal abortions. For live births, a gestational age of 38 weeks is used to estimate the age at conception. Thirdly, in calculating rates for young women under 20 and under 18, the population used for both numerator and denominator is women aged 15 years and over. This is because only a very small percentage of teenage conceptions occur at age 14 or under.

Using data at a local level is complicated by the method of allocation of births and abortions to the place where the young woman is resident at the time of the birth or abortion. The small numbers involved in some localities may mean that data cannot be published because of confidentiality. Nonetheless, where local data is available it is invaluable for the identification of 'hot spots' and the planning of interventions. At the other end of the scale, the complications that surround data collection mean that international comparisons are difficult to make and are often based on birth rates under the age of 20 years.

The Teenage Pregnancy Strategy

In response to the problem of teenage pregnancy, the government has adopted a strategy aimed at reducing the under-18 conception rate by 50% by 2010 from a 1998 baseline and at establishing a clear downward trend in the under-16 rate. The strategy is coordinated by the government's Teenage Pregnancy Unit. The Unit was launched in 1999 and is based in the Department for Children, Schools and Families. There has been a fall in the teenage pregnancy rate since the Unit was established, with the decline being greater in the under-16 age group.

A number of factors have been identified in areas that have achieved significant reductions in their rates and are recommended for wider implementation (Table 6.8).

ABORTION

Abortion is defined as 'the emptying of a pregnant uterus up to the 24th week of pregnancy'. Spontaneous abortion (often referred to a 'miscarriage') occurs in an estimated 9–15% of recognised pregnancies

Table 6.8 Key success factors in areas where teenage pregnancy is falling

- Active engagement of all of the key mainstream delivery partners who have a role in reducing teenage pregnancies – Health, Education, Social Services and Youth Support Services – and the voluntary sector.

- A strong senior champion who was accountable for and took the lead in driving the local strategy.

- The availability of a well publicised young-people-centred contraceptive and sexual health advice service, with a strong remit to undertake health promotion work, as well as delivering reactive services.

- A high priority given to PSHE in schools, with support from the local authority to develop comprehensive programmes of sex and relationships education (SRE) in all schools.

- A strong focus on targeted interventions with young people at greatest risk of teenage pregnancy, in particular with Looked After Children.

- The availability (and consistent take-up) of SRE training for professionals in partner organisations (such as Connexions Personal Advisers, Youth Workers and Social Workers) working with the most vulnerable young people.

- A well resourced Youth Service, providing things to do and places to go for young people, with a clear focus on addressing key social issues affecting young people, such as sexual health and substance misuse.

Source: Department for Education and Skills. *Teenage Pregnancy: accelerating the strategy to 2010.* London: DfES; 2006.

– usually for unknown reasons. A criminal abortion is one procured deliberately and unlawfully. A termination of pregnancy is the legal ending of a pregnancy.

The Abortion Act 1967 became law in April 1968 and covers England, Scotland and Wales but not Northern Ireland, where abortion remains illegal. It enabled the legal termination of pregnancy (by a registered medical practitioner) to take place in a National Health Service hospital or premises approved by the secretary of state for health. The current requirements are that two registered medical practitioners should certify that certain defined indications for abortion have been met (Table 6.9), that the abortion should be performed by a registered medical practitioner and that the procedure should be undertaken in a National Health Service hospital or other approved premises. The Abortion

Regulations require any terminations to be notified within 14 days to the chief medical officer of the Department of Health or to the chief medical officers of Wales and Scotland, according to where the termination takes place.

The factors that can influence the abortion rate in a population are diverse (Table 6.10). The proportion of terminations undertaken on non-residents of England and Wales reached a peak of 34% in the mid-1970s and by 2006 had fallen to less than a quarter of the number performed at the peak.

The proportion has fluctuated, however, being partly influenced by the liberalisation of abortion laws in countries from which a high proportion of non-resident abortions were drawn. The impact of these factors is well illustrated by the position of women from the Republic of Ireland (which prohibits abortion). Between the beginning of

Table 6.9 Grounds for abortion under the Abortion Act 1967 as subsequently amended

A legally induced abortion must be certified by two registered medical practitioners as justified under one or more of the following grounds:

- the continuance of the pregnancy would involve risk to the life of the pregnant woman greater than if the pregnancy were terminated

- the termination is necessary to prevent grave permanent injury to the physical or mental health of the pregnant woman

- the pregnancy has not exceeded its 24th week and the continuance of the pregnancy would involve risk, greater than if the pregnancy were terminated, of injury to the physical or mental health of the pregnant woman

- the pregnancy has not exceeded its 24th week and the continuance of the pregnancy would involve risk, greater than if the pregnancy were terminated, of injury to the physical or mental health of any existing children of the family of the pregnant woman

- there is a substantial risk that if the child were born it would suffer from such physical or mental abnormalities as to be seriously handicapped

- or in an emergency, certified by the operating practitioner as immediately necessary: to save the life of the pregnant woman or to prevent grave permanent injury to the physical or mental health of the pregnant woman.

Table 6.10 Some factors that can influence the rate of abortions in a population

- Prevailing legislation
- Social attitudes
- Contraceptive efficacy and usage
- Scope for diagnosis of foetal abnormalities
- Fertility patterns
- Age structure of female population

the 1970s and the start of the 1990s, there was a sixteen-fold increase in the number of women from that country having abortions in England and Wales. By 2007, Irish women (from both the north and south of Ireland) represented 85% of the non-residents of England and Wales having abortions.

Although there have been some dips in the abortion rate since legalisation took place in 1968, the overall trend has been upwards (Figure 6.12). In 2007 the age-standardised rate was 18.6 per 1000 women residents of England and Wales aged 15–44 years. This compares with a rate of 5.2 in 1969, the first full year of operation of the Act.

There is very substantial variation in the abortion rate in women of different ages, the highest rates being amongst 19-year-old women (Figure 6.13).

The proportion of conceptions overall that end in termination of pregnancy is around 22%. However, the figure is much higher for very young and older women: 60% (for the under-16s) and 32% (for the over-40s) respectively. The figure for the latter group reflects terminations undertaken as a result of screening for congenital anomalies – Down's syndrome in particular.

Critics of the abortion law have considered that liberal interpretation of the grounds for abortion has led to termination of pregnancy on demand. There is ample evidence from surveys of women who have had abortions that they do not regard it as a substitute for contraception but rather as a last resort in the case of failure or mistake.

INFERTILITY SERVICES

There are various formal definitions of 'infertility', most of which embody concepts of exposure to the risk of pregnancy over a certain period of time: for example, 'a failure to become pregnant over a period of two years whilst engaging in sexual intercourse without contraceptive use'.

There are a number of important influences on fertility. Factors both inherited and acquired, and of a short- or long-term nature, affect the physiological reproductive capacity of both males and females. Examples of acquired factors amongst women are infections such as gonorrhoea, chlamydia or other pelvic inflammatory conditions, which may prevent conception by causing scarring and blockage of the fallopian tubes. Acquired infertility in men is less well understood and less easy to treat. Female fertility declines with age, but the effect of age on male fertility is not as well understood. Women who smoke are likely to have reduced fertility, and there is an association between smoking in men and reduced quality of semen. Obesity is also likely to result in reduced fertility in both sexes.

Failure to conceive may produce as much distress as an unwanted pregnancy. Formerly, adoption was the sole resort of couples who were childless. The widespread availability and use of effective contraceptive methods, as well as changes in the law relating to termination of pregnancy, have had the effect of reducing the number of babies offered for adoption. This has, to some extent, been countered by the development of methods of assisted reproduction in couples of low fertility and by the acceptance of the use of donor sperm for men who are infertile.

With treatment, about a third of infertile couples can achieve a successful pregnancy (though success rates vary according to a woman's age, other clinical factors and the performance of the service). The investigation of subfertility and infertility should involve both partners. Approximately 35 to 40% of problems relate to the male partner and 35 to 40% relate to the female. In the remainder there is no apparent cause.

In general terms, infertility and subfertility are usually due to failure to produce sperm or to ovulate or to a mechanical blockage in the vas deferens or the fallopian tubes. Treatment of female subfertility and infertility may include drug-induced ovulation. This may result in multiple pregnancy.

The development of in vitro fertilisation (IVF) has dramatically altered the picture of treatment for infertility. It is regulated by the Human Fertilisation and Embryology Authority (HFEA), which was established

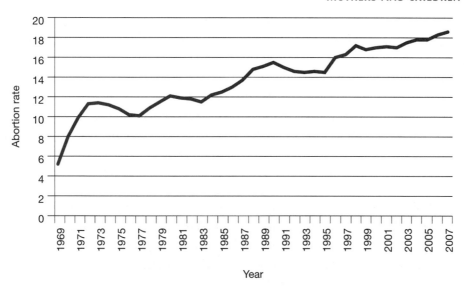

Figure 6.12 Age-standardised abortion rate per 1000 female residents aged 15–44 years, England and Wales, 1969–2007
Source: Department of Health. *Abortion Statistics, England and Wales: 2007.* London: DoH; 2008.

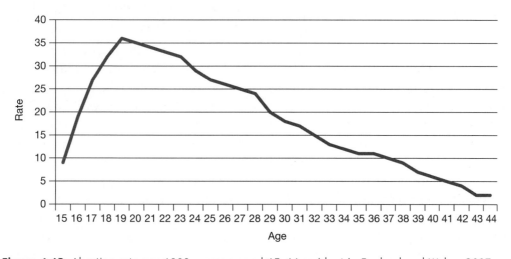

Figure 6.13 Abortion rate per 1000 women aged 15–44 resident in England and Wales, 2007
Source: Department of Health. *Abortion Statistics, England and Wales: 2007.* London: DoH; 2008.

in 1991 and was the first body of its kind in the world. The role of the HFEA is both to monitor and license facilities that carry out fertility treatments such as donor insemination and IVF. It also has a role in the regulation of the storage of eggs and sperm.

Childless couples may go to very considerable lengths to acquire a child. Recent years have seen the appearance of surrogacy, in which a fertile woman is willing to bear a child for one who is infertile. There are a number of ethical questions surrounding this issue that have still to be addressed, and there are differing legal situations between countries. Concerns arise particularly over the level of payments to surrogate mothers.

ANTENATAL CARE

The whole process of antenatal care is geared to a healthy outcome of pregnancy both for mother and baby. Increasingly, the traditional antenatal period is being extended to include the concept of preconception care. Women in their childbearing years are now encouraged to think about the prospect and implications of pregnancy before it happens. 'Well Women' clinics provide a focus for discussion about lifestyle, contraception and the timing of conception. The role of folate in preventing neural tube defects has been described earlier, and women planning a pregnancy are recommended to take an additional daily supplement.

It is important that a woman is enrolled into a programme of antenatal care as early as possible after pregnancy is confirmed. The most common model of antenatal care is a shared approach between the midwife, the general practitioner and the local hospital department of obstetrics and gynaecology.

Antenatal care encompasses a wide range of activities, including advice on lifestyle (for example, smoking, alcohol, drugs, diet); screening for maternal illness (for example, hypertensive disease, diabetes, infection); recognition and treatment of anomalies in pregnancy; detection of foetal anomaly; assessment of foetal size, development and well-being; psychological preparation for delivery (including antenatal classes); and education about the importance of breast-feeding and about parenting. The content of antenatal care has evolved over time as a development of medical and midwifery practice rather than on the basis of evaluation of the efficacy of specific interventions on the outcome of pregnancy. Increasingly, it is being recognised that a modern service must develop not on the basis of tradition but on evidence of what is proven to be effective, as well as on a parent's views and preferences.

THE PREVENTION AND RECOGNITION OF FOETAL ANOMALIES

There are certain groups of women who are at higher risk of foetal anomaly. Parents with a family history of certain genetically determined diseases or who have had a previously affected child, for example with cystic fibrosis, should be offered genetic counselling. They may decide to avoid pregnancy. In some cases it is now possible to determine whether a foetus is affected by the genetic/chromosomal anomaly by early chorionic villus sampling or amniocentesis. An increasing proportion of foetal anomalies can now be recognised by a variety of screening tests in the antenatal period. Parents can be counselled and offered termination. Although such decisions are difficult, an even more ethically challenging area is that of population screening of pregnant women for foetal anomaly – e.g., for neural tube defects and Down's syndrome (*see* below). The aim here is to offer the women a choice about screening which if accepted may lead to a diagnosis. Women can then be offered the opportunity to discuss all the options available to them, which could include termination of the pregnancy. Major questions arise about informed consent to testing, about health care professionals' ability to offer non-directive counselling and about guilt and distress caused by mid-trimester termination.

Some women are at higher risk of foetal anomaly due to their own health status. For example, women with diabetes require preconceptual care and planning and monitoring of the pregnancy and delivery. Prescribed drugs in pregnancy can cause anomalies, and women on long-term medication (for example, sodium valproate for epilepsy) require preconceptual advice and possible changes to their drug regime.

The effects of smoking and alcohol on foetal growth and development have been described earlier. An increasing problem is that of substance abuse in pregnancy and, to an extent related, HIV infection in pregnancy.

Rhesus Haemolytic Disease in the Newborn

This disorder arises from a genetic difference between a mother and her baby whereby they have different blood groups. Each member of the population belongs to one of four main blood groups, A, B, AB and O, but each person also falls into two other broad groups, rhesus-positive and rhesus-negative. In Britain 85% of the population is rhesus-positive, carrying the rhesus antigen (commonly the 'D' antigen) on their red blood cells. A rhesus-negative woman can conceive a rhesus-positive baby if the father is rhesus-positive.

If at some time during pregnancy or delivery foetal (i.e., rhesus-positive) red blood cells pass into the maternal circulation, the (rhesus-negative) mother may respond by producing antibodies against the rhesus antigen. The risk is that these antibodies (anti-D antibodies) can then cross back through the placenta and haemolyse the red cells of the foetus. The result is anaemia, jaundice, brain damage and even death in subsequent pregnancies where the baby is rhesus-positive. This kind of bleeding occurs most commonly at delivery. However, it is also associated with invasive prenatal diagnosis – amniocentesis, chorionic villus sampling, foetal blood sampling, antepartum haemorrhage, abdominal injury, intrauterine death and abortion.

In the 1950s, haemolytic disease of the newborn accounted for over 1000 stillbirths and neonatal deaths each year. The development of postpartum exchange transfusion, intrauterine transfusion and early induction of labour reduced the number of deaths to 708 by 1969. However, it was the introduction of postnatal anti-D (antibody to rhesus-D antigen) prophylaxis in 1969 that led to the major reduction in infant deaths attributable to rhesus haemolytic disease from 46 per 100 000 then, to 1.6 per 100 000 by 1990.

All rhesus-negative women currently receive intramuscular anti-D within 72 hours of delivery. This destroys any rhesus-positive foetal red cells circulating in the mother's blood before they can stimulate continuing maternal antibody formation. In addition, pregnant rhesus-negative women who have risk factors, invasive prenatal interventions or abdominal trauma during pregnancy also receive anti-D.

However, a small number of rhesus-negative women continue to develop anti-D antibodies during pregnancy. The most important cause in 1% of all rhesus-negative women without obvious risk factors is occult transplacental bleeding. There is good evidence from large studies that this could be reduced to 0.2% or less by giving two additional injections of anti-D routinely at 28 and 34 weeks of pregnancy. Guidance on antenatal care indicates that anti-D should be offered to all non-sensitised rhesus-negative women at 28 weeks.

The Detection of Neural Tube Defects

The possibility of early detection of open neural tube defects came in the 1970s, when it was noted that a substance called alpha-fetoprotein was present in increased amounts in the amniotic fluid of women carrying babies with anencephaly or spina bifida. A later discovery, that raised alpha-fetoprotein levels could be detected in the serum of mothers carrying foetuses with a neural tube defect, meant there was a potential for a screening test. Serum alpha-fetoprotein screening followed by amniocentesis for those with high levels has now largely been superseded by ultrasound scanning. The foetal anomaly scan at around 18 to 20 weeks' gestation is a safer method of detecting neural tube defects. If a neural tube defect is confirmed, parents are offered (with appropriate counselling) the choice of terminating the pregnancy.

The Detection of Down's Syndrome

Down's syndrome occurs in about one in a thousand live births. Screening for Down's syndrome using amniocentesis at 15 weeks pregnancy (or chorionic villus sampling before 15 weeks) has been offered since the 1980s to older mothers (over 35 years) or those who had a previously affected child or one partner with known chromosomal anomalies. These techniques look for abnormal cells. However, because most babies affected by Down's syndrome are born to women aged below 35 years, the screening of older women makes a limited impact on the overall number of affected babies born.

More recently, maternal serum screening for Down's syndrome has been developed using a variety of serum markers, and this is combined with ultrasound examination of the baby's neck area to form the basis of a first-trimester screening programme. The follow-on diagnostic test is either chorionic villus sampling or amniocentesis, depending on the gestational age. Again, women are then offered termination of pregnancy if the diagnosis is confirmed, with the principle of informed choice being key. Before screening of any sort commences, it is seen as important that the woman fully understands the possible outcomes of the screening process and gives her informed consent.

INTRAPARTUM CARE

During the second half of the twentieth century in Britain, there was progressive closure of smaller local maternity units, often on the basis that they could not fulfil professionally set standards for care during labour. This trend took place with medical professional support and accorded with Department of Health policy.

There will always be some mothers for whom underlying medical problems or complications of pregnancy mean that delivery away from immediate obstetric and paediatric assistance entails risk. There will similarly be many mothers whose delivery will be so straightforward as to entail virtually no risk at all. In between these two is a group of mothers who may face a higher risk of complications in labour because of, for example, their age or the fact that it is their first baby; it is these women who, were they to be given a free choice, would truly have to weigh up the risks and the advantages of either having their baby at home or in hospital.

Those in favour of home delivery argue that labour should take place in the more intimate atmosphere of their own home with those members of their family or friends who they might wish around them. They would also argue that the technology of a modern labour ward dehumanises what is an intense, emotional and essentially normal experience. There are others who would argue that the risk of something going wrong at very short notice is such that they are willing to trade the familiar and comforting environment for safety. Evidence can be produced on both sides to support the arguments advanced for both points of view. Unplanned home births occur either in very young mothers (concealed pregnancy) or because of too-rapid events in mothers who planned a hospital birth, and these have the expected very high perinatal mortality.

It seems unlikely that there will be any major shift away from the specialised obstetric unit as the main focus of care in the early decades of the twenty-first century. However, there is greater flexibility and choice in provision than in the past. When women do choose to have their baby in a specialist unit, it is essential that they receive the highest standards of care available. This includes, for example, the availability of epidural anaesthesia and access when needed, to the equipment necessary to detect foetal distress. In turn, this means ensuring that units are well equipped and staffed with highly trained personnel. Some large units now contain dedicated midwifery-led units, where women can opt for low-technology midwife-led care with the safeguard of adjacent high-technology services.

PAEDIATRIC SERVICES AT BIRTH

The majority of babies require no resuscitation at birth. Some will require temporary assistance with airway clearing. Others will require full resuscitation and transfer to special care. This includes premature babies, babies with congenital anomalies and congenital infections and those who are found, for whatever reason, to be asphyxiated at birth.

There are three categories of neonatal units providing care:

1   Level 1 units provide special care but do not aim to provide any continuing high dependency or intensive care. This term includes units with or without resident medical staff.

2   Level 2 units provide high dependency care and some short-term intensive care

as agreed within the network.

3   Level 3 units provide the whole range of medical neonatal care but not necessarily all specialist services such as neonatal surgery.

For very tiny and very pre-term babies, there is no doubt that the outcome is better if they are treated in units where long-term ventilation is a standard procedure. The development of such regional or sub-regional level 3 units has also led to the establishment of neonatal flying squads. These consist of an experienced junior paediatrician or consultant and an experienced neonatal nurse who go out with a fully equipped incubator to peripheral hospitals to stabilise and then supervise the transfer of the baby requiring high-dependency care back to the sub-regional centres.

While in the short-term, facilities need to be available to ventilate babies with respiratory distress in all hospitals offering an obstetric service, current evidence suggests that, given the medical and nursing expertise required to deal with babies who need long-term ventilation, high-dependency neonatal care should be provided in a smaller number of centres in each health region.

SERVICES FOR CHILDREN
HISTORICAL PERSPECTIVE

Services exclusively dedicated to the welfare of children developed slowly and sporadically in Britain during the eighteenth century. A dispensary for children of the poor was established in London in 1769, and as part of its service children were visited at home. A hundred years later, this feature was developed when a home-visiting service was established in Manchester and Salford. This service involved 'respectable working women' visiting homes to help and advise on child welfare matters. At the beginning of the twentieth century, a comprehensive health visiting service was established in Huddersfield to combat the high infant mortality rate. A local act made notification of birth to the medical officer of health compulsory so that a home visit could be made shortly after the birth. This pioneering service was followed by national legislation, which was permissive at first but was later made compulsory through the Notification of Birth Act 1915.

A few years later, local authorities were empowered to make arrangements for safeguarding the health of mothers and children, including the provision of free antenatal and postnatal clinics. Child welfare clinics provided by local authorities became more numerous, and a national scheme for training health visitors was inaugurated.

Universal compulsory education, introduced in 1870 and 1880, revealed the extent of poor hygiene, malnutrition and handicapping conditions prevalent amongst school children. Further legislation was soon passed to give powers to local authorities to make provision for blind, deaf, mentally handicapped and epileptic children. The first full-time school medical officer was appointed in London in 1890 and other places followed suit. However, it was the disquiet about the nation's health following the discovery of the poor physical condition of recruits for the Boer War that finally persuaded the government to introduce a school health service. Medical inspection of school children was made compulsory in 1907, and as there was no National Health Service, provision was also made for the treatment of school children. This arrangement continued until the National Health Service was established in 1948.

In the eighteenth and nineteenth centuries, young children were often admitted to women's hospital wards, usually accompanied by their mothers, who helped to care for them in hospital. In 1852, the Hospital for Sick Children in Great Ormond Street, London, was opened, and shortly afterwards many other children's hospitals were built. A register for 'sick children's nurses' was established in 1919, and the emerging new specialty of paediatrics assumed increasing importance during the late 1920s and early 1930s.

Over the past 150 years, social attitudes to children have changed. In early Victorian times, children were on the whole viewed as amoral beings who needed instruction and discipline in order to become 'civilised'. There was widespread and systematised abuse of children, both in working conditions in the developing industries and in child prostitution – particularly in the big cities. Understanding of the psychological and emotional needs of children developed over the first half of the twentieth century.

THE RIGHTS OF CHILDREN

It was only at the end of the 1980s that there was an international statement regarding the rights of children: the United Nations Convention on the Rights of the Child. The Convention was ratified by the United Kingdom government in 1991. The Committee on the Rights of the Child, which is under the auspices of the Office of the United Nations High Commissioner for Human Rights, monitors the implementation of the Convention. Countries that have ratified the Convention are obliged to submit a report every five years. Article 24 of the Convention states that countries:

> recognize the right of the child to the enjoyment of the highest attainable standard of health and to facilities for the treatment of illness and rehabilitation of health. States Parties shall strive to ensure that no child is deprived of his or her right of access to such health care services.

A further article, Article 23, deals with the rights of children who are mentally or physically disabled.

In 2007 the United Nations Children's Fund published a comprehensive assessment of the well-being of children in 21 developed countries. The health indicators were deaths under the age of one, low birth weight, immunisation status and deaths from accidents and injuries under the age of 19 years. The United Kingdom was ranked at the bottom of the league overall, and 12th out of the 21 countries in respect of the health indicators.

EVERY CHILD MATTERS

In the United Kingdom, following the inquiry into the murder in London in 2000 of a young child called Victoria Climbié, a series of major changes to the operation of children's services took place. The policy direction was established under the title

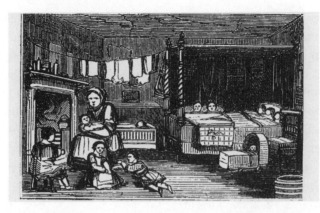

Figure 6.14 Woodcut: a mother and 10 children in a damp and dilapidated room; anon., c. 1864
Source: George Godwin. *Another Blow for Life.* London: WH Allen; 1864.

'Every Child Matters' and was based on the necessity of integrating children's services to ensure that children would be protected and cared for without the danger of them falling through the cracks between various statutory responsibilities and organisational boundaries.

The Children Act 2004 provided for the creation of the post of children's commissioner, whose task is to champion the interests of children and to report annually to parliament. The Act also changed the structures at a local level in England, creating statutory local safeguarding children boards and requiring top-tier local authorities to have a director of children's services and a lead member for children from amongst the elected members of the authority. Under the Act, appropriate local authorities are also required to prepare a 'children's and young people's plan' setting out their strategy for young people's services.

HEALTH SERVICES FOR CHILDREN

Children are major users of health services, and a high proportion of children come into contact with the health service every year in one way or another (Table 6.11).

Organisational arrangements within the health services and between agencies may create barriers to providing high-quality care for children. A large number of professionals may be involved in the care of one child, and without overall coordination and proper communication there can be real frustration for families.

The current model preferred by professional bodies in the United Kingdom is an integrated or combined child health service where community child health services are offered locally, including, for example, secondary-level care in outpatient and day-care investigation, with close relationships with the local hospital and tertiary centres where inpatient care is offered. The local focus is essential because it is at this level that proper relationships can be established between health services, local authority education services and children's social services.

The integration of children's frontline services is a central theme of the Every Child Matters cross-government policy approach in England.

CHILDREN'S MENTAL HEALTH

The incidence of behavioural and mental disorders amongst children is at a lower level than amongst adults, but it does represent a significant level of morbidity. This subject is discussed more fully in Chapter 7.

HEALTH PROMOTION IN CHILDHOOD

The subject of health promotion and the importance of developing healthy lifestyles and behaviours early in life is described fully in Chapter 3. It is important to recognise the opportunities available for health promotion as a result of the regular contacts with children and their parents that occur throughout childhood. This applies whether the child is presenting with a problem to the

general practitioner or to the hospital service or for routine child health surveillance.

The development of the Healthy Schools Programme in the 1990s has had a major effect. This programme was established in 1999 and revitalised in 2005, and since this time it has been effective in helping schools take a whole-school approach to the health and well-being of pupils. This is in contrast with the individual-pupil approach that was taken traditionally by the health services provided for schools. The four core themes of the programme are personal, social and health education; physical activity; healthy eating; and emotional health and well-being.

THE PROTECTION OF ABUSED AND NEGLECTED CHILDREN

Although injury to children inflicted by their parents is not a new phenomenon, it only became widely recognised in the early 1970s. The term 'battered child syndrome'

Table 6.11 Children's interaction with the health service in a typical year in England

- Around 25% of calls to NHS Direct will be about a child.
- A pre-school child will see their general practitioner (GP) about six times.
- A child of school age will see their GP two or three times.
- Approximately 10% of Walk-in Centre attendances will be children.
- Up to half of infants aged under twelve months and one quarter of older children will attend an emergency department.
- Approximately 25% of A&E attendances will be children.
- One in eleven children will be referred to a hospital outpatients clinic.
- One in ten to fifteen children will be admitted to hospital.

Source: Department of Health. *Tips for Quick Wins: improving responses for children and young people requiring emergency or urgent care*. London: DoH; 2005.

was first used in 1962 by an American paediatrician, Dr Kempe, and was taken up by
the media.

In Britain, widespread attention was
first focused on child physical abuse in
1974 following an inquiry into the death of
seven-year-old Maria Colwell. This inquiry
uncovered serious deficiencies in professional
practice and in the response of services. Its
main historical importance is that it acted
as a stimulus to the establishment of a procedure for dealing with the problem. A
series of major public inquiries have since
discovered a consistent pattern of failure of
professional practice, lack of communication and poor coordination of services.

Recognition of the widespread nature of
child sexual abuse was much slower in coming. Although it was recognised amongst
professionals who were dealing with the
issue, the public were largely unaware of it,
at least as a major problem. All this changed
in the late 1980s, when the sexual abuse of
children became a prominent issue for the
public, the media and politicians. The broadcaster Esther Rantzen launched ChildLine, a
free telephone counselling service for child
victims of sexual abuse.

In Cleveland in 1986, the admission to hospital of large numbers of children suspected
of being sexually abused led to an inquiry
chaired by Lord Justice Butler Sloss. The
subsequent report stated that there was not
only a lack of communication but also a lack
of understanding by the agencies involved
of one another's functions in relation to
child sexual abuse. There were also fundamental differences in approach amongst
professionals of the same discipline.

The crisis in Cleveland raised new issues.

Firstly, it brought into the open the fact that
child sexual abuse might be a much greater
problem than had previously been realised.
Secondly, it drew attention to the need for
a balance between the rights of parents and
the power of professionals to take action to
protect children. Although the Cleveland
Inquiry report was far-reaching and a force
for the introduction of much new guidance on the detection and management
of child sexual abuse, the lessons were not
fully learned.

The Children Act 1989 was framed
against the background of inquiries into
physical abuse occurring in the 1970s and
1980s and the ongoing issues in Cleveland.
Although the Act clearly established what
is often referred to as 'the paramountcy
principle' (i.e., that the welfare of the child is
paramount), there are also strong messages
about the need to care for children whenever
possible within their families and to seek to
avoid court orders when possible. Even in
the Act, which was on the whole welcomed
by all those involved in childcare, there was
expression of the intrinsic conflict between
the need to protect children and recognition of the importance to the child of his
or her family.

In an attempt to diminish the problems
of communication and cooperation that
have been behind many of the serious child-
protection failures, the Children Act 2004
created a wide-ranging legal duty to safeguard children (Table 6.12). It also created
'local children safeguarding boards' with the
function of developing the safeguarding of
children amongst partner organisations. The
Act also has the role of undertaking investigations of allegations against individuals

Table 6.12 Key persons and bodies covered by a duty under the Children Act 2004 to ensure that they act to safeguard and promote the welfare of children

- Local authorities, including district councils
- The police
- The probation service
- NHS bodies (Strategic Health Authorities, Designated Special Health Authorities, Primary Care Trusts, NHS Trusts and NHS Foundation Trusts)
- Organisations (currently the Connexions Service) providing services under section 114 of the Learning and Skills Act 2000
- Youth offending teams
- Governors/Directors of Prisons and Young Offender Institutions
- Directors of Secure Training Centres
- The British Transport Police

Source: Department for Education and Skills. *Statutory Guidance on Making Arrangements to Safeguard and Promote the Welfare of Children Under Section 11 of the Children Act 2004.* London: DfES; 2007.

and reviews of service failure. These boards came into being in 2006, and child death reviews became obligatory under their auspices in 2008. As well as considering the individual circumstances of each child death, the review process is mandated to identify any public health or safety concerns arising from a pattern of deaths in the area.

At any one time, some 60 000 children in England will be looked after (in the care of) local authorities, and in the year 2008, 56% of the children were boys. Almost 70% of the children will have been looked after for more than 30 months. Care in this context encompasses a wide variety of settings ranging from fostering through various types of residential care to secure institutions (Table 6.13).

Children need care of these kinds for a variety of reasons: for example, they may have been abused or neglected, their parents may not be able to cope with their upbringing, they may have severe behavioural or emotional disturbance or their family may have broken down and fragmented (Table 6.14).

A child being considered for care by the local authority should have a full assessment so that the choice of placement can be made in a way that reflects his or her individual needs. In the mid-1990s, concern was expressed about the delivery of health, social care and education services to 'looked after' children. A report commissioned by the government highlighted failures of care – in particular, for highly vulnerable children and those with challenging behaviour. Children with frequent changes of foster placement were not receiving continuous education and were not receiving basic health services such as routine immunisation. A number of children suffered further abuse in foster care or residential care.

Children leaving local authority care are

Table 6.13 Placement of children looked after by local authorities in England, 2008

Placement	Percentage
Foster placement	71
Placed for adoption	4
Placement with parents	8
Other placement in the community	3
Secure units, children's homes and hostels	11
Residential schools	2
Other residential settings	1
	Total = 100% (59 500)

Source: Department for Children, Schools and Families. *Children Looked After in England (Including Adoption and Care Leavers) Year Ending 31 March 2008.* London: DCSF; 2008.

Table 6.14 Children looked after by local authorities in England: category of need, 2008

Category of need	Percentage
Abuse or neglect	62
Child's disability	4
Parent's illness or disability	5
Family in acute distress	8
Family dysfunction	11
Socially unacceptable behaviour	2
Absent parenting	9

Source: Department for Children, Schools and Families. *Children Looked After in England (Including Adoption and Care Leavers) Year Ending 31 March 2008.* London: DCSF; 2008.

known to be at risk of becoming homeless and are also at risk of prostitution, drug addiction and criminal behaviour. Children looked after by local authorities are, by definition, a most vulnerable and needy group. Meeting their needs presents a real challenge to providers of services. In 2007 the responsibility for social services for children passed from the Department of Health to the Department for Children, Schools and Families, which is now seen as the lead department on children's issues across government in England. In respect of looked-after children, the challenge is to promote independence through enhancing the life chances of children who need social services and to ensure that those who need safeguarding are properly protected. Life chances for looked-after children are not good, and therefore a significant amount of attention is given in the initiative to improving outcomes for this group of children and young people.

CONCLUSIONS

The health of the children in any population is an important indicator of its overall health status. Over the last hundred years, the industrialised world has witnessed a major reduction in the number of babies lost around the time of childbirth. Despite the fact that a high proportion of pregnancies now have a successful outcome for mothers and babies, a minority of babies still die or survive in a damaged or impaired state. A small number of mothers also die because of pregnancy or childbirth. An important role for public health is to identify the scope for further reductions in this pool of potentially avoidable death, morbidity and disability.

Health services working alone or with other agencies have a responsibility to improve the health and well-being of children. This can be through the promotion of health; the application of preventive interventions (such as immunisation); the maintenance of good surveillance; the provision of high-quality diagnostic, treatment and rehabilitation services; or making available alternative forms of care, protection and support for children in need.

More than at any other time of life, health and disease in childhood encompasses emotional, psychological, environmental and social influences as well as specific risk factors. Responding to the health challenges of the future will involve a vigorous and imaginative public health approach to the needs of mothers, infants, children and adolescents. For it is amongst these groups that the foundations of a nation's health are laid.

CHAPTER 7
Mental Health and Learning Disability

INTRODUCTION

This chapter deals with the basic concepts of mental health, the extent and range of mental illness and learning disabilities found in the population, the needs of people who suffer from them and the spectrum of services available to meet those needs.

Mental health is not just the absence of mental disorder. It is a state in which a person is able to fulfil an active, functioning role in society, interacting with others and overcoming difficulties without suffering major distress or abnormal or disturbed behaviour.

While attitudes in society are changing, both mental illness and learning disability continue to carry a stigma for those who suffer from them and, to a lesser extent, for those who care for people who suffer from them.

MENTAL HEALTH AND NEED

The World Health Organization estimates that mental and behavioural disorders account for 12% of the global burden of disease (Figure 7.1), yet mental health service expenditure represents less than 1% of total health budgets. Around 30% of the world's population will develop a mental illness each year, but two-thirds will receive no treatment.

The World Health Organization has stated that 'there can be no health without mental health'. This mission statement for universal access to high-quality mental health services has been a powerful rallying call endorsed by a wide range of other international and national mental health bodies. The total costs to society of mental illness are great (Figure 7.2).

The spectrum of psychological disorders that can incapacitate people and interfere with their ability to function normally is very large. While distinctions are often made between major and minor mental illnesses, disorders of the mind can be distressing and disruptive even when they do not amount to a full-blown psychiatric illness. For example, a 30-year-old woman with three small children who develops uncontrollable panic attacks when she enters a shop can be so incapacitated by this problem that she is unable to go outdoors unaccompanied. Moreover, she may be so distressed that she needs to ask her husband to stay away from work to be with her, thus putting his employment position in jeopardy. Similarly, the teenage girl who develops an eating disorder at the time of school-leaving examinations can perform so badly that she may lose important career opportunities.

Many so-called 'minor' mental illnesses are treated in primary care settings or do not necessarily come to the attention of specialist services. Few routine data are available to enable them to be quantified within the population.

The psychoses in particular, such as schizophrenia and bipolar disorders, although rarer, are often accompanied by severe social disability during a relapse and so also have a major social impact. While some psychotic episodes resolve quickly and do not relapse, others can pursue a relapsing course, and some become long-term illnesses requiring medication, support and periodic episodes of hospital care during the course of many years. Most people who have developed psychosis over the last

20 years have been able to maintain a home outside hospital, but there is a group of people with chronic psychotic illness who were diagnosed at a time when modern drugs were not available. Many such people were long-term residents within large psychiatric hospitals, which, in effect, became their homes. Their social disabilities due to their illness were aggravated by a dependence on the routines and habits of institutional life developed over many years. With the advent of programmes of care that have

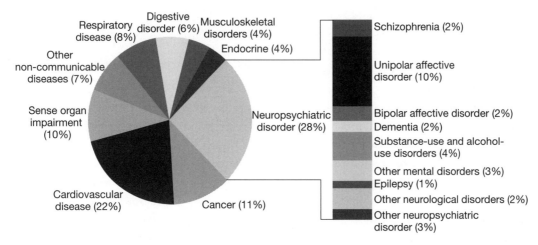

Figure 7.1 Contribution by different non-communicable diseases to disability-adjusted life years worldwide in 2005
Source: Prince M, Patel V, Saxena S, *et al.* No health without mental health. *Lancet.* 2007; **370**: 859–77.

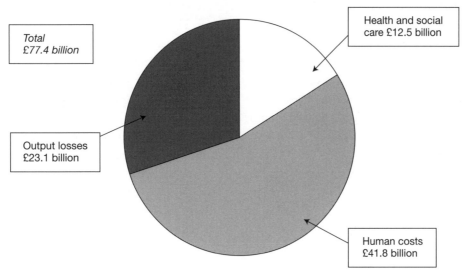

Figure 7.2 Total costs of mental illness, England, 2002/03
Source: Sainsbury Centre for Mental Health.

largely replaced the large long-stay psychiatric hospitals with more modern forms of
care, this group of people with long-term
mental illness must be considered as having
special needs. In addition, there is a group
of younger people with very severe mental
illness and complex social needs who tend
to be in and out of hospital and who would
benefit from intensive continuing NHS care
in small group homes in community settings
to prevent regular relapse and also to prevent
institutionalisation.

Amongst the more severe mental illness
problems within the population is the group
of people whose disorder of the mind leads
them to commit crimes such as assault,
rape, murder, theft and arson. Although the
numbers of mentally disordered offenders
is very small (probably no more than a few
thousand across the United Kingdom), they
pose problems that are complex to solve and
they have needs that require highly specialised forms of care.

Most forms of mental health disorder
amongst adults and children show a higher
concentration in the lower socio-economic
groups. An assessment of need should start
by recognising that more socially disadvantaged areas in a region and neighbourhood
are likely to need higher levels of mental
health service provision.

In addition to recognising the general
importance of factors such as poverty, unemployment and social isolation in assessing
need at the population level, a number of
specific indices of mental health status have
been developed. For example, the Mental
Illness Needs Index (MINI 2000) is designed
to predict mental illness levels in small geographical areas. It uses data on psychiatric

hospital admissions and social deprivation
analysed by Office for National Statistics
geographical areas. The index was developed from earlier versions and is still the
subject of research to refine and broaden
its use. Figure 7.3 shows how it can be used
to pinpoint areas of higher mental health
need in a region.

PREVALENCE OF MENTAL ILLNESS IN POPULATIONS

Describing the size and nature of the problem of mental illness in the population and
the range of needs experienced by people
with mental illness is very difficult. Not least
are the problems of diagnosis and disease
classification. While variation between psychiatrists in the use of disease labels is not
of major importance when addressing the
needs of individual patients, it is a problem
for aggregating diagnostic information to
produce estimates of the size of particular
pools of psychiatric morbidity at population
level. There is also a lack of routinely available population-based information.

Establishing the frequency of psychiatric morbidity in the general population
has been a major area of epidemiological
research since the 1960s and the subject of
important studies even before that. Early
studies concentrated on people already in
contact with mental health services, but it
was quickly realised that this represented
only a small proportion of total psychiatric
morbidity (Figure 7.4).

The Midtown Manhattan Study
One of the most influential early studies

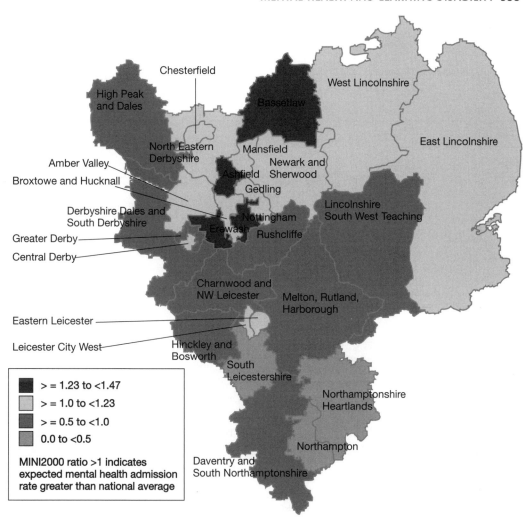

Figure 7.3 Mental Illness Needs Index: MINI2000 ratio, East Midlands region of England
Source: East Midlands Public Health Observatory. *Profile of mental health in the East Midlands.* Mansfield: EMPHO; 2006.

of mental illness in a population was carried out in New York in the mid-1950s. The Midtown Manhattan Study was based on a single home interview of a randomly selected sample of 1.7% of households to identify adults aged 20–59 years, together with information from searching records of hospitals and other agencies (to identify people who could have been missed in the household survey). The survey questions covered 120 manifestations of mental illness, mainly drawn from symptom-based psychiatric screening tools of the day. Psychiatrists then classified the responses gathered by the field interviewers.

The results were presented as a contin-

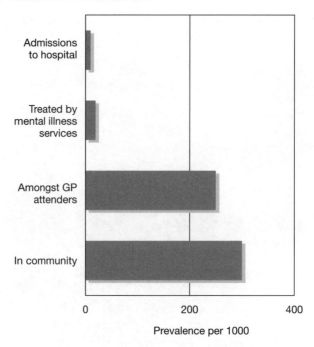

Figure 7.4 Annual period of prevalence of mental illness per 1000 population at risk
Source: Adapted from Goldberg D. *Indicators of Mental Health in the Population.* Department of Health Workshop; 1990.

uum of mental health (Table 7.1), not as a series of diagnostic categories. As a result, the prevalence of 'mental illness' appears quite high. For this reason, the study is often criticised by those who seek to establish the prevalence of mental illness in precise diagnostic groups. Yet it would have been impractical at the time to carry out a full psychiatric assessment on each member of the sample. Moreover, the variation in diagnostic approach between psychiatrists would have limited the extent to which the findings could be generalised.

In more recent years, views have differed as to the approach that should be used to establish the prevalence of mental illness in the population. Broadly, when the aim is to explore causation, disease categories

are more useful. When the aim is purely to examine need for services, functionally based measures are usually preferable.

Population Surveys

The Midtown Manhattan Study superseded early studies of mental health in the population that had used diagnostic labels applied by psychiatrists interviewing and assessing people in a clinical fashion. There had been no attempt to use standardised assessments in these earlier studies.

It is widely acknowledged that assessments of medical conditions, including psychiatric disorders, must be standardised in community surveys. Standardisation is the process of incorporating clinical assessment

Table 7.1 Classification of people's mental status in an early community study: Midtown Manhattan

Mental health	Percentage of sample
Well	18.5
Mild symptom information	36.3
Moderate symptoms	21.8
Marked symptoms	13.2
Severe symptoms	7.5
Incapacitated	2.7
N (100%) = (1660)	100

Source: Srole L, Langner TS, Michael ST, *et al. Mental Health in the Metropolis: the Midtown Manhattan Study.* New York: McGraw-Hill; 1962.

concepts on rules, and its purpose is to reduce between-observer variations and to allow comparability within and between studies. It is also important to contrast the needs of clinicians, for whom accuracy in the individual case is paramount, with those of a researcher, for whom reducing systematic bias or error also has a high priority. Reducing systematic bias is one of the most important advantages of standardisation. The decisions behind the choice of instruments will depend on the age group, the setting and the objectives of the survey, as well as on the resources available and the experience of the interviewers.

People with persecutory paranoid ideation are less likely to agree to take part in such surveys. Furthermore, since psychosis is a relatively rare condition (around 0.5%), a survey sample of 10 000 can only provide a small number of cases, from which it is not possible to produce small area estimates.

In this country, there has been a series of government-sponsored national psychiatric morbidity surveys that have supplied reliable data on mental disorders in the adult general household population (1993, 2000 and 2007); in people in institutional care (1993); in school children (1999 and 2004); in prisoners (1998); in carers; in the homeless; on prevalence; on risk factors; on consequences, including accompanying disability; and on service use. There have also been longitudinal follow-up surveys of adults and children, although so far, these have only been for one follow-up period – 18 months for adults and three years for children.

The most recently reported national sample survey of psychiatric morbidity of adults in private households in Great Britain was carried out by the Office for National Statistics in 2000. Interviews were carried out in two steps, initially by trained interviewers and a subset by clinical psychologists. The survey used a symptom-severity scale and provided estimates of the prevalence of psychiatric morbidity in internationally recognised diagnostic categories. Separate standardised assessment instruments were used, for example, to assess neurotic disorders, psychotic disorders or alcohol misuse.

Amongst the true mental disorders,

neurotic illness was the most common, though substance misuse (alcohol and drugs) was more common overall (Figure 7.5).

The Office for National Statistics has also carried out a follow-up study of the sample of people interviewed in the 2000 psychiatric morbidity survey in order to assess the degree of recovery and persistence of mental disorders.[1]

The prevalence of neurotic disorders shown in the national study of psychiatric morbidity is higher for women than for men, both overall and for individual conditions (Figure 7.6). The onset of common mental disorders was strongly associated with living in rented accommodation and with experiencing threatening life events. Unemployment and low income were important risk factors amongst men. Around half of men and women who had a common mental disorder in the original survey did not have it at the follow-up 18 months later.

A similar national survey of children's and young people's mental health was carried out in 2004. One in 10 children aged 5–16 years had a clinically diagnosed mental disorder (Figure 7.7).

Disorders of conduct were the most common (Table 7.2). Prevalence of mental disorder was higher in children in more disadvantaged circumstances or with weaker social networks.

Psychotic disorders were higher amongst young adults (Figure 7.8) and associated with higher levels of deprivation and isolation (Table 7.3).

Health Survey for England

Another source of information on people with mental health problems is the use of a standardised General Health Questionnaire (GHQ 12) as part of the Health Survey for England. This asks about factors such as general level of happiness, depression, anxiety and sleep disturbance. It identifies people with a mental health problem in general rather than applying a particular diagnostic label. A score of four or more on the General Health Questionnaire suggests possible mental health problems. In England, an estimated 13.2% of the population falls into this category.

The 'Russian doll' model

In Figure 7.9, the largest 'Russian doll' represents the people who present mainly in primary care with mental health problems. This group is estimated as between 10% to 25% of the population each year. Within this group are 'Russian dolls' representing the frequency of people in the population with severe mental illness and severe enduring mental illness. The inner 'Russian doll' represents the group with severe mental illness who are difficult to engage with services (for example, the homeless, those who are violent, those who are drug abusers, those who have complex social problems).

Health Service Usage Data

As with other groups of hospital patients, hospital episode statistics is the method by which statistics on psychiatric inpatients are collected from National Health Service psychiatric hospitals and psychiatric units

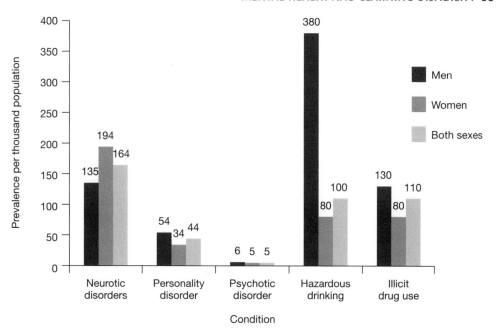

Figure 7.5 Prevalence (per 1000 population) of mental disorders and substance misuse amongst adults in Great Britain
Source: Singleton N, Bumpstead R, O'Brien M, *et al. Psychiatric Morbidity Among Adults Living In Private Households, 2000.* London: The Stationery Office; 2001.

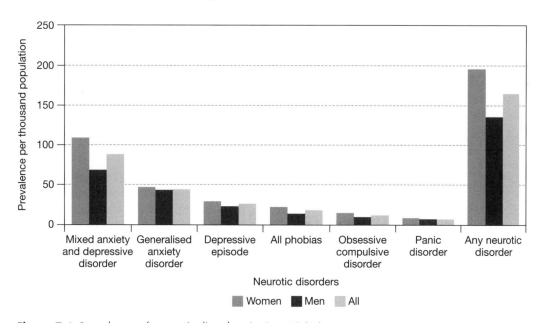

Figure 7.6 Prevalence of neurotic disorders in Great Britain
Source: Singleton N, Bumpstead R, O'Brien M, *et al. Psychiatric Morbidity Among Adults Living In Private Households, 2000.* London: The Stationery Office; 2001.

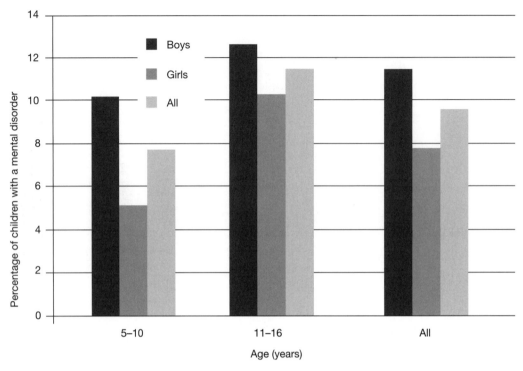

Figure 7.7 Prevalence of any mental disorder amongst children in Great Britain
Source: Green H, McGinnity A, Meltzer H, *et al. Mental Health of Children and Young People in Great Britain, 2004.* London: Office for National Statistics; 2005.

Table 7.2 Prevalence of mental disorders amongst children aged 5-16 years, Great Britain

Condition	Prevalence (percent)
Anxiety	3.3
Depression	0.9
Conduct disorders	5.8
Autistic spectrum disorders	0.9
Eating disorders	0.3
Other less common disorders	0.1
Any mental disorder	9.6

Source: Green H, McGinnity A, Meltzer H, *et al. Mental Health of Children and Young People in Great Britain, 2004.* London: Office for National Statistics; 2005.

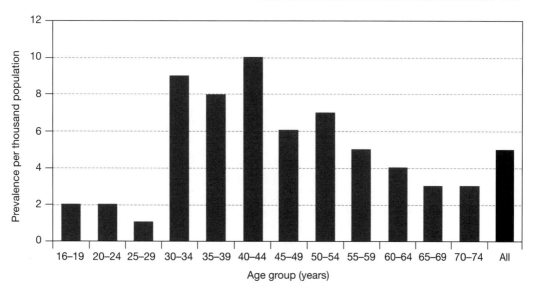

Figure 7.8 Prevalence of probable psychotic disorder in Great Britain
Source: Singleton N, Bumpstead R, O'Brien M, *et al. Psychiatric Morbidity Among Adults Living In Private Households, 2000.* London: The Stationery Office; 2001.

Table 7.3 Features of people with psychotic illness

More likely:

- to be separated or divorced and living in one-person household
- to have low educational qualifications
- to be in lowest socio-economic groups and be economically inactive
- to be in rented public housing and live in an urban area
- to have long-standing physical health problems.

Source: Singleton N, Bumpstead R, O'Brien M, *et al. Psychiatric Morbidity Among Adults Living In Private Households, 2000.* London: The Stationery Office; 2001.

in England and Wales. Detailed information is collected about each admission and discharge, and a notional census of all psychiatric inpatients is carried out once a year (*see* Chapter 1 for a fuller description).

Specialist providers of mental health services for adults are required to collect a Mental Health Minimum Data Set. This includes data on clinical condition, treatment, use of services and outcome.

The admission of fewer people with mental illness to hospital in one area than in another may reflect the availability of facilities, the policy for admission, the social stigma attached to mental illness in general or to a particular institution for its treatment, or the tolerance of the community towards abnormal behaviour. Other factors determining whether or not people with a particular psychiatric illness come to the

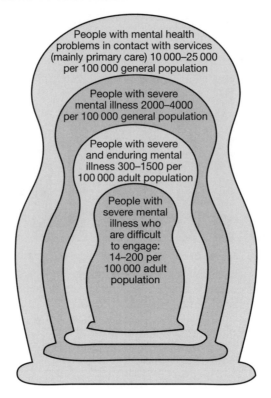

Figure 7.9 Estimated number of people with different degrees of mental health problem in the population
Source: Sainsbury Centre for Mental Health. *Keys to Engagement: a review of care for people with severe mental illness who are hard to engage with services.* London: SCMH; 1998.

attention of hospital-based services may be the extent to which they or their relatives perceive an abnormality and consider it necessary to make contact with services. This, in turn, may depend upon whether the abnormality interferes with social functioning, either in the person's job or in the discharge of other social responsibilities.

Health of the Nation Outcome Scales (HoNOS)

In the mid-1990s, the Royal College of Psychiatrists was commissioned to develop a scale to rate the level of health and social functioning of people with severe mental illness. The scale was initially intended to assess progress towards a target set in the *Health of the Nation*[2] public health White Paper: 'to improve significantly the health and social functioning of mentally ill people'. Over time this has broadened; the scale is now used for a much wider range of purposes: assessment of need, evaluating care and treatment interventions, resource allocation and planning of care and services more generally.

There are now 12 areas, with each rated

for the severity of the patient's problem (Table 7.4). There are a number of versions covering different groups, such as working-age adults (HoNOS), people with learning disabilities (HoNOS-LD) and people who have had brain injuries (HoNOS-ABI).

The Health of the Nation Outcome Scales are widely used by mental health services in the NHS and are part of the Minimum Data Set for Mental Health.

The Quality and Outcomes Framework

The Quality and Outcomes Framework (QOF) for general practice is described in Chapter 4. It provides a set of evidence-based clinical indicators for different groups of patients and conditions. General practices score points based on their achievement of these indicators and then are paid on their

scoring. As part of this system, prevalence information is held in registers by participating practices, including information on mental health problems. Data are limited to severe long-term mental health problems but nevertheless give an alternative and more regular source of prevalence estimates. There are limitations with the data, which are not a true measure of prevalence (i.e., if illness is not diagnosed, data are not recorded).

Comparing Sources of Data on Mental Health Problems

Each source of data on the frequency of mental health problems and the pattern of usage of services provides a different perspective, each with their usefulness and limitations (Table 7.5).

Table 7.4 The 12 areas covered in the Health of the Nation Outcome Scales (HoNOS) – severity is rated on each

- Overactive, aggressive, disrupted behaviour
- Self-harm
- Problematic drinking and drug-taking
- Cognitive problems
- Hallucinations or delusions
- Depressed mood
- Relationship problems
- Difficulties with activities of daily living
- Physical illness or disability
- Problems with occupation and activities
- Difficulties with living conditions
- Other mental and behavioural problems

Source: Wing JK, Curtis RH, Beevor AS. *Health of the Nation Outcome Scales: report on research and development.* London: Royal College of Psychiatrists; 1996.

Table 7.5 Information of value in assessing mental health needs of a population

Indicator(s)	Purpose	Comments
Population characteristics (e.g., age, deprivation)	General profiling of need	Broad-based and mainly contextual
Mental Health Minimum Data Set	Insight into who uses specialist mental health services and why, with information on outcome	Limited to users of specialist services
Hospital Episode Statistics	Information on mental health problems amongst general hospital admissions	Provides perspective on conditions that lead to hospital admission
Office for National Statistics Psychiatric Morbidity Survey	Population-level data on psychiatric illness	Good source of prevalence data but periodic only
Quality and Outcome Framework in primary care	Mental health problems in primary care	Limited to severe mental health problems and has variable data quality
Health Survey for England	Self-reported 'symptom'-based assessment	Does not attach diagnostic labels, therefore functional measure
Mental Health Needs Index (MINI 2000)	Mental health need in smaller geographical areas	Useful tool, methodological challenges still being addressed
Mental Health Act returns	Use of Mental Health Act	Limited insight on prevalence but important to monitor uses and abuses of Act

RISK FACTORS FOR SCHIZOPHRENIA

Schizophrenia is one of the psychiatric illnesses that has been most extensively studied using epidemiological approaches. Studies of risk factors have yielded a fascinating range of influences on the frequency of the disease (Table 7.6). The systematic reviews used in the study shown in Table 7.6 suggest a life-time risk of schizophrenia of seven individuals per 1000. Familial risk is now well established, and a great deal of subsequent work has been to elucidate whether this is due to genetic or environmental causes. Socio-demographic risk factors for schizophrenia have been classified into mutable (for example, marital status) and immutable (for example, ethnic origin). It must be remembered, however, that mutable risk factors may occur because of the disease and not vice versa. A good example of this kind of problem is the relationship between schizophrenia and social class.

One of the earliest and best-known examples of the use of hospital admissions to study mental illness was the investigation of the relationship between schizophrenia and social class carried out in the 1930s in Chicago.[3] First-admission rates to hospital for schizophrenia were used to pinpoint differences in its frequency between different parts of Chicago. The question of selection bias is not further raised here, except to say that first-admission rates for schizophrenia at that time are probably a fair approximation of incidence, since most people were hospitalised at some stage during their first episode of the illness.

It was observed that the mental hospital admission rates for schizophrenia were highest in the central slum districts, with much lower rates in the outer residential areas of the city. One interpretation of these observations was that since the poor areas contained many people of lower socio-economic status, it was therefore the environment, lifestyle and living conditions of people in the lowest stratum of society that predisposed them to the disease. This hypothesis seemed to be substantiated by a later study that looked at first-admission rates to all psychiatric services, including outpatients in a defined geographical area, New Haven, Connecticut.[4] The results

appeared to show that people in lower social classes had a higher incidence of schizophrenia. This phenomenon became known as 'the breeder hypothesis'; adverse social circumstances being seen as generating mental illness. Some doubt was shed on this reasoning by the observation that poor areas and social isolation do not necessarily go together, at least in European cities, and that schizophrenic patients quite often moved into isolated areas before admission to hospital.

British researchers then provided important new evidence. Their findings are presented in Table 7.7. They compared the social-class distribution of young male patients diagnosed with schizophrenia on first admission to mental hospitals with that of their fathers at the time of the patient's birth. It was found that although the patients had a marked excess of jobs in the lower social-class categories, they had been born

Table 7.6 Influence of sex, migrant status, urban status, secular trend, economic status, and latitude on the distribution of estimates from the systematic reviews of schizophrenia incidence, prevalence, and mortality

	Sex	Migrant status	Urban status	Secular trend	Economic status	Latitude
Incidence: core	Males > females	Migrant >native born	Urban > mixed urban and rural	Falling over time	No significant difference	High latitude > lower latitude (males only)
Prevalence: combined estimates	Males = females	Migrant > native born	No significant difference	Stable	Developed > least developed	High latitude > lower latitude
Standardised mortality ratio: all cause	Males = females	Not available	Not available	Rising over time	No significant difference	Not available

Source: McGrath J, Saha S, Chant D, et al. Schizophrenia: a concise overview of incidence, prevalence and mortality. Epidemiol Rev. 2008; **30**: 67–76.

Table 7.7 Social-class distribution of schizophrenic patients and their fathers (males, first admissions aged 25–34 years, England and Wales, 1956)

	Patients at admission		Fathers at patient's birth	
Social Class	Observed	Expected	Observed	Expected
I	12	12	14	8
II	21	44	42	42
III	178	203	192	192
IV	52	55	66	68
V	90	39	55	59
Total	353	353	369	369
Not stated	18		2	

Source: Goldberg EM, Morrison SL. Schizophrenia and social class. *Br J Psychiatry.* 1963; **109**: 785–802.

into families with a similar social-class distribution to that of the general population. The implication was that there had been a 'drift' downwards in the social classes of schizophrenic patients as a result of their illness. This contradicts the 'breeder hypothesis', which suggested that socioeconomic deprivation is of major aetiological importance. For a time, it was generally believed that the preponderance of lower-social-class patients with schizophrenia was due to the disabling effect of the illness (the drift hypothesis) rather than through poor environmental circumstances (the breeder hypothesis), but recent findings linking psychosis to living in cities has revived the view that social adversity is causal.

SUICIDE, SEVERE SELF-HARM AND HOMICIDE
SUICIDE

The classic work of the famous French sociologist Emile Durkheim (1858–1917) on suicides, conducted over a period of over 30 years, is a landmark in his own discipline and in social psychiatry.

Through studying statistics from various European countries and through analysing case records, Durkheim concluded that suicide was a relatively stable characteristic with a fixed rate for a given society that reflected its culture. He considered that factors in society, such as the degree of social cohesion, exercised a powerful effect on the individual and might predispose him to suicide. One of Durkheim's conclusions was that suicide rates were higher amongst Protestants and the well-to-do and lower amongst Catholics and poor people. He also found suicide more frequent in males than in females, with an increased rate in elderly people.

Although published statistics rely solely on officially confirmed suicides, misclassification is a problem. The potential sources of error should not affect the large, observed variations of suicide rates overtime.

The National Confidential Inquiry into Suicide and Homicide by People with

Mental Illness was established in 1990 and enables in-depth analysis of these occurrences and the identification of possible avoidable factors.

In the immediate post-war period, suicides in England and Wales increased to a peak in the mid-1960s and then fell until the mid-1970s. Thereafter, suicides increased to a peak in the early 1980s amongst women and in the late 1980s amongst men. From then until the late 1990s, suicide rates in both sexes fell (more so in women than men). These overall trends conceal contrasts between the age and sex groups.

Since 2000, suicide rates have fallen still further, reaching their lowest historical rate in 2006 (Figure 7.10). The majority of suicides are amongst young men, and across all age groups men kill themselves more often than women do (Figure 7.11). Overall, men kill themselves more often by hanging and suffocation, while women's preferred method is drug-related poisoning (Figure 7.12).

Particular risk groups are prisoners, mental health inpatients and those in contact with mental health services (Table 7.8). Prevention of suicide is multifactorial and encompasses the establishment of national strategies[5] relating to education of health and social care professionals about better diagnosis and treatment of mental illness, better assessment and management of suicidal risk and better support for high-risk groups. These high-risk groups are: people with severe mental illness, who have a one in six chance of killing themselves; those committing deliberate self-harm, who have a 100 times increased risk in the following 12 months; and certain occupational groups, such as doctors, vets, farmers, pharmacists and nurses. Other pertinent factors include the reduction in access to means of suicide, liaison with media to influence the way

Death rate per 100 000 population

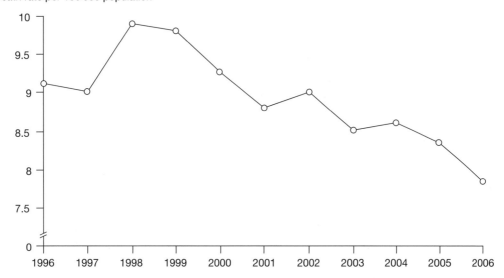

Figure 7.10 Suicide mortality in England
Source: Office for National Statistics.

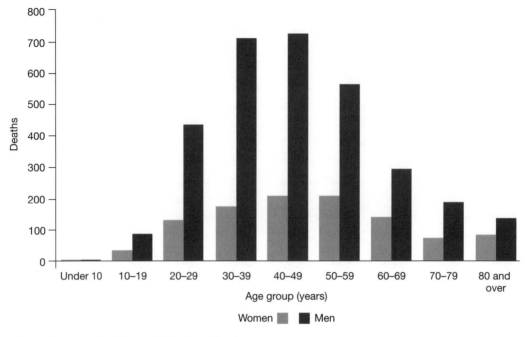

Figure 7.11 Deaths from suicide in England, 2006
Source: Office for National Statistics.

suicides are reported, research and continued audit of suicides.

SELF-HARM

Severe self-harm can be defined as a non-fatal incident in which a person causes self-injury or self-poisoning. The terms 'attempted suicide' and 'parasuicide' used to be applied to acts in which people tried to kill themselves but were not successful. While the socio-demographic characteristics of people who attempt suicide are somewhat different from those who complete suicide, there is great overlap between the two groups, and people who attempt suicide are 100 times more likely to kill themselves in the succeeding year. Thus all people who attempt suicide should be regarded as at risk from actual

suicide, and careful assessment and management is needed.

The frequency of severe self-harm in the population is difficult to define accurately. Estimates are usually based on cases of poisoning or self-injury attending an emergency department or admitted to hospital. However, from hospital admission data it is difficult to distinguish between accidents and deliberate acts of self-harm. Furthermore, it has been suggested that estimates based on hospital inpatient or emergency department statistics may miss between one-fifth and one-third of cases. Those who sought help from their general practitioner or did not seek help at all will not be included, nor will those who did not make contact with any medical authority. From hospital statistics, it is estimated that

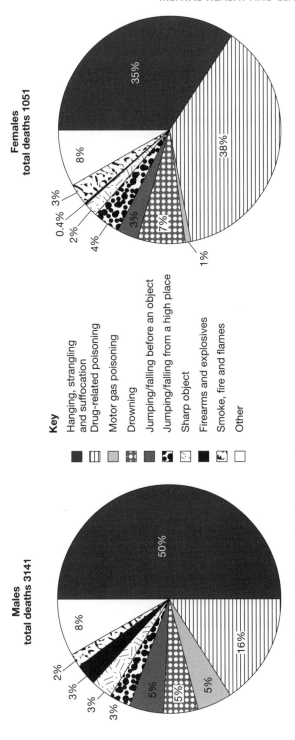

Figure 7.12 Deaths from suicide by method in England, 2006
Source: Office for National Statistics.

Table 7.8 High-risk groups for suicide in Britain

- Young men and men over 80 years
- Men from the Republic of Ireland and eastern Europe
- Unemployed people
- People who have been in local authority care during childhood and adolescence
- People who have suffered bereavement or loss
- People detained in prison, particularly young men
- Vets, farmers, pharmacists, doctors, nurses and others who have ready access to means of killing themselves
- People with a previous episode of deliberate self-harm
- People with severe mental illness

there are about 160 hospital admissions for self-harm per 100 000 population, while emergency department figures give estimates of 300–400 episodes per 100 000 population.

SUICIDE AND SELF-HARM: RISK FACTORS AND RISK ASSESSMENT

A number of risk factors predispose people to suicide or self-harm. The approach to the assessment of risk, and hence the prevention of suicide and self-harm, involves checking for the presence of risk factors and undertaking a careful clinical examination in which the person's history of previous incidents of self-harm and their ideas about suicide are explored. Having a plan to kill themselves and an intent to do so are strong predictors. Efforts have been made to improve risk assessment on the basis of what is now known about risk factors, but more research and training will be helpful.

Risks can be managed – much depends on the individual case, but the key to good risk management involves a multidisciplinary and multi-agency approach, well-trained staff and a great deal of direct contact with the patient. The annual incidence of suicidal thoughts is 4% (3% in men and 5% in women). Risk factors for onset of suicidal thoughts include: age (10% of 24-year-olds reported onset of suicidal thoughts); being single, separated or divorced; living alone; lower educational attainment; lower social class; unemployment; being long-term disabled; having several stressful life events; smoking; and illicit drug use. However, the strongest risk factor is high baseline psychiatric-symptom score (2% of people who score 0–5 symptoms reported onset of suicidal thoughts, compared to 23% of those with a score of 18 symptoms and above).

HOMICIDE AND VIOLENCE

When things go wrong in mental health services, they tend to attract considerable media attention. This is particularly so in

Table 7.9 Risk factors for self-harm

Variables	Higher risk	Lower risk
Age	Younger	Older
Sex	Female	Male
Marital status	Separated, divorced, widowed	Married
Living arrangements	Living alone, homeless	Others at home
Employment status	Unemployed	Employed
Physical health	Poor, especially terminal, painful, debilitating illness	Good
Mental health	Depression, schizophrenia, chronic sleep disorders, eating disorders	Good
Substance abuse	Alcoholism, illegal drug misuse	None

Source: *Learning materials on mental health: risk assessment.* Manchester: University of Manchester; 1996.

the case of homicides committed by people with mental illness. Currently, health authorities are required to set up independent inquiries into homicides committed by people who have been in recent contact with specialist mental health services, and the main findings and recommendations are made public. Aggregate data on suicide and homicide are also published together in five-yearly reports. The most recent is *Avoidable Deaths,*[6] a report by the National Confidential Inquiry into Suicide and Homicide by People with Mental Illness in December 2006.

In an analysis of homicides involving mentally ill people in Scotland carried out by the National Confidential Inquiry, the majority of perpetrators were male (sex ratio 13:1), young (median age 28 years), unmarried and unemployed or on long-term sickness benefit. These perpetrators were more likely to kill someone known to them (78%) rather than a stranger (22%). In

contrast to popular belief, the proportion of perpetrators with serious mental disorder is quite small, though a previous history of violence and drug misuse is common.

Hazardous drinking exerts the largest public health impact on serious and repetitive violence and versatility of violence. Estimates of the proportion of violent crimes that involve alcohol vary with type of crime and country, but an appropriate estimate is that over 50% of assailants have been drinking.[7] The socio-demographic characteristics of violent individuals who have been drinking are the same as those of violent individuals in general – being young, single, male and of lower social class.

The contribution to violence at the population level from persons screening positive for psychosis was very small, while by far the largest public health impact on serious and repetitive violence was exerted by hazardous drinking. A relatively small reduction in exposure to the risk factor of hazardous drinking at the individual level could result in a relatively large impact on violent behaviour.[8]

TRENDS IN THE CARE OF MENTALLY ILL PEOPLE
EARLY PRACTICES

In the Dark and Middle Ages, the treatment of mental illness was governed by ignorance and superstition. If the mentally ill had delusions of a religious nature, they were often revered; if their utterances were blasphemous, they were held to be possessed by demons and treated, in the first instance, through exorcism by a priest. If this was unsuccessful, they would be subjected to physical restraint, pain and degradation. This quasi-religious view of mental illness later gave way to the notion that insane people were practitioners of the 'black arts'. In Britain alone, thousands of women and children, many of whom must have had mental illnesses, were subjected to the ducking stool or burned at the stake as witches. The last woman to meet her death in this way did so in Scotland in 1722.

BRITAIN IN THE EIGHTEENTH AND NINETEENTH CENTURIES

In the early years of the eighteenth century, a number of singularly unpleasant fates could befall the person who was mentally ill, depending on the circumstances in which he found himself. There was then no organised service to provide care for the mentally ill.

The Pauper Lunatic

If the manifestations of his illness led him into the trap of poverty, the pauper lunatic became subject to the conditions of the Poor Law. Under the old Poor Law, which dated from Elizabethan times, the responsibility for paupers rested with individual parishes, each of which had an overseer who raised money by taxation to provide for them. The standard of poorhouses varied greatly from one part of the country to another, but in many of the larger cities the workhouse began to emerge as the principal type of provision.

A report by the Poor Law Commissioners that gave rise to the Poor Law Amendment Act 1834 saw the workhouse as the fulcrum of the state's policy on the poor. There was almost an obsession on the part of the authorities to prevent exploitation by malingerers. The workhouse, with its frugal and in many cases inhuman surroundings, was seen as the way to deter the lazy and work-shy and to extract the maximum productivity from the able-bodied pauper. The policy on the pauper lunatic was expressly to exclude him from the workhouse. Nevertheless, the majority found their way into it, although they were not recognised or treated as a separate category.

The law dealt with the vagrant very strictly, and thus the mentally ill who left their own homes to wander abroad as beggars would often find themselves in prison. Similarly, criminal insanity was not recognised. Hence if a person's mental condition led him to commit a crime, he would be judged by penal law and usually find himself in one of the already crowded prisons.

Because of the deep shame attached to

mental illness, many families of poor and well-to-do alike sought to conceal its presence amongst their relatives. This led to the practice of keeping 'single lunatics' in remote places. It was not uncommon for a family member to be secured in a cellar like an animal for years at a time.

The Private Madhouse

The wealthy escaped the indignity of the workhouse or the prison cell, but insanity brought confinement in one of the private madhouses that proliferated in England at the time. These were run for profit, and the fate of their inmates was scarcely better, and in many cases worse, than that of the pauper lunatic in the workhouse; shackling and deliberate ill-treatment were often the order of the day.

Bedlam

Originally founded in 1247 as a priory by the Order of St Mary of Bethlehem, Bethlehem Royal Hospital in London was the largest, and for some time the only, public hospital in England devoted to the care of the insane. It existed largely on public subscriptions. The treatment meted out to inmates was as harsh as that in the private madhouses. The mentally ill were chained in confined surroundings and often subjected to bizarre and whimsical therapies, such as bleeding, purging or the induction of vomiting. Towards the end of the eighteenth century, the general public could be admitted to the hospital and for the fee of one penny amuse themselves by watching the antics of the inmates. The name of the hospital,

corrupted in common parlance to 'Bedlam', gave the English language a new word that was synonymous with mindless disorder and chaos.

Discharged patients were given badges to allow them legitimately to exist as beggars without falling foul of the harsh vagrancy laws of the time. These 'Toms O'Bedlam' soon found their ranks swelled by impostors who had forged their badges.

The Humanitarian Movement

At the beginning of the nineteenth century, concern began to grow amongst a few enlightened reformers, and to a lesser extent in public opinion, about the appalling way in which the mentally ill were treated. In part, this came about through the existence of islands of compassion in the approach to mental illness. Outstanding in this respect was the Quaker William Tuke, who founded the Retreat at York where the mentally ill were not manacled and restrained but were treated humanely. The success of this venture made a deep impression on attitudes to mental illness and its treatment.

Equally important were the revelations made by various select parliamentary committees of the circumstances of those housed in public asylums and private madhouses. One of the most well-known examples is the visit made by Edward Wakefield, MP and his colleagues to Bethlehem Hospital. During their visit, they discovered one of the inmates, William Norris, who was half-naked and chained to the wall in such a way that he could stand up or lie down but not sit. This wretched man had been kept in this way for nine years and by the time he

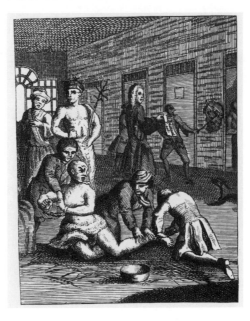

Figure 7.13 A ward in Bethlem, about 1745. From Tuke DH. *Chapters in the History of the Insane.*
London: Kegan Paul; 1882
Source: The Wellcome Institute Library, London.

became a cause celebre was in the terminal phase of tuberculosis.

Similar discoveries of conditions in private madhouses led to legislation bringing them under licence, although it must be admitted that conditions changed little at first. Another important advance was the County Asylums Act 1808, which recommended that local authorities should build asylums to provide treatment for the mentally ill. The programme was not compulsory, and consequently implementation was very slow in most parts of the country, and it was designed to cater mainly for the pauper lunatic, who would otherwise have found himself in the workhouse.

Under the Madhouse Act 1828 (with subsequent amendments), the Metropolitan Commissioners in Lunacy, consisting of medical practitioners, barristers and laypeople appointed by the Lord Chancellor, became the guardians of insane patients and made reports.

The culmination of the reform movement was the passing by parliament of the Lunatics Act 1845. In it, the power of the Lunacy Commissioners was greatly extended so that they were responsible for inspection, licensing and reporting on all places in which the mentally ill were housed or cared for. They were able to investigate and report the circumstances of the mentally ill in prisons and workhouses (which had previously been outside their jurisdiction), as well as in public hospitals, asylums, private madhouses and other licensed premises. Further measures introduced in the Act were the tightening up of procedures for certification of the mentally ill and the compulsory keeping of records by institutions treating them.

INTO THE TWENTIETH CENTURY: THE OPEN-DOOR POLICY

During the early years of the twentieth century, the mental hospital, closed and often situated in a remote locality, served a predominantly custodial role, with little attempt to treat mental illness or to forge links with the community. One of the first rays of light on this depressing scene was the widespread establishment of psychiatric outpatient clinics, which together with the move towards voluntary admission were by-products of the enlightened Mental Treatment Act 1930.

In 1948, mental hospitals, along with other types of hospital, became part of the National Health Service and were no longer the responsibility of the local authorities. The local authorities were given statutory responsibilities for providing community care, which comprised care and aftercare, as well as prevention.

Most of the hospital facilities for the mentally ill inherited by the National Health Service were in buildings erected during the last century and even earlier. These large mental hospitals had been designed to provide an isolated, self-sufficient community, often enclosed by high walls, with the objectives of protecting society from the patient and of protecting the patient from the outside world.

Few new mental hospitals had been built since the start of World War II, so serious overcrowding of existing hospitals reached crisis point by the mid-1950s. For instance, a typical large hospital designed to accommodate 1800 patients might contain 2700 patients, be serving a catchment population of about one million covering four or five different local authorities, and be staffed by three consultant psychiatrists. Thus serious thought was being given to the idea of building new hospitals.

The discovery of the psychotropic drugs, which helped to accelerate a trend in the reduction of psychiatric hospital inpatients (the open-door policy), arrested this development. A similar picture was seen in the United States and other countries. This more optimistic outlook in treatment led to changing attitudes to mental illness amongst professionals and the public. Locked doors were opened and many more patients left hospital to live in the community, where local authorities began to provide an increasing quantity of supportive services.

In a way, the Mental Health Act 1959 served as the legislature's imprimatur on a wagon that was already rolling. In a relatively short space of time, the mantle of isolationism fell away from mental hospitals and a real working partnership sprang up between hospital and community services. It was as if a latter-day Joshua had blown his trumpet and the high walls around the mental hospitals had fallen down.

The population of mental hospital inpatients reached a peak in England and Wales in 1954, at just over 152 000. By 1975 this figure had been reduced to 98 000, and by the beginning of the 1990s there were 59 000 mental illness beds.

From before the beginning of the century until the end of World War II, there was a slow increase in the number of admissions to mental illness hospitals and units in England. From the late 1940s until the early 1970s, there was an increase in annual admissions from around 25 000 to 160 000. During the course of the 1970s, admission rates remained stable, varying only slightly in an upwards or downwards direction. From then onwards, episodes of inpatient care have increased and lengths of stay have decreased. In other words, modern psychiatric inpatient facilities are now used much more intensively than they used to be, with a focus on treatment rather than a custodial approach to care.

CARE IN THE COMMUNITY: IDEALS AND CONCERNS

Current national policy on care of those with serious mental illness in Britain can be traced back to the famous speech by Enoch Powell in the 1960s when, as Minister for Health, he declared that the 'water tower' hospitals for those with mental illness had had their day and should be replaced with modern forms of local comprehensive care.

This policy was further developed in the White Paper *Better Services for the Mentally Ill*, which was issued in the mid-1970s. It proposed a reduced role for the large mental hospitals, many of which were the former asylums of Victorian times. In turn, there was to be development of a comprehensive range of locally based services, including inpatient facilities in district general hospitals. Greater emphasis on community care was seen as the best way to attain improved heath and social outcomes.

Considerable efforts have been made over the last few decades to implement the policy of local, comprehensive community-based care. The ratio of beds in larger psychiatric hospitals to those for the treatment of mental illness in district general hospitals fell from 8:1 in the mid-1970s to about 2:1 at the beginning of the 1990s.

The economic consequences of the closures of the large psychiatric hospitals should have been cost-neutral, as the capital sums derived from the sale of the land would have been enough to fund the new capital expenditure required, and the revenue costs of funding community teams were broadly similar to the revenue costs of funding institutional teams. However, the capital sums derived from the land sales were not generally hypothecated for mental health services, instead going elsewhere, and so new monies had to be found to fund the new local comprehensive services. Also, hospitals could not be closed until the last clients had left, so both institutional and community-based teams had to be resourced. However, the scale of the shift to community care can be seen by comparing the number of resident inpatients in 1954 (around 150 000) with the total number of beds in 2003, which was 71 000 (excluding private provision).

In some parts of Britain (especially the inner cities), a failure to provide a sufficient range of community services before the reduction of beds in psychiatric hospitals led to people with severe mental illness receiving inadequate care. Surveys at the time of homeless people with mental illness showed that people who had been discharged from long-stay psychiatric institutions were not generally represented in homeless populations (as they had generally been resettled with a dowry into a staffed hostel), but those homeless people who were mentally ill were people with new episodes of psychosis who had never previously accessed mental health services.

It has taken several decades to move from a largely institutional model of care to local comprehensive care, including acute hospital care in a general hospital setting, with associated day and outpatient facilities, together with smaller more local residential care and packages of community care tailored to individual needs. This is because of the resource implications of building up community provision; the need for political, managerial, professional and public commitment to the transition; and the timescales involved, amidst other competing priorities. Such a timescale is reflected in the experience of other countries.

The 1990s also saw the establishment of mental health as a key priority area. Two public health White Papers *The Health of the Nation* (1992) and *Our Healthier Nation* (1999) included targets to reduce morbidity and suicide; extended mental health policy to address the importance of systematic mental health information systems; promoted close intersectoral working between agencies; committed to user and carer involvement in the design and delivery of services. They also sought to achieve the integration of mental health into primary care; stressed the importance of mental health promotion and prevention in schools, workplaces and other settings; and expanded the mental health research and development programme.

CURRENT POLICY AND LEGISLATIVE CONTEXT

The National Service Framework for Mental Health was published in 1999 and has been implemented since then. It set clear standards for improvement in the quality and accessibility of mental health services, particularly in the following areas:

➣ mental health promotion
➣ access to services
➣ effective service models
➣ services for people with severe mental illness
➣ carer support.

A formal review of progress on the *National Service Framework* 10 years on showed expansion in community mental health services (crisis resolution teams, assertive outreach teams and early intervention teams); increased investment; expanded workforce (consultant psychiatrists, clinical psychologists, mental health nurses, primary care therapists); greater availability of more modern drugs with fewer side effects; and upgrading of buildings and facilities.

In the next phase of development, the key policies are promoting greater social inclusion for mentally ill people, expanding access to psychological therapies and improving services for ethnic minority communities.

The publication of the *National Service Framework* came at the same time as similar initiatives for coronary heart disease and cancer. Placing mental health on the same footing as these more glamorous and traditionally better-resourced disease areas has been a major step forward in giving mental health the priority status it deserves and hence mobilising resources and action to address the mental health needs of the nation.

MENTAL HEALTH LEGISLATION

At the beginning of the present century, the basis of legislation for people with mental illness was the Lunacy Act 1890. In this act, no distinction was made between mental illness and so-called mental deficiency. The main failing of the 1890 Act was, however, that it was deeply entrenched in a legal framework. Asylums could only admit patients who had been certified, and this was often performed only as a last resort. As a consequence, sufferers from mental illness were admitted only when the condition was severe, and this served to enhance the stigma attached to mental illness in the mind of the public.

Gradually, after World War I, a greater proportion of patients were admitted to mental hospitals without compulsory procedures being involved. This situation received legislative recognition in the Mental Treatment Act 1930, which had been preceded by the Royal Commission on Lunacy and Mental Disorder. Subsequently, the proportion of voluntary admissions to mental hospitals continued to increase. Compulsory admissions remained essentially a judicial procedure, with the final decision being taken by a magistrate. This situation continued until the Mental Health Act 1959 cleared the way for a more liberal approach. This Act was based on the report of a royal commission and embodied the basic principles of its recommendations, which were that the mentally disordered should be treated in the same way as those suffering from physical illness and that compulsory admission and detention should be used as infrequently as possible. The procedures became a mainly medical rather than a judicial affair.

Subsequent legislation removed much of the general provisions for the care and treatment of the mentally ill and handicapped. This has been incorporated in other acts. The Mental Health Act 1983 consolidated the Mental Health Act 1959, as amended by the Mental Health (Amendment) Act 1982. It is principally concerned with the grounds for detaining patients in hospital or placing them under guardianship, and it aims to improve patients' rights and to protect staff in a variety of ways. A code of practice under Section 118 of the Mental Health Act 1983 is prepared from time to time for the guidance of professional staff in the implementation of the Act.

In the late 1990s, the government decided to review the Mental Health Act 1983 to ensure that the current legislation was updated to support the effective delivery of modern patterns of care for people with mental disorders. This review aimed to ensure an appropriate balance of safety of communities against the rights of individual patients and the wider community.

Amendments to the Mental Health Act 1983 were made in the Mental Health Act 2007, which came fully into force in November 2008. The key changes made to the 2003 Act by the 2007 Act were:

➣ a new simple definition of mental disorder, renaming previous separate categories
➣ new criteria for detention on the basis of an 'appropriate medical treatment' test

- broadening of professional roles
- supervised community treatment after detention
- suitable environment for the under-18s
- advocacy arrangements.

LOCAL MENTAL HEALTH SERVICES: THE MODERN APPROACH

The cornerstone of the care for people with a mental illness or other mental health problems is a well-structured and coordinated system of care at local level. The precise pattern of care varies throughout Britain because different models of service have developed according to local circumstances.

A number of key principles should govern the approach to mental health (Table 7.10). The emphasis should be on moving 'upstream' to prevent as many mental health problems as possible and to promote positive mental health. Services and models of care should be integrated between health and social care and be focused on giving individuals with mental health problems, and also their families and carers, as much control as possible.

PROMOTING MENTAL HEALTH

The factors that influence positive mental health can be clustered into three key categories:

- *the structural level* – good living environments, housing, employment, transport, education and a supportive political structure
- *the community level* – a sense of belonging, social support, a sense of citizenship and participation in society
- *the level of the individual* – the ability to deal with thoughts and feelings and to manage life, emotional resilience and the ability to cope with stressful or adverse circumstances.

Belonging to a social network involving communication and supportive relationships is protective of good health and positive well-being: strong links between social support and mental health have been found in studies both of positive mental health and of mental ill health. Protective social factors for positive mental health include a culture of cooperation and tolerance between individuals, institutions and diverse groups in society; a sense of belonging to family, school, workplace and community; and a good network of supportive relationships.

In contrast, social exclusion damages both physical and mental health. For example,

Table 7.10 Key aims of mental health policy

- Overcome barriers to social inclusion.
- Improve the whole-life outcomes of those with experience of mental health problems.
- Improve whole-population mental health.

Source: The Future Vision Coalition. *A New Vision for Mental Health.* London: Sainsbury Centre for Mental Health; 2008.

perceptions of racial discrimination have been identified as a significant factor in the poor health of ethnic minorities, over and above the contribution of socio-economic factors. Populations at most risk from social exclusion include those with limited opportunities for employment, particularly women, racial and ethnic minority groups, refugees and sex workers; people living with disabilities, addictions or chronic illnesses; homeless people; the long-term unemployed; school leavers; and older people living on reduced income. Research on social capital has specifically pointed to important influences on mental health by community cohesion, involving levels of trust, reciprocity and participation.

Emotional well-being is a strong predictor of physical health and longevity, while sustained stress and psychological trauma increase susceptibility to physical illness. Physical exercise has a well-documented beneficial effect on mental health and on reducing depressive symptoms.

THE RANGE OF MENTAL HEALTH SERVICES

An indication of the diverse range of services required to provide a comprehensive service for a population is shown in Table 7.11.

The onset of mental illness is often accompanied by the inability of the individual concerned to participate fully in society. In severe mental illness, the resulting dislocation can be near total, with the loss of friends and employment and, in some cases, estrangement from family. Care will usually be directed towards integrating the individual into society, using services such as sheltered employment, day-care and accommodation in the community and creating opportunities for social contact. Ideally, a key worker will ensure that the mentally ill person is receiving and benefiting from the various elements of the care package.

The importance of a range of other components in a comprehensive network of services for people with mental health problems cannot be overstated. Such services will include community psychiatric nursing, social work services, day resource centres and supported employment projects to help mentally ill people regain the ability to earn a living. In time, the development of such a comprehensive range of services will reduce the need for acute admissions, as people's conditions will be monitored and stabilised in the community.

Primary Care

Most minor mental health problems and less severe mental illness (for example, some forms of anxiety and depression) are managed throughout their natural history in primary care settings. The balance in the work undertaken by the general practitioner, the community psychiatric nurse or another health professional will depend on the nature of the patient's problems, the clinical skills of the various practitioners in the primary health care team and the philosophy of care adopted. Many patients with longer-term enduring mental illness will also receive their continuing support (including monitoring of their medication and their social functioning) from members of the primary care team.

Table 7.11 Range of services for people with severe and enduring mental illness

Community support	Primary care
	Crisis intervention
	Community-based alternatives to acute care
	Assertive outreach
	Support with daily living
	Generic community mental health services
24-hour care, residential provision and housing	Ordinary housing with intensive support
	Sheltered accommodation
	Group homes/shared housing
	Medium-support hostels
	Residential homes
	High-support accommodation
	24-hour nursed accommodation
	Acute inpatient care
	Low secure units
	Medium secure units
	Special hospitals
Day-care and daytime activities	Ordinary employment
	Supported employment
	Adult education
	Employment rehabilitation places
	Clubhouse
	Day centre
	Day hospital
	Drop-in centre
Financial support	Welfare advice centre

Source: Sainsbury Centre for Mental Health. *Keys to Engagement: a review of care for people with severe mental illness who are hard to engage with services.* London: SCMH; 1998.

The close integration of primary care services with specialist mental health services and with other agencies (both statutory and voluntary) providing care, help and support for people with a mental health problem is a particularly important component of good local services.

The Care Programme Approach

The Care Programme Approach (CPA) was introduced in England in 1991 to provide a framework for the care of mentally ill people. Similar approaches are in place in the rest of the United Kingdom. The requirements of the Care Programme Approach are relatively simple: all people receiving specialist mental health services will be assessed, will have a named key worker and will have a care plan agreed with them, which will be subject to regular review. The approach requires strong cooperation between health and social care services and full involvement of the patient and his or her carers.

The Care Programme Approach has been strengthened, most recently in 2008, as a result of evaluation and user and professional feedback. New measures have included a single tier of assessment for those with complex needs, replacing the previous 'enhanced' (in contrast to 'standard') level of care; inclusion of crisis plans; more emphasis on risk management; and regular audit.

Mental Health Teams Operating in the Community

In most parts of Britain, community mental health teams have been developed to serve the needs of local communities. They deal predominantly with people who have more severe mental health problems. The precise model of service varies, but the best are made up of staff from all relevant local agencies, who deliver multidisciplinary care in a way that is 'seamless' as far as the user is concerned. Teams can comprise, for example, psychiatrists, community psychiatric nurses, clinical psychologists, specialist social workers, psychotherapists, counsellors, occupational therapists and welfare rights and benefits advisers. Their strength is that they enable users of services to be dealt with through a single point of delivery, avoiding some of the fragmentation and lack of coordination of the past. They liaise closely with primary care services and provide assessments as well as continuing care.

Assertive Outreach Teams

Assertive outreach is a way of managing the care of people with severe mental illness while enabling them to continue living in the community. It is particularly valuable for patients who were traditionally high users of hospital inpatient services.

Assertive outreach is delivered by a multidisciplinary mental health team. The teams work best when there is good leadership that is stable over a period of years and when team members retain a clinical role rather purely working in an organisational or management capacity. It is also important that teams do not take on too large a caseload.

Assertive outreach teams build relationships with other key agencies and organisations in a locality (such as housing associations, police, local authorities, leisure facilities and employment offices) so that they are able to address a wide range of their clients' needs. Regular team meetings enable patient needs and risk assessments to be discussed and problems to be surfaced and resolved. Risk management is particularly important, since failure in this area would undermine the credibility of, and public and professional confidence in, the assertive outreach model of care.

Residential Care

Many types of residential care exist for people who would in the past have been in long-stay hospitals. Services and projects vary. Some provide specialist staff (such as nurses) living with residents, and others provide a measure of independent living with back-up support. The range needs to include capacity for intensive support in order for it to be provided over the longer-term as well as round the clock if necessary.

People with severe and enduring mental illness are sometimes described as the 'new long stay', and although they are a relatively small group (about 5000 in England), they can end up occupying acute inpatient beds inappropriately. They need access to 24-hour care and support and recognition of the fact that they are chronically ill. The concept of 24-hour staffed accommodation is not new and is a key component of effective comprehensive mental health services.

Continuing care facilities will always be needed for those people whose illnesses are too severe in impact and chronic in nature to allow them to live on their own. Rather than being provided in traditional hospital wards, these services should be available in more intimate and community-based care settings, such as hostels, group homes and supported lodgings. Services provided in this way not only reduce the dislocation of the individual from society but also, when provided in a comprehensive network, allow easier progression to more independent forms of accommodation as the person's condition permits.

The spectrum of care for people with mental illness living in the community is quite wide. It ranges from independent living accommodation (for example, single flats in shared accommodation), to shared group accommodation (with or without support), to living as part of a family (including fostering), to hostels and staffed housing schemes.

Acute Inpatient Care

Many people with acute mental illness or severe and relapsing conditions will need to be cared for in an acute inpatient unit. Increasingly, most inpatient units also have small psychiatric intensive care units (PICUs) as part of their range of services.

QUALITY OF MENTAL HEALTH SERVICES

Individuals with mental illness have quite complex pathways of care over their lifetime (Figure 7.14). The quality of mental health services tends to be formally assessed mainly by inspections and reviews by the main health and social care regulator, the Care Quality Commission (a number of reports in the public domain were produced by one of its predecessor bodies, the Healthcare Commission).[9]

Individual services can assess their quality in a variety of ways: for example, through using the Health of the Nation Outcome Scales (described in an earlier section), through taking account of user and carer views and experience or through examining outcomes of care. International bodies have drawn together more global indicators of service performance. An example in Table 7.12 was produced by international consensus under the auspices of the Organisation for Economic Co-operation and Development (OECD).

SECURE ACCOMMODATION AND OFFENDERS WITH MENTAL ILLNESS

A small group of people with mental health problems need secure accommodation because they are a danger to themselves or others. Such services exist within a range of levels of security, which are dependent upon the degree of risk posed by the patient. At the lower end of the spectrum are locked

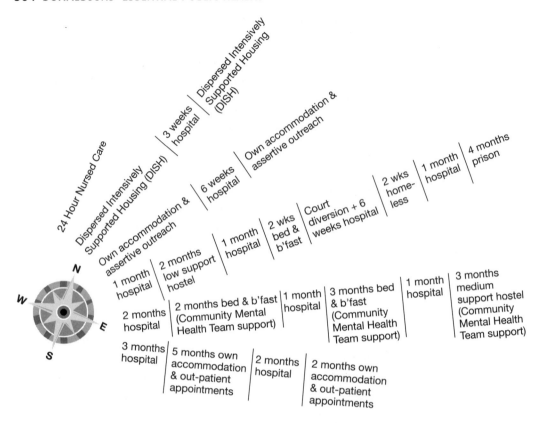

Figure 7.14 Examples of the diversity in pathways of care for people with mental illness
Source: Sainsbury Centre for Mental Health. *Keys to Engagement: a review of care for people with severe mental illness who are hard to engage with services.* London: SCMH; 1998.

wards within mental health units, while as more security is required to cope with the patient's problems (often associated with offending behaviour), medium-secure care (within what were previously called regional secure units) is available. The small number of patients deemed extremely dangerous can be cared for in high-secure hospitals. It is accepted that all patients should be cared for in the condition of the lowest security that can prevent danger to themselves or others.

Many patients need help when they become embroiled in the criminal justice system as a result of their mental illnesses. It has for some years been recognised that those who commit crimes as a result of mental ill health should receive care rather than custody. Although many mentally disordered offenders still end up in the prison system due to the still patchy nature of services for this difficult group of people, there has been a considerable growth in services to divert them away from the criminal justice system. Such initiatives include education and training for police officers, lawyers and those involved in administering criminal justice within the courts. This enables the

Table 7.12 International expert panel-recommended indicators for mental health care

Area	Indicator name
Continuity of care	Timely ambulatory follow-up after mental health hospitalisation
	Continuity of visits after hospitalisation for dual psychiatric/substance-related conditions
	Racial/ethnic disparities in mental health follow-up rates
	Continuity of visits after mental health-related hospitalisation
Coordination of care	Case management for severe psychiatric disorders
Treatment	Visits during acute phase treatment of depression
	Hospital readmissions for psychiatric patients
	Length of treatment for substance-related disorders
	Use of anti-cholinergic antidepressant drugs among elderly patients
	Continuous antidepressant medication treatment in acute phase
	Continuous antidepressant medication treatment in continuation phase
Patient outcomes	Mortality for persons with severe psychiatric disorders

Source: Organisation for Economic Cooperation and Development (OECD). *Mental Health Care Panel: selecting indicators for the quality of mental health care at health systems level in OECD countries.* Paris: OECD, 2004.

recognition of mental illnesses and hence referral to teams of mental health specialists who can formally diagnose whether mental illness is present and arrange for an admission into hospital. It is likely that there will be further growth in such initiatives as well as still greater liaison and cooperation between agencies such as the police, probation, social services and mental health services.

GROUPS WITH SPECIAL NEEDS

The needs of certain groups requires particular attention if services are to be truly comprehensive.

Homelessness is a precipitating factor in poor mental health (especially for diseases such as anxiety and depression) and can also be a result of the social dislocation that often accompanies major mental illness, which can easily lead to loss of accommodation.

Services have traditionally struggled to engage with mentally ill people who have no fixed abode and often only come into contact with them via the criminal justice system or following a major crisis such as a suicide attempt. In certain of the inner city areas of Britain that tend to have a larger than average proportion of homeless people, specialist multidisciplinary teams have been established to maintain contact and thus to attempt to prevent a crisis. More generally, the provision of adequate housing for previously homeless patients discharged from acute psychiatric care is a key issue in maintaining future mental health. Projects that bring together local authority housing departments, housing associations, social services and the NHS are particularly important.

Making services appropriate for, and acceptable to, minority ethnic communities is also a challenge. Issues such as varying cultural norms of what constitutes acceptable behaviour may have contributed to the over-representation of people from certain minority ethnic groups within those groups that are diagnosed as suffering from mental illnesses and those groups that have a greater than average proportion of their admissions to hospital being subject to the compulsion of law (as opposed to voluntary). The focused effort of the statutory mental health services working in conjunction with local minority communities is essential if services are to be fully effective.

Children and adolescents who have mental illnesses require specialist services. Apart from the fact that children's mental ill health can manifest itself in ways different from that of adult illnesses, there is a need for a different range of agencies to be involved in child and adolescent mental health. Of these, the most notable is the education services, in whose settings disruptive or disturbed behaviour is often first noticed and who have a statutory duty to provide education to the child throughout their illness. Other involved services include child psychiatry, child psychology, education welfare services, special educational services (including special schooling for children with severe emotional and behavioural difficulties who cannot be managed within the mainstream) as well as (where appropriate) the input of the probation service and the voluntary sector.

People who misuse substances (whether legal or illegal) to the extent that it adversely affects their social functioning may have a recognised mental illness. However, most do not and cannot be defined as mentally ill. For those without concurrent mental illnesses, services include inpatient or community-based detoxification, specialist counselling from drugs teams, and needle exchanges. Those patients with concurrent mental illnesses (the so-called 'dual diagnosis') require not only these services but also the input of mainstream psychiatric services if their care is to be optimised. The quality of this liaison between specialist drug and alcohol services and mainstream mental health services is of key importance for this numerically quite small but challenging group of patients.

USERS' VIEWS, ADVOCACY AND CARERS' NEEDS

All services for people with mental illness must share the aim of allowing maximum autonomy. It is increasingly recognised that people should have influence over the care that they receive and that when this is encouraged by services, a positive outcome from treatment is more likely. Mechanisms like patients' councils have been established to facilitate this process. Advocacy and other schemes to involve users can help people with mental illness express their views on services. User-led services are an increasingly common development.

Mental illness, particularly when it first develops in an acute form, can be extraordinarily stressful and difficult for families and friends of the affected person. As with other groups with special needs, the role of informal providers of care is of fundamental importance in the planning and delivery of services. Needs assessments of mentally ill people must also include an appraisal of their carers' needs. Statutory services must seek to involve carers in planning the response to an individual's problems and also provide support to the carer. The absence of such support can lead to the collapse of the informal caring arrangement and the consequent admission of the mentally ill person to the statutory services.

THE MENTAL HEALTH REVIEW TRIBUNAL

The basic function of the Mental Health Review Tribunal is to consider applications for discharge of patients who are compulsorily detained in hospital or under guardianship orders and to ensure that no patient is detained compulsorily without good reasons. The appointment of the Mental Health Review Tribunal is the responsibility of the Department of Health. Three categories of members (legal, medical and lay) are recognised, and each tribunal comprises at least three members, one from each category, with the legal representative acting as chairman. An application for discharge may be made by the patient himself, his next of kin, the secretary of state for health or the home secretary, depending on the section of the Mental Health Act under which the patient is detained.

THE CARE QUALITY COMMISSION

The Care Quality Commission subsumed the functions of the former Mental Health Act Commission from early 2009. Its role is described more fully in Chapter 4. The Commission has a wide brief. It can investigate complaints and keep under review all aspects of the care and welfare of detained patients. Second independent medical opinions can be given by doctors appointed by the Commission. Furthermore, it can submit proposals for change to the secretary of state for health.

THE NEEDS OF PEOPLE WITH LEARNING DISABILITY

Accurate and respectful descriptions of this subgroup of the population have proved difficult to establish. Early legislation used and defined terms such as mental defective, idiot, imbecile and feeble-minded, which, although they were felt to be scientifically valid descriptions at the time, have subsequently become terms of abuse. The Mental Health Act 1959 introduced the term 'subnormal', and the definition encompassed both subnormality of intelligence and the concept of social incapacity. The term was traditionally confined to those individuals who were cognitively impaired from childhood. It excluded those who acquired their learning disability in later life, such as people with permanent and severe impairment of the central nervous system caused by road accidents after the age of 18 years.

There was much debate about whether to include people with learning disability in the 1983 Mental Health Act at all. Thus it was something of a compromise that the concept of 'abnormally aggressive and seriously irresponsible conduct' deliberately limited inclusion to the minority of people with learning disability who needed some sort of legally supervised care because of their behaviour. The 2007 Act that amended the 2003 Act (see earlier) 'declassified' learning disability as a mental disorder.

The Education Act 1981 introduced the term 'learning difficulties', but this was a definition of educational progress and thus did not recognise the social aspect of mental handicap. Internationally, both scientific study and health service practice have yielded a bewildering diversity in terminology, conceptual frameworks and classification of this group of conditions. Different approaches are based on, for example, causes, disorder or injury to the brain, low intelligence on formal testing, socially maladaptive behaviour and personality dependency. It is important to establish what taxonomy is being used. Without this, it is impossible to establish which people are being counted in epidemiological studies or in needs assessment of populations.

Three approaches have been used for classification in this context (Table 7.13). The intellectual impairment approach, widely used in the past, is based upon the idea of low intelligence. Intelligence is measured by intelligence tests and usually expressed as the intelligence quotient (IQ). The IQ measure is distributed within the population in a way that has some similarities with other characteristics of people (such as height). Although much criticised, this approach to classification has remained popular precisely because it is so readily measurable and can be expressed in terms of severity (based upon IQ scores). Thus 'severe intellectual impairment' is the term used to describe people with an IQ less than 50, while the term 'mild intellectual impairment' is used

Table 7.13 Taxonomy: different approaches

Intellectual impairment	
• Criteria	*Intellectual:* intelligence or development tests
• Main categories	*Severe:* IQ <50 (or 'severe and moderate') *Mild:* IQ 50–69

Learning difficulty	
• Criteria	*Usually educational:* e.g., reading or numeracy tests, but should reflect learning dysfunction, not merely achievements
• Main categories	*Various,* according to legal, administrative and professional contracts

Mental handicap/retardation	
• Criteria	*Social:* e.g., dependency or maladaption scales
• Main categories	*Severe:* coextensive with severe intellectual impairment, if IQ <50 is used as a necessary criterion *Mild:* many factors in selection, varying in different communities

Source: Adapted from Fryers T. Epidemiology and taxonomy in mental retardation. *Paediatr Perinat Epidemiol.* 1992; **6**: 181–92.

for people with an IQ between 50 and 69 (Table 7.14).

The second approach to classification is to view the problem through the resulting disability, principally in learning. Thus the concept of 'learning disability' has emerged in the United States ('specific learning difficulty' in the United Kingdom), which is not synonymous with mental handicap.

Recently, a third approach has gained currency. This attempts to assess the effects of the individual's disability on daily living skills and on their social functioning and the support they will need to live ordinary life. In this approach, the quantified intellectual level of a person is held to be less relevant than its results as expressed in these terms. A wide range of tools are now available to assess individuals on this basis. Typically, this model can offer benefits when planning services to meet an individual's personal needs.

At the beginning of the 1990s, the Department of Health in England formally adopted, for use within the health and social services, the term 'people with learning disabilities', instead of 'mental handicap'. In some other countries, the term 'mental retardation' is used, despite its negative connotations, and the term 'intellectual disability' is accepted internationally in scientific and policy fora. The officially used definition of learning disability in the United Kingdom derives from a government White Paper on services for people with learning disability (Box 7.1). For the remainder of this chapter, the term 'learning disability' is used.

FREQUENCY IN THE POPULATION

Assessing the size of the problem in a population and making comparisons between different places or over time is particularly difficult because of the complexity surrounding definition and classification.

Despite the limitations of measuring IQ and of relating intellectual impairment

Table 7.14 Differences between severe and mild learning disability*

	Severe (IQ below 50)	Mild (IQ 50–70)
Social class distribution	Evenly distributed	Strongly aggregated in Social Class V
Prevalence	Four per 1000; almost all are in contact with services	Ten per 1000; only one-third are in contact with services
Education	School for severe learning difficulties	School for mild learning difficulties, but many in ordinary schools
Employment	Most attend training/education centres, but supported work has become an option for more people	Some in open employment, in poorly paid jobs
Physical disability	High proportion have additional physical and/or sensory impairment	Most do not have an additional physical disability

* Traditional 'mild'/'severe' categorisation on IQ not always used.

BOX 7.1 DEFINITION OF LEARNING DISABILITY

- A significantly reduced ability to understand new or complex information, to learn new skills (impaired intelligence), with;
- A reduced ability to cope independently (impaired social functioning);
- Which started before adulthood, with a lasting effect on development.

— *Source:* Department of Health. *Valuing People: a new strategy for learning disability for the 21st century.* London: Department of Health; 2001.

---

to disability, the most comprehensive epidemiological data relate to the frequency of people in populations with an IQ of less than 50 (severe intellectual impairment, but often also referred to in older studies or those from other countries as 'severe mental handicap' or 'severe mental retardation'). Reasonably reliable estimates are also available for the more clear-cut syndromes that are associated with learning disability (for example, Down's syndrome).

The two measures used most often to express the frequency of learning disability in the population are the birth prevalence (number of affected infants per 1000 births) and age-specific prevalence (number of affected people in particular age groups expressed per 1000 people of that same age living in the population concerned).

Most data on the frequency of learning disability in the population are derived from epidemiological surveys. Routinely available health service data are not generally useful sources. Notifications of congenital abnormalities (*see* Chapter 6) can provide estimates of the population frequency of only some conditions that cause learning disability.

Using data from various sources to estimate the frequency of learning disability, it is clear that the numbers involved are very substantial, both of children and adults and of the severe and mild/moderate forms of the disability (Table 7.15).

When considering the frequency of severe intellectual impairment, it is important to examine rates of occurrence within birth cohorts (children born in the same year) as well as within different age groups of the population. The prevalence of severe intellectual impairment varies between similar birth cohorts in different populations, both nationally and internationally. Similarly, birth prevalence shows changes over time. For example, it was relatively low in many developed countries of the world for birth cohorts of the early 1950s (1.8–4.0 per 1000) and higher for birth cohorts in the early 1960s (3.5–5.5 per 1000). Factors likely to affect birth prevalence at different times include survival of impaired infants due to better neonatal intensive care, detection of foetal abnormalities through screening and subsequent termination of affected pregnancies, and changes in maternal age. Differences in birth prevalence then work through to be reflected in age-specific prevalence ratios as the cohort concerned grows older.

Changes in survival of affected children and the prevalence of disabilities caused in later life to otherwise unimpaired people

Table 7.15 Prevalence of learning disability: some key numbers

- 2.5% (1.5 million people) in the United Kingdom have a learning disability.
- 3% of children and 2% of adults have a learning disability.
- 1.2 million people have a mild to moderate learning disability.
- 210 000 people have severe and profound learning disability (65 000 children, 120 000 working-age adults, 25 000 older people).
- Prevalence of learning disability will rise by 10% by 2020 (and become more complex).

Source: Derived from Michael J. *Healthcare for All.* London: Department of Health; 2008.

(such as head injuries) are the other main factors that affect such age-specific prevalence figures. It is predicted that the prevalence of learning disability will increase by 1% per year over the next 10 years.

People with learning disabilities often have complex needs. In addition to cognitive disability, they may have physical and sensory impairments and associated complications or coexisting mental health problems. They are also likely to have shortened life expectancy (Table 7.16).

AETIOLOGY OF LEARNING DISABILITY

Causes of learning disability are mostly multifactorial processes. It is important to recognise that the precise mechanisms of causation of many forms of learning disability are not established, even though there may be a principal causal agent. For example, alcohol intake during pregnancy causes foetal alcohol syndrome (which can include learning disability). However, the amount of alcohol that will induce damage is not well established, nor are the predisposing maternal or foetal characteristics. The causes of learning disability at population level must be viewed more broadly. The

influences on the population frequency of learning disability in different places or over time can be diverse. For example, learning disability resulting from foetal alcohol syndrome will depend on pricing of alcohol, on the availability of alcohol in the society concerned and on attitudes to pregnancy and childbearing.

Causes of neurological impairment (i.e., organic causes of learning disability) can be classified as pure primary disorders, primary disorders with secondary neurological damage and pure secondary disorders.

Pure Primary Disorders

Some disorders resulting in learning disability arise from abnormal chromosome formation. The nuclei of normal human cells contain 23 pairs of chromosomes; one of each pair is derived from either parent. There are two types of chromosome: one pair that determines sex (sex chromosomes) and the other 22 pairs, which are called autosomes. Males have 44 autosomes and one X and one Y sex chromosome; females have 44 autosomes and two X sex chromosomes.

Chromosome abnormalities may involve either the sex chromosomes or the

Table 7.16 Health aspects of learning disability: some key facts

- People with learning disabilities are 58 times more likely to die before 50 years than the general population.
- Half of the people with Down's syndrome have congenital heart problems.
- Around a third of people with learning disabilities have a physical disability (e.g., cerebral palsy) that predisposes them to other problems (e.g., chest infections, osteoporosis, incontinence).
- A third of people with learning disabilities have epilepsy.
- Mental health problems, autism, attention deficit disorders and challenging behaviour are more common amongst people with learning disabilities.

Source: Derived from Michael J. *Healthcare for All.* London: Department of Health; 2008.

autosomes and may be due to abnormalities in chromosome number (more or less than the usual complement) or to abnormalities in their structure. Specific chromosomal abnormalities are associated with particular diseases.

Down's Syndrome

The physical characteristics of Down's syndrome (although each is not present in all cases) include narrow, slanting eyes with prominent epicanthic folds; short stature; small ears; short, broad neck; furrowing of the tongue and a tendency for the mouth to hang open; a single transverse palmar crease; and prominent and characteristic skin ridges on the palms of the hand, fingers and soles of the feet. Congenital abnormalities of the heart and intestinal tract occur more frequently in these children than in other infants.

There is a range of cognitive ability within the spectrum of Down's syndrome, but the IQ usually lies somewhere between 20 and 55, with a small proportion of affected people having an IQ greater than 50. People with Down's syndrome are usually described

as humorous, cheerful and affectionate. While it would be wrong to accept this as a stereotype, many people involved in the care of children with Down's syndrome would agree with this description of their personalities.

People with Down's syndrome always possess extra chromosomal material in the cells of their bodies. The presence of an extra discrete autosomal (i.e., non-sex) chromosome is called 'trisomy'. In 94% of cases of Down's syndrome, all or part of an extra chromosome resembling the normal number 21 pair of chromosomes is present in the cell; this most common variant of Down's syndrome is called 'trisomy 21'. It arises because of a failure of separation of chromosomes (non-disjunction) during cell division in the formation of the ovum. The foetus developing from this ovum, when it is fertilised, has 47 chromosomes rather than the usual 46.

In a less common form of Down's syndrome (3–5% of cases), the extra chromosomal material becomes joined to another chromosome: the so-called 'translocation type'. These are familial, with a high risk of recurrence in families, so there are opportunities for prevention through genetic counselling.

In a third rare form (1–3% of cases), non-disjunction occurs after fertilisation, so only some of the cells of the body are abnormal (mosaicism) and people show some signs of Down's syndrome but not all. They may be of normal intelligence.

The birth prevalence of Down's syndrome in the absence of screening is of the order of 1.3–1.8 per 1000 live births. The precise aetiology of Down's syndrome is unknown, but the most striking feature is the strongly increased risk of trisomy 21 with increased maternal age. However, the majority of babies with Down's syndrome are born to younger mothers, and screening has little impact on birth prevalence if restricted to mothers over 35 years.

Many cases of Down's syndrome can be detected prenatally if screening is used between 15 and 20 weeks of pregnancy. Ultrasound screening is used routinely in pregnancy to assess the foetus, and some of the features of Down's syndrome can be evident. Maternal blood testing can detect levels of certain markers (for example, alpha-fetoprotein and human chorionic gonadotropin) that are suggestive of Down's syndrome. Blood testing and ultrasound are screening rather than diagnostic tests, and they only assess the risks of an abnormal baby rather than providing a definitive diagnosis. The latter involves moving on to amniocentesis and various forms of sampling. For a full description of the principles of screening, *see* Chapter 3.

Fragile X Syndrome

This is a sex chromosome disorder that can result in severe intellectual impairment, although only in a minority of males and almost never in females. About 80% of affected boys will have an IQ less than 70, and a smaller proportion of girls will have cognitive impairment, mostly in the mild category. Boys are more seriously affected because they only have one X chromosome, and when that is faulty it has a big impact.

This is a sex chromosome disorder in which one gene, FMR1, becomes elongated and as a result does not produce one of the body's essential proteins. Some individuals with a less pronounced defect of the FMR1 gene are said to have a 'pre-mutation' and can be carriers for the condition. Fragile X is inherited and affects about one in 4000 males and one in 6000 females. Most fragile X syndrome children have behaviour disorders and about a fifth have autism. Epilepsy is common. Older children and adults often have a characteristic facial appearance: a long, flat face with prominent ears and jaw. Mitral valve prolapse can also be present.

Fragile X syndrome can be confirmed with a blood test in childhood, but it can only be detected prenatally by amniocentesis and chorionic villus sampling.

Primary Disorders with Secondary Neurological Damage

A second group of disorders do not affect the constitution of the individual per se, but a genetic abnormality leads to abnormal or arrested development.

Phenylketonuria

This is a rare recessively inherited condition (birth prevalence is 0.05–0.2 per 1000 births) in which the absence of a specific enzyme leads to a failure in the ability of the body to convert the amino acid phenylalanine to tyrosine. Normal diet thus becomes a direct hazard to the child. Phenylalanine accumulates in the blood and tissues and has a toxic effect on the brain, leading to convulsions and, if untreated, severe damage. The deficiency of tyrosine leads to paucity of melanin formation and thus lack of pigmentation, giving rise to the other characteristics of the syndrome: blonde hair, blue eyes, pale skin and a tendency to infantile eczema.

The treatment is to eliminate phenylalanine from the diet until the central nervous system is mature. This cannot be done completely because it is an essential amino acid, but if a special diet is instituted as early as possible, there is a chance of limiting the degree of damage resulting from the condition. This has led to the practice of screening all newborn babies by taking a few drops of blood and testing for excess phenylalanine (the Guthrie or 'heel prick' test), which has been very effective.

Sporadic Congenital Hypothyroidism

Congenital hypothyroidism occurs sporadically within the population (birth prevalence is 0.1–2.0 per 1000). It is important to realvise that this results from a mutation, not from iodine deficiency (see below). Thyroid failure ensues, and if the condition is not recognised early and treated with thyroid replacement therapy, severe intellectual impairment can result.

Pure Secondary Disorders

A third group of disorders arises because of an environmental factor interacting with a normal foetus after conception. The mechanisms are not understood fully in all cases, but the range of factors that can lead to learning disability is wide.

Infections

Maternal exposure to the rubella (German measles) virus, particularly during the first trimester of pregnancy, puts the developing foetus at risk of congenital rubella syndrome. The manifestations include congenital heart disease, deafness, blindness and learning disability. This has been largely eliminated by vaccination, but it can still occur if population vaccine coverage falls (*see also* Chapter 9).

Many other infections of the mother during pregnancy, in particular cytomegalovirus and toxoplasmosis, can cause learning disability in the offspring. Congenital syphilis acquired by the mother and passed to the foetus was in the past an important cause of learning disability as part of a general multisystem disorder. Infections acquired post-natally can also lead to learning disability: for example, meningitis, encephalitis and malaria.

Alcohol Intake in Pregnancy

Learning disability can arise from consumption of alcohol during pregnancy, usually as part of foetal alcohol syndrome (*see also* Chapter 6).

Rhesus Incompatibility

The problem of rhesus incompatibility and its prevention is discussed in Chapter 6. The cerebral damage caused by jaundice (kernicterus) may result in cerebral palsy and learning disability, though this condition is now largely preventable.

Exposure to Radiation

Excessive use of diagnostic X-rays in pregnancy has, in the past, led to radiation being identified as a risk factor for learning disability. This is not an important cause today, and the use of ultrasound has in any case superseded X-rays as a diagnostic technique in pregnancy.

Perinatal Factors

During the process of birth, there are two factors of particular importance that may lead to injury of the brain and some degree of neurological impairment: hypoxia and birth injury. Hypoxia in the foetus may occur for a variety of reasons, such as pre-eclamptic toxaemia, antepartum haemorrhage, anaesthetic complications, excessive sedation during labour, respiratory distress in the infant, pressure on the umbilical cord or prolonged labour. Trauma during delivery is particularly likely to occur with abnormal presentation of the foetus or with instrumental delivery. Fortunately, with modern obstetric care and the tendency towards early Caesarean section in difficult cases, birth trauma is probably less common today.

Prematurity with low birth weight is strongly associated with the later development of learning disability. It is unlikely, however, that the relationship is one of direct cause and effect; it is probably explained by the fact that babies in this category are much more susceptible to adverse factors during delivery and afterwards. Indeed, intellectual impairment, epilepsy and cerebral palsy are sequelae of the same processes and problems.

Iodine Deficiency

When considering learning disability worldwide, iodine deficiency disease is an important cause of severe intellectual impairment. Other features may be associated, including the full syndrome of cretinism. In parts of the world where iodine is not present in sufficient quantities in water or in the diet, the solution is population-based prevention strategies, including dietary supplementation or injection (this lasts several years).

Neural Tube Defects

Learning disability can be a feature of the group of disorders called neural tube defects, which are described fully in Chapter 6.

After Birth

A wide variety of elements of the post-natal environment may lead to neurological impairment and learning disability. In the early post-natal period, hypoglycaemia is a serious problem that, if uncorrected, can cause convulsions and cerebral injury. Infectious diseases have already been discussed. Head injury, either accidental or deliberate (as part of child abuse), may have similar repercussions. One of the effects of excessive exposure to inorganic lead, either as a result of pica (ingestion) or environmental pollution, is varying degrees of intellectual impairment. There is no evidence of lead causing damage to a degree resulting in identified learning disability, but it probably does cause slight reduction in children's IQs at all levels of exposure.

General Factors

Causes not associated with an underlying organic process are a complex interrelationship between genetic endowment, deprivation and educational under-functioning. In general, these factors are relevant to mild degrees of learning disability.

The number of people with IQ scores in the range 50–69 is a reflection of the statistical distribution of IQ within the population. Whether they are then labelled as intellectually impaired or suffering from a learning disability (in effect 'abnormal') is a socially determined phenomenon. Factors that influence this are the structure and orientation of services; professional attitudes and training; employment and training practices; social and cultural expectations; family and kinship structures; and legislation in relation to health, welfare, education and employment.

PREVENTION OF LEARNING DISABILITY

Preventive strategies can be grouped into three categories directed at processes before conception, processes during foetal life and birth, and processes after birth.

PROCESSES BEFORE CONCEPTION

If social attitudes lead to reduced births in older women or lowering of maternal age overall, this would reduce the frequency of Down's syndrome. The birth prevalence of a range of disorders could be reduced by minimising inherited disease in identified families by use of genetic counselling and screening and by offering parents the choice of termination of pregnancy. Examples of causes of learning disability that can be addressed by these kinds of strategies include genetic counselling after one child (for example, translocation Down's syndrome), screening for carriers and preconceptual counselling (for example, Tay-Sachs disease) and population screening. This is a rapidly moving field, and as technologies advance new opportunities for prevention will open up. The mapping of the human genome is of major significance. Other preventive measures directed at processes before conception include reduction of hazardous factors in the environment (such as drugs, chemical exposures and industrial radiation).

PROCESSES DURING FOETAL LIFE AND BIRTH

Preventive approaches at this stage include targeting the nutritional status of pregnant women; providing folate supplementation to avoid neural tube defects; minimising harm to the foetus (for example, reducing alcohol intake and smoking during pregnancy or taking measures to prevent rhesus haemolytic disease); the use of ultrasound and other screening methods to detect foetal abnormalities and offering parents termination of the affected pregnancies;

and generally good obstetric and neonatal care.

PROCESSES AFTER BIRTH

Preventive measures after birth include protection (as far as possible) against communicable diseases which can cause intellectual impairment, early recognition of problems such as kernicterus, hypothyroidism and phenylketonuria and strategies to reduce accidents and their impact.

SERVICES FOR PEOPLE WITH LEARNING DISABILITY

The philosophy of service provision for children and adults with learning disability must be based on a clear set of values that seeks to place individuals at the centre of a care process that regards their particular needs as paramount. At its heart is a responsibility placed on all statutory and other agencies, under the lead of the social services authority, to identify individuals with special needs (such as those who have a learning disability) and to design an appropriate service response to meet those needs, whether it be a placement in the community or in a residentially-based setting. All agencies must work together and all professionals must collaborate to provide appropriate care. It is also important that services identify the needs of carers of those with a learning disability and provide help and support to them.

Running through the modern approach to care is the concept of normalisation, in which, as far as possible, the person with learning disability is given the same rights and entitlements as other members of society.

In 2001, a White Paper, *Valuing People*,[10] set out a philosophy of care and a range of commitments for the care and support of people with learning disabilities. It aimed to achieve equality of citizenship, advocacy and person-centred care for this important group of the population, so often neglected and shunned. It has been developed further and priorities have been issued in the late 2000s (Table 7.17).

Despite the strong policy framework, serious concern arose as a result of a number of major failures in standards of care for people with learning disabilities. The Healthcare Commission (one of the predecessor bodies to the Care Quality Commission) investigated concerns about poor standards of care and abuse of people with learning disability in the Cornwall Partnership NHS Trust in 2006.[11] It found poor practice, an

Table 7.17 Priorities for service development for people with a learning disability

- Personalisation: real choice and control over their lives and services
- What people do during the day: included in communities and paid work where possible
- Better health: equal access to high-quality health services
- Access to housing: emphasis on home ownership and tenancies
- Making change happen: clear accountability

Source: Department of Health. *Valuing People Now.* London: Department of Health; 2007.

unacceptable care environment and physical abuse of people with learning disabilities.

A year later, the learning disabilities charity MENCAP publicised six case studies of avoidable death, which it alleged pointed to institutionalised discrimination against people with learning disabilities in the NHS.[12] This led to *Healthcare for All*, an independent inquiry into access to health care.[13] The report made some clear recommendations to be implemented throughout the NHS to ensure that the Disability Discrimination Act is not breached and that 'reasonable adjustments' as required under the Act are made to enable people to have equal access to health services. Examples of reasonable adjustments are the use of pictorial information and the provision of liaison nursing staff in acute hospitals. Firstly, NHS organisations need processes in place to identify people with learning disabilities, recognising the difficulties with definition that were discussed earlier in this chapter. The report also asked for annual reporting by the boards of NHS organisations.

Overall, the population of people with different service needs adds up to large numbers in the population as a whole (Table 7.18). Children and adults with a learning disability can successfully live in their own home or in their family home, only being admitted to residential or hospital care when serious problems develop with their health or behaviour.

SUPPORT FOR PARENTS

Parents of a child with a learning disability will need a great deal of counselling and practical support to help them come to terms with the birth of an affected baby. Thereafter, as the child grows older, many will continue to require emotional support, advice and practical help, including welfare benefits. The presence of a person with a learning disability can give rise to special problems in a family.

Both day services and respite care provide some relief for parents. There are some schemes for placing carers in the family home to give parents an opportunity to get away for a break. Aside from short-term care, support for a family can be given by a health visitor, a community learning disability nurse, a social worker or a voluntary worker. Usually this takes the form of advice and information about service availability. Families are often helped by being put

Table 7.18 Services for people with learning disabilities in England: key facts

• There are 134 000 people with learning disabilities known to social services.
• 103 000 people with learning disabilities receive community-based services.
• 3600 people with learning disabilities live in non-health care residential settings.
• 5500 people with learning disabilities receive direct care payments.
• 6708 care homes are registered as providing care to people with learning disabilities.
• 9400 people with learning disabilities are in inpatient facilities provided by the NHS.

Source: Healthcare Commission. *A Life Like No Other.* London: Healthcare Commission; 2007.

in contact with other parents with similar problems. Practical assistance with transport or workload (for example, nappy service) is usually very valuable. The provision of adequate and suitable housing can often ease the problems of caring for a person who has a learning disability.

A frequently voiced concern amongst parents is the future for the son or daughter when the parents die. Some voluntary-sector initiatives attempt to meet part of the problem with trustee schemes. Help for families in considering the future and options for continuing support needs is vital.

COMMUNITY TEAMS

Most health localities in England have at least one multidisciplinary community team for people with learning disabilities, usually under social services management. Such teams are made up of people from a variety of professional backgrounds, but most have a social worker, a community learning disability nurse, a psychiatrist, a psychologist and usually one or two therapists (physiotherapists, occupational therapists or speech therapists).

Teams provide a domiciliary service to people with learning disability and their families. Core team members make routine visits to clients' homes. They provide advice and assistance with current day-to-day problems and they advise on welfare benefits, arrange respite care and advise or assist with any problem behaviours. They have an important role in coordinating domiciliary services and can also be helpful in breaking down the organisational barriers that sometimes exist between agencies. On the other

hand, they have to deal with issues relating to the blurring of professional boundaries while maintaining their own professional identities and, at the same time, sharing their skills.

The range of services available to people with learning disabilities who do not or are no longer able to live in their family home is very wide and varies in type around the country. Such arrangements will usually be supported by a community team. Supported living arrangements to enable people to live in their own home, or with a peer or a small group, are developing, increasingly with the help of direct payments (individual budgets).

EDUCATION OF CHILDREN

A key issue for families with a child with learning disability is education. Schools and local education authorities are under a duty to identify and make suitable provision for all children with special education needs. Around 20% of children will be identified as having special needs at some time in their school careers, with around 3% having sufficiently severe and complex needs to require a 'statement' of special needs for their local education authorities.

A child with learning disability may attend an ordinary preschool playgroup or one for children with special needs similar to theirs. A playgroup gives the child an opportunity of benefiting from contact with other children and learning through play as well as providing a period of relief to the parents. A child with learning disability may be admitted to a nursery class in an ordinary school. This is usually at the discretion of the head teacher and often for a trial period. Problems can arise because of lack of staff to cope with the extra requirements necessary for a child with special needs.

Children with a 'statement' of special educational needs can be exempted from some or all of the demands of the national curriculum as laid down by the Education Reform Act 1988. The exemption from, or modification of, the national curriculum is detailed in the child's statement of special educational needs. This is a legal document that sets out the child's individual needs and the ways in which the local education authority will meet them.

Specialised provision is made at schools for children with moderate, severe or profound and multiple learning difficulties. These children often also have severe physical and sensory disabilities. A small number of children are educated in residential schools. The vast majority of children live at home and go to school on a daily basis. Transport is often provided for them.

Many young people with severe learning disabilities remain at school until they are 19 years of age. Others attend local colleges of further education, where specialised courses are made available. A small number of young people attend special residential colleges, run either by the voluntary or the private sector. Whichever type of college is chosen, the aim of the course is the same: a successful transition to adult life and the maximising of social functioning. There is a range of government employment and training measures that help people with learning disabilities to access employment.

It is recognised that many children with learning disabilities benefit from early educational intervention. In some parts of the country, peripatetic teachers visit the home and work with parents. Parents are encouraged to stimulate their children and teach them skills. A number of different schemes for use by parents in teaching their children are in operation in Britain.

Education and training centres for adults, formerly called adult training centres, are run by local authority social services departments to provide a place for adults with learning disabilities to go during the daytime. Their main activity was originally light assembly work, which was subcontracted by local firms. The centres are now called social educational centres or resource centres, which more accurately reflects their modern purpose. Over the years, the emphasis has switched to the development of social and personal skills, further education and work experience, with a focus on individualised learning programmes and clients going outside the centre into community resources for much of the week.

While social education centres remain part of the network of provision, there has also been a trend to encourage and support people with learning disability to take paid employment within the general workforce where appropriate.

RESIDENTIAL CARE

Local authorities now provide directly only about one-third of non-health service care. The type of residential care that can be provided by the local authority social services departments varies with the degree of social competence of the individual. Social services authorities arrange residential and nursing home care, much of which is organised by other providers (from both the voluntary and the private sector).

The person with a learning disability may be placed with foster parents, in lodgings, in a home or a hostel specifically for people with learning disabilities or in an unstaffed home or hostel supervised by supporting social work staff. Increasingly, individual arrangements are being made for semi-independent living.

The typical local authority hostel of early community care developments had about 25 beds and attached staff accommodation. Such hostels are now often divided into smaller units, and few new hostels of that type are being built. An increasingly common form of community accommodation is that provided by independent trusts.

Voluntary organisations dedicated to the interests of people with learning disabilities also operate community housing. Most of these houses are ordinary dwellings in ordinary streets. They have staff support during the daytime and some will have a member of staff awake during the night. Others may have a member of staff sleeping in the house at night. These support arrangements are also provided to people living in their own individual homes.

While the average home in the average street is where most people with learning disability live and always have lived, there are those who disagree that this should be the only model. An alternative view is provided by the supporters of special villages and residential communities. It is suggested that residential villages have the advantage of containing various-sized residences, all with a domestic home-like atmosphere, and at the same time provide ready access to a wide range of services. There is a view that people with severe forms of learning disability feel less isolated and more protected in a village setting than in the general community.

A pragmatic case has been made in some parts of the country for the re-use of hospital sites for large settlements but with modern style accommodation. However, the geographic remoteness and the perceived stigma attached to those sites could militate against this, and this model of care remains controversial amongst professionals in the field and amongst self-advocates.

The private sector has emerged as a major provider of community services for people with learning disability. Many of these homes cater for rather large numbers of people, and there is concern because they do not necessarily fit the ordinary life model with its emphasis upon family-sized groups living together. Family placement schemes, where the person with learning disability lives with a family in a private household, gained popularity during the 1990s. These can provide either a permanent home or be used for respite care on a regular basis.

SECONDARY CARE SERVICES

At the end of the 1960s, there were 7400 children and 52 000 adults aged 16 years or older in hospitals for the mentally handicapped. The White Paper published in 1971 called *Better Services for the Mentally Handicapped*[14] envisaged that by the beginning of the 1990s hospital beds for mentally handicapped people would be reduced to 33 000.

At the end of the 1990s, there were some 6000 people with learning disabilities living in old long-stay hospitals. As part of the *Valuing People* White Paper published in 2001, the government committed to closing all these establishments in order to give people with learning disabilities the opportunities and support they need to live in the community. On 1 October 2008, just one old long-stay hospital, accommodating 32 residents, remained open, with full closure expected in 2009.

The government also made a commitment to close all NHS campuses (residential inpatient accommodation) by 2010. An estimated 3000 people with learning disabilities were living in this type of NHS accommodation in 2006, and by October 2008 this figure had fallen to around 1000. Suitable alternatives to campus accommodation will continue to be developed with the aid of government grants.

There are many people with learning disability who live with elderly parents, and provision will eventually have to be made for these people. Comprehensive community services must respond to the questions of where, how and with whom the person will live and how they wish to spend their time (work- and leisure-related activities). They must also provide specialised services as necessary, preferably well in advance of the death of parents.

A range of specialist services are now available (Table 7.19).

Challenging Behaviour

Some people with learning disability exhibit very disturbed behaviour. If the behaviour is such as to place the physical safety of the person or others in serious jeopardy or make impractical the use of community facilities, the term 'challenging behaviour', originally meaning behaviour that challenges service providers, is applied. The disruptive behaviours are usually aggression and self-injury. It has been estimated that 10–15 people with learning disability per 100 000 of the total population demonstrate behaviours that present a serious challenge to current services.

There is a view that people demonstrating seriously aggressive or self-injurious behaviours should be cared for, wherever possible, by specialists visiting them in their own homes, as that is the environment in which the behaviour has been manifest.

Table 7.19 The range of secondary care services available for people with learning disability

Acute assessment and treatment (inpatient services)
Specialist residential and day provision (complex needs)
Forensic services (low, medium, high security)
Adolescent services
Short breaks
Community learning disability teams
Specialist teams providing support in peoples' homes

Source: Healthcare Commission. *A Life Like No Other.* London: Healthcare Commission; 2007.

Another view is that 'challenging behaviour units' should be planned for a health locality or on a shared basis between several health localities. Such units can operate as part of an assessment and treatment unit, with the expectation that individualised care plans will enable people to return to community living once the reasons for their behaviour have been understood.

Secure (Forensic) Units

People with a moderate or severe learning disability who have committed crimes (such as arson, assault or rape) may be admitted to one of the special hospitals in England or they may be admitted to a regionally based secure unit for treatment. It is a general view that this group should be treated in specialised units, not as part of the general forensic psychiatric services.

VOLUNTARY ORGANISATIONS

There is a range of voluntary organisations solely or partly orientated towards the needs of people with a learning disability. Many have a long tradition of providing care and support for this group. This can include the provision of residential accommodation, day nurseries and playgroups, social clubs and recreational centres, holiday homes, outings and toy-lending libraries.

ADVOCACY

The desire to involve people with learning disability in decisions about their own lives has resulted in a need for advocacy services. A system of citizen advocacy is one way of ensuring personal representation. A citizen advocate is often a volunteer who has had some training for the role and who works on a one-to-one basis with the individual. Self-advocacy is being promoted amongst disabled people themselves and aims to equip them with the skills and self-confidence to make their voices heard in relation to service providers.

CONCLUSIONS

The mental health status of a population is an important component of its overall health, though it is difficult to conceptualise and measure. By careful study design, including giving particular attention to defining terms and ascertaining cases, important information can be yielded on the patterns of mental illness and learning disability in the population. This in turn can enable ideas about disease causation to be generated, trends over time to be monitored and health needs assessments to be carried out.

Methods for the promotion of mental health and the prevention of mental illness in the population are not well developed. This is partly because of the complexity of describing mental health and partly because the aetiology of many mental illnesses has not yet been elucidated. In the field of learning disability, the scope for prevention is greater and is likely to grow as techniques advance in antenatal detection and treatment of foetal abnormalities, as well as in genetic-risk identification.

Services for people with mental illness and learning disability must be wide-ranging in nature. Although they are very different in kind, these two groups must be characterised by teamwork at the level of the professionals providing the care and by strong partnership and coordination at the level of the agencies organising the care. Increasingly, high-quality care is seen as that provided in non-institutional surroundings within, or close to, the community. Its hallmark is that the type of service should be based upon, and matched to, an assessment of the individual's needs. At the same time, protection of the public from the small number of mentally ill people who pose a risk to society is a vital part of modern services.

REFERENCES

1 Singleton M, Bumpstead R, O'Brien M, *et al. Psychiatric Morbidity Among Adults Living in Private Households, 2000.* London: Office for National Statistics; 2001.

2 Department of Health. *The Health of the Nation: a strategy for health in England.* London: HMSO; 1992.

3 Faris REL, Dunham HW. *Mental Disorders in Urban Areas: an ecological study of schizophrenia and other psychoses.* Chicago: University of Chicago Press; 1939.

4 Hollingshead AB, Redlich FC. *Social Class and Mental Illness.* New York: John Wiley; 1958.

5 Department of Health. *National Suicide Prevention Strategy for England.* London: Department of Health; 2002.

6 University of Manchester. *Avoidable Deaths: a five-year report of the National Confidential Inquiry into Suicide and Homicide by People with Mental Illness.* London: The Stationery Office; 2006.

7 Coid J, Yang M, Roberts A, *et al.* Violence and psychiatric morbidity in the national household population of Britain: public health implications. *Br J Psychiatry.* 2006; **189**: 12–19.

8 Coid J, Yang M, Roberts A, *et al.* Violence and psychiatric morbidity in a national household population: a report from the British Household Survey. *Am J Epidemiol.* 2006; **164**: 1199–208.

9 Healthcare Commission. *Survey of Users 2005: mental health services.* London: Healthcare Commission; 2005.

10 Department of Health. *Valuing People: a new strategy for learning disability for the 21st century.* London: Department of Health; 2001.

11 Healthcare Commission. *Joint Investigation into the Provision of Services for People with Learning Disabilities at Cornwall Partnership NHS Trust.* London: Healthcare Commission; 2006.

12 MENCAP. *Death by Indifference.* London: MENCAP; 2007.

13 Michael J. *Healthcare for All. Report of the Independent Inquiry into Access to Healthcare for People with Learning Disabilities.* London: Independent Inquiry; 2008.

14 Department of Health and Social Security. *Better Services for the Mentally Handicapped.* London: HMSO; 1971.

CHAPTER 8
Health in Later Life

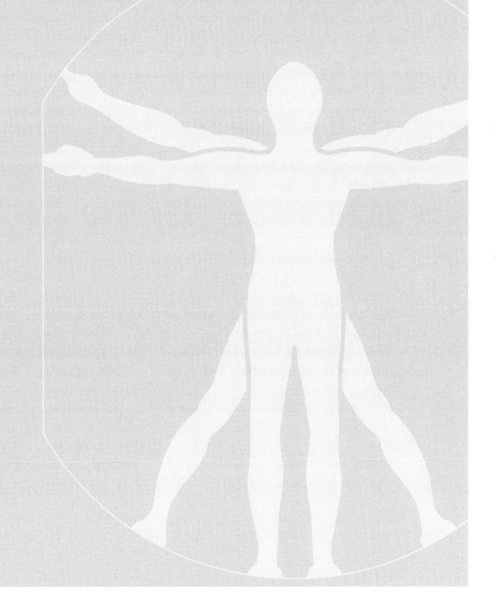

INTRODUCTION

At one time, descriptions of the problems of old age would have dwelt little on what group constituted the elderly of a population. The definition would have been based solely on age and would have had a cut-off point of 65 years (sometimes 60 years for women). In Britain these ages would have also coincided with the normal times of retirement from work.

Today the concept of old age is much more fluid, with considerable diversity in the perspectives taken to describe it. On the one hand, it is well recognised that chronological age is only a rough guide to the biological age of an individual. There are alert and active octogenarians, as well as people who have appeared to age prematurely. It has been suggested that we should think only about biological age, as measured by the abilities and performance of the individual. On the other hand, for most record-keeping and administrative purposes, the convenient label of chronological age is still necessary.

Improvements in the general health of the population have meant that higher levels of dependency are now found at later years of age. Many health and welfare services view the age of 70 years, or even 75 years, as the start of the elderly age groups for planning purposes, rather than the traditional 65-years-old watershed.

The concept of a fixed age of retirement fundamentally changed in Britain and many industrialised countries during the 1980s and 1990s. The transition to old age, if viewed through retirement, may be entered by some people today as late as 70 years (for example, the radio broadcaster who

has continued to work and may even have fathered a second family). For others, the transition may be quite early, perhaps in their 50s (for example, the primary school headmistress who married young and has grown-up children who has decided to opt for early retirement as part of a restructuring of the teaching profession).

Health and social policy discussions about the elderly in the population are likely to adopt a more flexible and functional way of defining the later years of life, for example in the use of a social life cycle (Table 8.1). For characterising the later years of life, it is the Third and Fourth Ages that are important. Some definitions regard the Third Age as beginning after full-time work has ended. However, this fails fully to take into account the position of women. Some women may not have worked during the period of their life when they were responsible for bringing up children but have chosen to work when their children left home. The definition of the Third Age shown in Table 8.1 encompasses these issues in a more subtle notion of a period of life free from the formal structures and constraints of full-time work and career-building, as well as a time in which family responsibilities do not include dependant children. The Fourth Age is the final period of life, in which dependency and disability occur. However, this kind of conceptualisation does not capture certain aspects of social exclusion, including unemployment. It must not be seen as a classification that conveys wider significance about the circumstances of later life.

In this chapter, the demographic origins of the present older population are described. So are the adverse physical, mental, social and financial factors that are frequent accompaniments of advancing years. The spectrum of services available to attempt to meet the problems of people in later life is also examined. Some special health problems are dealt with in a separate section of the chapter.

HEALTH AND NEED IN LATER LIFE

The onset of mental and physical frailty and the advent of chronic diseases (most of which occur more commonly in old age) lead many older people to have multiple, rather than single, reasons for needing help, support or care. These considerations make it particularly important that a clear picture is built up of the health and social needs of the older population if the best kinds of services are to be developed to meet its needs. As with many other fields of care, no single measure or source of data can be relied upon to provide a comprehensive picture of the health and social status of an older population and the extent to which this translates into needs.

Older people are not a homogeneous group. For planning purposes in health care, it can be helpful to think about three broad categories. There are many older people who remain in reasonably good health and do not require services for age-related needs, other than for age-based disease-prevention activities such as vaccination programmes and cancer screening. At the other end of the spectrum, there is a small minority of older people, mainly in their seventies and eighties, who would be regarded as frail or who have one of the major disabling illnesses that are associated with later life, such as dementia or a severe stroke. These people are major users of acute hospital services and of long-term care services in residential and domiciliary settings. In the middle are a large number of older people who are starting to experience age-related health problems, including falls, early memory loss and sensory deficits, that put them at risk of losing independence and experiencing reduced well-being. There is a challenge in primary health care to identify these often-unmet needs at an earlier stage.

To describe the characteristics of such a population in the depth required to plan effectively to meet its needs, it is necessary to draw upon a wide range of sources of information. Even then, in many places relevant information will not be routinely available. In such circumstances, it may be necessary to consider conducting local surveys.

Table 8.1 The social life cycle and ageing

First Age	The period of childhood and socialisation
Second Age	The period of work and family raising
Third Age	The period free of the formal structures of full-time work and dependant children
Fourth Age	The period of eventual dependency and disability

Source: Derived from Carnegie Institute. *Life, Work and Livelihood in the Third Age: final report of the Carnegie Inquiry into the Third Age.* Fife: The Carnegie United Kingdom Trust; 1993.

DEMOGRAPHIC AND SOCIAL FACTORS

DEMOGRAPHIC IMPLICATIONS OF AN AGEING POPULATION

In the United Kingdom in 1901, there were 1.8 million people over the age of 65 years out of a population of 38.2 million – representing 4.7% of the total. There were only half a million people 75 years and older, or 1.3% of the total population. By the middle of the first decade of the twenty-first century, the situation had changed dramatically: an estimated 16% of the population were aged 65 years and over, and 8% were aged 75 years and over.

It is a popular misconception that these population changes were due to advances in medical science, new drugs and high technology allowing older people to live longer. The real explanation lies before the turn of the nineteenth century. At that time, most deaths occurred in infancy and childhood. When mortality started to fall, more children survived into adult life and younger age groups were predominant in the population. As mortality rates fell further and birth rates also started to decline during the twentieth century, the older age groups began to make up a much greater part of the population than they had done earlier.

The age structure of any population is often represented graphically by so-called 'population pyramids'. The age structure of the population of Britain at the beginning of the twentieth century, when plotted graphically, did indeed resemble a pyramid. There were large numbers of young people at its base and very few elderly people at its peak. In this respect, it resembled that of some present-day developing countries. By near the middle of the first decade of the twenty-first century, the age structure of Britain's population causes the graph to look more like a chimney than a pyramid, with a relative shrinking in the numbers of young people and a larger proportion of elderly people (Figure 8.1).

Changes in population age structure are part of what is called the demographic transition. The pattern can be seen not just in historical comparisons but also in different countries of the world today. Broadly, populations start in a position where mortality and fertility are high and move to a point where both are low. The demographic transition (Table 8.2) started to gather pace in Britain and other industrialised countries during the late nineteenth century and the first half of the twentieth century. This didn't happen in many developing countries until the last third of the twentieth century.

In exploring the reasons for the demographic transition in Britain's population, it is necessary to identify the time at which improvements in mortality started to occur and why. Relatively little improvement in mortality occurred from the sixteenth century through to the latter part of the nineteenth century (Figure 8.2). For most of the period of several hundred years before the graph in Figure 8.2 starts, a person could expect to live on average until their mid-30s. Such fluctuations as there were coincided with periods of famine and epidemics of infectious diseases. Better agricultural methods and food distribution during the eighteenth century enabled higher levels of nutrition to be achieved by more people. The major impact on mortality was made by the measures taken by the public

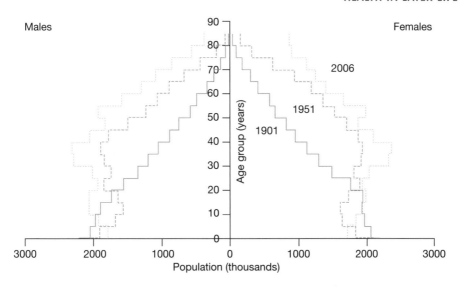

Figure 8.1 Age and sex structure of the United Kingdom population by quinary age group
Source: Office for National Statistics.

Table 8.2 Stages of demographic transition

Fertility	Mortality	Population
High birth rate	High mortality in early life	Predominantly young
High birth rate	Mortality falls in early life	Still predominantly young
Birth rate falls	Mortality falls further	Proportion of adults increases
Birth rate low	Mortality falls across all ages	Proportion of elderly sharply increases
Birth rate low	Mortality falls further, especially in later adult life	Proportion of very elderly rises

health and social reformers during the late nineteenth century. Proper disposal of sewage, purer water supplies and less-crowded, higher-quality housing all helped to reduce the incidence, spread and consequences of the major infectious diseases of the day. As has been previously mentioned, the big improvement was for mortality in infancy and childhood.

By the beginning of the twentieth century, a male child could expect, on average, to live a further 48 years, whereas a male child born in the middle of the first decade of the twenty-first century could expect on average to live into his late 70s (Figure 8.3). Even greater improvements in survival have taken place amongst women. This is a result of a complex relationship between behavioural, social, environmental, economic and genetically linked factors. The excess male-over-female mortality can be largely accounted for by higher mortality for men from coronary heart disease, lung cancer, cirrhosis of the liver and fatal accidents.

Life expectancy for people who have already lived to the middle and later years of their lives has also increased during the twentieth century. A man aged 60 years in 1901 lived an average of 13 further years. By the middle of the first decade of the twenty-first century, the comparable figure was almost 21 years (Figure 8.3). Thus, while the major changes in the age structure of the population of Britain in the twentieth century were due to changes in birth rates and improvements in expectation of life, more recently, additional ageing of the population has been produced by falling mortality rates in old age. When a population is already ageing but has relatively low fertility and low mortality rates, changes in death rates in the older age groups are the major determinant of further population ageing.

Expectation of life at birth varies greatly between countries. Japanese women have the greatest life expectancy at birth. However, the gap between industrialised countries and some developing countries is still marked (Figure 8.4). In some African countries, the impact of HIV and AIDS on life expectancy is profound. The demographic transition that occurred in many developing countries in the late twentieth century (and is still occurring) has had slightly different origins. Social, public health and economic improvements have been important. These populations have also benefited from immunisation programmes in childhood, modern birth-control methods and more advanced medical care. None of these technological influences were available to assist the speed of the demographic transition in Victorian and Edwardian Britain or the other industrialised countries of the northern hemisphere. The relative speed of these demographic transitions is illustrated by examining the time it has taken for populations to age (Figure 8.5).

In many developing countries, the numbers of elderly people occupy a relatively small proportion of the total population, but the annual growth in numbers of older people in these countries is exceeding that of their developed counterparts. Population ageing is thus becoming an issue for the world population, as well as for developed countries such as Britain, other countries of western Europe, the United States and Japan. These changes are illustrated in comparisons of the distribution of deaths and population by age group in the world's population (Figure 8.6).

DEMOGRAPHIC AND SOCIAL FACTORS AFFECTING INFORMAL SUPPORT

Much of the care and support given to older people in the population is still provided informally by their children or other relatives. Therefore, it is important in considering their needs to take account of the size of the pool of potential informal carers, as well as the numbers of economically active people necessary to sustain a more dependent older population. A broad indication is provided by comparing the extent to which the numbers of older people within a society are balanced by those in adult age groups prior to conventional retirement age.

An important demographic indicator is the number of inactive elderly people as a ratio to the number in the workforce: the

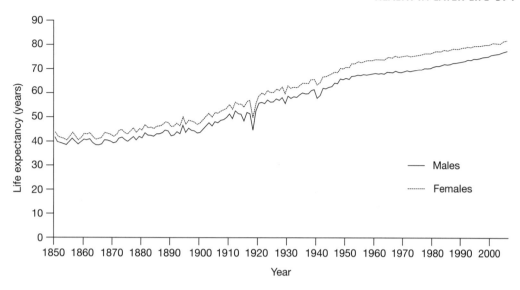

Figure 8.2 Life expectancy at birth, England and Wales
Source: Office for National Statistics.

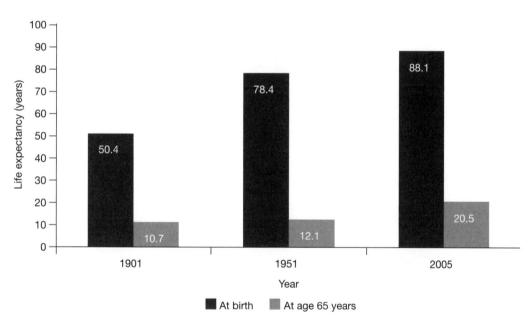

Figure 8.3 Life expectancy (cohort data) for males in England and Wales
Source: Office for National Statistics.

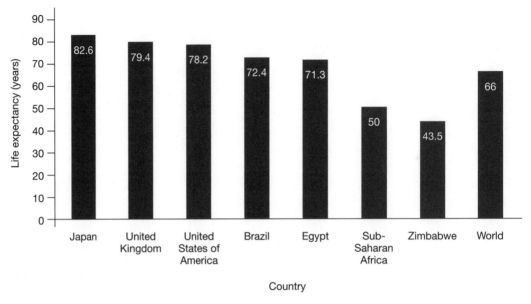

Figure 8.4 Life expectancy at birth for selected countries
Source: United Nations Population Database.

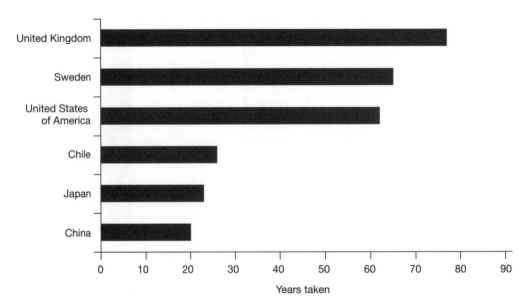

Figure 8.5 Number of years required for population aged 65 years and over to move from 10% to 20% of population
Source: Calculated from United Nations World Population database; 2006.

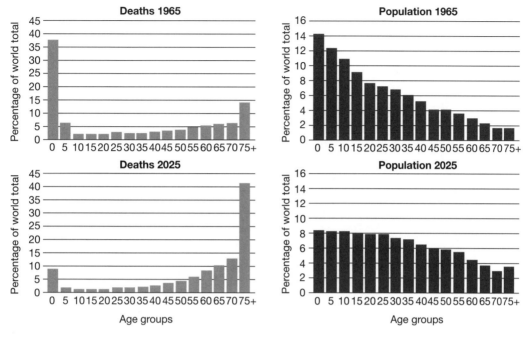

Figure 8.6 Deaths and population in the world by age: 1965 and 2025
Source: World Health Organization. *The World Health Report.* Geneva: WHO; 1997.

so-called aged-dependency ratio. Although this increased only slightly between 1971 and 2006 in the United Kingdom (Figure 8.7), this was because the population of working age was swelled by the large number of 1960s 'baby boomers' who started work in the late 1970s. When the ratio of older people to children (the ageing index) is examined instead, the rise is sharper: 64.0 in 1971 compared to 97.8 in 2006 (Figure 8.7). Moreover, population ageing will rise faster once the baby boomers move into the over-65 groups and are replaced by much smaller numbers in the working age population.

Similar trends will occur in many other developed countries. The impact will be less in countries with high birth rates (for example, Mexico, Iceland and Turkey) or with high levels of immigration (for example,

New Zealand and Canada). However, in countries such as Spain, Japan and Italy, the aged-dependency ratio is projected to be very high.

Such population ageing indices can only give a general indication of the potential support available to older people in a population. A fuller impression is given by information on family size and structure, patterns of geographical mobility and cultural attitudes to family life.

Family size fell during the twentieth century. The change away from the Victorian tendency to have large families has meant that there are fewer children available to give support to parents as they become old and frail. However, in more recent times, the proportion of women who never married, and therefore would not have children

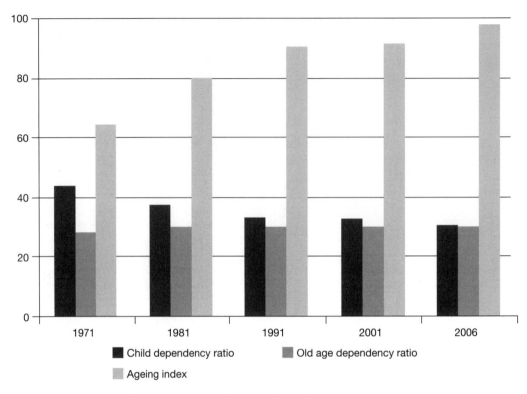

Figure 8.7 Indicators of age structure in the United Kingdom
Source: Office for National Statistics.

potentially available to give support as they grow older, has declined and is projected to fall still further, thus counteracting some of the earlier trends. The extent to which very elderly women are likely to have no surviving children (and hence less potential source of support) is also projected to fall. These higher marriage rates mean that more women will have the potential support of a spouse and one or more children.

Other factors relating to marriage and family-building have potential implications for the informal support available to people as they grow old. If, for example, there were more marriages in which both partners agree not to have children (perhaps to enable the woman to pursue a full career), there would be implications for future generations of older people. Moreover, the increased divorce rate that has been such a feature of the later decades of the twentieth century in Britain will also have an impact. Firstly, divorced elderly people who have not remarried will not have the support of a spouse when they begin to develop the problems associated with old age. Secondly, younger people who become divorced (whether or not they remarry) will have more complex family relationships, which may weaken their capacity for or commitment to providing tangible support to their elderly parents when it is needed. On the other hand, complex family structures associated with divorce and finding new partners has created extended family networks, which in some cases provides additional contact between older people and younger generations.

Increased geographical mobility also affects the pool of potential supporters of older people. Older people can be left behind in the inner cities. In addition, older people themselves often move following retirement to more rural locations or to coastal communities. Many northern Europeans move to the Mediterranean. There are nearly one million older United Kingdom citizens who have moved on retirement to continental Europe, particularly to Spain and France. This has put a strain on care services in these countries and has reduced access to family caregiving networks.

It is difficult to fully discern the implications of all these factors on the actual support given to people in later life. However, of equal importance to the numerical assessment of potential supporters in the light of socio-demographic changes of the kind described above is the actual response made by grown-up children and other relatives of old people when they do need help. Many men and women who are in their middle years of life, with dependent children of their own, will at some time be faced with the problem of how to respond when one or more of their surviving elderly parents or parents-in-law becomes too frail, too ill or simply too lonely to maintain an independent way of life. Sometimes this will be precipitated by the sudden death of a spouse, but more often it will be a situation that builds up gradually.

Depending on the extent of need of the older person, the type of support provided by families varies enormously, ranging from a regular telephone call from a son or daughter through periodic or regular visits to them actually taking up residence with children and grandchildren.

The way in which such situations are resolved depends upon a complex interaction of factors, including geographical proximity of the families; the nature of the housing of the older person and of the family; the quality of family relationships; the attitude of the older person towards independent living; and financial considerations. Informal care is extensively provided to older people.

FUTURE POPULATION CHANGES AND IMPLICATIONS

The immediacy of the problems encountered by the older population is highlighted by a simple demographic fact. Disproportionate increases in the very elderly (Figure 8.8) produce higher levels of dependency and greater needs and demands for health and social services.

The very elderly also tend to be proportionally highly represented in the most intensive forms of non-home-based care, such as hospital inpatient care. In addition to their having the highest rate of hospital admission, this group also have a much longer average duration of stay in such care when compared to other sectors of the older population.

Thus, overshadowing the more subtle factors that determine the need for care within the elderly population are some stark

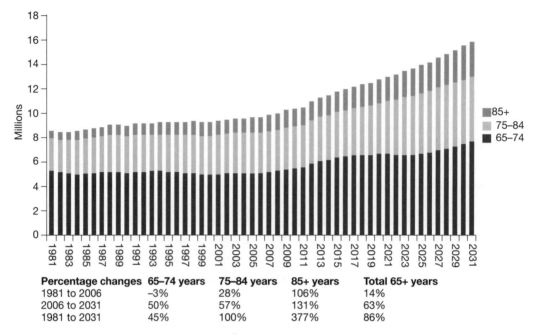

Percentage changes	65–74 years	75–84 years	85+ years	Total 65+ years
1981 to 2006	–3%	28%	106%	14%
2006 to 2031	50%	57%	131%	63%
1981 to 2031	45%	100%	377%	86%

Figure 8.8 Changes in composition of elderly population of United Kingdom
Source: Office for National Statistics.

and simple facts. Well into the twenty-first century, there will be an inexorable increase in the numbers of people who are in the oldest age groups. These are the people who are the frailest, sickest, poorest and most likely to be living on their own. The most dramatic manifestation in the growth of the very old in the population is the increase in the number of centenarians (Table 8.3).

ILL HEALTH, LOSS OF FUNCTION AND NEED

One of the characteristics of any ageing organism is that the older it becomes the greater is the risk of impairment, disease or death. In most organisms, including human beings, the risk of death fluctuates during the early years of life before beginning to rise

progressively with time. Ageing is related to disease in three main ways:

1 *altered response to disease* – some diseases are overcome less easily in elderly people than they are in younger people (for example, pneumonia and fractures)

2 *diseases associated with ageing* – some diseases are so closely associated with ageing that they occur to some extent in all individuals as they age (the best example of this is arteriosclerosis)

3 *increased risk with ageing* – many diseases, although not exclusive to ageing individuals, occur much more commonly when old age is reached (examples of these are many of the common cancers).

The hallmark of the occurrence of disease in older people is the presence of multiple

Table 8.3 Number of centenarians in the United Kingdom

Year	Number aged 100 years or more
1961	600
1981	2600
2006	9800
2031	59 000

Source: Office for National Statistics.

pathology with decreased physiological reserve. Very old people rarely suffer from a single disease; instead they suffer several chronic degenerative processes, some of which surface for the first time in old age, while others are carried over from middle age. In addition to multiple pathology, there are other properties of ill health in later life that are important when designing medical care responses (Table 8.4). Very old people often display impaired adaptability to disease, so their health problems manifest themselves in atypical ways, such as falls and confusion, making the problems difficult to diagnose. Rapid deterioration and a relatively high incidence of complications are also features of disease in very old age. The importance of rehabilitation in recovery is much more important than it is in younger age groups. So is the environment in which care is provided.

Assessment of specific diseases has a place in evaluating the health status of an elderly population, but this approach is not as relevant as examining the way in which pathological processes interfere with the old person's level of functioning (in relation, for example, to particular aspects of self-care) or produce disability.

Activities relevant to the limitation of function in later life are broad. They include self-care (for example, washing, dressing, eating and using the toilet); walking and other movements; mobility in the wider sense (for example, the ability to move from house to shops); the performance of socially allocated roles; and self-determination. Some data on activities of daily living amongst older people are available through national surveys and some are available from study of local populations. Such data can be invaluable in assessing the needs of older people in a locality and planning the response of services. All information on functional capacity shows a strong relationship between increasing age and loss of independence in such functions (Figure 8.9).

The use of a functional capacity perspective of elderly people's needs has led to the formulation of the concept of active life expectancy. It separates the years of relatively healthy life from those characterised by disability, major illness or dependency. As has been discussed in Chapter 3, one of the aims of public health is not just to enable more people to live into late old age but to 'compress morbidity' so that active life expectancy is as close as possible to the number of years lived per se (Figure 8.10).

It is likely that information on functional

Table 8.4 Some features of illness in later life

- Multiple pathology
- Risk of dependency
- Presentation of problems often not typical
- Side effects and complications frequent
- Limited resilience
- Care environment important
- Multidisciplinary care essential

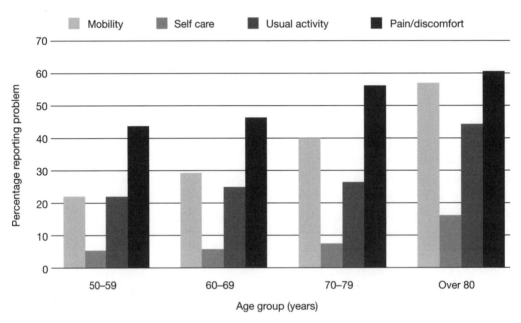

Figure 8.9 Self-reported limitation of function and pain, United Kingdom
Source: Derived from Kind P, Dolan P, Gudex C, *et al.* Variations in population health status: results from a United Kingdom national questionnaire survey. *BMJ.* 1998; **316**: 736–41.

capacity will become a predominant feature in assessing the needs of older populations. This approach has many attractions (Figure 8.11). Defining, for example, the help an elderly woman requires against an assessment of her ability to wash, dress, cook and go out to the shops is of relevance to most caring professionals. It gives a focus for a multidisciplinary approach to care. In addition, assessments of functional capacity provide a common currency that enables the aggregation of data to population level so that it is possible, for example, to describe the proportion of a local elderly population with incontinence of urine and then organise an appropriate service response.

There is a growing problem of isolation amongst elderly people, particularly in the

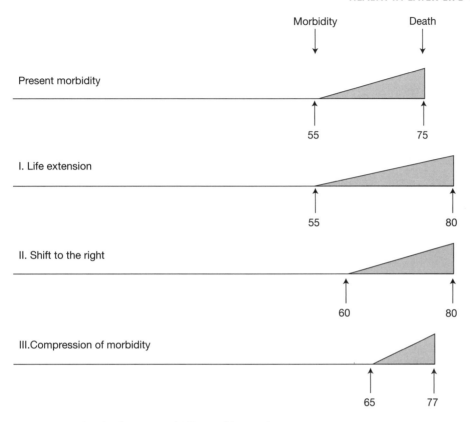

Figure 8.10 Scenarios for future morbidity and longevity
Source: Fries JF. Physical activity, the compression of morbidity, and the health of the elderly. *J R Soc Med.* 1996; **89**(2): 64–8.

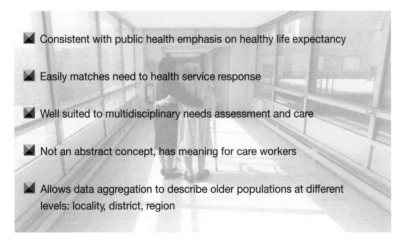

Figure 8.11 Advantages of using functional capacity measures to describe the health of older populations

inner-city areas from which the young have migrated. Loneliness can be a major factor in many of the problems of the elderly. It can cause apathy and lack of interest. It can lead to problems such as malnutrition, hypothermia and general self-neglect.

Older people's social networks are a vital aspect of their need for care as they age. It does not automatically follow that an elderly person living alone is socially isolated. It does raise, however, the importance of the nature of social contacts (as opposed to their number) in the lives of elderly people. For most, their main social contacts are either with those with whom they live or with relatives outside their home. The potential impact of social and demographic changes related to these issues was discussed earlier in the chapter. Much less is known about the extent to which other societal changes have influenced elderly people's own perceptions of the importance of social networks. For example, an old person living alone in an inner-city area who enjoys regular social contact with relatives and friends may be so fearful of personal attack that she would much rather be resident in a sheltered housing scheme than remain in her own home any longer.

The social networks of older people will be based heavily on relatives, but friends and neighbours are also important. The number of social contacts that people maintain in later life is very variable and depends upon their social and educational background, their ethnic group, the type of community they live in and their personal attitudes and outlook. There is some research evidence suggesting that health and mortality in later life are both affected by the strength of older people's social networks.

Changes in the position of older people in society are also closely related to the economic effects of growing old. Retired people who are mainly dependent on a state pension have lower income than other groups, as might be expected (Figure 8.12). State pensions and other welfare benefits provide the main source of income for elderly people. Older people spend a higher proportion of their income on basics – housing, fuel and food – than do younger people.

A key issue may well be the distribution of income among the older age groups. There is evidence that this distribution widened considerably during the latter part of the twentieth century, with major differences in standard of living between those dependent upon state benefits for their income and the smaller number with other income such as investments and occupational pensions.

ETHNIC MINORITY ELDERS

In the last few years of the twentieth century, ethnic minority communities made up about 7% of Britain's population. The proportion was much higher in certain conurbations. The relatively young age structure of these communities reflects a high birth rate (in some groups) and the waves of immigration that occurred in the 1960s and early 1970s and (for those who came from Caribbean countries) in earlier years still.

While the numbers of older people belonging to ethnic minority groups are as yet small compared to the indigenous elderly, their numbers will increase as the structure of the minority populations begins to resemble that of the majority (Table 8.5).

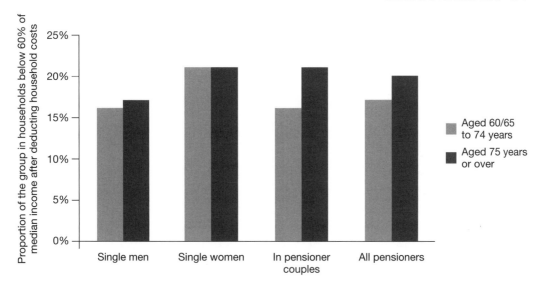

Figure 8.12 Single female pensioners and older pensioner couples are most likely to have a low income, United Kingdom
Source: New Policy Institute. The Poverty Site. Available at: www.poverty.org.uk. Palmer G, Kenway P, MacInnes T. *Monitoring Poverty and Social Exclusion.* York: Joseph Rowntree Foundation; 2007. Data are derived from the Department of Work and Pensions and are average for 2003/4 to 2005/6.

Relatively little information is available on the health of older people in the ethnic minority populations, and it is important not to fall into stereotypic assumptions about the needs of ethnic minority elders. For example, it is widely believed that old age is a greatly revered state in some ethnic minority communities within Britain. Hence it is assumed that an elderly person will enjoy the warmth, support and care of an extended family, so little attention should be given by statutory services to meeting the needs of this group of elderly people. While this may be the ideal shared by people in some ethnic minority communities themselves, patterns of geographical mobility and other factors will mean that it is unlikely always to be realised. Contrasts between this cultural ideal and the social reality may give rise to problems for elderly

people belonging to ethnic minority groups as well as leading to false assumptions amongst those responsible for providing services.

A population survey of the health and social status of elderly people of 'Asian' descent in Leicestershire (described as an example of a public health investigation in Chapter 2) was one of the earliest to provide objective data on need amongst the ethnic minority elderly in Britain. It showed similar levels of incapacity to the indigenous population but a greater direct involvement with the extended family. Wider social contact was seriously limited, however, by lack of literacy and language skills, which may also limit contact with the helping agencies in the health and social care arena.

In responding to the needs of older people from ethnic minority communities, it is

Table 8.5 Proportion of older age groups amongst different ethnic populations in the United Kingdom, 2007

Ethnic Group	Percentage aged (years)		
	45–59	*60–74*	*75+*
White British	20.4	15.3	8.0
Other White	17.1	12.1	6.3
White and Black Caribbean	3.5	0.9	0.5
White and Black African	8.9	1.6	1.0
White and Asian	4.6	2.0	0.9
Other mixed	7.2	3.0	0.7
Indian	17.8	8.7	2.4
Pakistani	11.9	4.7	1.3
Bangladeshi	8.9	5.1	1.1
Other Asian	15.4	5.4	1.2
Black Caribbean	17.9	11.3	4.3
Black African	10.2	2.5	0.5
Other Black	7.4	6.9	2.2
Chinese	16.5	4.3	1.5
Other	14.4	5.2	2.1

Source: Office for National Statistics. Estimates are based on small sample sizes and should be treated with caution.

especially important for health services to ensure that they are aware of and work with varying cultural norms. Knowledge of and sensitivity to issues such as diet, religious practice and observance and the role of the older person in his or her own community is of particular significance.

SOME SPECIAL HEALTH PROBLEMS OF LATER LIFE

A number of specific health problems of later life that are amenable to prevention or that have major medical care implications are considered briefly in this section.

Cardiovascular disease and cancer, which are particularly important causes of illness and disability in older people, are discussed in Chapter 3. Respiratory infections, which are a common cause of emergency admission to hospital amongst older people, are considered in Chapter 9. Sensory impairment (loss of vision and hearing) is discussed in Chapter 5.

HYPOTHERMIA AND EXCESS WINTER DEATHS

Accidental hypothermia is said to be present if a deep body (core) temperature falls to below 35°C. The term 'accidental' is used to distinguish this type of hypothermia from that which might be induced deliberately for therapeutic purposes. The diagnosis of hypothermia must be confirmed with a special low-reading thermometer inserted rectally. Such instruments are becoming an increasingly common part of the equipment of doctors and nurses working in the community. It is estimated that 3–4% of people aged 65 years and over who are admitted to hospital have a core body temperature below 35°C. Over 90% of cases of accidental hypothermia occur indoors.

The older person with hypothermia does not usually shiver or complain of being cold because of an impaired perception of temperature change. However, the skin is pale and cold to the touch and consciousness is clouded, leading to drowsiness, disordered thought and speech. Coma is more likely the lower the body temperature becomes. Movement and reflexes are sluggish. Speech may be slurred, the hearing and respiratory rates are slow and characteristic changes in an electrocardiograph may be present. The blood pressure may fall. Some patients with hypothermia may become agitated and restless, and if tranquillisers are prescribed, this can complicate their serious condition.

Fatality amongst patients with hypothermia is high. Treatment, usually in hospital, consists of gradual rewarming (if conducted too rapidly, this may be fatal) and other supportive measures, such as administration of oxygen, intravenous fluids and broad-spectrum antibiotics.

The main causes of accidental hypothermia are defective thermoregulatory mechanisms (a consequence of ageing) and exposure to cold through low environmental temperature. Other factors, such as immobility due to general infirmity, mental impairment, strokes, falls, effects of medicines or certain illness (for example, infections, endocrine disorders) may be superimposed.

Reducing the occurrence of accidental hypothermia in later life can be addressed through community programmes directed particularly at the homes of older people living alone. Living accommodation can be reviewed to ensure that there is an adequate indoor temperature. This can be maintained by a combination of heating, draught reduction and insulation measures. In addition, health education advice to older people should emphasise moving around (if possible) to increase body heat by metabolic activity and also ensuring adequate nutrition and clothing, especially in advanced age. Financial support through the benefits system for heating, insulation and cold weather payments are particularly important.

All health and social care professionals and informal carers should be made aware of, and be vigilant for, the danger signs of hypothermia, especially in cold weather. It is also valuable to ensure a basic knowledge of these issues amongst members of the general public (such as postal workers) who come into regular contact with older people.

Hypothermia has been discussed in detail because deaths from this cause in later life are a tragedy that effective public health action can help to avoid. However, the issue of death due to cold weather is a much more complex question, which has been subjected to extensive epidemiological study.

Measuring mortality in the winter months (usually December–March) as a proportion of mortality at other times of year yields an index called excess winter deaths. The excess winter mortality index (Table 8.6) is calculated as the number of excess winter deaths divided by the average non-winter deaths expressed as a percentage. While this index fluctuated during the twentieth century, it has persistently showed an excess of winter deaths in older age groups. The excess mortality is due to circulatory illness (ischaemic heart disease and stroke), respiratory disease (particularly influenza), accidents and violence (including hypothermia) and a range of other causes. The excess winter mortality rises sharply with age in the older age groups (Table 8.6) and is worse in the years with influenza epidemics.

HEATWAVES

Until recently, the effect of weather and environmental temperatures on the health of older people was always viewed in the context of the risks of exposure to the cold. Recent alterations in summer weather patterns (attributed to climate change) in western Europe have raised the risks of extreme heat. This came to prominence in France in August of 2003, when very high temperatures led to nearly 15 000 excess deaths. The majority were women aged 75 years or older. There were major recriminations for the French government.

In the United Kingdom there is now a Heatwave Plan[1] that provides advice and contingency plans to protect older and vulnerable people. The plan is triggered by different ambient temperature thresholds.

FALLS

An older woman is more likely to die from the complications of a hip fracture than from breast cancer. Accidents are a common cause of death, disability and hospital admission in later life. Falls are the single most important cause of accidental death in older people, the remainder resulting from road traffic accidents, burns and a variety of other causes. The economic costs are high, with fractured hips alone estimated to account for nearly £2 billion of expenditure in the health and social care system.

The propensity of older people to fall over has long been recognised. Many falls in the elderly produce no injuries. However, partly because of the increased fragility of bones in old age, a fracture is a common

Table 8.6 Excess winter mortality index for women

Cause	Age group (years)		
	65–74	75–84	85 and over
Circulatory disease	13.9	22.2	24.4
Respiratory disease	63.4	64.1	76.2
Injury and poisoning	19.8	29.1	28.8
Cancer	2.7	3.5	4.7

Source: Office for National Statistics. Data relate to 2004/05.

outcome of a fall. Fracture of the neck of the femur is a particularly serious example that can result from seemingly quite trivial falls or no apparent trauma (for example, rising out of a chair). Even with the modern approach of immediate operation (to pin the fracture or replace the hip joint) and early mobilisation, fatality can still be as high as 25%. A less serious fracture, such as Colles' fracture of the wrist, may still be a considerable handicap for an elderly woman attempting to cook her meals and do her housework with an arm immobilised in plaster.

The types of falls have been classified into four categories:

1   *intrinsic* – in most older people who have fallen, there are underlying causes such as disorders of vision, disorders of balance (e.g., vestibular disorders), neurological problems (e.g., Parkinson's Disease) and/or cardiovascular disorders (e.g., carotid sinus syndrome)

2   *drug-induced* – about 7% of acute hospital admissions amongst older people are related to drug side effects, the most common of which is drug-induced falls; drugs that are particularly dangerous include sedatives and drugs with anticholinergic properties, including some anti-depressants, which induce postural hypotension

3   *extrinsic* – environmental factors such as poor lighting and loose rugs are thought to contribute to about 40% of falls.

Approaches to the prevention of falls and their consequences are targeted at three levels. In the general population, throughout life, increasing the level of exercise, particularly weight-bearing activity, reduces the risk of falls and fractures in later life. In primary care, many older people will report a history of a fall. It is not possible to offer everyone a full multidisciplinary assessment and treatment programme, nor is there evidence that this would be cost-effective. Nevertheless, older people who have fallen should be reviewed within primary care to encourage weight-bearing exercise, review vision, enquire about the home environment and review medications. Older people who suffer recurrent falls or have been admitted to hospital with a major fall or a fall-related fracture should be reviewed by a multidisciplinary falls and bone health service. There is now good evidence for the cost-effectiveness of screening for and treating osteoporosis in people who have had a fragility fracture.

URINARY INCONTINENCE

Urinary incontinence is a common problem in the elderly; estimates suggest that the overall prevalence is around 10% in older adults. It is perhaps the most embarrassing, distressing and ultimately humiliating problem of old age. Moreover, its onset is often the reason why the elderly person is judged as no longer fit to remain in his or her home, rejected in a family or friend's home or considered an unsuitable candidate for certain forms of residential care. Urinary incontinence has been defined by the International Continence Society as '. . . the involuntary loss of urine which is objectively demonstrable and is a social or hygienic problem.'

The causes of urinary incontinence are

many and may arise from local factors, for example, bladder-neck obstruction (most often due to prostatic enlargement), stress incontinence (usually due to weakening of pelvic-floor musculature following childbirth) or urinary tract infections. General factors in the elderly that may lead to incontinence are often multiple and not clear-cut. A common reason for urinary incontinence is loss of inhibition of need to void when the bladder is partly full. This mainly occurs at night and may be associated with early brain failure. Emotional upsets resulting from bereavement, accidents or illnesses can give rise to incontinence of either a transient or permanent nature. Confusion arising from organic cerebral disease (including stroke) or side effects of sedatives or psychotropic drugs can also lead to incontinence. Other drugs, such as rapidly acting diuretics, may also contribute. Incontinence may be a feature of limitation of mobility, with the elderly person being unable to reach the toilet in time to avoid an accident.

In order for continence of urine to be maintained, five conditions need to be fulfilled (Table 8.7). Approaches to management need to identify which of these factors is contributing to the loss of continence in the individual concerned and then address the problem.

The cornerstone of management of urinary incontinence in the elderly is making a correct diagnosis of the cause, together with a sympathetic and understanding attitude on the part of the professionals. This means good assessment – for example, by a continence adviser with expertise and experience in this field. Incontinence is seldom the result of a single underlying cause. It cannot be over-emphasised that the presence of incontinence is a deeply emotional issue, both for the elderly people who have it and for relatives, friends and neighbours who are in contact with them.

In some cases, operative treatment of an enlarged prostate or of a gynaecological disorder, treatment of an underlying urinary tract infection or review of a long-standing drug regime may solve the problem. Aside from these measures, probably the most important step in treating urinary incontinence is bladder training. For incontinent patients already in an institutional setting, episodes of incontinence are recorded on a fluid chart, and nursing staff ensure regular toileting of the patient to re-educate the bladder. Such bladder training may be supplemented by physiotherapy in the form of

Table 8.7 Factors necessary to maintain urinary continence

- Adequate function of the lower urinary tract to store and empty urine
- Adequate cognitive function to recognise the need to urinate and to find the appropriate place
- Adequate physical mobility and dexterity to get a toilet and use it
- Motivation to be continent
- Absence of environmental barriers to continence

Source: Ouslander JG. The efficacy of continence treatment. In: Kane RL, Evans JG, MacFayden D, editors. *Improving the Health of Older People: a world view.* Oxford: Oxford University Press; 1990.

exercise for the pelvic-floor muscles. Despite such measures, some people will continue to experience episodes of incontinence.

A wide variety of support is possible for older people with incontinence who are living in the community. In many parts of the country, specialised continence advisers (often with a nursing background) visit old people and make assessments, as well as providing help to those whose problem has been diagnosed. The use of specialised underclothes and pads are a particularly important part of a support strategy once specific interventions have been tried or as an accompaniment to other therapies. The range of available products is quite wide and makes use of disposable pads with highly absorbent materials.

MENTAL ILLNESS

Mental illness in later life can take many different forms. Some degree of depression is the commonest disorder and affects approximately 15% of the population aged 65 years and over. In addition to the causes of the disease amongst younger people, depression amongst older people can be precipitated by any of the major life events that are common in this age group: for example, the loss of a spouse, retirement or the onset of physical illness associated with pain.

The manifestations of depression can be quite wide-ranging and include apathy, social withdrawal, neglect of personal appearance, tearfulness, sleep disorders, loss of appetite and suicide. For many older people, the episode of depression may resolve with professional help, but in others the condition becomes chronic.

Another serious mental illness of later old age is dementia, a disorder of brain functioning that leads to deterioration in the capacity of the mind. It affects areas such as memory, decision-making, understanding and the use of language to communicate with others. Old people with dementia can also have disturbances of normal behaviour that lead them to wander, to sleep irregularly and fitfully and to exhibit disruptive and antisocial behaviour. Another practical aspect of the effect of dementia on elderly people is the extent to which they are able to care for themselves. Progressive loss of function in this respect is an important feature of the disease. Dementia varies in the way in which it affects the mental, physical and social functioning of any individual elderly person, but it is capable of affecting all such areas of functioning (Table 8.8).

Minor degrees of memory impairment and temporary confusion may not necessarily threaten an old person's capacity to maintain an independent existence in the community. However, more severe and sustained problems of this kind, especially when coupled with disturbed or erratic behaviour and an inability to perform basic activities of daily living, will lead rapidly to a state of dependency.

Dementia affects around 5% of people aged 65 years and over, while closer to 20% of over-85s will exhibit some signs of it. Thus ageing of the population is strongly linked to increasing numbers of people with dementia.

Dementia is of two main types. The first and most common is Alzheimer's disease, in which there are permanent changes in the brain characterised by loss and severe abnor-

Table 8.8 Practical features of dementia

Progressive impairment of intellectual functioning
● Memory problems
● Loss of sense of time
● Loss of sense of where or who they are
● Speech difficulties
Personality and behavioural changes
● Neglect of personal care and hygiene
● Incontinence
● Emotional instability
● Loss of social inhibitions

malities of nerve cells and their processes. In particular, nerve cells that produce important chemical substances for brain activities are lost. Alzheimer's disease accounts for about half of all cases of dementia amongst the over-65s. Dementia is much less common in middle age and early old age, but when it does occur here, Alzheimer's disease is commonly found. The second type of dementia is associated with disease of the arteries of the brain, causing death of small or large areas of brain tissue. This is called multi-infarct dementia.

Aside from these two main types of dementia, there are other less common forms, including Lewy body dementia, dementia associated with neurodegenerative disorders such as Huntingdon's chorea, Parkinson's disease and Creutzfeldt-Jakob disease. In addition, the symptoms and signs of dementia can be produced by vitamin B12 deficiency, brain tumours, thyroid disease and chronic alcoholism.

Anti-cholinesterase inhibitor drugs are now available and moderately effective in delaying decline in mental function for people with Alzheimer's dementia of moderate severity. Reduction in cardiovascular risk factors reduces the incidence of both multi-infarct dementia and Alzheimer's disease. Extensive investigation by the pharmaceutical industry into the pathophysiology of Alzheimer's disease is likely to yield new and more effective approaches to treatment in the next decade.

Other groups of elderly people with mental illness are important and need services. Many of those with psychotic illnesses such as schizophrenia have grown old within large, old-style psychiatric hospitals. With the policy of phasing out such long-stay institutional-type facilities, these patients have particular needs that must be matched by appropriate community services if they are to leave what has effectively become their home over many years. Amongst elderly people admitted to hospital for treatment of acute medical, surgical or orthopaedic conditions, so-called 'confusion' (more properly 'delirium') is common. Many cases can be managed clinically if identified at an early stage and underlying factors are treated.

SERVICES FOR PEOPLE IN LATER LIFE

It often surprises people to learn that the majority of older people are able to lead an independent existence in their own home. However, with advancing age and the impact of the negative forces of old age, this independence is less easily maintained. The main categories of need were discussed in the previous section and are summarised in Table 8.9. When older people are no longer able to manage on their own, a wide range of services may be available to provide help, support and advice.

The overall aims should be maintaining health and independence for as long as possible and ensuring that when services are provided, they give the best possible outcome and experience of care for the older person.

NATIONAL SERVICE FRAMEWORK

Chapter 4 has described the concept of a national service framework. This is a new planning mechanism introduced in 1999 that sets out standards for particular fields of care and models of service organisation that represent good practice. A *National Service Framework for Older People* was produced in 2001.[2] Its ambitions were to reduce age discrimination, improve personalisation in care, invest and reform community services, particularly those that bridge the gap between hospital and home. It also set standards of care for people with stroke, falls and fractures, mental health problems in old age and to promote healthy active life. The *National Service Framework* was refreshed in 2006 with the publication of *A New Ambition for Old Age*,[3] which stressed the importance of ensuring dignity in care for older people, and with the development of national strategies for stroke and for dementia.

THE MAINTENANCE OF HEALTH IN OLD AGE

The main conditions that contribute to incapacity and dependency in old age are heart disease; stroke; joint disease and fractured neck of femur; diabetes mellitus; cancer (particularly of the breast, lung, prostate, colon and rectum); dementia and depression; and eye disease (cataract and glaucoma). Measures to promote health and prevent disease earlier in life can help to improve health in later life by delaying the onset of some of these chronic diseases. However, action in old age itself can also have an impact. More effective management of chronic diseases in old age can prolong independence, maintain good quality of life and prevent unnecessary hospital admission. Health promotion strategies addressing factors such as good diet, exercise, smoking cessation and the control of high blood pressure and high blood cholesterol can also be effective, even when used for the first time in later life.

A wider perspective on the promotion of health would also include programmes that prepare older people psychologically for retirement and address their social welfare in ways that prevent problems and crises occurring.

Table 8.9 Key features that determine health need in later life

- Social networks and support
- Income level
- Presence of disease or illness
- Mobility and capacity for self-care
- Housing quality and neighbourhood environment
- Sensory impairment
- Personal security
- Access to services

PRIMARY AND COMMUNITY CARE

The majority of older people will continue to live in the community, either with their spouse, with their children, with other members of their family or, increasingly as they grow older, alone. For some considerable time, the central objective of policy for care in old age in the United Kingdom has been to enable elderly people to remain in the community for as long as possible. For most people in later life, their ability to reside in their own home is a potent symbol of autonomy, independence and self-determination.

The nature of services provided in the community is critical in determining successful outcomes of care for old people who do have needs. Whether organised around the primary care trust directly, based within a community health service unit or located within a hospital's services (as an outreach function), health professionals other than doctors are an essential element of the network of health care delivered to older people in the community. For example, occupational therapists, district nurses, home helps and health visitors are vital professionals whose input to the care of housebound old people can help to convert their tenuous hold on independent living into a well-supported daily routine enhanced by social contacts.

A major challenge for primary health care is the early identification and response to old-age-related health care needs and the sharing of assessment information with social care services. There is recognition of the need for shared record systems to avoid duplication in recording information and to ensure that there is a common understanding of the range of needs and problems faced by the older person.

Community nurses have a major role in caring for the elderly. Of all the patients treated at home by nurses in the United Kingdom, almost half are elderly. Increasingly, in many parts of the country, although overall responsibility remains in the hands of a qualified nurse, nursing auxiliaries assist with some duties such as bathing, washing hair, cutting toenails and generally performing home nursing tasks. The role of the fully trained nurse is in the assessment of older people and the delegation of the personal care to nursing auxiliaries and care assistants whom he or she supervises.

Community nurses have become members of multidisciplinary health and care teams, which have been established to support early discharge from hospital and to provide alternatives to admission. These intermediate care services offer short-term support of up to six weeks. Other members of the team include physiotherapists, occupational therapists and social care practitioners, and there is medical involvement from general practitioners or hospital specialists. Additional staff, including specialist mental health practitioners, are sometimes involved. There was a 70% reduction in delayed discharge from acute hospitals in England in the five years following the introduction of these services in the year 2000.

The availability of day and respite care backed up by good transport to provide widespread access can be another key ingredient of support for the vulnerable elderly. Services that are available on a 24-hour, seven-day-a-week basis to provide, for example, night nursing, toileting, bathing or sitting services will often make the difference between a hospital or residential care admission and sustaining an old person with a reasonable quality of life at home.

Specialist nursing services such as community psychiatric nurses (for example, for older people with severe depression or dementia) or palliative care nurses (for example, for elderly people with end-stage cancer) are a valuable adjunct to these general community services.

Local authorities in England with social services responsibilities have a statutory duty to assess the needs for social care of any person who requires it and commission the provision of services for those who are eligible. The process of assessment is standardised, but individual local authorities can set their own eligibility criteria. Some, for example, will limit the provision of care only to those with acute care needs.

The largest category of people receiving state-funded social care is people aged 65 years and over who have been assessed as having physical disability, frailty or sensory impairment. A substantial number of older people are assessed as needing and eligible for social care by virtue of their mental ill health.

The range of domiciliary social care includes home care, day care, meals on wheels, equipment and adaptation to the home environment.

Domiciliary Social Care

Because most older people wish to remain in their own homes for as long as possible, priority has been given to providing intensive packages of social care support. This has resulted in a higher proportion of older people with high levels of need being able to stay at home rather than moving into a care home. However, less money has been available to support the larger numbers of older people with lower levels of need, for example through home help services. The introduction of direct payments and personal budgets for social care has given increasing numbers of older people and their carers more control over their care.

Day Centres and Recreational Clubs

Many older people will attend a day centre or be a member of a club (often organised by a voluntary organisation or in some places by a church). Such facilities are places where they can interact with their peers and with staff. This can help to counteract loneliness and social isolation. A hot meal is often provided midday, and this helps to meet the overall nutritional needs of the older people concerned. Day centres like these can also help to relieve some of the burden of care for informal carers and allow them time and space to unwind, to go shopping or to get on with household tasks.

Respite Care

Respite care can be of major importance in allowing dependent older people to remain in their own homes. There are a variety of models of respite care, which are designed to meet a range of individual needs of older people and of carers. There is still a clear role for the health service in providing hospital inpatient respite care. Other forms of respite care are provided by local authorities or the independent sector. Respite care does not always mean that individuals leave their homes. Given the importance of familiar surroundings to many older people (especially those with mental illnesses of old age, such as dementia), some models of respite care involve care workers looking after the person in their own home.

Voluntary Organisations

In Britain, voluntary organisations have traditionally played a vital role in the care of older people in the community. While their role will vary according to the philosophy and infrastructure of the organisation concerned, it will invariably include raising public awareness of the issues involved and providing information to older people and their carers. Many voluntary organisations will additionally have a service-provision role, which can encompass the delivery of specialist advice on state financial benefit entitlements, the running of day-care centres, counselling, advice and home visiting.

CARING FOR CARERS

Understanding the full spectrum of care needs (Figure 8.13) requires an understanding of the needs of those who look after others, many of whom are themselves in middle age.

Carers must be given practical support as partners with professionals in giving care (Table 8.10 and 8.11). This should be based on an assessment of their individual needs separate from their dependants. Above all, they should have access to high-quality, up-to-date information about the availability of facilities, services, rights and entitlements. They must be recognised as having needs of their own, requiring support and care. There might be a need for counselling and emotional support or for training in particular aspects of disease management, or they might have health care needs of their own. Support to enable them to take regular breaks or continue in employment (if they want to) is a particularly important part of supporting carers. Much of this work is anticipatory, to prevent a breakdown of the caring relationship.

Assessment of need

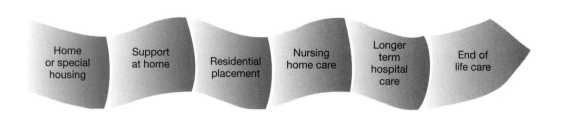

Planning of care

Figure 8.13 Continuing care needs in later life: key components

OLDER PEOPLE WITH LONG-TERM CARE NEEDS WHO CANNOT MANAGE AT HOME

Sometimes, even with a high level of support from services, it is just not feasible or humane to allow an older person to remain at home. Through multi-agency assessment, local authorities with social services responsibilities are the lead agencies that commission care for such people, unless they meet health service eligibility criteria or if they have sufficient funds to buy private care. The choice of care will be that which best suits their needs from within the range of facilities in a locality.

In addition to assessing the individual's need for long-term care, the local authority is also required to evaluate the older person's income and assets (including the value of any property that he or she owns). In England, local authorities must then adhere to a nationally determined charging system in which only people with assets below a certain level are eligible for local authority-funded care. Others must contribute to the costs of care or fund themselves entirely.

Only a minority of residential care is now provided by local authority-staffed and managed facilities (which is a major shift since the 1970s and before). Local authorities are largely commissioners of care, organising placements for older people (who need and are eligible for funded care) in independent-sector residential homes or nursing homes.

NHS responsibilities for long-term care include the commissioning and provision of nursing care in people's homes and in nursing homes. Some older people have such high levels of need that they are judged to require NHS-funded continuing health care. In England, the costs of continuing health care and the nursing contribution to long-term care are paid for by the NHS. Personal care is commissioned by local authorities and is means tested. In Scotland, personal care costs are not means tested.

There has been a growing realisation of the importance of the nature of the institutional environment and regime of long-stay accommodation. Places where the interior fabric is drab and decaying, where furnishing

Table 8.10 Characteristics of carers in the United Kingdom

- At any time, one in 10 is a carer
- Women are more likely to provide personal care
- Bangladeshi and Pakistani groups have the highest rate of carers amongst ethnic minorities
- More than 20% of 50–59-year-olds are carers
- 175 000 young people under 18 years provide care (16% between 20 and 50 or more hours per week)

Source: Department of Health. *Carers at the Heart of 21st-Century Families and Communities.* London: The Stationery Office; 2008.

Table 8.11 Strategy for carers: key elements

- Information and advice
- Funded breaks from caring
- Expanded NHS services, including annual health checks
- Flexible working opportunities and increased training provision
- Emotional support
- Targeted support for young carers

Source: Department of Health. *Carers at the Heart of 21st-Century Families and Communities.* London: The Stationery Office; 2008.

is uniform, where there is a permanent smell of urine and where privacy is limited, coupled with regimes that are organised and regimented to facilitate the tasks of the staff rather than the needs of the individual resident or patient, can be destructive. This lack of self-determination encourages an apathy and indifference amongst people with special or long-term care needs that may lead not only to poor quality of life but to poor outcome of care. Such long-stay institutions are also often characterised by poor staff morale, high staff turnover and problems with recruitment.

There are two major groups of older people who require these forms of long-term care: those who need care for considerable parts of a 24-hour period from staff with nursing training and those who need staff to give help or assistance in carrying out some of the activities of daily living, such as washing, dressing, getting to the toilet and feeding themselves.

In the past, these types of care have been regarded as discrete entities, developed to a level within the population determined by the agencies that control them and with admission and care policies that were similarly individual-agency orientated. The advent of the changes to the organisation and funding of community care at the beginning of the 1990s helped to achieve a greater degree of integration.

The aim of all facilities that care for older people should be to allow the individual to have maximum dignity and self-determination. While in practice the daily routine for elderly patients or residents can often seem dull and monotonous, there is much that can be done to ensure that the regime does not develop the adverse features of an institution. Older people in continuing-care facilities should not spend extended periods of the day bedridden or chairfast unless their condition dictates that this must be so. Older people should receive personalised care and should not be subjected to set regimes in relation to toileting, bathing or feeding. Each continuing care facility should pursue a personalised clothing scheme to encourage the maintenance of self-respect and individuality. Residents should be encouraged to bring as many of their personal possessions with them as is feasible.

The older person's environment should provide a sense of security and cheerfulness. Therefore floors should be safe to walk on and appropriate furniture, including a wide variety of chairs, should be provided. The layout and furnishing of the hospital or home should be designed to avoid confusion, as this is particularly important for the elderly with dementia. Decoration should be in a non-institutional manner, with soft furnishings and colour schemes of homely appearance. The communal rooms should be arranged to allow each resident to pursue their own hobbies and interests. With positive attention to building design, environment, regimes, individual care plans and staff training, adverse factors of institutional life can be reversed.

HOSPITAL-BASED SERVICES

A central part of a comprehensive system of care for older people is the capacity to provide specialist assessment and treatment for older people with acute medical problems. Older people with acute illnesses present a particular challenge for the service seeking to provide the most effective clinical management of their condition and to maximise their level of independence. Older people will often have several problems coexisting that require skilful assessment and treatment, but, as already mentioned, their functional capacity, such as mobility and continence, will be equally as influential in determining both recovery and future living status. Moreover, the acute presentation will often bring to light issues of family and social support that have previously not been addressed but that require resolution as part of the care plan.

Inpatient Care

The appropriate organisation of acute medical care to provide prompt and accurate assessment, treatment and rehabilitation, and ultimately a return to the community or other care facility, is a constant source of discussion amongst health policy-makers and clinicians providing services. Attention has also centred on what kind of hospital bed the older person with an acute illness should be admitted to and what the relationship should be between geriatric medicine and general medicine as specialties of clinical practice. It is now widely acknowledged that care of the acutely ill elderly person is best provided within a bed in a general hospital setting, where there is access to the full range of diagnostic and therapeutic facilities. Reduced age discrimination since publication of the *National Service Framework for Older People* has meant that older people have been the main beneficiaries of improved access and quality of acute and elective general hospital services.

Many older people present to hospital as emergencies with acute illnesses (such as pneumonia, heart failure or stroke) or after falls or fractures. Others are admitted for planned treatments (such as hip- or knee-joint surgery). Care of older people is a large part of the work of acute hospitals – some 70% of acute hospital beds are occupied by people aged 65 or older.

The focus in acute hospital care should be ensuring the best possible outcome while keeping the older person's length of stay as short as possible. Prolonged hospital stay amongst older people greatly increases the risk of complications such as infections and falls. It is also potentially wasteful of health service resources. The key to this focus is accurate early diagnosis and ensuring that older people receive the most appropriate specialist care for their needs. Achieving early discharge from hospital means planning and coordinating support in the home whenever possible.

Many residential and nursing home placements arise from acute hospital admissions. Some of these are unnecessary. Proper assessment and rehabilitation can enable many older people to return, with support, to their own homes rather than entering long-term care. This is best undertaken in step-down intermediate care services in more homely environments or in the person's own home rather than in the acute setting.

Assessing older people in acute hospital beds and planning their discharge is a crucial test of the success of multidisciplinary multi-agency working in the care of older people. If it is done badly, discharge is delayed, and older people occupy acute beds unnecessarily. This can lead to reduced social functioning due to learned dependence and may well therefore end up in more intensive forms of care than would otherwise have been the case.

The nature of services for the treatment of non-emergency problems of the elderly within the acute care sector is also of great importance. Many elderly people's lives are impaired by the presence of conditions that are potentially correctable. For example, many elderly women with chronic pain and severe limitation of movement caused by osteoarthrosis of the hip could have their level of independence and quality of life immediately improved by a hip-joint replacement. Similarly, the lives of old people with very poor eyesight due to cataracts can be transformed by a simple operation.

SPECIALIST OLD AGE MENTAL HEALTH SERVICES

Specialist old age mental health services have provided expertise in managing age-related conditions such as dementia and in managing mental health problems amongst older people with multiple co-morbidities. There is increasing emphasis on early intervention and on providing integrated or liaison services with primary health care, social care and acute hospital care.

CONCLUSIONS

An ageing population brings with it increasing need for help and support from society – medical, social, emotional and financial. The ultimate aim of public health is to increase the period of later life that is free of poor health, incapacity and dependency. This will mainly be achieved by measures taken to promote health and prevent disease earlier in life, but action taken in old age itself can also make an important contribution.

Greater health expectancy will make old age a time of continuing participation in the life of the community and of personal fulfilment for many more older people. However, with ever-advancing years, the need for support for old people who become frail, ill, incapacitated or socially isolated becomes increasingly important. Early identification and response to health and social care needs by primary health care teams, community health practitioners and social care staff is essential to reduce the progression to frailty as people develop old-age-related health problems.

For people who have become frail, the key is to assess individual need on a multidisciplinary, multi-agency basis and then organise an appropriate response. Improved systems of anticipatory care planning and end-of-life care are important for ensuring choice control and dignity for frail older people.

While the planning and commissioning of support and care is undertaken by social care and health services, the independent sector increasingly plays the major part in the actual provision of care. Much, if not the majority, of the care provided to old people is given by informal carers (families and friends), and this must be recognised by all care agencies. Practical and emotional support for such carers is a vital part of the infrastructure of support for older people themselves, and it is important that they and their carers are fully involved as part of the care process.

If these services work well, many older people with problems will be able to remain in the community, well supported, close to family and friends. Throughout, however, emphasis must be placed on setting and maintaining high standards of care, whether this is to be provided in the community, in a hospital or in a residential care facility. In these ways, quality of life and dignity for people in the final years of their lives will be sustained.

REFERENCES

1 Department of Health. *Heatwave Plan for England*. London: Department of Health; 2008.

2 Department of Health. *A National Service Framework for Older People*. London: Department of Health; 2001.

3 Department of Health. *A New Ambition for Old Age: next steps in implementing the National Service Framework for Older People*. London: Department of Health; 2006.

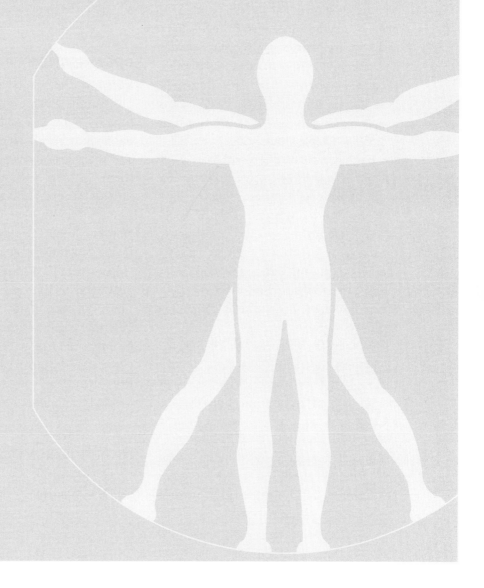

CHAPTER 9
Infectious Diseases

INTRODUCTION

The threat posed to human health by infectious diseases is still potent even towards the end of the first decade of the twenty-first century. The century dawned with the spectre of new dangers arising from bioterrorism in the wake of the attacks on New York City and Washington, DC on 11 September 2001 and the subsequent anthrax incidents involving government buildings in the United States.

In addition to this unanticipated and sinister challenge to public health systems, Nature has shown that she can continue to generate new and unexpected threats. Early in the twenty-first century, a coronavirus that had never previously caused illness in people produced an outbreak of a respiratory illness that was given the name SARS (severe acute respiratory syndrome). Transmission of SARS in China, Hong Kong, Canada and some other parts of the world had caused 8000 illnesses and 774 deaths by the time the outbreak subsided in the summer of 2004. The infection was not that easily transmissible, but it led to huge public concern across the world, major economic damage as stock markets in the Far East responded, and a great deal of soul-searching in the countries affected about the weaknesses in their public health systems.

The folly of the words of a US Surgeon General in the 1960s ('it is time to close the book on infectious diseases') is shown year in, year out as new infectious diseases emerge and old, established ones renew their assault on health and well-being. Chronic diseases have been the global rising tide of the twentieth and early twenty-first centuries, but infectious diseases remain the rocks on which human health frequently founders.

Combating infectious diseases depends upon high levels of vigilance, strong surveillance systems, good prevention (including vaccination where possible), robust control measures and excellent science and research.

This chapter outlines the services and methods involved in the prevention, investigation and control of infectious diseases and provides a detailed account of some of the main infectious disease problems encountered in the United Kingdom.

ORGANISATION OF SERVICES

Infectious diseases do not respect geographical or administrative boundaries, and efforts to prevent, control and treat them depend upon input from a variety of local, national and international bodies. Key amongst them are local authorities, the National Health Service, the Health Protection Agency, Health Protection Scotland, the National Public Health Service for Wales, DHSS Northern Ireland and the Central Government Department of Health. Other national agencies (e.g., the Health and Safety Executive, the Water Authorities and the Veterinary Laboratories Agency) also play an important role, as do international agencies such as the European Centre for Disease Prevention and Control (ECDC) and the World Health Organization.

LOCAL GOVERNMENT

Local authorities are empowered to take action to control notifiable diseases within their boundaries. They are required to appoint a proper officer for this function, who is usually a public health physician nominated from within the local health service to provide medical advice relating to communicable disease control. The person concerned is usually the consultant in communicable disease control (CCDC). Sometimes it is the director of public health or another consultant in public health who also has other duties within the primary care trust's department of public health. The local authority can appoint more than one proper officer and can define the limits of their responsibilities, so it does not follow that all proper officers of this function have the same powers. In Scotland, the designated medical officer to the local authority may be the health board's consultant in public health medicine (communicable diseases and environmental health) or the chief administrative medical officer, who is usually the director of public health. The role of public health doctors in the National Health Service is described more fully in Chapter 4.

The structure of local government varies, but the department concerned with communicable disease control is that containing environmental health services. Its function is usually led by a chief environmental health officer. Local authorities have a wide range of duties covering most aspects of environmental protection. The duties include the registration, inspection and investigation of food premises; involvement in the investigation of outbreaks of certain infectious diseases (mainly those which are food-borne); monitoring and dealing with other environmental hazards; and

responding to concerns and enquiries from the public about environmental food-quality matters. Legal powers of enforcement and prosecution with respect to the control of communicable diseases rest mainly with local authorities and their proper officer.

HEALTH SERVICES

In addition to the formal infectious disease control responsibilities, local health services and health boards have an important role in promoting health, preventing disease and securing care to meet the population's needs. Thus surveillance of infectious diseases, the identification of particular problems and the planning of preventive measures are key roles.

Health services also have responsibilities for the treatment and care of people with illnesses caused by infectious diseases and parasites. The general practitioner, with the support of the primary care team, is the person who treats the majority of cases in the community. Only serious cases or those with complications are admitted to hospital. The fall in the incidence of serious infectious diseases over the years has led to fewer hospital beds being required for treatment. Many general hospitals are able to provide only limited isolation facilities, but specialist advice and care is provided by specialist infectious disease physicians or physicians with a special interest in infectious diseases, as necessary.

Since 2004, all NHS bodies in England (including primary care trusts, acute hospital NHS trusts, mental health NHS trusts and ambulance NHS trusts) have been required to appoint a director of infection prevention and control (DIPC). Each major hospital or group of hospitals has a hospital infection prevention and control committee consisting of senior professional staff and reporting to the director. The committee meets at regular intervals and keeps problems in relation to infection in the hospital under review. The day-to-day work is carried out by an infection control team comprising an infection control doctor, usually a consultant medical microbiologist on the hospital staff, and infection control nurses, generally led by a nurse consultant. They are responsible for surveillance and feedback on the levels of infection (for example, in intensive care units and other high-risk areas, as well as general wards), and they deal with outbreaks when they occur and monitor compliance with infection prevention and control procedures and protocols. Reports from the committee and the director of infection prevention and control are standard agenda items for NHS trust board meetings.

THE HEALTH PROTECTION AGENCY

The Health Protection Agency (HPA) was created in 2003. It is an independent agency with the following main functions, some of which are UK-wide:

- to advise the United Kingdom government and devolved administrations on public health priorities, policies and programmes
- to deliver services and support the NHS and other agencies to protect people from infections, poisons and chemical and radiation hazards
- to respond to new threats to public health and provide a rapid response

- to provide important and authoritative information and advice to the public and professionals.

The Agency was created initially through the merger of four existing organisations – the Public Health Laboratory Service, the National Focus for Chemical Incidents, the National Radiological Protection Board and the Centre for Applied Microbiology and Research – with the addition of the consultants in communicable disease control and health protection units that were formerly part of the NHS public health provision in primary care trusts. Subsequently, a fifth element, the National Institute for Biological Standards and Control, was added.

The Health Protection Agency plays a major role in protecting the health and well-being of the population of England. It also provides some services to Wales, Northern Ireland and Scotland, though detailed additional arrangements for health protection are provided separately in these other United Kingdom countries.

The creation of the Health Protection Agency was an important development because for the first time it combined functions for the surveillance, prevention and control not just of infectious diseases but also of other public health threats (such as radiation and chemical hazards). It also carries out a range of scientific, laboratory and technical functions, such as the detection, identification and typing of micro-organisms; vaccine development; and assessment of radiation contamination.

The Health Protection Agency deploys public health experts in local and regional teams called health protection units. The teams work closely with primary care, and hospital NHS trusts, foundation trusts, strategic health authorities, regional directors of public health and local authorities.

During the first decade of the twenty-first century, the Health Protection Agency used its new capability successfully in responding to a number of public health emergencies, including the international outbreak of severe acute respiratory syndrome (SARS), the poisoning of a Russian with the radioactive substance polonium-210 and contingency planning for pandemic influenza. It also played a major role in developing the mandatory surveillance system for health care-associated infections in England in support of the government's programme to reduce these infections.

The Health Protection Agency and its senior staff and scientists are extensively networked across Europe, where they have had a prominent role in the establishment of the European Centre for Disease Prevention and Control, and across the rest of the world. The Agency plays a major role in developing international health protection plans and policies.

HEALTH PROTECTION SCOTLAND

The Health Protection Agency does not provide general health protection and infectious disease control services to Scotland, which has its own surveillance system and independent network of reference laboratories as part of Health Protection Scotland (HPS). A national surveillance centre (the Scottish Centre for Infection and Environmental Health) had existed since 1969 and was established following a public inquiry into a large outbreak of typhoid in Aberdeen in 1964. This has responsibility for the surveillance and control of communicable and non-communicable environmental hazards, and thus its remit is equivalent to that of the Health Protection Agency in England.

THE DEPARTMENT OF HEALTH

The Department of Health has overall responsibility in England for national policy matters in relation to infectious diseases, for example:

➤ ensuring that adequate and suitable hospital accommodation is available for infectious disease cases
➤ securing adequate infection prevention and control provision
➤ promoting adequate immunisation levels, not just at the time of outbreaks
➤ assuring microbiological laboratory support for public health from the NHS
➤ maintaining international communication networks on infectious diseases matters.

The chief medical officer for England is the United Kingdom government's principal adviser on infectious disease matters. The chief medical officers for the other United Kingdom countries advise their ministers directly (although in practice efforts are made to ensure that advice is consistent between them). This is particularly important with devolved parliaments and assemblies responsible for health service provision in three of the United Kingdom countries. In turn, the chief medical officer will seek advice from a wide range of sources, including experts within and outside the Department of Health and from the chief executive of the Health Protection Agency (and specialists on its staff).

It is important to remember that the chief medical officer advises government as a whole, not just the Department of Health. Hence other relevant departments, such as the Department for Environment, Food and Rural Affairs (DEFRA) or the Department for Children, Schools and Families (DCSF), may seek or receive advice from the chief medical officer.

THE FOOD STANDARDS AGENCY

The Food Standards Agency was established by an act of parliament in 1999, having been discussed widely as a concept following the bovine spongiform encephalopathy (BSE) epidemic. A proposal was set out by the leading academic in nutrition policy, Professor Philip James of the University of Aberdeen.

The Food Standards Agency is an independent government agency with its own non-executive chair and board. It seeks to protect the public interest and the consumer and to be free of the undue influence of the food or farming industry. The Food Standards Agency is responsible for the Meat Hygiene Service, which inspects and regulates slaughterhouses, meat-cutting plants and other facilities and premises.

The Food Standards Agency also has a major role in promoting healthy nutrition. It has major programmes, for example, in relation to reducing salt intake, enhancing cookery and catering skills, food labelling

and detailed consumer research.

The role of the Agency in preventing food-borne illness is described in a later section.

THE EUROPEAN CENTRE FOR DISEASE PREVENTION AND CONTROL

In May 2005, a new international body – The European Centre for Disease Prevention and Control (ECDC) – was established by the European Parliament to identify, assess and provide information about threats from infectious diseases. The Centre, based in Stockholm, Sweden, gives a formal annual assessment of current and emerging threats (Table 9.1). It works with European Union member states and other international bodies to encourage action to prevent and control a wide range of infectious diseases.

THE WORLD HEALTH ORGANIZATION

The World Health Organization, established in 1948, is a United Nations agency with its headquarters in Geneva, Switzerland. It is responsible for providing leadership in global health, setting norms and standards, providing technical support to countries and assessing trends in health and disease. Its remit is much wider than infectious diseases, but it does have a key role in surveillance, coordinating action and identifying new and current threats. It works closely with national governments and other international health bodies.

LEGISLATION

A range of legislation relates to the control

and spread of infectious diseases. Until recently, much of this was fragmented and related to the early part of the twentieth century and to the 1980s. In 2008, as part of a wide-ranging Health and Social Care Act, new and more flexible health protection powers were brought in. These included measures directed at spread of infections through international travel (*see also* the section later in this chapter on international health regulations), imposing restrictions on infected persons and various emergency procedures. Separate legislation, passed in 2006, relates to health care infection (*see* p. 512).

GENERAL PRINCIPLES OF COMMUNICABLE DISEASE CONTROL

When describing the spread of an infection and its control, three aspects should be considered. These are source, mode of transmission and susceptible recipient (Figure 9.1).

THE SOURCE

This is the person, animal, object or substance from which an infectious agent is transmitted to a host. Most communicable diseases in Britain are caused by either bacteria or viruses, and some of these pathogens have human beings as their sole host. There are numerous exceptions. The *Salmonella* group of organisms have reservoirs in many domestic and wild animals. Other examples are brucellosis in cattle and leptospirosis in rats and other species. Viruses multiply only in living cells, never in inanimate substances. Certain fungi may cause infection, but most,

such as candida (thrush), are mild and not life-threatening except in circumstances where immunity is impaired. Medical parasitology includes the study of pathogenic protozoa, worms and insects. The first two groups often have reservoirs in wild or domestic animals, sometimes with insect vectors and complex life cycles involving several hosts.

THE MODE OF TRANSMISSION

There are three main mechanisms through which infection can enter the body:

1 *Direct transmission* involves the direct transfer of micro-organisms to the skin or mucous membranes by touching, biting, kissing or sexual intercourse. Diseases that spread in this way include scabies (touching), rabies (biting), glandular fever (kissing) and syphilis or HIV infection (sexual intercourse). Some infections spread from pregnant mothers to their babies, for example, rubella and HIV infection.

2 *Indirect transmission* involves an intermediate stage between the source of infection and the individual. The infection may be vehicle-borne (for example, by infected food or water) or vector-borne (by animals or insects). Vehicle-borne infections include food poisoning, while malaria is vector-borne.

3 *Airborne transmission* involves inhaling aerosols containing micro-organisms. Smaller droplets can penetrate right down to the alveoli of the lungs and be retained there. The micro-organisms in the aerosols can remain suspended in the air for a long time. Legionnaires' disease is a good example of an infection

Table 9.1 Major infectious disease threats in the European Union

- Health care-associated infection
- HIV infection
- Pneumococcal infection
- Influenza
- Tuberculosis

Source: The European Centre for Disease Prevention and Control. *Annual Epidemiological Report on Communicable Diseases in Europe.* Stockholm: ECDC; 2007.

due to airborne transmission, and so is tuberculosis.

Measures directed at the route of transmission are key control measures for many communicable diseases. For example, typhoid and cholera may be controlled by the efficient disposal of sewage and the by supply of uncontaminated drinking water.

THE SUSCEPTIBLE RECIPIENT

Whether a person develops an infectious disease after contact with any given causal agent is governed by a number of factors, such as the virulence and dose of the organism; previous exposure to the organism or to an antigenic component, as in vaccination conferring immunity; the age of the individual (babies up to six months have natural immunity to some infections from their mothers); the nutritional state of the person; the presence of other diseases; and whether the individual is receiving immunosuppressive therapy.

INFECTIOUS DISEASE SURVEILLANCE

A strong system of surveillance of infectious

diseases is essential to their prevention and control, to the investigation of outbreaks, to tracking disease trends and spread of epidemics, to evaluating the impact of vaccination programmes and other control measures and to identifying new and emerging threats to the public health.

Surveillance is the systematic collection, collation and analysis of data with dissemination of the results to those who need to know so that appropriate control measures can be taken. A number of systems, both formal and informal, exist to enable information about communicable disease occurrences in the population to be gathered and analysed (Figure 9.2).

Notification of Infectious Disease

A legal duty rests on all registered medical practitioners who are attending people suspected of having certain specified infectious diseases (Table 9.2) to notify the names and addresses of these patients. It should be noted that the list of notifiable diseases in Scotland differs slightly from that for the rest of the United Kingdom.

Notification is supposed to take place on the basis of clinical suspicion. According to

Transmission route

Airborne
    e.g. viral exanthemata
        tonsillitis
        tuberculosis
        meningococcal disease

Ingestion – person to person; faecal-oral;
food/water borne
    e.g. salmonellosis
        Campylobacter
        E. coli 0157

Direct contact
    e.g. impetigo
        scabies
        anthrax

Sexual contact
    e.g. herpes genitalis
        gonorrhoea
        HIV

Injection
    – by insect
        e.g. malaria
    – by animal
        e.g. rabies
    – iatrogenic
        e.g. Hepatitis B, C

Congenital
    e.g. rubella
        syphillis

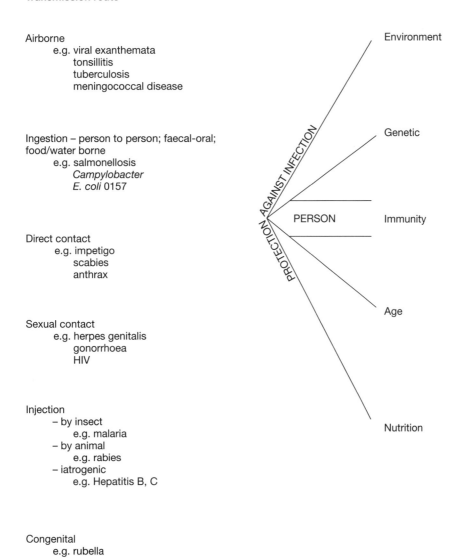

Figure 9.1 Major methods of transmission of infection

the legislation, a diagnosis does not have to be laboratory-confirmed for notification to take place. This makes sense when considered in the context in which the legislation was drawn up. The purpose of notification is to allow public health action to be taken within the incubation period of the disease in question, thus the system needs a sensitive trigger. Waiting a couple of days for a diagnosis to be laboratory-confirmed might

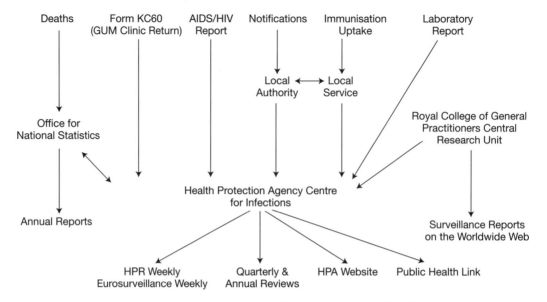

Figure 9.2 Flow of information about communicable diseases, England and Wales

Table 9.2 Notifiable diseases in England and Wales

Anthrax	Plague
Cholera	Acute poliomyelitis
Diphtheria	Acute encephalitis
Dysentery (amoebic or bacillary)	Relapsing fever
Rabies	Rubella
Food poisoning	Scarlet fever
Leprosy	Smallpox
Leptospirosis	Tetanus
Malaria	Tuberculosis (all forms)
Measles	Typhoid fever
Mumps	Typhus
Meningitis	Viral haemorrhagic fevers (including dengue fever, Ebola virus and Lassa fever)
Meningococcal septicaemia (without meningitis)	Viral hepatitis
Ophthalmia neonatorum	Whooping cough
Paratyphoid fever	Yellow fever

This list is under review as part of the regulations for the implementation of the Health and Social Services Act 2008.

mean that secondary spread has already taken place. The notification system should, therefore, be a sensitive, although not a specific, indicator of communicable disease in a community.

Notifications in England and Wales are made to the proper officers of the local authorities. The proper officers submit this information (not names and addresses, only anonymised aggregated data) to the Health Protection Agency Centre for Infections, which collates the information on behalf of the Office for National Statistics. In addition to the weekly returns, the proper officers submit returns at quarterly intervals, which enable corrections to be made to the data gathered weekly. The Health Protection Agency publishes weekly, quarterly and annual reports of notifications of infectious diseases in England and Wales.

In Scotland and Northern Ireland, notifications are sent to the chief administrative medical officer (CAMO) of the appropriate health board. Notification data in Scotland are collated by the Information and Statistics Division (ISD) of the NHS National Service Scotland and published in a weekly report produced by Health Protection Scotland.

Unfortunately, the effectiveness of the notification system is variable because there is a serious degree of under-notification of these statutorily notifiable diseases by medical practitioners. Part of the reason for this may be the fact that many doctors perceive notification simply as a means of gathering statistics and not as a tool for public health action. This is compounded by the fact that the list of notifiable diseases contains conditions that rarely occur in Britain but which appear by international agreement.

Nevertheless, notifications remain a key source of information about the incidence of certain communicable diseases in the population.

Laboratory Reports

The other major source of epidemiological information is reports of positive laboratory isolates. In England, laboratories report a range of microbiological results to the Health Protection Agency Centre for Infections and to local and regional health protection units. The collated laboratory reports are published weekly by the Health Protection Agency in the *Health Protection Report*, which is the national electronic public health bulletin for England and Wales. Laboratories providing these reports include the Health Protection Agency regional microbiology laboratories, NHS trust departments of microbiology and virology, and a small number of private laboratories. In addition, there are specialist reference laboratories that undertake detailed typing, molecular analysis, virulence investigation and detection of toxins in relation to particular organisms or sources of infection. Similar arrangements apply in the other United Kingdom countries.

Routine laboratory reporting is not a statutory requirement, but rather a voluntary system. It complements the notification system by providing specific data about the occurrence of a wider range of infectious organisms in a community. However, the Health and Social Care Act 2008 requires laboratories to notify positive results on those infections in the list of notifiable diseases (or other highly pathogenic infections) to complement the notification by the medical practitioner responsible for the patient. This enables the specific microbiological diagnosis (including typing information) to be ascertained.

Sentinel Surveillance in Primary Care

In England and Wales a sentinel scheme for reporting disease in general practice, under the auspices of the Royal College of General Practitioners (RCGP), includes some infectious diseases. Returns from a number of selected spotter practices are made on a weekly basis to the Royal College of General Practitioners Research Unit. The sentinel practice scheme involves some 60 general practices covering a population of approximately 425 000 people. In Scotland there is a much larger system involving 124 general practices collecting information about almost 700 000 patients. In addition, there are various 'tailor-made' enhanced surveillance schemes at both local and national level that aim to link clinical and laboratory data to provide analysis of risk groups, trends and outcomes.

Other Sources of Surveillance Data

Other sources of surveillance data include the special confidential reporting system for HIV infection and AIDS. In addition, genitourinary medicine clinics make returns to the Health Protection Agency Centre for Infections on a quarterly and annual basis about the incidence of sexually transmitted infections.

Data on vaccination coverage are collected by a local immunisation coordinator.

In England and Wales these data are collated centrally and published by the Health Protection Agency Centre for Infections. In Scotland there are similar arrangements. The system is referred to as COVER (Coverage of Vaccination Evaluated Rapidly).

The Royal College of Paediatrics and Child Health houses the British Paediatric Surveillance Unit, which carries out a small number of time-limited surveillance projects, some of which might include infectious disease topics, e.g., the United Kingdom and Republic of Ireland survey of haemolytic uraemic syndrome in children.

In addition to these usual routes, information can be gleaned about previously unsuspected cases of infectious diseases from death notifications, from reports of sickness absence (e.g., during an influenza outbreak) or from hospital episode statistics. Informal communications between the local public health doctors or other professionals are of paramount importance. A telephone call from a general practitioner, a practice nurse, a microbiologist, an environmental health officer, an official in one of the water companies or a school nurse can yield rapid information. In an attempt to speed up the passage of information, many health organisations are linked directly with their reporting laboratories by means of an electronic network.

The Health Protection Agency Centre for Infections is also linked electronically to most NHS laboratories for automated reporting of laboratory results.

European Surveillance Schemes

A number of European networks for the

surveillance of infectious disease have been funded by the European Commission, including Enter-net (for the surveillance of salmonellosis and *E. coli* O157) and the European Working Group on Legionella Infections (EWGLI).

Feeding Back Surveillance Data

At local level, regular bulletins are distributed from health protection units to local general practitioners, laboratories and environmental health departments. Regular surveillance bulletins are also produced at regional and national level. Information is fed back by means of an electronic weekly report containing, amongst other things, the notification data and details of isolates derived from hospital laboratories, the Health Protection Agency regional laboratories and their Welsh equivalents. In addition to the weekly report, quarterly and annual reviews are also produced for various infections. Surveillance data are also posted on the Health Protection Agency website. In Scotland a weekly report is produced by Health Protection Scotland.

INVESTIGATION OF COMMUNICABLE DISEASE OCCURRENCES

The accounts of individual communicable diseases given later in this chapter illustrate the importance of thoroughly investigating people with symptoms suggestive of an infectious cause. In this way, the organism responsible can be identified (wherever possible), the most effective treatment can be instituted and other potential cases or contacts can be traced (if appropriate for

disease control). The rapid identification of organisms that cause illness is also essential for good surveillance of communicable diseases in the population to enable control measures to be instituted.

The key to successful communicable disease control in the population is prevention. However, when cases occur, either singly, in small or in large numbers, everything possible should be learned from such occurrences. In this way, control measures can sometimes be strengthened so that new incidents or outbreaks can be ended rapidly, thus minimising the numbers of people affected.

While the circumstances of communicable disease occurrences will differ in practice, a number of general principles apply when approaching an investigation. The most common reason for starting an investigation is because of an outbreak. Whatever the circumstances, the aims must be to act quickly, to establish clear operational principles and to perform a sound investigation.

How Problems Come to Light

The way in which occurrences of communicable diseases prompt investigation varies. With good surveillance systems, a sudden upsurge in the incidence of a particular disease, clustering of several cases in a certain geographical area or the occurrence of one or two cases of a very rare disease or unusual strain type will be rapidly detected and could be the starting point for an investigation.

Some incidents will come to light in other ways. For example, a call for help may be received from a hotel after a large number of guests have developed vomiting and diarrhoea. Similarly, enquiries from the media may be made to a health organisation's press office after people in a locality have reported being ill. Outbreaks reported from abroad might have implications for United Kingdom citizens. A publication by a research team may draw attention to the unusually high incidence of a particular disease or a previously unrecognised causation.

Steps in an Investigation

Broadly, investigation of an outbreak involves three tasks. These are to describe the incident, analyse the data and give public health advice. The objectives of an investigation include:

➤ to identify the source and mode of transmission
➤ to put in place control measures which will interrupt the chain of transmission
➤ to prevent secondary spread
➤ to provide advice that will prevent a further outbreak occurring under similar circumstances.

It should be borne in mind that the outcome of any outbreak investigation might result in a perpetrator being prosecuted. While this is rarely a primary objective of an outbreak investigation, it might be a consequence of it. This means that notes need to be kept assiduously, meetings including decisions need to be formally recorded and evidence needs to be gathered correctly. The decision to prosecute rests with the enforcing authority – usually the local authority environmental

health department (or equivalent) – and not with health officials.

Information needs to be collected that *describes the outbreak* (i.e., the nature and timing of the illness, where people acquired the disease and the characteristics of the affected people). This descriptive information often yields clues to the source of an infection and its means of spread, thereby allowing early intervention. When the source is not readily apparent, a more detailed analytical approach needs to be undertaken. This will often involve comparing the exposures of people who became ill with those who did not. A variety of statistical techniques are used in such analyses. The results help to draw out inferences concerning transmission and exposure to disease.

The logical sequence of action in investigating an outbreak or epidemic is outlined in Figure 9.3.

The first requirement is to *confirm the existence of an epidemic or outbreak* and to *verify the diagnosis*. This involves the collection of as much information as possible about the disease and its characteristics. Information also needs to be assembled about the expected level of such an infection under normal circumstances and about the population that is primarily affected. This preliminary exercise will help to determine the extent of any subsequent investigation and the urgency with which it is carried out.

It is important to involve microbiological experts at a very early stage. A microbiologist can ensure that the most appropriate arrangements are made for the collection and rapid processing of clinical and environmental specimens. Environmental health

1. Confirm the existence of an epidemic or outbreak

2. Verify the diagnosis

3. Identify and count cases or exposure – create a case definition

4. Tabulate and orient data for time, place and person

5. Formulate hypotheses

6. Test hypotheses

7. Plan additional studies if necessary

8. Evaluate control measures by continued surveillance

9. Communicate findings – write report, publication

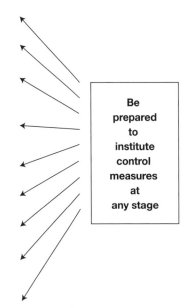

Be prepared to institute control measures at any stage

Figure 9.3 Steps in a communicable disease investigation
Source: Adapted from Goodman RA, Buehler JW, Koplan JP. The epidemiologic field investigation: science and judgement in public health practice. *Am J Epidemiol.* 1990; **132**: 9–16.

officers of local authorities play a key part in the investigation process, particularly of food-borne outbreaks. Their areas of expertise include inspection of premises; knowledge about food hygiene and food preparation; collection of environmental and food samples for microbiological testing; and education (of food handlers, for example). The environmental health officer will also be able to judge the relevance and quality of any risk assessment systems (Hazard Analysis Critical Control Point (HACCP), for example) and the adequacy of record keeping as well as examining policies on, for example, pest control. Environmental health officers are also empowered to interview people under caution, i.e., to collect evidence that might be used later in court if a prosecution ensues.

The next step requires the *identification of the number of people affected and what they have been exposed to*. In order to do this, a working case definition must be created. A case definition will usually contain personal (clinical and/or demographic), temporal and geographical characteristics. When an outbreak presents, the investigators might have a shrewd idea about the causative organism from a combination of the event that took place and the average incubation period. When constructing the case definition, the incubation period range should be used in order to take account of what might appear to be unusually swift or late presentations.

It is surprising how often constructing a case definition is overlooked, but without it highly misleading conclusions can be drawn from an investigation. For example, in an outbreak of food-borne illness in which people have presented with symptoms of vomiting, are people who report feelings of nausea to be counted as cases or not? In outbreaks of illnesses with ill-defined symptoms, several case definitions may be used to test an association between illness and exposure, but great care must be taken to ensure that whichever case definition is used it is rigorously adhered to.

Case-finding methods will vary according to the severity or importance of the suspected disease and the setting in which the outbreak or epidemic has occurred. In a hospital outbreak, there is likely to be a clearly identifiable risk group. However, in a community outbreak this is likely to be far more complex because people are widely dispersed. Cases are usually found either by locating other people who were exposed to the probable risk factor (for example, people on an affected aeroplane flight) or by contacting local doctors or hospitals. For diseases that do not have a clear presentation (for example, atypical pneumonia), extensive checking of possible cases, which may be recorded under a different diagnosis, on a local surveillance system or in clinical notes will need to be undertaken. This ensures that case ascertainment is as comprehensive as possible.

Once data have been collected, they are arranged by time, place and person in the same *descriptive* epidemiological terms that are described in Chapter 2. When graphs of the occurrence of cases over time (an *epidemic curve*) are plotted, it is frequently possible to distinguish different types of epidemic such as a *common or point source*

(Figure 9.4) and a *propagated source* or person-to-person transmission (Figure 9.5). In the former, there is a rapid upsurge to a peak and then a rapid fall-off. With the latter, the curve is much less steep and the period over which people develop symptoms is much longer, either because people continue to be exposed to the infected source or because secondary cases occur.

Plotting data geographically can often provide a clue to the source of an infectious agent or the nature of exposure. This has proved particularly useful in determining the source of *Legionella pneumophila* in outbreaks of Legionnaires' disease. Arranging data by patient characteristics such as age, sex or occupation may point to a particular risk group or mode of spread.

By this time, the investigators may have a very good idea about the organism responsible and its source and mode of spread. It is still necessary, however, to determine the most likely exposure that caused disease. It is at this stage that hypotheses are formulated, and those concerning causation are then tested by using appropriate *analytical epidemiological techniques*.

Care is required in choosing appropriate controls if either a *case-control* or a *cohort study* is undertaken. This reduces the risk of inadvertent biases. A discussion of the use of controls in studies of chronic diseases is in Chapter 2.

The precise method of gathering information from cases and controls will again depend upon the incident being investigated. With a group of tourists who are leaving shortly for their next travel destination, the chosen method may be a simple listing of case details along one side of a grid and exposures down the other side. Where there is less urgency, the chosen method may be administration of a detailed, carefully constructed questionnaire. Whichever method is chosen, it is important that the interviewers ask questions in the same way so that one group of people is not prompted to remember more details than others, thus

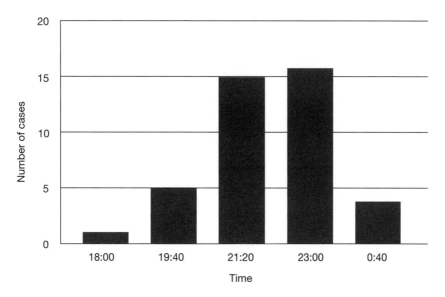

Figure 9.4 Point source of outbreak

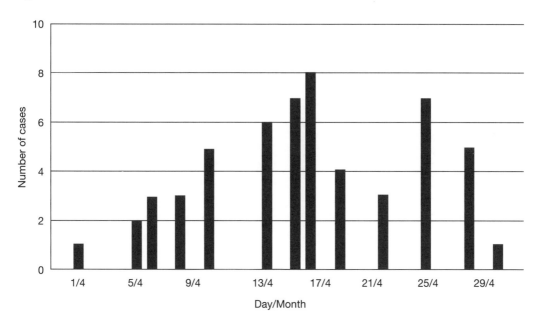

Figure 9.5 Propagated source outbreak where person-to-person transmission occurs

introducing an element of bias.

When investigating outbreaks of food-borne illness, it is usual to compare exposure to different foodstuffs in those who developed illness and those who did not. This is illustrated in the following example of an outbreak of food-borne illness amongst hotels guests in Brighton. The results of the investigation are shown in Table 9.3.

An outbreak of gastrointestinal symptoms occurred amongst a party of 136 elderly people who stayed in a hotel over the six-day Christmas period. Sixty-eight people were ill. The authorities were notified about the outbreak after the guests had left.

A guest list was obtained. The guests were contacted and a standard questionnaire was administered to them asking them about foods eaten and about symptoms. Stool samples were obtained from the 68 guests who had symptoms and from the nine food-handlers on duty over the Christmas period. The hotel kitchen was inspected and information was obtained about food-handling practices, food supplies and cooking methods. Samples of food were taken, but little remained from batches used over the period concerned.

Analysis of the food items revealed three that showed an independent, statistically significant association with the illness: chocolate mousse, lemon mousse and creme caramel (Table 9.3). All had been made with fresh eggs. The preparation of the mousse involved the heating of raw egg yolks over a low heat for two minutes. The creme caramel was baked in the oven for half an hour. *Salmonella enteritidis* was isolated from the stools of 29 of the 68 cases. A high proportion of these were submitted to phage typing and found to be phage type 4. Stool samples from food handlers were negative. No organisms were grown from the food samples that were taken. Kitchen practices were found to be good.

The investigators concluded that it was probable that the organism responsible for the outbreak was introduced into the kitchen via the eggs in the dishes containing raw eggs.

The report described is a good example of a practical investigation of a communicable disease outbreak. It should be noted that controls were members of the same hotel party. Some investigations would require controls to be chosen from other sources.

Investigations establish associations; deciding whether the association is causal or otherwise is a separate process. The same rules of attributing causality apply in communicable disease investigation as in chronic disease investigation (*see* Chapter 2).

In outbreak investigation generally, having identified the probable source, it is important to revisit the facts and ask the following question: does the hypothesis fit with the natural history of the disease in question? The clinical, laboratory and epidemiological results together with those of any environmental investigations should provide a logical, biologically plausible

Table 9.3 An investigation of an outbreak of *Salmonella enteritidis* associated with the consumption of egg dishes

Food	Cases		Controls	
	Ate	*Did not eat*	*Ate*	*Did not eat*
Chocolate mousse	66	2	21	14
Lemon mousse	60	4	25	12
Creme caramel	55	9	24	13

Note: People who were unsure of what they ate are excluded from this analysis.
Source: Franks CR, Harding BH, Jeffrey PA, *et al. Communicable Disease Report.* 1990; **47**(3). (Internal publication of the Public Health Laboratory Service.)

explanation of the events that have taken place.

At this stage, the investigation may be complete or the decision may be taken to conduct additional systematic studies. In any event, communicating the findings of an outbreak investigation is extremely important, and the final report should contain details of the investigation, the findings and any recommendations.

Once control measures have been implemented, continuing surveillance must be put in place to monitor their effects. If the surveillance data suggest that the outbreak is continuing despite the control measures implemented, the facts must be revisited and some, or all, of the steps described above must be repeated.

Instigating Control Measures

The question of when to instigate control measures during a communicable disease investigation can be very difficult. However, it is important both to investigate quickly using sound methodologies and to have the best possible information available when taking such decisions. When in doubt, the

balance should always lie with protection of the public.

Organisation and Management of an Investigation

All investigations involve teamwork, so coordinating the various team members is an integral part of the investigation. The exact composition of a team will depend upon the disease under investigation, although core members will include the local consultant in communicable disease control (or equivalent), who is likely to lead the team, a microbiologist and an environmental health officer. All local health services have plans for dealing with outbreaks of communicable disease in the community. Similar plans exist in NHS trusts for coping with an outbreak of hospital-acquired infection. These plans include:

➢ a description of the roles and responsibilities of the organisations and individuals concerned

➢ arrangements for liaising with others outside the local health service, including the Department of Health, the strategic health authority, reference laboratories, the Health Protection Agency or equivalent (in the other United Kingdom countries), the NHS headquarters and neighbouring authorities

➤ the circumstances under which the outbreak control team (OCT) will be convened

➤ the facilities required for an incident room

➤ the arrangements in place for convening a group out of hours.

A plan will contain details of suggested membership of an outbreak control team, although allowing it to be tailored to individual situations, and will describe the terms of reference of the team. Many plans also contain a model agenda.

Good communication, both within the outbreak control team and between the team and others, is vitally important. Investigations flounder when communication is poor, and this may have a detrimental impact on public confidence. An important point to bear in mind, particularly when dealing with a larger outbreak, is the relationship with the media. Possibly because of a fear of sensationalism by the local press, radio and television, many health professionals are apprehensive about having contact with the media. A single spokesperson who is acceptable to both health and local authorities should be appointed, and he or she should be available to the media at appointed times only. If either organisation has a press officer, he or she might be the right person to act as a spokesperson, although members of the press often prefer to discuss such matters with someone who is medically qualified. In any case, it is essential that factual information is reported in an unbiased way. Reporters are quick to realise when relevant information is being withheld. They will not expect personal details about patients to be divulged. Experience shows that a more accurate report is much more likely to result when the fullest possible information is released to the media. It is wrong to regard the media as a nuisance. Indeed, if good relations are established, particularly with local press, radio and television, this contact can be a great asset, helping, for example, to trace contacts or give health education advice.

Time is of the essence when investigating an outbreak or epidemic. The longer it takes to mount an investigation, the slimmer the chances of success. People's memories fade. The greater the time between the incident and the investigation, the lower the chances of confirming a diagnosis microbiologically. Depending on the infecting agent and the existence of a serological test, vital environmental evidence might have been lost or destroyed.

Finally, outbreak investigations always provide the opportunity to learn for all concerned.

INTERNATIONAL HEALTH REGULATIONS

In the summer of 2007, a new set of International Health Regulations agreed by the World Health Assembly (the governing body of the World Health Organization) came into effect. They had not been reviewed since 1969. The earlier Regulations had applied mainly to three infectious diseases – cholera, plague and yellow fever. The current International Health Regulations are much broader and require member states of the World Health Organization to report 'any public health emergency of international concern', whether this is biological, nuclear or chemical, irrespective of origin or source. The new Regulations strengthen the ability to reduce global health risks and prevent national outbreaks or incidents spreading internationally. In England, they are incorporated into the Health and Social Care Act 2008 (described earlier).

Each country has to designate a focal point to be accessible 24 hours a day and to notify the World Health Organization if any two of the following four criteria for assessment and notification are fulfilled:

➤ Is the public health impact of the event serious?
➤ Is the event unusual or unexpected?
➤ Is there a significant risk of international spread?
➤ Is there a significant risk of restrictions on international travel or trade?

NEW AND EMERGING DISEASES

The category of infectious diseases that continues to attract most interest internationally is new and emerging diseases. This is a very broad range of diseases that covers infections that have never previously been seen or documented and problems that, having once been controlled, are showing a resurgence. The reason that such infections cause concern is because a new threat to human health requires a new response to combat it. Before the threat can be mitigated, it often

takes time to understand the nature of the infectious agent and the way that it behaves. Also, the return of a disease previously well-controlled suggests a breakdown in public health measures and is an equally important reason for concern.

Viewed over a decade or more, the number of new and emerging disease outbreaks is surprisingly large (Figure 9.6). Many are contained in the part of the world in which they originate and do not pose any immediate threat to a wider population. Sadly, outbreaks in remote parts of the developing world attract little coverage by Western media, so the general public knows little of them. From time to time, however, a new infection poses a threat to the population of a major developed country or even becomes a worldwide threat. Then the 'fear factor' is very prominent and the media coverage is extensive, sometimes disproportionate to the true nature and scale of the threat.

Some of the key considerations when dealing with a new or emerging infectious disease are the laboratory identification and characterisation of the infectious agent, establishing its mode of transmission and the groups within the population most at risk, setting up a system of surveillance to track the disease's progress, formulating the criteria for making a clinical diagnosis and working out what treatments are likely to be effective and what public health measures will control its spread or eradicate it.

There are no hard and fast rules for deciding when to stop classifying an infectious disease as 'new'. When the human immunodeficiency virus (HIV) emerged in the early 1980s, causing AIDS, it was to all intents and purposes a new infection. Nearly

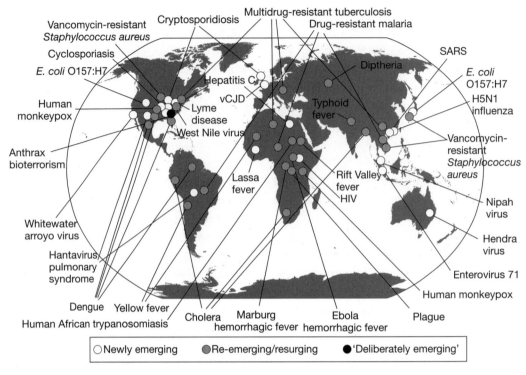

Figure 9.6 Global examples of emerging and re-emerging infectious diseases
Source: Dr Jeremy Farrar, personal communication.

three decades on, it is still 'emerging' in some parts of the world and at a global level remains one of the twenty-first century's greatest threats to health, societal cohesion and economic prosperity.

Bearing in mind that experts will differ on the diseases that should be covered in a list of new and emerging infections, in this section the ones that are commonly discussed in the United Kingdom or reflect the general principles of this category are described.

HUMAN IMMUNODEFICIENCY VIRUS (HIV)

An estimated 60 million people worldwide

have been infected with the human immunodeficiency virus (HIV) and 25 million have died of acquired immune deficiency syndrome (AIDS) since it emerged as an apparently new disease in the 1980s.

In the United States during 1981, increasing numbers of cases of opportunistic infection (particularly *Pneumocystis carinii* pneumonia) and unusual tumours (for example, Kaposi's sarcoma) were reported in previously healthy men who have sex with men or bisexual men. The presenting clinical features are often general: weight loss, fever, malaise and lymphadenopathy. The fully developed AIDS syndrome involves opportunistic infections or patterns of malignancy infrequently seen in people with normal immune systems, although any one of a wide range of infections or malignancies can occur.

HIV belongs to the retrovirus group, and by infecting a subset of the T-lymphocyte population (so-called CD4 cells) it gradually destroys the normal immune response mechanism. The first virus to be discovered was type 1 (HIV-1), and in the late 1980s a second variant, HIV-2, was isolated in West Africa. HIV-2 is uncommon outside this part of Africa.

People who are HIV positive can remain asymptomatic for long periods of time. The precise proportion of such people who will eventually develop AIDS is not fully established.

The Global Position

The disease is rampant in many parts of the world, with an estimated 33 million people living with HIV/AIDS in 2007. The worst affected area is sub-Saharan Africa, which accounted for three quarters of the world's AIDS deaths in 2007 (Table 9.4).

Over the last 10 years, the rate of new infections has fallen in some parts of the world but has increased in others (for example, Russia and Indonesia). Globally, the number of AIDS deaths has declined, partly as a result of better access to therapy. In sub-Saharan Africa, the predominant means of spread is heterosexual intercourse. Elsewhere in the world, injecting drug users, men who have sex with men and sex workers are the major risk groups.

The twin challenges of HIV prevention and improving access to treatment are formidable given the scale of the problem worldwide. In parts of the world, there are profound cultural barriers – fear, superstition, stigma and denial – which seriously restrict the scope for preventive action. It is vital to address these. Strong, enlightened commitment from the most senior levels of government as well as from local community and civic leaders is the key to successful action. Basic health education programmes are important for modifying people's (especially young people's) attitudes and behaviour towards issues such as condom use and avoiding multiple partners. A particularly difficult problem is communicating with and influencing the harder-to-reach groups – injecting drug users and sex workers.

The evidence base for the effectiveness of different preventive strategies has expanded

Table 9.4 HIV and AIDS: key facts

- An estimated 33 million people are living with HIV worldwide.
- 67% of all people living with HIV are in sub-Saharan Africa.
- 15–24-year-olds make up 45% of new infections worldwide and two million under 15 years are living with HIV.
- Heterosexual intercourse is the main risk factor in sub-Saharan Africa, while men who have sex with men, sex workers and injecting drug users are the main risk groups elsewhere in the world.
- The epidemic is slowing in some parts of the world but increasing in others.

Source: UNAIDS.

in the last decade. For example, male (and to some extent female) condoms are very effective. More recently, male circumcision has been shown to reduce transmission. There are many good examples around the world of successful local programmes based on health education and community engagement.

Good prevention, like successful treatment programmes, cannot be easily delivered without a strong health system in the country concerned. This is a problem in many of the worst-affected parts of the world; a great deal of resources have been invested in strengthening health care systems in the developing world, but there is still a long way to go.

The emergence of antiretroviral drugs has revolutionised the treatment of HIV infection and AIDS. In developed countries, they have prolonged survival for those infected by a decade or more so that HIV has in effect become a chronic disease. Treatment is not always effective, can produce side effects and needs careful monitoring.

In the developing world, the challenges are funding the drugs required, distributing them effectively and then achieving long-term compliance with therapy. Stories of successful treatment in sub-Saharan Africa are truly inspiring, as people have been rescued from 'death's door'. However, the challenge is to reach the larger proportion who have no access to life-saving therapy (Figure 9.7).

A number of international organisations are important in combatting the HIV pandemic.

➤ UNAIDS started work in 1996 as a pooling of functions amongst a variety of United Nations agencies. It sets policies and priorities and implements action plans.

➤ The World Health Organization, as part of its wide range of functions, assesses progress in the fight against HIV and AIDS, sets standards and coordinates action within its regions and member states.

➤ The Global Fund to Fight AIDS, Tuberculosis and Malaria was created as a vehicle to attract, manage and distribute funds to fight the three diseases of its name. It works closely

Table 9.5 Preventive strategies for HIV worldwide

• Strong governmental leadership and active local communities
• Positive culture: reducing stigma, fear and denial
• Widespread male and female condom use
• Reducing numbers of sexual partners
• Male circumcision
• Better control of sexually transmitted diseases
• Greater access to HIV testing and counselling (including in pregnancy)
• Strengthened health care systems

Source: Partly derived from UNAIDS documents.

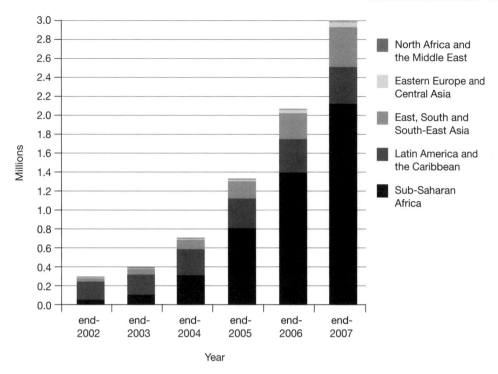

Figure 9.7 Number of people receiving antiretroviral drugs in low- and middle-income countries, 2002–07
Source: Data provided by UNAIDS and WHO, 2008.

with other multilateral and bilateral international organisations, individual countries and other donors.

Other bodies, such as the World Bank, are important and so too are the international development departments within governments (for example, DFID in the United Kingdom) and non-governmental organisations (for example, the Bill and Melinda Gates Foundation).

The United Kingdom Position

The United Kingdom government ran a major public education campaign between 1986 and 1987, relatively early in the occur-

rence of the epidemic. The campaign made heavy use of mass media: television, radio, cinema and posters. A leaflet was delivered to every household in the country giving information about HIV infection and AIDS. A telephone line, the National AIDS Helpline, was also established.

The *'AIDS: Don't Die of Ignorance'* campaign was judged to be remarkably successful, and many consider it, along with the early introduction of needle exchange schemes for injecting drug users, as responsible for helping to keep the prevalence of HIV infection in the United Kingdom relatively low: approximately 0.2% of the population is affected.

However, the position is far from reassuring, as can be seen from the following:

➤ the number of people with HIV infection was estimated at 73 000 in 2006, and almost a third (31%) were undiagnosed

➤ almost half the new diagnoses of HIV in 2006 were in Black Africans – a five-fold increase in a decade

➤ a high proportion of people leave a genitourinary medicine clinic (a high-risk group) being unaware of their HIV infection.

The group most at risk of acquiring HIV infection in the United Kingdom is still men who have sex with men, but heterosexuals with HIV as a whole now exceed them (Figure 9.8). Particularly prominent is the risk group of heterosexual people born in sub-Saharan Africa, most of whom have probably acquired infection there. HIV diagnoses in intravenous drug users have remained low and relatively stable in recent years, while a small number of cases occur amongst children by vertical (from an infected mother) transmission and in past recipients of blood transfusion.

Too many HIV infections in the United Kingdom are diagnosed late, and in these circumstances therapy is less successful and death more common. In the early

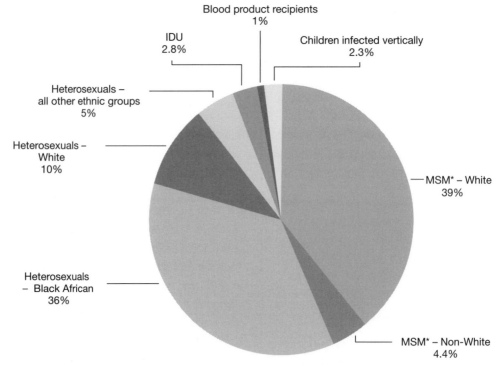

Figure 9.8 HIV-infected persons accessing care by prevention group, United Kingdom, 2006
Source: Health Protection Agency.

1990s, most people who were diagnosed as HIV positive lived (or received services) in London. By the late 2000s, 50% were receiving their care outside London. Overall, half of the HIV positive men who had sex with men had been infected for more than six years before they were diagnosed. Amongst Black African heterosexuals, the figure was 70%.

Early diagnosis of HIV infection is crucial because it reduces the risk of transmission to others and because it allows the infected individual to start treatment early, giving them a much better prognosis. Failure to provide HIV testing to someone who attends a genitourinary medicine clinic with another sexually transmitted disease is a major lost opportunity for HIV control.

The network of genitourinary medicine clinics is a key element of HIV services, and ensuring that there is open access and very short waiting times is important. Unless resources are invested in this area, the risks of an explosive increase in HIV infection in this country is ever present.

One of the problems for public education programmes for HIV infection in a country like Britain is that a number of target groups are being addressed simultaneously. Thus, the health education initiative must continue to target the sexual behaviour of men who have sex with men. The emphasis must not lead the heterosexual population to believe that HIV infection is not a risk for them. Campaigns and programmes must be appropriately targeted for gay/bisexual men, intravenous drug abusers, sex workers and travellers to high-risk areas of the world.

Public education, while a vital element

of programmes to prevent and control HIV infection in the population, is only one part of a comprehensive range of measures that have been adopted. For example, well-organised needle-exchange schemes are particularly important in reducing risk amongst intravenous drug abusers. Free, open-access genitourinary clinics provide the main entry point for most HIV patients. Other key elements of the overall programme include training of staff in the care of infected people and in the risks of transmission during the process of patient care.

Surveillance

Information on the prevalence of HIV infection and AIDS in Britain is reported on a voluntary and confidential basis by clinicians and laboratories to the Health Protection Agency in England and Wales and its counterpart in Scotland. Other information on the prevalence of HIV infection includes data from unlinked anonymous surveys that use blood left over after completion of diagnostic testing. These surveys provide essential public health information about the prevalence of HIV in high-risk groups (genitourinary medicine clinic attendees and injecting drug users) and in the general population (pregnant women).

SEVERE ACUTE RESPIRATORY SYNDROME (SARS)

In March 2003, the World Health Organization alerted the world to a new disease. The disease did not have a name and was given one based on the symptoms it produced – a severe respiratory illness with atypical pneumonia. The infectious agent could not be identified initially.

The SARS Story

The first case of severe acute respiratory syndrome (SARS) occurred in the Guangdong Province of China in November of 2002. Other cases occurred in China through the autumn of 2002 and into the first two months of 2003. In this early phase, a number of key events occurred. Firstly, a SARS victim hospitalised in Guangzhou, China, transmitted the virus to 50 hospital staff and 19 relatives. Secondly, a serious outbreak occurred in Hong Kong, signifying the beginning of international spread.

A medical professor from Guangzhou with respiratory symptoms travelled in mid-February 2003 to attend a wedding at the Metropole Hotel, Hong Kong. He stayed only one night, but at least 16 other guests and one visitor were infected as a result. The professor was admitted to hospital and died 10 days later.

Another man who became infected at the Metropole Hotel was admitted to hospital but recovered. The importance of his condition was not recognised, and as a result he infected 143 people, including health care workers. Meanwhile a woman who had stayed at the Metropole Hotel had travelled back to her home in Toronto, Ontario. She passed the infection to four members of her family. This was to be responsible for a large outbreak in Canada.

During March of 2003, outbreaks occurred in Singapore, Vietnam and Taiwan. Cases continued to occur in these and other countries, as well as in China, through April of 2003.

There were further high-profile outbreaks. A housing complex in Hong Kong – Amoy Gardens – was the focus of one. A man from the Guangdong Province of China who visited Hong Kong twice a week for kidney dialysis stayed with his brother in an Amoy Gardens apartment. He was infected with SARS, and an outbreak affected 329 residents of the housing complex, 42 of whom died.

In the Toronto area of Canada, more than 250 people fell ill, 44 died and 10 000 people were put in quarantine. A particularly serious aspect of the outbreak was in-hospital transmission: 100 staff at the Scarborough Hospital, Ontario, caught SARS.

In total, there were more than 8000 cases of SARS worldwide, with 774 deaths and reports of the disease in 29 countries and areas before the disease was stopped from spreading.

Lessons learned from the SARS experience

The SARS epidemic caused massive upheaval, not just economically and socially but also in the scrutiny that it brought to bear on international public health systems. Within countries and areas such as Canada and Hong Kong, there were major independent reviews of the public health infrastructure, policies, governance and accountability arrangements for the prevention, investigation and control of infectious diseases. Across countries, attention focused on the gathering and exchange of surveillance and laboratory data so that the world could have early warning of such outbreaks in the future. Efforts have been made subsequently to remove barriers to reporting of data (especially a tendency in some countries toward inappropriate secrecy) and to strengthen laboratory links between countries.

The exact source of the SARS virus, a coronavirus, has not been proven, but could be yet another example of transmission from animals to people. The use of a wild, exotic animal (the civet cat) for food is a strong possibility, and in turn this animal may have acquired the virus from a bat (as its natural reservoir).

The SARS story is a modern classic of an apparently new disease emerging suddenly and unexpectedly. Important lessons that must be applied in the future have been learned from the SARS experience (Table 9.6).

TRANSMISSIBLE SPONGIFORM ENCEPHALOPATHIES (TSEs)

Creutzfeldt-Jakob disease (CJD) was first described in the 1920s. It is one of a group of fatal diseases that are characterised by spongy degeneration of the brain. As a group, they are called transmissible spongiform encephalopathies (TSEs), and they can occur in both people and animals.

CJD in its classical (or sporadic) form is the commonest of this group of diseases, but it is still rare, with an annual incidence across the world of 0.5 to 1.0 cases per million population. In Britain there are between 50 and 80 cases per year. The average age of onset of classical CJD is between 55 and 75 years. Classical CJD has no known cause and is thought to arise spontaneously. However, a minority (about 14%) of other CJD cases run in families and appear to result from gene mutations. About 1% of CJD cases are a result of transmission via medical treatments such as brain surgery, human-derived growth-hormone injections and corneal transplants. A new form of CJD emerged in 1996, variant CJD (see below), which was related to bovine spongiform encephalopathy (BSE) in cattle (see below). In the summer of 2008, a new subtype of CJD was reported from the United States in 11 patients. These patients had an average age of 62 years and in many cases had a family history of dementia, and work is underway to further investigate this condition.

The most highly publicised of the animal

Table 9.6 Key lessons from SARS

- Early sharing of surveillance data between countries and with the World Health Organization is vital.
- Getting virus isolates to specialist laboratories quickly is essential.
- 'Never say never' about the possibility of animal-to-human transmission.
- Strong public health systems and clear accountability within countries is important.
- Travel restrictions and advisories are always controversial and need careful consideration.
- Early, accurate public information and regular updates are key to retaining public confidence.
- Global coordination of response is pivotal to success.

transmissible spongiform encephalopathies in recent years has been bovine spongiform encephalopathy (BSE), and this is because of its links to variant Creutzfeldt–Jakob disease (vCJD) in humans. It is a progressive, lethal central nervous system disease of cattle, which exhibit changes in behaviour, loss of weight and loss of coordination. There is no effective treatment. The first case in cows in the United Kingdom was recognised in 1985, and BSE was first identified as a new disease in 1986. The number of cases reached a peak of 36 000 in 1992, and the annual number has fallen steadily since. At the height of the epidemic in British cattle, the incidence of BSE was almost 1000 cases per week, and by mid-2008 more than 181 000 cases of BSE had been confirmed in British cattle.

The precise nature of the agent that causes BSE and other transmissible spongiform encephalopathies is not known, but the main theory implicates an abnormal protein particle called a 'prion'. Prion proteins are distributed throughout nature in normal circumstances. For example, they are found in the tissues of healthy people, animals and even yeast. When normal prion proteins alter in shape, folding in an abnormal way, they are associated with disease, though the exact relationship between cause and effect is unknown. The abnormally shaped prion protein influences normal protein to copy its shape and is associated with destruction of nervous tissue, particularly in the brain, giving it a 'spongy' appearance under the microscope. The abnormal type of prion protein is heat stable, less soluble than the normal form and more resistant to enzyme action. It is therefore very difficult to destroy or remove by normal decontamination processes.

A sheep-transmissible spongiform encephalopathy, scrapie, has been an endemic disease in the United Kingdom for more than 200 years. Goats are also affected. There is still uncertainty about sheep disease and whether BSE may have transmitted to sheep. Other transmissible spongiform encephalopathies have been found in domestic cats, mink, captive cheetahs and other exotic cats as well as in captive antelopes and wild deer.

It is generally agreed that the BSE epidemic in cattle was exacerbated by feeding rendered-meat-and-bone meal to cattle. The probability that BSE could be transmitted between cattle emerged in 1991 when, following a ban on such feed for ruminants (cattle, sheep and goats), a case of BSE occurred in a calf. Measures to control the BSE epidemic in cattle were first introduced in 1988, and these measures included the ban on feeding meat-and-bone meal to ruminants and a policy of slaughtering infected cattle. During the summer of 1989, the European Union banned the export of cattle from the United Kingdom. A wide range of measures to reduce the risk of cattle products infected with BSE entering the human food chain were subsequently introduced.

In 1990 the United Kingdom's National CJD Surveillance Unit was established in Edinburgh, and in 1996 the Unit identified a new form of CJD. Variant CJD (vCJD) is distinguishable from the classical (sporadic) form in a number of ways. It tends to affect younger people, with an average (median) age of onset of around 26 years (median age at death is 28 years). The predominant initial clinical symptom is of psychiatric or sensory problems, with brain changes (shown as coordination problems, dementia and muscle-twitching) occurring later. The illness usually lasts between six months and two years before death (the median is 14 months). The definitive diagnosis of vCJD can only be confirmed by looking at brain tissue, usually at post-mortem, and it requires the exclusion of sporadic and familial CJD.

From the time it was first described up until July 2008, there have been 164 deaths from definite or probable cases of vCJD in the United Kingdom. (Table 9.7). The peak year of deaths was 2000, since when numbers of cases have fallen.

The government's independent committee advising on all transmissible spongiform encephalopathies, the Spongiform Encephalopathy Advisory Committee

Table 9.7 Deaths from definite and probable cases of Creutzfeldt-Jakob disease in the United Kingdom*

Year	Sporadic	Iatrogenic	Familial	GSSS	vCJD	Total Deaths
1990	28	5	0	0	–	33
1991	32	1	3	0	–	36
1992	45	2	5	1	–	53
1993	37	4	3	2	–	46
1994	53	1	4	3	–	61
1995	35	4	2	3	3	47
1996	40	4	2	4	10	60
1997	60	6	4	1	10	81
1998	63	3	3	2	18	89
1999	62	6	2	0	15	85
2000	50	1	2	1	28	82
2001	58	4	4	2	20	88
2002	72	0	4	1	17	94
2003	79	5	4	2	18	108
2004	50	2	4	2	9	67
2005	66	4	8	5	5	88
2006	68	1	6	3	5	83
2007	62	2	7	1	5	77
2008	44	4	1	3	1	53
Total Deaths	**1004**	**59**	**68**	**36**	**164**	**1331**

*Figures as at August 2008. Note: GSSS = Gerstmann-Sträussler-Scheinker syndrome.
Source: National CJD Surveillance Unit.

(SEAC), concluded that the most likely explanation for the emergence of vCJD was that it had been transmitted to people who had eaten cattle meat, organs or tissue infected with BSE. There is strong epidemiological and laboratory evidence for a causal link between vCJD and BSE. In the late 1990s, new research provided further evidence that the agent that causes BSE is the same as that which causes vCJD.

Sporadic CJD has been transmitted by instruments used in brain surgery. Abnormal prion protein is very difficult to remove from instruments. Abnormal prion protein has been found in the tissues (brain, spleen, tonsils) of patients who have developed vCJD. There is therefore a possibility that vCJD might be transmitted by medical procedures. Guidance is in place to ensure that precautions are taken when dealing with known or suspected cases, with people at possible risk of CJD and with the disposal of instruments used in their care. A detailed account of all relevant guidance and action is beyond the scope of this book, but such guidance is very extensive.

Additional precautionary actions for blood and blood products were introduced from the late 1990s, including reducing the level of white cells (which may carry a significant risk of transmitting vCJD) in blood for transfusion and importing some blood products from countries outside the United Kingdom. This precautionary action proved well-founded because, in 2003, the first of four cases of vCJD infection associated with blood transfusion were identified. As a result, further controls on blood transfusion have been introduced. In particular, individuals are excluded from donating blood if they themselves have received a transfusion since January 1980.

It cannot be firmly asserted that the vCJD epidemic is tailing off, because so many uncertainties still surround the behaviour of the agent that causes vCJD. Until recently, all known cases of vCJD have occurred amongst people with a particular sequence of genes that is found in only 40% of the United Kingdom population. In December 2008, a clinically diagnosed case of vCJD with the other genotype was found. It is entirely possible that the remaining 60% of the population are susceptible but have longer incubation periods. In that case, there may be a second wave of cases to come. Or, alternatively, the 60% may carry the disease and not develop clinical signs but still be able to transmit the infection through blood transfusion or surgery.

There is currently no effective treatment, nor is there a blood test for vCJD, though research is ongoing.

There are still many imponderables about vCJD, including the number of people who may be infected but show no clinical symptoms, the continuance of the current decline in cases, a possible future epidemic and the possibility of secondary spread via blood or surgery. Therefore, there is no doubt that BSE and vCJD are likely to be of concern for the foreseeable future.

TUBERCULOSIS

Tuberculosis has been recognised since antiquity but has undergone a resurgence since the second half of the twentieth century. In earlier centuries, its transmission was enhanced by overcrowding in urban settings and by malnutrition. Known as the 'white plague' or simply 'consumption', it was much feared, especially in Victorian England. Mortality rates were high and there was no specific treatment for it until streptomycin was discovered in 1943. Until then poor people often died from tuberculosis, while the wealthy received treatment in sanatoria, where purer air, sunshine and a good diet sometimes arrested the disease. An account of the world of sanatoria can be found in Thomas Mann's novel *The Magic Mountain*.

Tuberculosis is caused by bacteria of the *Mycobacterium tuberculosis* complex. The commonest form of active tuberculosis infection affects the lungs when an uninfected person inhales *M. tuberculosis* during contact with someone who is infected and coughing up the bacteria. Non-respiratory tuberculosis is also important, particularly amongst immigrants to the United Kingdom. It can affect any part of the body – particularly the lymph nodes, genitourinary tract and bone – and is becoming more common. The non-respiratory form is not generally infective to another person.

Mycobacterium bovis is a bacterium that has a reservoir in animals – particularly cattle. In the early decades of the twentieth century, rates of tuberculosis in cattle approached 40%, but surveillance, tuberculin testing and slaughter of cattle and pasteurisation of milk controlled the disease and reduced the risk of transmission to people.

By 1980, the rate of tuberculosis in cattle in the United Kingdom was very low. Transmission of *M. bovis* to people (via unpasteurised milk and milk products or via aerosol) was uncommon (17–35 cases per year) and has remained so. However, the incidence of tuberculosis in cattle has been increasing again over the last two decades. The role of badgers as a source of bovine tuberculosis infection remains a subject of scientific debate, but tuberculosis in cattle can spread easily. Compulsory testing of cattle is the key control measure, but concern remains about the size of the problem. Scientific opinion differs on the potential for large-scale culling of badgers to control the disease.

The Resurgence of Tuberculosis

There was a dramatic decline in the number of notifications of and deaths from tuberculosis in the United Kingdom during the twentieth century, with improvements in sanitation, better-quality housing and the advent of effective antibiotic treatment. By the mid-1980s this trend began to plateau. Since then the annual rate of new cases has increased steadily. This trend of resurgence of tuberculosis has also occurred in other developed countries. In the United Kingdom, resurgence has happened for a number of reasons:

- ➢ increased immigration of people born in countries that have a high prevalence of tuberculosis (more than two-thirds of all cases fall into this category)
- ➢ the emergence of HIV and consequent co-infection
- ➢ impaired immunity due to chronic disease or drug treatments that reduce resistance to infection.

The worldwide spread of tuberculosis led

to the disease being declared a global emergency by the World Health Organization in 1993. It is estimated that a third of the world's population is infected with tuberculosis – one in 10 have active disease and about two million people die from it each year. The highest rates are in sub-Saharan Africa, but the populations of India, Pakistan, Bangladesh, China and Russia are also seriously affected. Overall, 22 countries account for 80% of the world's tuberculosis cases. The disease is strongly linked to poverty, and international initiatives to combat it often also target HIV and malaria.

The rate of tuberculosis varies across the United Kingdom, with more than 40% of all cases and the highest rate being in London. Most cases in the United Kingdom are amongst 15–44-year-olds, and over 70% of people with the disease were born outside the country.

Drug Resistance

The challenge of stopping the march of tuberculosis in the developing world and its resurgence in the United Kingdom is made all the more difficult by the emergence of strains of *M. tuberculosis* that are resistant to drugs. So-called multi-drug-resistant tuberculosis (MDR-TB), resistant to the two most important first-line drugs, rifampicin and isoniazid, began to emerge in the 1980s. In the middle of the first decade of the twenty-first century, cases of resistance to both first- and second- line drugs (extensively drug-resistant TB, XDR-TB) had emerged.

Death rates are much higher for patients with multi-drug-resistant tuberculosis, and many ideally require treatment in inpatient isolation settings to ensure full supervision of treatment, to allow regular testing and monitoring and to reduce the risks of onward transmission. This is impractical in many developing countries but good practice in developed countries.

Control Measures

The risk of a contact of someone with tuberculosis becoming infected depends on the nature and duration of their exposure, ranging from a one in 100 000 risk from casual social contact to a one in three risk if living at home with the infected person. BCG vaccine is effective against the more severe forms of the disease (such as meningitis) but not very effective in preventing the respiratory form of tuberculosis. The vaccine is administered in a risk-based approach and offered to:

➤ all infants living in high prevalence areas of the United Kingdom
➤ all infants and unvaccinated children with a parent or grandparent born in a high prevalence country
➤ previously unvaccinated tuberculin-negative contacts of cases of respiratory tuberculosis
➤ individuals at occupational risk.

In some of these groups, a tuberculin skin test must be carried out prior to BCG vaccination.

The key elements of a tuberculosis control strategy are:
➤ maintaining high levels of awareness of the disease amongst the public and health professionals
➤ promptly recognising and treating

people with the disease, including screening of recent immigrants

➤ ensuring that people with the disease complete their treatment

➤ establishing high-quality surveillance of the disease at local, regional and national level, including the rapid investigation of outbreaks

➤ screening and actively case-finding amongst high-risk groups (such as asylum seekers and refugees, prisoners and homeless people)

➤ running an appropriate and effective tuberculosis-testing and BCG vaccination programme.

Outbreaks

There are around 300 local reported incidents (for example, an infected school teacher) or outbreaks of tuberculosis each year in this country. These occur most commonly in health care settings, such as hospitals and nursing homes, but may also occur in a range of other settings, such as schools and prisons. Some have involved multi-drug-resistant strains of tuberculosis. The Health Protection Agency is almost always involved, bringing its expertise in investigation, diagnosis and control measures to bear in addressing the problem.

HELICOBACTER PYLORI

Helicobacter pylori is one of a growing number of infectious agents being linked with chronic disease causation, in this case peptic ulcer disease and gastric cancer. *H. pylori* is a spiral-shaped bacterium related to *Campylobacter* (*see* below), and it is found either adherent to the gastric epithelium or in the gastric mucous layer.

It is estimated that about two-thirds of the world's population is infected with *H. pylori*. Although most people who are infected are unlikely ever to suffer symptoms, infection can be associated with chronic active, chronic persistent and atrophic gastritis in both children and adults. The organism is said to be responsible for approximately 80% of gastric ulcers and 90% of duodenal ulcers. It has been demonstrated that people infected with *H. pylori* are between two and six times more likely than uninfected people to develop gastric cancer and mucosal-associated lymphoid-type (MALT) lymphoma. Gastric cancer is the second most common cancer globally.

Diagnosis of *H. pylori* infection is either by serology, by a urease breath test or by upper gastrointestinal endoscopy with biopsy. In the latter case, the organism can be cultured from biopsy specimens.

Treatment of *H. pylori* infection is by means of antibiotics in combination with acid-suppressing medication, and eradication is successful in between 70% and 90% of patients, depending upon the drug regimen used. The two major reasons for treatment failure are antibiotic resistance or patient non-compliance.

The source of *H. pylori* and its routes of transmission are not yet known. It has been suggested that faecal–oral or oral–oral spread might be implicated and that contaminated water sources may serve as an environmental reservoir. Iatrogenic spread has been documented, occurring via contaminated endoscopes. This can be prevented by cleaning equipment properly.

Until the source and routes of transmission of *H. pylori* are better understood, it is difficult to give advice to the public about how to prevent infection. In the absence of specific control measures, however, it is important to reinforce the general principles of good personal and food hygiene.

HEPATITIS C

Hepatitis C is a blood-borne virus that is a leading cause of liver disease worldwide. An estimated 170 million people have chronic hepatitis C infection. Most acute hepatitis C infections produce no symptoms. Some people may feel briefly unwell, and jaundice is rare. In many of those with chronic infection, which develops in about 60–80% of those infected, symptoms will be uncommon. When symptoms do occur, they include fatigue, loss of appetite, weight loss, abdominal pain or discomfort, poor memory or concentration and depression. Chronic hepatitis C infection progresses over about 20–30 years to liver cirrhosis and liver cancer in a proportion of people affected. In some cases, liver transplantation is required.

Size and Nature of the Problem in the United Kingdom

In the United Kingdom, the majority of hepatitis C infections have arisen amongst people who are or have been injecting drug users. Some infected people may have experimented with injecting drugs for a short time many years ago. 'Hippie era' recreational drug users have particularly attracted professional attention because many are unaware of the risk they were exposed to and many have had undiagnosed chronic infection. The late Anita Roddick, founder of The Body Shop, was a high-profile individual who tested positive for hepatitis C and played a role in raising public awareness of the infection. She was diagnosed with hepatitis C in 2005, but caught it from a blood transfusion during childbirth in 1971. As with many people, she harboured the infection silently for many years.

The true prevalence of hepatitis C infection within the population aged 15–59 years in this country is unknown, but it is estimated that around 0.72% are antibody positive and 0.53% are chronically infected. The number of people with chronic hepatitis C infection in the United Kingdom is estimated at around 250 000, the majority of whom have probably not been formally diagnosed.

Infection is more common in men (the male:female ratio is about 2:1). There is an increased risk of hepatitis C infection amongst people who are HIV positive. High-risk sexual behaviour amongst men who have sex with men is an area of concern in which co-infection (HIV and hepatitis C) is increasing. Those who received blood products before 1986 and blood transfusions before 1991 are also at increased risk. A small proportion of cases occurs through mother-to-baby transmission. There is also a risk from medical or dental treatment abroad in countries where infection control is inadequate and infection is common. Tattooing and body piercing using unsterile equipment is another risk factor.

Deaths from liver failure or cancer caused by hepatitis C have been rising since the mid-

1990s, and there have been similar increases in the numbers scheduled for liver transplants because of the infection. The future burden of disease from chronic liver damage or cancer is likely to be considerable.

Treatment, Disease Control and Prevention

In England, as many as three out of every five people with hepatitis C infection may be unaware that they have it. This necessitates strong public-awareness-raising campaigns coupled with the offer of testing to reduce the number of undiagnosed infections. In addition, it is important to increase testing amongst high-risk populations such as those in specialist drug-treatment centres, prisons and genitourinary medicine clinics.

A combination of pegylated interferon and ribavirin is the currently recommended drug therapy for chronic hepatitis C infection. Treatment has an overall success rate of 55% in those treated, varying from about 40–80% depending on the virus genotype. Not everyone is suitable for treatment (because of medical contraindications, for example), and there may be unpleasant side effects that are intolerable for some. The aim of treatment is to reduce the 'viral load' in the body to undetectable levels in order to prevent progression to serious liver disease. New drugs are being researched and may offer more-effective, less-toxic treatment in the future, although the development of drug resistance may be a problem.

Preventive measures are aimed at reducing ongoing transmission of hepatitis C, particularly amongst injecting drug users and other at-risk populations. Key activities include increased drug education (particularly in schools), drug intervention programmes, provision of needle exchange schemes, safe disposal of drug-injecting equipment, distribution of disinfection tablets in prisons and sex education programmes.

Special control measures are needed to ensure that the small number of health care workers who are infected with hepatitis C do not pass the infection on to their patients. In the United Kingdom, there is detailed guidance to the NHS with particular emphasis on restricting infected health care workers from carrying out 'exposure-prone' procedures (such as surgical operations).

CAMPYLOBACTER

It might be argued that, with an annual incidence of around 70 000 cases in Britain, *Campylobacter* has 'emerged'. It is, however, still regarded as an emerging infection. The importance of *Campylobacter* as a cause of gastroenteritis has been recognised relatively recently, with the development of improved laboratory techniques for diagnosis. *Campylobacter jejuni* is a Gram-negative vibrio-like organism. *Campylobacter coli* is a similar organism that also causes illness in people. Since it was first described in the late 1970s, the incidence of campylobacter infection in Britain has risen so much that it is now the most common bacterial cause of gastroenteritis.

The incubation period for *Campylobacter* ranges between 1 and 10 days (usually 2 to 5 days), and infection results in a range of symptoms. Characteristically, profuse diarrhoea (occasionally blood-stained) occurs and is associated with very painful colicky abdominal pain. This can be alarming for those concerned (and often results in hospital admission), but usually it subsides and the person affected makes a full recovery. Guillain-Barré syndrome has been linked with *Campylobacter* infection, occurring rarely as a late complication of infection.

The source of the organism is probably the gastrointestinal tract of poultry, cattle and pets. The mode of transmission is by food (undercooked poultry, for example), milk or contaminated water. Because the infectious dose is low, cross-contamination of ready-to-eat foods may also be a significant mode of transmission. Cases have occurred after drinking milk that has been pecked on the doorstep by wild birds (such as jackdaws). Unlike *Salmonella* (*see* p. 463), *Campylobacter* does not grow on food. Like *Salmonella*, it is heat-sensitive, so adequate cooking should destroy it. Animal-to-person transmission (by direct contact) is generally regarded as an established route of transmission, whilst person-to-person transmission is much less common.

One of the tantalising epidemiological conundrums relating to *Campylobacter* is the fact that outbreaks of infection are seldom recognised. In part, this might be due to the absence, until recently, of a discriminatory laboratory typing scheme.

VEROCYTOTOXIN-PRODUCING *E. COLI* O157

Most strains of *Escherichia coli* live in the gut of people or animals without producing ill effects. Some strains can produce serious illness, amongst them the organisms that produce toxins called verocytotoxins. The name for an *E. coli* serotype that produces such toxins is verocytotoxin-producing *E. coli* O157 (VTEC O157).

This *E. coli* strain was first identified in 1982 and has caused outbreaks in many parts of the world ever since. The main reservoirs are cattle and sheep. It is unusual in requiring a relatively small number of organisms (less than 100) to cause infection. The comparable infective 'doses' for *Campylobacter* are 500 and for *Salmonella* 100 000 to one million.

Infection results in a spectrum of illness ranging from mild diarrhoea through profuse diarrhoea to bloody diarrhoea (this is a key feature). Some cases are complicated by the development of haemolytic uraemic syndrome. This usually affects children and may necessitate them undergoing renal dialysis. A proportion of these children will develop long-term renal damage.

Outbreak investigations in Britain have shown that, while food-borne transmission is an important route of infection (particularly undercooked ground beef, cold sliced meats, raw milk and untreated water), person-to-person and animal-to-person transmission are also significant. The increasing vogue for children visiting open farms and city farms has brought outbreaks in its wake. The whole question of waste management in farming and the use of farmland for leisure purposes is also important. Good personal hygiene, particularly ensuring hand cleanliness for children, is vital in preventing transmission.

While the incidence of VTEC O157 is still low compared with that of other gastrointestinal pathogens, there is no room for complacency given the very severe consequences of infection. There have been large, serious outbreaks of VTEC O157 infection in many parts of the world, including, notably, an outbreak in Central Scotland in November and December 1996 that affected around 500 people and claimed 20 lives. Other outbreaks have been associated with schools and nurseries, school field trips and the consumption of raw milk and cheese.

WEST NILE VIRUS

West Nile virus belongs to the flavivirus family. Other infections caused by this group of viruses include St Louis encephalitis and Japanese encephalitis. West Nile virus was first discovered in Uganda in 1937, when a woman developed an unexplained fever. Until the end of the twentieth century, the virus was confined to tropical and subtropical areas of the world (such as Africa, Israel, India and Egypt). There it caused occasional outbreaks: for example, in Israel in the 1950s and in South Africa in the early 1970s. During the mid-1990s there were signs of a changing pattern of disease. Outbreaks of infection with the virus occurred in Romania, Morocco, Tunisia and Russia.

The first sinister signs of a major shift in the geographical occurrence of West Nile virus infection came in the summer of 1999 when a number of dead crows were found in New York City. That same year, 62 people fell ill with viral encephalitis and seven died from it. Colder weather and mosquito spraying ended the outbreak in New York City that summer, but West Nile virus was now established in the United States.

The natural host for West Nile virus is birds, but it is usually transmitted to people and some other mammals (including horses) by mosquitoes. It can also be transmitted from person to person through blood transfusion, organ transplantation, breast milk and laboratory accidents.

Many people who are exposed to West Nile virus will not develop symptoms. When illness does occur, it often results in mild flu-like symptoms. Some people develop serious illness, including encephalitis, and for those who do, around 12% will die.

Since its unexpected emergence beyond its traditional geographical boundaries, West Nile virus has spread extensively in North America and is now endemic in that continent. West Nile virus activity in people, birds or mosquitoes has now been reported from all states in the United States of America except Hawaii, Alaska and Oregon.

The main factors that influence the transmission of the virus are:
- climatic conditions
- population density and species of mosquitoes
- presence of susceptible birds.

In affected areas, a number of measures are important in prevention and disease control. The first is to establish enhanced systems of surveillance for the virus, not just identifying and testing people with encephalitis and unexplained fevers but tracking the occurrence of the virus amongst birds, mosquitoes and animals (particularly horses). The second measure is advising the public to take action to reduce their risk by covering skin with clothing (particularly at dawn and dusk when mosquito bites are more common), using skin insect repellents and nets and draining pools of water around houses and yards. The third is environmental control measures, mainly directed at mosquito breeding (eliminating areas of standing water) and mosquito populations (pesticide spraying). The fourth action is aimed at reducing person-to-person transmission and includes treatment of blood products and restrictions on blood donations from individuals who have been at risk. Blood is screened in the United States, as the disease is more common there.

The risk of West Nile virus occurring or becoming established in the United Kingdom is currently low because climatic conditions do not support it, nor does the spectrum of endemic mosquito species favour it. However, it is important to maintain a high level of vigilance, and as with all such new and emerging infection, 'never say never'.

ANTIMICROBIAL RESISTANCE

The issue of antimicrobial resistance is of global concern. Not only is antimicrobial resistance accumulating worldwide in many bacteria, but it is also emerging amongst viruses (*Herpes simplex* virus, influenza and HIV) and fungi (*Candida* sp.). Some of the issues of major concern in Britain are listed here.

Meticillin-resistant *Staphylococcus aureus* (MRSA)

Staphylococcus aureus is classically a cause of superficial or deep-seated wound infections. In 1944, when penicillin was introduced, over 95% of isolates were susceptible, but this proportion has subsequently diminished

to about 10%. During the 1950s, resistance to penicillins and tetracyclines became a huge problem in hospitals. In order to overcome this, beta-lactamase-stable penicillins were introduced in the 1960s (including methicillin and flucloxacillin), and shortly thereafter, the first MRSA was recognised. Having sought therapeutic refuge with the aminoglycosides (e.g., gentamicin), gentamicin-resistant strains developed by the 1970s. Strains then emerged that had a peculiar ability to spread very easily in the hospital environment (so-called epidemic MRSA, or EMRSA), and some of these are highly invasive.

A very worrying recent development has been the emergence of strains showing intermediate resistance to glycopeptides (e.g., vancomycin) in Japan, the USA and France. These strains show some resistance to all the available antimicrobial agents. Unlike most other pan-resistant organisms, they pose a threat to patients who are immunocompetent, not only those who are immunocompromised (*see also* section on health-care-associated infection).

Streptococcus Pneumoniae

Streptococcus pneumoniae is a leading cause of community-acquired pneumonia, septicaemia and bacterial meningitis. When penicillin was first introduced, these organisms were highly susceptible. Low-level resistance to penicillin was first reported in the 1960s, with high-level resistance emerging in the late 1970s. High-level resistance has important therapeutic consequences, especially for the treatment of meningitis, where alternative antibiotics do not necessarily penetrate into the cerebrospinal fluid as efficiently as penicillin.

Penicillin resistance reached a peak in 2000, when almost 7% of bacteraemia-causing isolates were resistant; this figure fell to 3% by 2007. There are also significant levels of macrolide (erythromycin) resistance (9% in 2007). There is considerable variation in levels of resistance to penicillin and macrolides in this country, with the highest levels in London. The introduction of a seven-valent pneumococcal conjugate vaccine to the childhood vaccination programme should provide immunity to infection with many antibiotic resistant strains (*see also* section on vaccination).

Enterococci

Part of normal gut flora, enterococci, which are usually harmless, pose a threat to immunosuppressed patients in hospital settings such as transplant units. The clinical spectrum of illness caused is broad, but in serious infections like septicaemia and endocarditis, enterococci prove very difficult to treat because of their high degree of antimicrobial resistance. They are intrinsically resistant to some antibiotics and readily acquire resistance to others.

Penicillin and aminoglycosides (e.g., gentamicin) were used successfully in combination to treat infections due to enterococci until the mid-1980s, when aminoglycoside resistance emerged. This left only the glycopeptides (e.g., vancomycin). Glycopeptide-resistant enterococci (GRE) first appeared in the United Kingdom in the late 1980s and have rapidly spread in the hospital setting. Vancomycin resistance rates in isolates in 2007 were around 20% for *Enterococcus faecium* and 2–3% for *Enterococcus faecalis*.

Hospital-acquired Gram-negative Rods

The significance of Gram-negative rods is usually as opportunistic pathogens in immunocompromised patients in hospital, and they cause considerable problems on intensive care units. Recent rapid rises in cephalosporin resistance in *Escherichia coli* since 2003 reflect the emergence of strains producing extended-spectrum beta-lactamases (ESBLs) (Figure 9.9). *E. coli* have also shown significant increases in resistance to ciprofloxacin and gentamicin.

Worrying patterns of resistance have also been noted in *Klebsiella* (to cephalosporins, aminoglycosides and quinolones) and *Acinetobacter* species, particularly *Acinetobacter baumannii*, which is developing significant resistance to carbapenems.

Salmonella

Concern about antibiotic resistance in *Salmonella typhimurium* dates back to the 1960s, when a series of epidemics occurred in both cattle and people, a feature of which was increasing antimicrobial resistance. Following these epidemics, an expert committee recommended that certain agents should only be available on prescription for veterinary use and that they should not be added to animal feed as growth promoters. For a while after this, the level of antibiotic resistance in *S. typhimurium* from both animals and humans subsided. However, a substantial increase in multi-resistant *S. typhimurium* from food animals, particularly cattle, occurred over a decade from the mid-1970s, and this coincided with an increase in multi-resistant isolates from humans. It followed the introduction of therapeutic antibiotics into veterinary practice that were very similar to those used in people.

In the early 1990s, a further upsurge in resistance occurred, due in large part to the epidemic spread of *S. typhimurium* DT104, which at its peak was widely distributed amongst food-producing animals, not just cattle. This was quickly reflected in the human population; in 1996, 80% of isolates of *S. typhimurium* from humans were multi-resistant. Fortunately, the most common *Salmonella* found in people, *S. enteritidis*, remains generally sensitive to antibiotics.

Campylobacter

Campylobacter is demonstrating increasing

levels of resistance to quinolones, and also to macrolides for *C. coli*. (*see* p. 455 for more information on this infection).

Gonococci

By 1944 the use of sulphonamides for the treatment of gonorrhoea was all but defeated by the development of resistance (sulphonamides had only been introduced in 1937). Penicillin resistance has developed much more slowly, but there are now strains with the ability to produce penicillinase (designated PPNG), and these account for roughly 50% of *Neisseria gonorrhoeae* in the developing world. High levels of azithromycin resistance were detected in England and Wales for the first time in 2007 by the Gonococcal Resistance to Antimicrobials Surveillance Programme (GRASP).

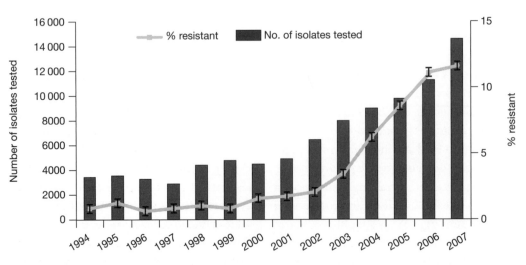

Figure 9.9 Resistance to ceftazidime in *E. coli* from bacteraemia, England, Wales and Northern Ireland

Source: Health Protection Agency Centre for Infections. *Antimicrobial Resistance and Prescribing in England, Wales and Northern Ireland, 2008*. London: HPA; 2008.

Influenza

Influenza viruses are responsible for the seasonal outbreaks of flu seen each year and also have the potential to cause a pandemic. National pandemic preparedness plans in the United Kingdom and many other countries include the use of antiviral drugs to reduce the spread of infection. Recent surveillance data have highlighted increasing rates of oseltamivir resistance in the seasonal influenza virus across Europe, demonstrating that antimicrobial resistance is not limited to bacteria alone (*see also* section on influenza).

Combating Antimicrobial Resistance

Combating antimicrobial resistance has become a major priority for governments and for the National Health Service. Several high-level committees have published reports detailing concerns about antimicrobial resistance. Measures to tackle this important public health problem include stopping the use of antibiotics as growth promoters in animal husbandry, agriculture and aquaculture; responsible prescribing by both the medical and veterinary professions; and educating the public not to expect antibiotic treatment for viral conditions such as the common cold and simple sore throats.

The Advisory Committee on Antimicrobial Resistance and Healthcare Associated Infection (ARHAI) currently has a central role advising on work in this area in the United Kingdom. Large-scale public information campaigns aimed at decreasing demand for antibiotic prescribing in other European countries, notably France, have demonstrated that they can be successful in reducing antibiotic prescribing rates.

Data from the European Antimicrobial Resistance Surveillance System (EARSS) and European Surveillance of Antibiotic Consumption (ESAC) have demonstrated the correlation between antimicrobial prescription rates and resistance rates at a national level (Figure 9.10)

An illustration of the range of measures that need to be addressed in combating antimicrobial resistance is set out in Table 9.8.

GASTROINTESTINAL INFECTIONS
FOOD-BORNE ILLNESS

Examples of diseases that can be transmitted by food are discussed throughout this chapter. This particular section deals with the specific causes of food-borne illness (sometimes called food poisoning) that result in the acute onset of symptoms, predominantly vomiting and/or diarrhoea. The causal agents that are responsible for food-borne illness are bacterial (these will be considered in detail in this section), viral, parasitic and, relatively infrequently, other substances (for example, heavy metal or mushroom and shellfish toxins).

Five major organisms are the source of the majority of reported cases of food-borne illness: *Salmonella*, *E. coli* O157, *Campylobacter*, *Listeria monocytogenes* and *Clostridium perfringens*. Two of these, *E. coli* O157 and *Campylobacter* have been dealt with in the section on new and emerging infections. The remaining members of the 'big five' and other causes of food-borne illness are described in this section.

The estimated cost of food-borne illness (in England and Wales) is high, around

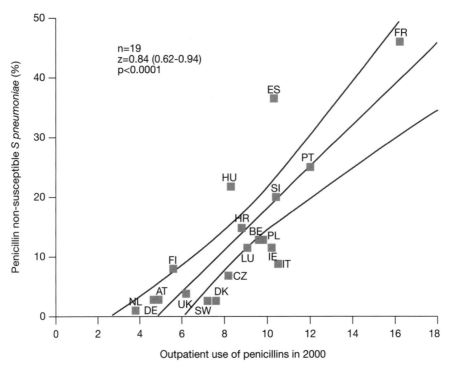

AT, Austria; BE, Belgium; HR, Croatia; CZ, Czech Republic; DK, Denmark; FI, Finland; FR, France; DE, Germany; HU, Hungary; IE, Ireland; IT, Italy; LU, Luxembourg; NL, The Netherlands; PL, Poland; PT, Portugal; SI, Slovenia; ES, Spain; UK, England only.

Figure 9.10 Outpatient penicillin usage is correlated with penicillin resistance across European countries

Source: Goossens H, Ferech M, Vander Stichele R, *et al.* Outpatient antibiotic use in Europe and association with resistance: a cross-national database study. *Lancet.* 2005; **365**: 579–87.

Table 9.8 Key measures to reduce antibiotic resistance

- Keep antibiotics as prescription-only medicines.
- Adhere to infection-control policies in hospitals and other health care facilities.
- Raise professional, public and farming awareness.
- Promote high-quality prescribing of antibiotics (and reduce their unnecessary use).
- Reduce use of antibiotics in farm animals.
- Establish good surveillance of antibiotic resistance.

£1.5 billion on the economy in 2006 (comprising costs to the NHS, loss of earnings and a factor for pain and suffering).

Food-borne illness rose throughout the 1990s, but after 2000, with the work of the Food Standards Agency, it fell substantially. Rates began to flatten out by 2007 (Figure 9.11). Periods of increasing notifications may reflect a greater tendency for the public to seek help when they have symptoms related to food poisoning, or more decisions by medical practitioners to investigate and report cases that present to them. In addition, major changes have occurred in people's eating habits. With more women working outside the home, and the development of a more leisure-orientated society, there is a greater tendency for people not to cook at home.

Salmonella Infections

There are some 2200 *Salmonella* serotypes that can cause illness in people. In the United Kingdom, the reported occurrence of Salmonella food-borne infections increased sharply in the 1980s but began to fall from 2000 onwards, stabilising around 2005. One of the principal *Salmonella* organisms associated with illness in Britain is *Salmonella enteritidis*. Illnesses due to this one organism showed a very large increase in Britain in the mid-1980s.

Illnesses caused by *Salmonella* organisms in food vary in severity. Common symptoms include fever, headache, abdominal pain, diarrhoea and vomiting. Illness usually lasts between one and seven days. However, infections can be fatal, particularly in the elderly or the very young.

Foodstuffs commonly implicated in outbreaks of *Salmonella* infection include

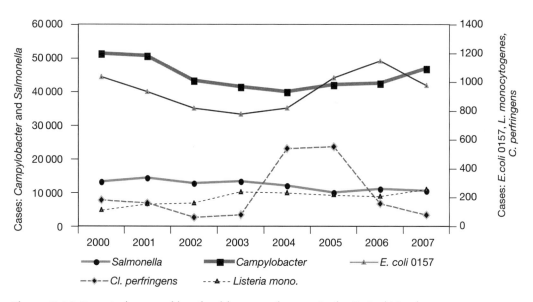

Figure 9.11 Reported cases of key food-borne pathogens in the United Kingdom
Source: Food Standards Agency.

undercooked poultry, eggs (particularly dishes prepared with raw eggs), milk and milk products.

Clostridium Botulinum Infections

Toxin produced by the organism *Clostridium botulinum* (a Gram-positive, anaerobic bacillus that produces spores that are very resistant to destruction by heat) is the cause of an uncommon but potentially fatal illness called botulism. The toxin affects the nervous system and can cause double vision, respiratory (and more generalised) paralysis, vomiting and diarrhoea. The time between ingestion of toxin and the onset of symptoms is typically between five and 36 hours, but symptoms can occur as early as three hours or as late as eight days.

Classically, the illness is associated with the toxin accumulating in anaerobic conditions (for example, during home bottling or canning of vegetables), but it also occurs with smoked or preserved meats and fish. In the United States, outbreaks of botulism in infants have been associated with contamination of honey by spores of *C. botulinum*, subsequent multiplication of the organism within the intestine and toxin formation (this is an unusual mechanism of acquiring botulism compared with primary ingestion of the toxin). In Britain, cases of botulism have been associated with foodstuffs as diverse as duck pâté and hazelnut yoghurt.

Treatment involves the administration of antitoxin and intensive care, including respiratory support. If such care is instituted promptly and effectively, the case fatality rate can be reduced. Some people will still die from what is a very serious food-borne illness.

Bacillus Cereus Infections

Bacillus cereus is an aerobic Gram-positive bacillus that produces spores and occurs widely in nature (for example, in soil and dust). It produces two main types of illness, both of which are self-limiting, almost always leading to a full recovery within a day or so. The first, called the diarrhoeal type, usually takes longer for symptoms to appear (between eight and 16 hours) and gives rise to severe abdominal pain and profuse diarrhoea (often there is no vomiting). It arises from an enterotoxin that the organism releases into the bowel following infection. The second main presentation of *B. cereus* infection, called the emetic type, presents with sudden onset of vomiting relatively early (one to six hours) after ingestion of the suspected foodstuff. It is caused by a toxin produced by the organism and accumulated in the contaminated foodstuff prior to ingestion. Diarrhoea is much less common with this presentation.

The diarrhoeal-type infection is associated with foods such as cornflour, sauces, soups and meat dishes that have been insufficiently heated. The emetic type infection is classically associated with rice that has been cooked, stored and reheated later.

Staphylococcus Aureus Infections

Staphylococcus aureus is a very commonly occurring Gram-positive coccus that causes a range of infections, including superficial skin infections (such as boils) and wound infections following surgical operations. It is a cause of food-borne illness by virtue of the production of a toxin (for example, after it has accumulated in a foodstuff following contamination by a food handler with an infected finger). Ingestion results in sudden onset (usually within one to six hours) of abdominal pain, vomiting and diarrhoea.

Foods commonly incriminated include those left at room temperature for the organism to multiply, such as cakes, trifles, sandwiches and cold meats. Outbreaks are frequent in the summer, when salad lunches and cold buffets are served out of doors, in marquees or pavilions at fetes, weddings or sporting events.

Clostridium Perfringens Infections

An illness with sudden onset of abdominal pain, nausea and diarrhoea (but not usually vomiting or fever) anything between eight to 24 hours after ingestion of a suspected foodstuff is characteristic of infection with *Clostridium perfringens*. This is an anaerobic, Gram-positive bacillus that produces spores and is widely distributed in nature (in soil and the gut of animals). It requires special tests to confirm the diagnosis, so the reported cases are likely to seriously underestimate the problem.

It typically occurs when poultry or meat dishes are inadequately cooked in the first place or when they are reheated. The spores change into the vegetative form, which multiplies during slow cooling, storage at ambient temperature or inadequate reheating. The organism then produces a toxin when in the intestine. The illness usually lasts about 24 hours and is very seldom fatal (except occasionally in the elderly).

Yersinia Infections

Yersinia enterocolitica is a small Gram-negative bacillus that is found amongst wild and farm animals (particularly pigs), in water and sewage. It produces an illness with abdominal pain, diarrhoea and fever, most commonly in children. The clinical picture can closely mimic acute appendicitis or mesenteric adenitis. Erythema nodosum can be a complication in up to one-third of adults.

The most common routes of transmission are contaminated milk or water or various foodstuffs. Another species of *Yersinia, Yersinia pestis,* whose reservoir is rodents, causes plague. Although a scourge of the past, it no longer occurs in Britain. It is still found in some parts of the world.

Protozoan Parasites

Protozoan parasitic organisms can cause illness if they are ingested with food or water. Four in particular are commoner than the others and are described in this section – Cryptosporidium, Giardia, Toxoplasma and Cyclospora.

Cryptosporidium

Cryptosporidium is a protozoan organism with a number of species, the most common being *Cryptosporidium parvum*. It has a parasitic life cycle that causes illness after the ingestion of the oocystic stage. It is a relatively commonly reported cause of diarrhoeal illness (there are between 3000 and 5000 cases in England and Wales per year), and it usually produces watery diarrhoea that lasts up to a month. In immunocompetent individuals it can last much longer. There is no effective drug treatment.

Waterborne transmission occurs, and outbreaks have happened when treatment of the public mains water supply has failed. A large outbreak in the home counties in England occurred after drinking water from a borehole supply became contaminated. Expert committees have, amongst other things, reviewed the risks from domestic water supplies and have made recommendations for the control of cryptosporidiosis, which may be transmitted either by direct animal-to-human spread or via contamination of water. The organism can also be spread from an infected person to others. Contact with farm animals along with poor personal hygiene is a cause. For example, one outbreak that occurred in Britain resulted from a party of schoolchildren visiting a farm and eating food without first washing their hands.

Giardia

Giardia is a parasite with a two-stage life cycle. It produces a cyst, which lodges in the duodenum after ingestion and releases trophozoites that multiply and occupy the small bowel. There are a number of *Giardia* species that infect people, including *Giardia intestinalis*, *Giardia lamblia* and *Giardia duodenalis*. *Giardia* causes acute and chronic symptoms (such as diarrhoea, abdominal pain and bloating).

The organism is found in the faeces of wild and domestic animals (sometimes pets), and its cyst is quite environmentally resistant. It can be water or food-borne or contracted because of poor personal hygiene when in contact with animals or animal pastures. Although the classic occurrence is amongst backpackers drinking from mountain streams, in some parts of the world it can be contracted from public water supplies. Notably, the cysts are resistant to chlorine disinfection (a method of water purification in some jurisdictions).

If the initial acute episode of diarrhoea is passed off by the individual as 'traveller's diarrhoea', the chronic symptoms can become insidious – malaise, weight-loss, flatulence, abdominal pain – and the diagnosis may not be suspected. Moreover, it is notoriously difficult to detect on stool samples. In such cases, the affected person may soldier on for a long period of time being investigated for persistent and vague bowel symptoms or even for more sinister causes, such as malignancy.

Treatment with high doses of appropriate antibiotics is usually effective but may need more than one course. The key is to have a high awareness of the possible diagnosis in returning travellers, even from developed countries where it may be thought public water supplies are safe.

Toxoplasma Gondii

Toxoplasma gondii is a coccidial protozoan parasite found in the tissues of many animals, as well in people. Only in the cat is there a stage of development in the intestine. Hence the cat excretes *T. gondii* as oocysts, which when ingested by other animals cause the disease. It may also result from the ingestion of contaminated uncooked meat.

Toxoplasmosis is found in all parts of the world, both in animals and people. In Britain up to 50% of adults have antibodies to *Toxoplasma*, indicating previous infection, even though the vast majority show no symptoms.

The primary infection rarely causes symptoms that are severe enough to be reported. In its acute form, the patient has fever and enlarged lymph glands. In immunocompromised individuals, primary infection can cause a much more severe illness affecting the brain, lungs and heart, invariably leading to death. Cerebral toxoplasmosis is recognised as a serious consequence of infection with HIV. Infections in pregnancy can cause foetal damage and resulting congenital malformations.

The incubation period is thought to lie somewhere between 10 and 23 days. Person-to-person infection only occurs in the intrauterine infection. The oocysts excreted by cats become infective after one to five days and can remain viable in moist conditions for up to a year.

The definitive hosts are members of the cat family. The cat becomes infected by eating infected mammals (such as rodents) and birds. The parasite then undergoes a complex process of development in the epithelial cells of the cat's intestine. For a short period of time, the cat passes oocysts, a stage of the parasite that can remain potentially infective in the environment for long periods. However, despite the fact that two-thirds of the cat population have been infected, only 1% are likely to be passing oocysts at any one time.

It is not known how often people become infested by these oocysts. It is thought that they acquire the infection either directly by injecting oocysts from soil (for example, during gardening) or by eating raw or insufficiently cooked pork, mutton or beef that contains the parasite. Transplacental infection occurs in humans when the pregnant mother acquires a primary infection. The foetus can be affected at any stage of pregnancy, but is most at risk during the first trimester, when infection can lead to foetal death. Congenital infection may also give rise to chorioretinitis, cerebral calcification and hydrocephalus in up to 60% of survivors. These severe consequences have led to a call for a national screening programme to combat this disease.

The most important means of preventing toxoplasmosis are the thorough cooking of meat, fruit and vegetables and advising pregnant women to avoid handling cat litter, especially with bare hands.

Cyclospora Cayetanensis

Cyclospora cayetanensis has been responsible for producing large outbreaks of food-borne disease in North America, notably associated with transmission by fresh raspberries from Guatemala. The life cycle of *Cyclospora* is not as well understood as some of the other food-borne and waterborne parasites described in this section. It does produce oocysts, which are the way that the infection is acquired. Infection probably occurs via human sewage contamination, since no animal reservoir has yet been identified.

Escherichia Coli Infections

Escherichia coli is a Gram-negative bacillus that is frequently found in the intestine of humans and animals. *E. coli* organisms are usually classified into broad groups, in each of which there are many serotypes. Most strains of *E. coli* are harmless, but some can cause severe disease.

➤ Enteropathic *E. coli* (EPEC) cause outbreaks of diarrhoea in infants and are a particular problem when they occur in hospital neonatal or paediatric wards.

➤ Enteroinvasive *E. coli* (EIEC) are very similar in their modes of infection to *Shigella* bacteria and occur in sporadic cases and outbreaks in similar circumstances to the latter.

➤ Enterotoxigenic *E. coli* (ETEC) produce toxins and watery diarrhoea rather like that which occurs in cholera. They are a common cause of diarrhoeal illness amongst infants in tropical countries and in adults visiting tropical countries. They are one of the causes of 'traveller's diarrhoea' and are acquired by contaminated food and water.

➤ Verocytotoxin-producing *E. coli* (VTEC) were described in the section on new and emerging diseases.

Listeriosis

Listeria (more correctly, listeriosis) made headline news in Britain during the late 1980s when it was one of a number of food hygiene issues which aroused public concern and which led to urgent government action. The causative organism is a Gram-positive bacillus, *Listeria monocytogenes*, which is widely distributed in nature.

The organism can grow at temperatures as low as those maintained in refrigerators, which is unusual for a micro-organism. It is usually transmitted to people via foodstuffs such as some mould-ripened soft cheese, pâté, cold meats, and cook-chill recipe dishes.

It is mainly a danger to people whose immune system is impaired or to unborn and newborn babies, pregnant women and the very old. It is an important cause of neonatal septicaemia and meningitis and can spread from mother to foetus, either in utero or through direct contact with the mother's infected genital tract. Listeria infection in pregnant women can also cause abortion. There are about 250 confirmed cases each year, and this began to increase from the early 2000s, mainly in the over-60 years age group.

Non-bacterial Toxins

In addition to the many food-borne illnesses caused by toxins produced by bacteria, some toxins of non-bacterial origin can be ingested in foods (Table 9.9).

The Prevention and Control of Food-borne Illness

A major reduction in the occurrence of food-borne illness could be achieved if well-established control measures were even more rigorously applied. In practice, this means enforcing safeguards and taking preventive action at all points in the food chain, from the rearing of animals that are to be consumed by people to the process of food production, storage, distribution, sale and preparation for eating, commercially and in the home. Concerted, coordinated action is, therefore, needed from 'farm to fork', and this requires the cooperation of producers, the food and catering industries, several government departments and non-governmental bodies, the National Health Service and local government. The need to tackle the prevention of food-borne disease across the whole food chain, from producer to consumer, was a major reason for the establishment of an independent Food Standards Agency. Since its creation, the Agency has led change in this area.

There are control measures that are particular to individual organisms described in this section, but the majority of measures are common to all. Good animal husbandry, careful attention to the content of animal foodstuffs, the raising of *Salmonella*-free flocks of poultry, high standards of slaughterhouse hygiene and a range of other measures are essential steps in ensuring that when food and drinks are consumed, they are free of harmful micro-organisms and their toxins.

It is also important to ensure that strict control measures operate during the manufacture of food. Increasingly, food in Britain is bought in processed form. Whether this is as joints of meat or poultry, canned or frozen products or more elaborate heat-and-serve recipe dishes, measures to prevent food-borne illness must be built in at all stages of the production process.

This has implications for the design of food-processing plants and for the building materials used in them: for the type of equipment used and how it is maintained; for heat and other treatments given to various types of food; for the type and content of packaging materials; for operating practices for, and training of, staff; and for inspection and quality-control procedures. Many of the same considerations apply to storage and distribution chains, which should maintain the food in a hygienic condition in the interval between it leaving the production plant and reaching the shop, supermarket or catering outlet.

Enormous expenditure and extensive research and development takes place in these aspects of food technology, particularly on the part of the major producers and suppliers. Food hygiene and safety are an integral part of the food industry, but the fact that there is such a large number of producers and suppliers, and the fact that even a small lapse can lead to a serious outbreak of food-borne illness, means that the task is one of constant vigilance and improvement of standards.

The storage, handling and preparation of food in the home, in institutions (such as hospitals and schools), and in restaurants, cafes and other catering outlets is a vital issue for the prevention and control of food-borne illness. This will be evident from the accounts of individual causes of food poisoning earlier in this section of the chapter. The following list details important principles and practices.

➢ High standards of personal hygiene must be maintained by those handling food (for example, washing hands before and after handling food, between stages of preparation and after going to the toilet).

Table 9.9 Some causes of non-bacterial food poisoning

Toxin	Source	Comments
Muscarine	*Amanita pantherina*, *Amanita muscaria*	Toxin found in two of the more common poisonous fungi, which can easily be eaten in error. Incubation period <6 hours. Symptoms include diarrhoea, vomiting, abdominal pain, sweating, twitching, diplopia and convulsions.
Amanitine	*Amanita phalloides* ('death cap')	Incubation period 6–24 hours. Symptoms include diarrhoea and vomiting, abdominal pain, jaundice and acute renal failure. Mortality 50–90%.
Solanine	*Solanum tuberosum* (potatoes)	Incubation period a few hours. Leads to headache, fever, abdominal pain, diarrhoea and vomiting. The alkaloid toxin is water-soluble, so peeling and soaking potatoes before cooking alleviates the problem.
Scombrotoxin	Scombroid fish – tuna and mackerel. Also pilchards, herring.	An increased histamine level in the fish leads to facial flushing, urticarial rash, nausea, diarrhoea and vomiting. Incubation period usually within 1–2 hours.
Ciguatera fish poisoning	Toxin produced by dinoflagellates and accumulates within flesh of fish which feed on them	Incubation period usually within 1–2 hours. Causes nausea, diarrhoea, paraesthesia of mouth and feet, weakness of legs. Seen increasingly because of tendency to holiday in exotic locations. Barracuda is one of the fish implicated.
Paralytic shellfish poisoning	Toxin produced by dinoflagellates that are eaten by shellfish. Toxin does not harm the shellfish but accumulates in the flesh.	Incubation period 30 minutes to 12 hours. Symptoms include circumoral paraesthesiae, numbness of limbs, incoordination, dizziness and drowsiness. In extreme cases may cause respiratory muscle paralysis. Has been a problem in the last few years off the northeastern coast of Britain.
Tetramine*	Red whelks	Incubation period often less than 1 hour. Causes headache, dizziness, diplopia, incoordination and drowsiness.
Nicotinic acid	Along with ascorbic acid added to minced beef to keep it pink.	Dose-related incubation period. Causes rash and tingling of face and extremities.

Source: Christi AB. *Infectious Diseases*. London: Churchill Livingston; 1987. (Except * which is additional material.)

- Avoid cross-contamination from raw meat (which should always be regarded as potentially contaminated) to cooked meat and other foodstuffs by storing it apart (store raw foods below other foods to avoid dripping if they have to be in the same fridge) and by using separate cutting tools and other utensils for each.
- Clean and disinfect equipment used for food, such as kitchen utensils, chopping boards and worktops. The widely accepted meaning of ' cleaning' in food safety is the removal of dirt and grease. This may not kill harmful bacteria, so disinfection chemicals are usually applied afterwards. Different (and often incompatible) chemicals and practices are used for each stage.
- Avoid transference of infection from the nose and throat by the fingers to food. When cuts and sores occur, ensure they are covered.
- Exclude people with symptoms of food poisoning from food handling based on Food Standards Agency guidance.
- Store food at the right temperature. Fridges and freezers should be kept at the correct temperatures: best practice is below 4°C for cold food, above 63°C for hot food and below –18°C for frozen food. This will greatly restrict the growth of almost all food-poisoning bacteria. Food businesses may have to follow different temperature requirements; the Food Standards Agency provide guidance. Chilled foods should not be maintained at room temperature for any length of time. Frozen food, especially poultry, should be completely defrosted before cooking.
- Special care should be taken when cooking food for later use and when reheating it. Cooling should be undertaken quickly and can be speeded up by dividing into portions. Reheating should not be undertaken more than once and should be thorough.
- Shoppers should take chilled or frozen food home quickly and store it in the fridge or freezer, rather than letting it stand in the car or office. It is good practice to use cool boxes, especially in the summer.
- Food should be allowed to stand for the recommended periods of time before serving after microwave cooking.
- Pets should be kept out of, and pests and insects should be eliminated from, food storage, display and preparation areas.

Ensuring proper adherence to these measures in all situations in which food is stored, prepared and served is vitally important. In the commercial context, it requires that senior management is fully committed to food hygiene and safety and that all relevant staff are effectively trained, although there is no legal requirement for qualifications. With the kind of transient workforces that exist in the catering and hotel industries, this requires special effort. Environmental health officers play a key role in education and in protecting the public.

Careful preparation of food in the home is just as important as it is for large-scale catering concerns. Even if foodstuffs are contaminated when they are bought, the measures listed above can be taken in the home to help ensure that micro-organisms do not cause illness, either directly or through being spread to other foods.

It is also important for the public to receive information on specific issues as they arise, such as the risk of botulism in home bottling of vegetables (described earlier). Another example is the risk of *Salmonella* transmission from eggs; current Food Standards Agency advice to the general public is that it would be prudent not to eat raw eggs or uncooked foods made with eggs. To pregnant women, to the very young, to the elderly and to the sick, the advice is that eggs should be cooked until the white and the yolk are hard before they are eaten.

The Law Relating to Food-borne Illness

In addition to general legislation relating to infectious diseases, there is a large body of legislation relating to food hygiene and safety, an important element in the range of control measures for food-borne illness.

Most food legislation is based on European Union law, which applies in all European Union member states. European Union food law also imposes conditions on the import of food from non-European Union countries that wish to trade with the European Union. In the UK, the legislation applies to over 600 000 food businesses, from slaughterhouses at one end of the food chain through to retail and catering businesses at the other end.

Under the legislation, it is a requirement that almost all food businesses should be registered or approved, depending on the nature of their trade, and failure to do so is an offence. This provides local authorities and other food enforcement bodies with information to carry out inspections and enforce the law.

With its focus on consumer protection, food legislation places obligations on food business operators to ensure the safety of food. It is an offence, punishable by fine or imprisonment, to place unsafe food on the market. The legislation also provides a range of powers to take enforcement action to ensure food business operators meet these obligations.

In the case of a large-scale food poisoning outbreak or evidence of widespread food contamination, where it is necessary, the Food Standards Agency issues food alerts. These provide local enforcement bodies with information or advice necessary for action to investigate problems and ensure unsafe food is not sold to the public. Where appropriate, such action is undertaken in parallel with advice issued at local or national level to alert consumers.

OTHER INFECTIVE CAUSES OF VOMITING AND DIARRHOEA

Illnesses characterised by vomiting, diarrhoea and associated symptoms are common in the population, and not all are food-borne. Many are transmitted from person to person by the faecal–oral route or by droplets. Some of the organisms that can be transmitted in this way can also be food-borne.

This section of the chapter describes organisms that cause illness mainly through person-to-person spread, though the fact that they are not described in the previous section does not mean that some of them cannot also be spread by ingestion of food contaminated with the organism.

Viruses

A variety of viruses regularly cause diarrhoea and vomiting. A spectrum of gastrointestinal symptoms in which viruses have been implicated has been recognised for many years and was often referred to as winter vomiting disease. Characteristics of viral gastroenteritis are that symptoms are sometimes severe but short-lived, lasting 24 to 48 hours, and the incubation period is usually fairly short. Fatalities are rare but can occur in the elderly and the very young.

Viruses are much more difficult to identify from specimens such as faeces than are bacteria, and they are only present at the beginning of the acute stage of the illness, so reported cases undoubtedly grossly under-represent the true size of the problem. People do not always present to medical care for these self-limiting illnesses. General practitioners treat symptomatically and do not collect samples. Viruses are difficult to isolate from human and food specimens. All this means that the frequency of these viruses in the population and other aspects of their epidemiology are not well understood.

Rotaviruses are RNA viruses that cause vomiting, diarrhoea and fever, mainly amongst children under five years of age. Rotavirus infection is a major cause of diarrhoea in children. The incubation period ranges from 24 to 72 hours, and symptoms typically last for 4 to 6 days. The profuse watery diarrhoea in infants can lead to severe dehydration and death, and rotavirus infection is a major cause of admissions to paediatric units during the winter months. Adults are less frequently affected. It is estimated that 18 000 children in England and Wales are hospitalised with rotavirus infection each year. Efforts to produce a vaccine against rotavirus are underway in order to combat this important cause of childhood morbidity and consequent hospital usage. Adenoviruses cause similar symptoms.

Another group of viruses that cause symptoms of diarrhoea and vomiting are the so-called 'small round structured viruses' (SRSVs), of which the most well known is perhaps the Norwalk virus. The incubation period is usually 24 to 48 hours, and symptoms typically last for about 48 hours. It is characterised by the sudden onset of diarrhoea and explosive vomiting. Symptomatic patients shed millions of virus particles into the environment. These contaminate surfaces and appear to remain viable for some time, infecting others who pick them up on their hands.

They are an important cause of outbreaks in institutional settings such as hospitals and nursing homes. They are also becoming an increasing problem for the leisure industry. Outbreaks in hotels or on cruise liners can be very difficult to control, especially when susceptible people (as new guests) continue to be introduced at regular intervals, setting up the chain of transmission over and over again. The mainstay of control in all these settings is prompt and thorough cleaning of body-fluid spillages and isolation of affected individuals. Even with rigorous regimens in place, the chain of transmission can be very difficult to interrupt. Sewage pollution of shellfish is an important means of food-borne spread. A classic scenario is an outbreak following a romantic dinner on St Valentine's Day because of the consumption of raw contaminated oysters.

Dysentery: Bacillary

Shigella is a group of Gram-negative bacilli of which there are four species: *Shigella sonnei*, which accounts for the great majority of cases of dysentery occurring in Britain; *Shigella flexneri*, which is only an occasional cause of infection in Britain, but was found most frequently historically in hospitals for the mentally ill or those with learning disabilities; *Shigella boydii*; and *Shigella dysenteriae*, which is very seldom the cause of dysentery in Britain.

The disease has a worldwide distribution. In the United Kingdom, epidemics of *S. sonnei* occur amongst young and school-age children every seven years or so. During the last major epidemic, over 17 000 cases were notified in England and Wales in one year (1992). In inter-epidemic years, the number of notifications can drop approximately ten-fold. There were just over a thousand laboratory-confirmed isolates of *Shigella* species in 2006. The most common was *S. sonnei*. Outbreaks of *S. sonnei* dysentery are often associated with day and residential nurseries and with nursery and infant schools. The laboratory diagnosis of Shigella infection is made by isolation of the organisms from the faeces.

There are many mild cases of this disease, while others have few or no symptoms. When the full clinical picture occurs, it is typified by diarrhoea of acute onset (with mucus, blood and pus in more severe cases), abdominal pain and fever.

The incubation period ranges between 12 to 96 hours (usually 1 to 3 days) but can be up to seven days for *S. dysenteriae*. Patients are highly infectious during the acute stage of the illness and continue to excrete the organism for about four weeks after recovery. In a minority of cases, a chronic carrier state may develop.

The reservoir for infection is the human gastrointestinal tract, and transmission is by the faecal–oral route, either directly or indirectly. The direct method is probably quite common. Young children carry the infection on their hands and pass it to other children or members of the family. Indirect transmission by ingestion of contaminated food or drink is also quite common.

In an established case, control measures include instituting standard precautions, including care in the handling of excreta from the patient. Bacteriological screening of well contacts is usually not necessary unless the contacts are food handlers, work in the health care field or in outbreak situations.

General preventive measures include hand washing after using the toilet, the use of disposable paper towels, regular cleaning of lavatory door handles and seats and extra precautions in the preparation of food. Food handlers with bacillary dysentery should be excluded from work until three negative specimens have been obtained. In the event of an outbreak in a day nursery, all new admissions should cease and all infected children should be excluded. Three negative specimens are required before affected children may be readmitted. Once an outbreak is established in an infant school or nursery, it is difficult to control the spread of *S. sonnei* dysentery, even with the measures recommended. General environmental measures are less important in Britain but include adequate disposal of sewage and the control of fly populations.

Dysentery: Amoebic

Amoebic dysentery is caused by *Entamoeba histolytica*, a protozoan that can become a cyst with a tough, resistant membrane. In the human intestine it can emerge from the cyst in its active form and cause symptoms. It is most commonly found in the tropics and subtropics. Most of the cases occurring in Britain each year are people who have contracted the disease in an endemic area overseas. A small proportion, possibly 2% of the population, are carriers.

The clinical presentation varies, with many people remaining asymptomatic while others proceed to ulceration of the bowel and hepatic involvement. The classical clinical picture of amoebic dysentery is abdominal pain and recurrent attacks of diarrhoea containing blood or mucus. There are periods of remission and the cycle may continue for years. From this primary colonic site, in a small proportion of cases, the infection can spread to involve other organs (most often the liver). It is important to exclude amoebic dysentery when making the diagnosis of ulcerative colitis. The diagnosis of amoebic dysentery is made by observing large amoebae-containing red blood cells on microscopic examination of specimens of faeces. Tests on sera are available but are positive in only a proportion of cases and, most importantly, do not identify the carrier state.

The incubation period is variable, most often two to four weeks, but it can extend to months. Cysts may continue to be passed in the faeces for many years. Man is the sole reservoir, either as symptomless excreter or with the chronic disease. The infection is transmitted by the cysts through faecal–oral spread. The usual vehicle is contaminated water or food – especially salads and raw fruit.

Provided proper precautions are taken in nursing the patient, no isolation is necessary, nor is there any need for surveillance of contacts except to ensure that fellow travellers have not contracted the disease. The maintenance of good standards of personal hygiene and the exclusion of cases from food handling are important in preventing this disease, as is the provision of a pure water supply and an adequate sewage disposal system.

Enteric Fever

Enteric fever is caused by either *Salmonella enterica serovar Typhi* (typhoid fever) or *Salmonella enterica serovar Paratyphi* types A, B and C (paratyphoid fever). These are Gram-negative rods identical in appearance and only distinguished by different reactions in laboratory tests. An enteric fever-like illness can also be caused by other members of the *Salmonella* family that usually cause gastroenteritis.

The diseases occur in all parts of the world, but endemic typhoid and paratyphoid has been virtually eliminated from northwestern Europe, North America and Australasia. The majority (approximately 90%) of the nearly 500 or so cases of typhoid (a similar number of paratyphoid) in the United Kingdom each year are contracted abroad, by people visiting India, Pakistan or Bangladesh.

The clinical picture of typhoid fever varies. Symptoms can include pyrexia, headache, anorexia and constipation (occasionally diarrhoea). A classical rose-spot rash may appear on the trunk, and enlargement of the spleen may also occur. Rarely, intestinal ulceration and perforation may occur. Paratyphoid fever has similar but milder symptomatology, with a lower fatality rate. Clinical symptoms depend on the dose of the organism, and a much larger dose is required to cause paratyphoid fever than to cause typhoid fever. Subclinical cases of paratyphoid fever also occur.

The laboratory diagnosis of the enteric fevers is made by isolating the organisms from blood culture (which is usually positive in the first week of illness) or from culture of faeces or urine (usually in the second and third weeks of the illness). Antibodies can be detected from the second week (Widal test), and a sharply rising titre in serial samples of sera confirms the diagnosis. Phage typing is also important.

The incubation period for typhoid fever is usually one to three weeks but can vary from three days to three months depending on the dose of organism. Paratyphoid infections have a shorter incubation period (one to ten days). Cases remain infectious for as long as the person excretes the organism, usually from the early stages of the illness until some weeks or even months after recovery. Up to 5% of typhoid fever cases become permanent carriers.

The reservoir of infection is human. Usually the organism is found in the faeces, but it can also occur in the urine. Considerable antibiotic resistance is evident in both typhoid and paratyphoid organisms. A permanent residue of infection is the gall bladder, and in extremely persistent carrier states where antibiotic therapy has failed, surgical intervention to remove it may be considered. The mode of transmission of infection par excellence is by food and drink that have been contaminated by faeces of the case or carrier. Particularly implicated are those substances on which the organism can multiply: pastries, meat, milk, milk products, ice cream and raw fruit and vegetables. Contaminated water supplies have also been responsible for typhoid outbreaks.

Cases should be isolated and particular care should be taken when handling the patient's urine and faeces. Contact tracing is generally limited to identification and screening of contacts in risk groups – particularly food handlers. If the contacts are food handlers or work with vulnerable groups of people (as is the case with health care workers), they should be excluded from work during this period.

Typhoid vaccine gives around 50–70% protection and is recommended for travellers to areas where typhoid is endemic, but it is important that travellers are aware of the risks, take precautions with their choice of food and do not drink local tap water. Other environmental control measures include adequate sewage disposal, the provision of a pure water supply and the control of flies and rodents. A high index of suspicion should be maintained in returning travellers from the regions described. Non-travel associated cases should be intensively investigated because they may have acquired the disease from a carrier in the community (he/she could then infect others).

Cholera

The causative organism is *Vibrio cholerae*, a slightly curved and twisted (comma-shaped), motile, aerobic Gram-negative rod. The O1 serogroup includes two biotypes of *V. cholerae*: classical and El Tor. The two types produce illnesses that are indistinguishable, but they differ in laboratory haemolysis tests. The O139 serogroup has recently been recognised as a cause of outbreaks of cholera.

During the last several hundred years, classical cholera has been endemic in the basins of the rivers Ganges and Brahmaputra, from which it has spread repeatedly as pandemics to many countries of the world. Fatality rates have been high, especially amongst the poor. A pandemic of the El Tor variant started in Indonesia in the 1960s and reached western Europe. Britain was virtually free of cholera during the twentieth century, except for the occasional imported case.

Evidence of the devastating effects that epidemics of the disease can still have in many parts of the world are seen from time to time on the television screens of the West when there are natural disasters (such as floods or earthquakes) or war. In such circumstances, sanitation can break down as people are displaced from their houses into makeshift and overcrowded camps. Cholera outbreaks then occur, often associated with huge loss of life, especially in the very young. It is most liable to happen when the sanitary infrastructure breaks down. For example, in Iraq in 2007, 3300 cases of cholera were reported. In that country, sewage works have been targeted by insurgents and water supplies are polluted. Similarly late in 2008, an outbreak initially affecting more than 10,000 (and increasing) people began in Zimbabwe, triggered by the breakdown of the country's infrastructure.

The characteristic clinical features of cholera are very severe diarrhoea with copious watery stools ('rice water') accompanied by vomiting and rapid dehydration. The latter causes death in a high proportion of untreated cases. The organism can be identified in cultures from specimens of vomit or faeces or in rectal swabs. A rise in antibody titre in paired samples of sera is helpful in confirming the diagnosis.

The incubation period is usually two to three days, although it may be as short as a few hours and as long as five days. The organism is excreted during the illness and for a few days after recovery. The carrier state is uncommon and usually lasts only a few months – in contrast to typhoid fever.

Humans are the only known mammalian host, although recent observations from America, Bangladesh and Australia demonstrate that environmental reservoirs exist. Transmission is mainly by faeces-contaminated water and also by food – particularly shellfish. Flies are not generally regarded as a significant vector, although fly control is regarded as important in the epidemic setting or in cholera wards. Direct spread from cases, carriers or contaminated objects is much less important. Gastric acid acts as a protector against infection.

Acutely ill patients require hospital treatment with careful management to replace lost fluids and electrolytes. Surveillance of contacts is important, and their stools should be examined for *V. cholerae* for five days following the last exposure. Contact surveillance is of limited value, unless they have been exposed to the same source of infection.

Vaccination gives low protection and short-lived immunity and is therefore of limited value. No vaccine is currently available in the United Kingdom. People travelling to areas where cholera is known to be present should take precautions with drinking water, salads and other uncooked foods.

The main environmental control measures are the protection of water supplies and the supervision of disposal of sewage. Health education of food handlers and measures to protect food against flies are also important. In a country with modern water supply and sewage disposal systems, cholera is of almost no public health importance (aside from recognising occasional imported cases).

RESPIRATORY INFECTIONS

Acute upper respiratory infections are still the commonest manifestation of illness caused by infectious disease in the population of the United Kingdom. They include colds, coughs, ear infections, bronchitis and pneumonia. A wide range of organisms are responsible, most of them viruses. Although such illnesses occur throughout the year, most display a marked seasonal variation.

Some common examples of viruses that cause respiratory infections are the common cold (for example, rhinoviruses, myxoviruses, picornaviruses, coronaviruses); those causing sore throats (for example, ECHO virus, Coxsackie virus, adenoviruses); the Epstein-Barr virus, which causes infectious mononucleosis (also called glandular fever); the respiratory syncytial virus, which causes coughs, ear and chest infections; parainfluenza viruses, which cause croup in children and other respiratory infections; and influenza itself.

There are no fully effective control measures for this group of infections, and action is directed at minimising the complications of the clinical syndrome by prompt diagnosis, symptomatic treatment and treatment of complications. However, better population hygiene (covering the mouth and nose when coughing and sneezing) and better hand hygiene do make an impact. Vaccine for influenza is the exception where there is scope for preventing the seasonal form of the disease.

STREPTOCOCCAL INFECTIONS

Streptococci are Gram-positive, spherical bacteria that tend to form chains when they grow. An important feature that determines their classification is whether or not they produce haemolysis when grown on a medium containing red blood cells: complete haemolysis (beta-haemolytic streptococci), partial haemolysis (alpha-haemolytic streptococci) or no haemolysis at all. A further classification is made on the basis of antigenic differences in the components of the cell wall. On this basis, beta-haemolytic streptococci are divided into a number of serological ('Lancefield') groups (A to G).

Group A beta-haemolytic streptococci are the most important of them and often cause sore throats and tonsillitis. Scarlet fever is now, fortunately, infrequent. More rarely, the organism can result in a number of other infections: erysipelas, impetigo, puerperal fever, necrotising fasciitis or bacterial endocarditis. After a delay of several weeks, infection with the beta-haemolytic group A streptococcus may result in acute nephritis or rheumatic fever. These delayed manifestations are probably hypersensitivity reactions, not infections. They were much more common in the past, but it is possible that they will again become problematic if virulence of the causative organism changes.

Haemolytic streptococci also cause other infections. Groups A, B and G cause several thousand cases of bacteraemia each year in Britain. The infection occurs in all age groups but is particularly serious when it occurs in babies – especially premature babies. Much less commonly, the same groups of organism cause bacterial meningitis. Again, all age groups are affected but the disease is a particular problem in neonates.

Streptococcal infection occurs in most parts of the world but is more common in temperate zones. Streptococcal throats are characterised by sudden onset of sore throat, fever and inflamed tonsils, with exudate and enlarged lymph glands. The tongue may have a strawberry-like appearance in the early stages of the disease. The main differential diagnosis is with viral infections of the upper respiratory tract, which are often clinically indistinguishable. If, in addition, an erythematous rash appears several days later, scarlet fever is likely. At the beginning of the twentieth century, this disease was a major cause of death of children, but it is now a milder, treatable illness.

The more serious complications – bacteraemia, nephritis, meningitis, endocarditis and rheumatic fever – are identified by the clinical manifestations characteristic of these conditions. The organism can be cultured from throat swabs, where the beta-haemolytic streptococcus will be seen surrounded by its characteristic zone of haemolysis. Blood cultures are taken where bacteraemia is suspected. Rising serum antibody titres may be helpful in aiding diagnosis.

The incubation period is usually one to three days. Most patients cease to be infective 24 hours after starting treatment with antibiotics, although in some a persistent carrier state may develop.

The reservoir of infection is human, and transmission is by direct contact, droplet spread and via articles freshly contaminated with nasopharyngeal secretions. In the past, outbreaks have occurred through infected milk.

Isolation is unnecessary, because the patient becomes non-infective shortly after treatment is started, but it is usual to keep close contacts under surveillance for a few days. In closed communities of children, prophylactic antibiotics should be considered.

PNEUMONIA

Pneumonia is a common cause of illness and death amongst the very young, elderly people and those with suppressed immune systems. A wide range of organisms can be responsible, the most important being *Streptococcus pneumoniae* (the pneumococcus).

Pneumonia is much less common in younger, previously healthy people. When it does occur in such circumstances, the common organisms are *S. pneumoniae*, which may cause classical lobar pneumonia; *Mycoplasma pneumoniae*, which can cause pneumonia but is also much more commonly responsible for milder respiratory illnesses; and Legionnaires' disease. In Britain pneumonia tends to occur in small winter epidemics every four years or so.

A pneumococcal polysaccharide vaccine has been shown to prevent invasive pneumococcal infection and is recommended for those over 65 years and those at high risk of pneumococcal infection by virtue of underlying disease or immunosuppressive treatment, including those with an absent or dysfunctional spleen. A conjugate pneumococcal vaccine is now part of the childhood immunisation programme (see later in this chapter).

LEGIONNAIRES' DISEASE

This illness derived its name from 183 cases of pneumonia that occurred amongst nearly 4000 delegates attending an American Legion convention in Philadelphia in July 1976. The episode attracted wide publicity, particularly in view of the 15% fatality rate, and it was intensely investigated. Many agents were suggested as being responsible for the outbreak, some of them fanciful, but it was eventually established that the disease was caused by a small, previously unrecognised

Gram-negative bacillus (named *Legionella pneumophila*), which was isolated from the water in the air-conditioning system in the hotel. In all, some 35 species of Legionella and about 45 serogroups have been identified. The predominant human pathogen is *Legionella pneumophila* serogroup 1.

Between 300 and 500 cases are reported in England and Wales each year, mostly sporadic or in small groups. About half the known affected people have acquired the infection abroad. A number of outbreaks have occurred. An outbreak in which 101 people developed Legionnaires' disease (28 died from it) was associated with a hospital cooling tower in Stafford in 1985. The subsequent committee of inquiry made recommendations that form part of present policy to control the disease. Another outbreak affecting over 90 people in central London in 1988 was associated with a British Broadcasting Corporation (BBC) building. In November 2003, 28 cases occurred in Hereford. The outbreak was eventually traced to a cooling tower.

Other than sources that affect a resident population in an area, such as cooling towers, the disease can be acquired in a range of other settings, including hotels, nursing homes, cruise ships, shopping malls and even car washes. A typical small-scale 'outbreak' occurred amongst three United Kingdom travellers on a European coach tour to France, Switzerland and Italy in August 2007. Two people developed the disease and survived, and one died from it. The group of 42 passengers had stayed in seven hotels in a 13-day tour.

The disease is most common in adults, and while anyone can acquire the infection, those who smoke heavily or who have a chronic disease appear to be at higher risk. Clinically, the condition is rarely distinguishable from other causes of pneumonia. Early symptoms are non-specific, with fever, malaise, myalgia, headache and often diarrhoea. As the illness progresses, the patient develops a high fever and non-productive cough, which becomes productive. Chest signs are often unimpressive and not in keeping with the marked changes observed on chest X-ray. The overall case fatality rate in patients admitted to hospital is about 10–15%.

In addition to history and clinical features, diagnosis is made by culture of the organism from secretions, by serological testing or by detection of urinary antigen (for *L. pneumophila* serogroup 1). Culture of the organism is difficult. Detection of urinary antigen is therefore a very useful diagnostic test, since the antigen can be detected early in the illness (during the first 10 to 14 days), long before serology becomes positive. This speeds up considerably the ability to mount a public health investigation.

The incubation period is usually between 2 and 10 days (usually 5 to 6 days) but has been reported to be as long as 18 days. Person-to-person spread has not been demonstrated.

The bacterium is widely distributed in nature and often found in soil and water. Although not usually found in mains water supplies, it may become established in complex water systems in large buildings such as hotels, hospitals and office blocks. Surveys have shown that the organism is commonly present in systems of such buildings. The likelihood of this is increased by stagnation and water temperatures between 20°C

and 45°C. Water-cooled air-conditioning systems and the towers associated with them are another common source of the organism.

The presence of *L. pneumophila* in a system does not necessarily lead to an outbreak of Legionnaires' disease. Nevertheless, the main route of infection when it does occur seems to be via inhalation of contaminated aerosols from, for example, cooling towers or from spa baths.

Since Legionnaires' disease was first recognised, and since the larger outbreaks occurred in Britain, a wide range of regulatory and standard-setting guidance has been put in place. This will continue to be updated as research into the organism and the disease continues. The key to control lies in preventive measures taken by those involved in the design, operation, supervision and maintenance of water systems and cooling systems – particularly in large buildings. Detailed codes of practice are available. Important aspects include regular inspection, cleaning and disinfection, as well as careful temperature regulation. A cooling-tower registration scheme is now in operation to assist monitoring compliance and outbreak investigation.

A non-pneumonic infection with *L. pneumophila* also occurs: so called 'Pontiac fever'. It has a much shorter incubation period (5 to 66 hours), and although the attack rate is much higher (approximately 95% in outbreaks compared with 0.1% to 5% for Legionnaires' disease), it is a much less severe illness from which patients recover spontaneously in about two to five days. Pontiac fever appears to arise as an allergic reaction to inhaled antigen, possibly from dead bacteria, rather than as a result of bacterial invasion.

INFLUENZA

Influenza viruses are divided into three main groups: influenza A, B and C. Most outbreaks and epidemics of influenza are caused by type A viruses. Influenza B and C viruses infect people only. Influenza A virus can also infect birds and other animals (pigs and horses, for example). The ability of the virus to jump between species is important in the way that it evolves into new strains capable of producing large-scale outbreaks or even pandemics of influenza. Influenza viruses are passed easily from person to person through the air when someone who is infected with the virus coughs or sneezes (droplet infection) or when someone touches a surface contaminated by the virus.

Influenza viruses usually have an incubation period of between one and three days and cause symptoms of variable severity, such as headache, sore throat, cough, aches and pains, running nose, weakness and fatigue.

Virology

Influenza viruses have two glycoproteins on their surface – a haemagglutinin and a neuraminidase. They are the antigens that characterise the particular strain of influenza virus. There are 16 different haemagglutinins and nine neuraminidases. They produce an antibody response when someone is infected.

The convention is to give each influenza

A virus an 'H' number and an 'N' number to define the subtype. The numbers refer to the particular haemagglutinin and neuraminidase involved. A name is used to define the variant (which differs antigenically between subtypes). Thus the influenza A virus that caused the pandemic in 1957 was an H2N2 subtype, and the variant was called 'Asian influenza'.

Influenza viruses are very unstable antigenically, frequently becoming transformed into new variants and less often into new subtypes. When a new variant occurs that is different antigenically to the currently circulating subtype, antigenic drift is said to have occurred. This happens periodically with influenza A viruses that cause seasonal or winter influenza. Larger outbreaks then tend to occur because fewer people have immunity to it. The size of the outbreak and the severity of symptoms varies greatly and depends on the degree of cross-infection by (or vaccination against) the previous variant as well as environmental and other factors.

A second and more dramatic type of transformation of the protein structure of the influenza A virus is the so-called antigenic shift. This happens when an entirely new subtype is formed. The population has very little immunity since the subtype is so different to circulating seasonal influenza strains. As a result, the virus spreads widely and usually causes a pandemic (a worldwide epidemic).

These transformations of the influenza A virus occur in one of three ways. The most common way for antigenic drift to occur is through adaptation of the virus during the normal process of viral replication. The most common way for antigenic shift is through a process of reassortment – an exchange of genetic material between two different influenza viruses, often a human and an animal one. A person or an animal (such as a pig) can act as a 'mixing vessel' for the two viruses.

Less commonly, an antigenic shift is caused by genetic adaptation of a bird (or other animal) influenza virus to a human influenza virus. This route of transformation is thought to have created the 1918 'Spanish influenza' pandemic, and it generally results in a virus that causes more severe infections and more deaths than a virus resulting from reassortment.

Key Distinction: Seasonal, Avian and Pandemic Influenza

It is important to distinguish clearly three different influenza situations. *Seasonal influenza* is an illness caused by influenza viruses of a subtype that has been around for a number of years and to which the population has a relatively high level of immunity (either because they have had an influenza illness caused by the virus or been vaccinated against it). When people get it, many illnesses are mild, though some people get serious complications, and in some sections of the population (the very young, the very old and those with chronic diseases) there are deaths.

Avian influenza is an illness of birds (wild and domesticated). It transmits easily from bird to bird but can only infect people with difficulty (typically those who are in close contact with infected poultry). Avian influenza viruses are, however, 'candidates'

to reassort with human influenza viruses to generate an antigenic shift (a new subtype of influenza causing a pandemic).

Pandemic influenza is an illness of people caused by the emergence of a new influenza virus subtype to which the population has no (or little) natural immunity. This happens by reassortment or mutation (as discussed above). Large numbers of people became ill, and the number of deaths is substantially above the excess deaths in normal flu seasons.

Pandemic Influenza: Past and Future

Three past pandemics of influenza have been well documented. All were in the twentieth century (Figure 9.12). The first was caused by the H1N1 subtype of influenza A and emerged in 1918 as the 'Spanish influenza'. The prospect of any similar event to the Spanish influenza pandemic is much feared because of its severity. Between 1918 and 1919, the influenza virus responsible infected an estimated 20% of the world's population and killed 40–50 million people. A significant feature was that it affected young adults (20–40-year-olds) disproportionately.

To some extent, the severity of the Spanish influenza pandemic was accentuated because it fell in an era when levels of general population health and nutrition were much poorer than they are today and when there was an absence of the benefits of modern medicine (such as antibiotics and intensive care units). Nevertheless, there is evidence that the virus itself was capable of producing much more serious illness than occurred in later pandemics. This was probably because it produced a much greater and

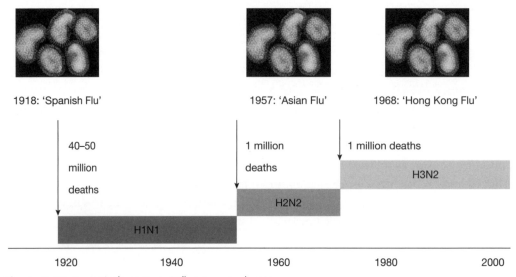

Figure 9.12 Twentieth-century influenza pandemics

earlier viral invasion of the lungs rather than the upper respiratory tract.

Studies of the influenza virus recovered from bodies frozen and preserved in the permafrost in Alaska have allowed scientists to genetically map the Spanish influenza virus. It is almost certain that it arose through mutation (genetic adaptation) from an avian influenza virus rather than through reassortment. This could explain its virulence and the high mortality it induced.

The second pandemic of influenza in the twentieth century happened in 1957–58. It was caused by the H2N2 subtype of influenza A virus and was dubbed 'Asian influenza'. While, as expected, it caused much more widespread and serious illness than seasonal influenza, it was a much milder pandemic than the Spanish influenza 40 years previously.

The Asian influenza pandemic began in the Far East in May of 1957. The first cases in Britain were seen in June of that same year in limited outbreaks. When the schools opened in September, there was a major surge to epidemic levels. There was a second wave at the beginning of 1958. During the autumn and winter of 1957–58, there were approximately 50 000 influenza-related deaths.

The third influenza pandemic of the twentieth century came a decade later, in 1968–69. It was caused by a H3N2 subtype of the influenza A virus and was called 'Hong Kong influenza'. The first isolation of the new virus in Britain was in August 1968. Throughout the autumn of 1968, into the winter and to the spring of 1969, there were more cases and local outbreaks, but there was no large-scale epidemic in Britain. This was in marked contrast to the situation in the United States that same year, where there was a large epidemic with high attack rates and many deaths. North America was unusual compared to other temperate parts of the world in suffering a high impact from

Hong Kong influenza during the winter of 1968–69. It was the following winter of 1969–70 that major epidemics took place in Britain and other European countries. This pattern of spread was very different to the Asian influenza pandemic and illustrates how unpredictably influenza viruses behave.

Given the regular cyclical occurrence of pandemics, the first twenty-first century pandemic of influenza is regarded by experts as inevitable ('when not whether'). This serious threat to the public health has moved to the top of the agenda of national governments and the international community. This is for a number of reasons: firstly, there has been a realisation of the potential of a pandemic to produce large numbers of deaths and major economic damage and a desire to find a way to mitigate these effects; secondly, the mobilisation of international leaders to address the threat of terrorism (including bioterrorism) led to the scrutiny of other risks; thirdly, there is sensitivity amongst politicians – in the light of SARS and Hurricane Katrina – that they lack competence and have been complacent in responding to major emergencies.

Most attention has focused on the spread of a particular avian influenza virus (H5N1) that emerged in China in 1997, causing outbreaks of illness and death amongst poultry and wild birds. A particular incident in May 1997 in Hong Kong involved the transmission of the virus from poultry to people. The first death was a 13-year-old boy, and a further 17 people were affected. The Chinese carried out a large-scale slaughter of poultry and the outbreak was controlled. Since then, H5N1 has spread widely in the wild bird population around the world. There have been many outbreaks in different countries amongst domesticated birds. There have been cases of illness and death amongst people.

This H5N1 avian influenza virus is regularly and repeatedly linked in media coverage to pandemic influenza. This leads to great misunderstanding of the relationship between them. It is important to understand the context.

➤ H5N1 is an avian influenza virus that primarily affects birds.

➤ The H5N1 avian influenza virus can infect people but crosses the species barrier with difficulty and almost always involves those who have had close contact with infected birds.

➤ The poor ability of the H5N1 avian influenza virus to infect people is illustrated by the relatively small number of human infections as against the large viral load amongst birds in circumstances where they are in close contact with people.

➤ The H5N1 virus could mutate or mix and reassort with another influenza virus and become associated with the initiation of the next influenza pandemic.

➤ Alternatively, an entirely different subtype of the influenza virus could emerge that is unrelated to H5N1.

Planning and Preparedness

It is difficult to predict precisely the impact of any future pandemic, but assumptions have to be made if planning and preparedness are to be effective. Previous pandemics provide a useful basis for impact assessment because their epidemiology is quite well documented.

Key elements are the proportion of the population who become infected, the severity of the illness and the proportion who will die. In the United Kingdom, up to half the population might fall ill with influenza and between 50 000 and 750 000 additional deaths could occur. Apart from the direct effects on health, a future pandemic will have much wider impact – disruption to public services, business and the economy will result from high sickness absence levels.

Planning to mitigate the impact of the next influenza pandemic is a high priority for the United Kingdom government and the governments of many other countries of the world. There is a great deal of international cooperation, led by the World Health Organization.

No one can be sure what influenza virus subtype will emerge in the new pandemic nor what its severity will be. Planning must therefore be based on a range of assumptions. Good statistical modelling is a key element in that it can use data from past pandemics and other sources to give a range of predictions, for example, on numbers of people who will be affected and number of deaths. Modelling data can also be used to assess different possible interventions. For example, how much is to be gained by border controls? Should antivirals be given only when people have symptoms or also prophylactically? Should schools be closed, and if so, at what point in the pandemic? Working out policy on these matters in advance is essential to good preparedness.

As far as the key countermeasures are concerned, there is nothing that can turn back the pandemic of influenza when it emerges. This is because a vaccine needs to be subtype- and strain-specific against the virus, and this cannot be known in advance. Modern science cannot yet provide a broad-spectrum influenza vaccine that protects against all known and unknown subtypes and strains of the influenza virus in advance. When a vaccine is raised, it is likely to take three to six months to produce, by which time the pandemic will be well underway in many countries. Nevertheless, it will still be worth having in order to protect those who have not yet been affected.

Research is ongoing to develop pre-pandemic vaccines. The consideration here is based on whether the pandemic will arise from a reassortment or mutation involving H5N1 Avian influenza (the 'bird flu' that has

Table 9.10 Potential impact of pandemic influenza in the United Kingdom

• 25–50% of people with symptoms
• 50 000–750 000 deaths
• 80 000–1.15 million people needing hospital care
• 15–20% of people absent from work during peak
• Duration 15 weeks
• Cost to society up to £1.24 billion

dominated the last decade), in which case a degree of cross-protection may be possible against an eventual human strain derived from it. Alternatively, if the pandemic influenza virus that eventually emerges is completely unrelated to H5N1, massive resources will have been wasted on the pre-pandemic vaccine. However, research is ongoing to devise a vaccine that could provide broader–spectrum protection.

The main countermeasure that can be prepared in advance is antiviral drugs. In many countries, including the United Kingdom, these have been stockpiled for distribution when the pandemic comes. Antiviral policy is not straightforward. Firstly, the drugs must be given in the first 24–48 hours of symptoms developing, otherwise they will not be effective. Secondly, they do not 'cure' influenza, they simply shorten the duration of the attack and possibly its severity. Thirdly, drug resistance can develop. Fourthly, antivirals have never been used in a mass or epidemic situation, so there may be unforeseen consequences.

Other elements of preparedness include raising public awareness, educating about the benefits of good hygiene (which does have an impact on slowing spread) and having good public messaging in place to use at different phases of the pandemic when it hits the country. Local health and social care services also need to have their own plans that assess capacity and contingencies and are well rehearsed. In the United Kingdom, central guidance from the departments of health of the various governments assists local services. Business and essential service continuity is very important, and awareness of the need for this and for detailed plans needs to be put in place.

It is important to recognise that planning for an influenza pandemic is not just a matter for health. All sectors of society and all government departments must be involved. In the United Kingdom, a subcommittee of the Cabinet under its emergency planning machinery coordinates action across all government departments to ensure that proper contingency plans are in place (such as disposal of the dead or policy on school closures) and that key policy positions are hammered out and agreed. Regular scenario planning exercises that cover the main national and international bodies are also essential to test the robustness of plans and highlight weaknesses and omissions (Table 9.11).

INFECTIONS FOR WHICH COMPREHENSIVE VACCINATION PROGRAMMES ARE AVAILABLE

When the NHS was founded in 1948, most children were offered vaccination against just two diseases: smallpox and diphtheria. Smallpox vaccination was eventually phased out as the disease became eradicated globally. During the first half of the twentieth century, vaccines were developed against the common infectious diseases of childhood. In the early years, there was no official programme to offer the vaccines, and population coverage rates were not high enough to stop the diseases spreading. For 'herd immunity', it is necessary to hit vaccine coverage rates of well over 90% for the most infectious diseases (such as measles).

The establishment in the mid-1980s of 'call and recall' systems based on child health

Table 9.11 Pandemic influenza: planning and countermeasures

- Global cooperation and coordination (particularly on policy, surveillance, and laboratories)
- Statistical modelling
- Antiviral stockpiles and distribution
- Pandemic vaccine (fast-tracking production)
- Guidance given to health and social care system
- Business and essential service continuity plans
- Regular exercises and scenario planning
- Hand and respiratory hygiene campaigns
- Public preparedness and communication

records supported by computerisation enabled appointments and reminders to be sent to parents when children reached the appropriate age for vaccination. This, together with targets and incentive payment for general practitioners, has enabled much higher levels of coverage to be achieved.

The childhood vaccination programme has, without doubt, been one of the most successful public health interventions in modern public health, bringing about huge reductions in morbidity and mortality from a range of infectious diseases in childhood, many of which were still major killers in Britain as late as the 1950s. This section describes those infections for which large-scale immunisation is available (Table 9.12). It should not be used as a practical guide for immunisation. Details of individual vaccines and their indications and contraindications can be found in a Department of Health publication on immunisation against infectious disease that is regularly updated.[1]

PUBLIC ATTITUDES AND ACCEPTANCE OF VACCINATION

The success of vaccination programmes has been remarkable. Generations of children are alive who would otherwise have died from the infectious disease scourges of the past. Many others would have suffered the misery of these illnesses or sustained a disability as a result.

The folk memory of many of these diseases now rests in the mind of older grandparents and great-grandparents. The 'fear factor' for younger parents is missing. As a result, many parents worry instead about the possible complications of vaccines. This was the climate into which the unfounded scientific claims about autism, bowel disease and measles-mumps-rubella (MMR) vaccine were made. Most medical authorities considered the claim at the outset to be unsound and misleading to parents, but it dominated media coverage. Needless anxiety and distress were caused to millions of families, and the repercussions were felt in the falling MMR uptake rate. MMR has been a highly

Table 9.12 Routine childhood immunisation programme

At what age to immunise	Diseases protected against	Vaccine given
At birth (to babies who are more likely to come into contact with TB than the general population)	Tuberculosis	BCG
At birth (to babies whose mothers have hepatitis B)	Hepatitis B	Hep B
Two months old	Diphtheria, tetanus, pertussis (whooping cough), polio, *Haemophilus influenzae* type b (Hib), pneumococcal infection	DTaP/IPV/Hib Pneumococcal conjugate vaccine (PCV)
Three months old	Diphtheria, tetanus, pertussis, polio, *Haemophilus influenzae* type b (Hib), meningitis C (meningococcal group C)	DTaP/IPV MenC /Hib
Four months old	Diphtheria, tetanus, pertussis, polio, *Haemophilus influenzae* type b (Hib), meningitis C, pneumococcal infection	DTaP/IPV/Hib MenC PCV
Around 12 months old	*Haemophilus influenzae* type b (Hib), meningitis C	Hib/MenC
Around 13 months old	Measles, mumps and rubella (German measles), pneumococcal infection	MMR PCV
Three years and four months or soon after	Diphtheria, tetanus, pertussis, polio, measles, mumps, rubella	DTaP/IPV or DTaP/IPV and MMR
Girls aged 12 to 13 years	Cervical cancer caused by human HPV papillomavirus types 16 and 18	HPV
13 to 18 years old	Tetanus, diphtheria, polio	Td/IPV

effective vaccine used for over three decades, and it has an excellent safety profile.

Ten of the 13 authors of the original scientific paper that unfairly discredited MMR formally retracted some of the paper's conclusions, saying: 'We wish to make it clear that in this paper no causal link was established between (the) vaccine and autism, as the data were insufficient.[2] However, the possibility of such a link was raised. Consequent events have had major implications for public health. In view of this, we consider now is the appropriate time that we should together formally retract the interpretation placed on these findings in the paper.'

The MMR story has important lessons. Firstly, the public must be made constantly aware of the dangers of the diseases that vaccines protect against. It is not a risk-free decision to refuse a child a vaccine. Secondly, health professionals who advise parents on vaccines need the most up-to-date information on any claims of risks so that they can answer any questions from parents. Thirdly, the government must continue to be open about the information it has and offer it freely for independent scientific scrutiny. Finally, health and medical authorities should not allow themselves to be intimidated or vilified by those pressure groups ideologically opposed to vaccines. They should speak up objectively in defence of vaccines when it is appropriate to do so.

MEASLES

The measles virus is a paramyxovirus. Measles occurs in all parts of the world. In developed countries, it is usually a mild disease with a low mortality rate, although a complication rate of 10% can be expected. In developing countries with poorly nourished inhabitants, childhood mortality can be 10% or more.

Until the introduction of mass measles vaccination, few people in Britain reached adult life without having had the disease. The use of the vaccine has altered the previous classical pattern of two-yearly epidemics, and the number of notifications in England and Wales has fallen substantially (from nearly 140 000 in 1980 to 3700 in 2007, of which 971 were confirmed). However, the fall in uptake of the MMR vaccine has reduced the level of herd immunity, so outbreaks of measles are now becoming more common in the United Kingdom.

Infection with the virus produces a prodromal illness with upper-respiratory symptoms, pyrexia and spots (Koplik spots) on the buccal mucosa. Classically, the maculopapular rash appears on the fourth day of the illness, but this is variable. The blotchy rash starts on the face and spreads over the body. Secondary bacterial infection of the respiratory tract and otitis media are common complications, and encephalitis is rare. A very rare complication is subacute sclerosing panencephalitis, which develops late (approximately seven years after infection) and results in death within a few months. The frequency of cases proceeding to complications has remained unchanged since the introduction of the vaccination programme. The diagnosis is made initially on clinical grounds and confirmed by salivary antibody testing.

The incubation period is 7 to 18 days, usually 10 days. It is a very infectious illness, particularly in the prodromal phase, and the patient is infectious for four to five days after the appearance of the rash. The reservoir is human. Transmission is via droplet spread and directly by objects freshly contaminated by secretions from the nasopharynx.

PERTUSSIS (WHOOPING COUGH)

Pertussis is caused by *Bordetella pertussis*, a small, ovoid, Gram-negative coccobacillus that is difficult to culture and grows only on special media. It occurs throughout the world, and epidemics of pertussis tended to occur every four years. Since the early 1950s, when pertussis vaccine was introduced, the size of epidemics has progressively lessened, although the periodicity of epidemics remains. There were three major epidemics in the late 1970s and early 1980s that were a consequence of the reduction in the uptake of pertussis vaccination. Loss of public confidence in the vaccine occurred when it was suggested that vaccination caused brain damage, a claim that was subsequently shown to be invalid. Although the occurrence of the disease is now at very low levels, it has followed four-yearly cycles in peak incidence with an underlying downward trend.

Pertussis begins with a slow onset of an irritating cough that progresses to paroxysmal attacks over a period of a few weeks, and these may last for many months. The coughing attacks are accompanied by 'whooping' and vomiting. Pulmonary atelectasis and bronchopneumonia are common complications during the paroxysmal phase. Persisting low-grade infection encourages the development of chronic lung damage, bronchiectasis, but fortunately this has become a rare occurrence. Convulsions may occur in infants. Fatality rates are highest in children under six months.

Pertussis can be difficult to diagnose, and diagnosis depends on the history given by the mother. Similar clinical syndromes can be produced by viral respiratory infections. Organisms can be cultured from carefully taken pernasal swabs if there is no delay in getting them to a laboratory, although the organism is isolated in less than half the swabs taken. Since 2007 the Health Protection Agency has been undertaking enhanced surveillance for pertussis, including oral fluid analysis.

The incubation period is usually between 6 and 20 days. The patient is highly infectious during the catarrhal stages of the illness and for about three weeks after the onset of paroxysmal coughing. If the patient is treated with antibiotics, however, the infectivity period only lasts for about five days after the onset of therapy. The reservoir is human, and transmission occurs mainly by droplet spread but also indirectly from objects contaminated by fresh discharges from the upper respiratory tract.

The main control measure is prevention through the use of pertussis vaccine, which is a key element of the childhood vaccination programme in Britain. Pertussis control requires vaccine uptake in excess of 90%. Although rates in Britain remained well below this level for many years in the 1980s and 1990s, in part reflecting parental and health professional concern about the safety of earlier vaccines and litigation brought on the basis of allegations of neurological damage caused by them, vaccination uptake in the middle of the first decade of the twenty-first century was above 90%.

The major concern is the protection of unimmunised and therefore susceptible infants, although the introduction of an immunisation schedule starting at two months of age helps to alleviate this problem. Although it is often advised that babies should be isolated from infected children, such a measure is rarely, if ever, successful. There is an argument for protecting a vulnerable baby with a two-week course of antibiotics to stop them developing the infection. The child with the disease should be treated at the same time, since erythromycin rapidly eliminates the organism, although it has little effect on the clinical course unless given in the catarrhal phase of the disease. There is increasing awareness of pertussis as a disease of adults, often responsible for infecting young unimmunised children.

POLIOMYELITIS

Poliomyelitis is caused by poliovirus (three serological types), which belongs to the enteroviruses. Type 1 is the most virulent, most commonly causes epidemics and is most often isolated from paralytic cases. There has been a concerted worldwide effort to eliminate poliomyelitis by means of vaccination, and worldwide eradication is now within reach. By 2008, the last United Kingdom case arose in the year 2000 and was vaccine-associated.

Most people who are infected with the virus remain asymptomatic, while some develop an acute pyrexial illness in which the person affected may have a fever accompanied by headache, stiffness of the neck and gastrointestinal upset. A minority of patients develop paralysis through involvement of the motor neurones. The diagnosis may be suspected on clinical grounds, but every effort is made to confirm on laboratory evidence (such as viral cultures or antibodies). As we approach eradication of poliomyelitis, the occurrence of a case of acute flaccid paralysis warrants detailed investigation in order to exclude wild poliomyelitis as the cause.

The incubation period is commonly 7 to 14 days, although it has been as short as 3 days and as long as 35 days. Poliovirus can appear in throat secretions as quickly as 36 hours after infection and in faeces about three days after infection. The virus is excreted in the faeces for three to six weeks or more, although it can be isolated from the throat for only about a week after onset. The reservoir is human.

The faecal–oral route is the major mode of transmission, especially in areas of poor sanitation. In areas of good sanitation, spread by direct contact with pharyngeal secretions becomes much more significant. Oral polio vaccine remained the mainstay of polio control and eradication in endemic countries. Vaccine-associated poliomyelitis can occur – that is why the vaccination recommended in the United Kingdom is now the inactivated polio vaccine given by injection.

The World Health Organization has the aim of eliminating polio worldwide, but this is not yet accomplished, with cases still being reported from India, Pakistan, Afghanistan, Nigeria and other parts of Africa.

RUBELLA

The rubella virus is a member of the Togaviridae family of viruses. In 2007, there were 34 cases in England and Wales.

The virus produces a mild febrile illness with upper-respiratory symptoms, a fine macular rash and enlargement of the posterior cervical and occipital glands. The incubation period is usually 16–18 days, with a range of 14–23 days. It is a highly infectious disease: the patient is infectious a week before and a week after the appearance of the rash. Rising antibody titres can be demonstrated in paired sera with 10–14 day intervals during the 2–4 weeks following infection, and specific immunoglobulin can be detected for a month or so. The disease is easily confused with other viral infections and in many cases is subclinical. The reservoir is human and transmission is mainly by direct contact with droplets and respiratory secretions.

The public health importance of rubella lies in the risk of congenital rubella syndrome, which affects infants whose mothers had the disease during the first trimester of pregnancy. Defects are rare in children born to women infected after the twentieth week of pregnancy. At birth the infant can have a variety of defects, including cataracts, deafness, neurological damage and cardiac abnormalities. In some cases these are mild and not detected for some years after birth, at which stage it is too late to make a definitive diagnosis. Babies affected by congenital rubella may shed the virus for months or years.

Prevention includes avoidance of contact with cases of rubella by pregnant women, but any pregnant woman who is in contact should undergo serological screening. There is a possible risk in giving the vaccine in the early stages of pregnancy, hence it is not recommended when there is a possibility of pregnancy, although no cases of congenital rubella syndrome have so far arisen by this means.

The main thrust of United Kingdom policy is to eliminate the disease. The original strategy of protection of women of childbearing age by rubella immunisation was augmented in 1988 by the use of MMR vaccine given to young children. The live-attenuated rubella vaccine is combined with mumps and measles as part of the MMR (measles, mumps, rubella) vaccine given

to all children. Staff working with pregnant women should also be vaccinated (for example, nursing staff, medical students and ambulance personnel).

DIPHTHERIA

Diphtheria is caused by *Corynebacterium diphtheriae*, which is a slender, Gram-positive rod. The organism produces a powerful exotoxin. The disease has a worldwide distribution but is more common in temperate climates. It is seen in Britain from time to time in imported cases.

The disease is an acute upper respiratory-tract infection that may affect the tonsils, pharynx, larynx or nostrils and also the skin. The characteristic feature is the presence of a greyish membrane in the throat, firmly attached and surrounded by inflammation, with enlarged cervical lymph glands. The main hazards (which may cause death, particularly in an untreated case) are local obstruction of the respiratory passages (by the membrane) and the effects of the exotoxin on the myocardium and on the peripheral nervous system (most seriously leading to paralysis of the respiratory muscles). Throat or nose swabs are taken from the suspected case, carrier or contact, and the organism is identified after culture on a suitable medium. Once isolated, the *Corynebacterium* should be tested for toxigenicity by injection into guinea pigs or by in vitro diffusion techniques. Serum anti-toxin levels may further assist in diagnosis. Treatment and control measures should be taken without waiting for laboratory confirmation.

The incubation period is two to five days,

although it is occasionally a little longer. Cases are seldom infectious beyond four weeks, especially with effective treatment, but rarely a chronic carrier can shed organisms for six months or more. The reservoir is human. Transmission is by direct contact with another person or carrier, usually by the airborne route, may be spread indirectly by discharges or fomites (inanimate objects).

In order to control the spread of diphtheria, the patient is isolated and treated with antitoxin and suitable antibiotic therapy. Close contacts should have nose and throat swabs taken and be kept under surveillance for seven days. The non-immune are immunised with the toxoid, and prophylactic antibiotics may also be of value. Nose and throat swabs may identify carriers, who are then also isolated and treated with antibiotics until the carrier state no longer exists. Articles that have been in close contact with the patient should be disinfected, especially those that may have been contaminated with nasal or oral secretions.

Vaccination is an important control measure, so non-vaccinated children should be given a full course at once and others should be given a booster dose. The key control measure is the maintenance of a high level of immunity in the child population by means of an effective immunisation programme.

TETANUS

This serious illness is now relatively rare in England and Wales, largely due to active immunisation of children. The causative organism, *Clostridium tetani*; a Gram-positive, anaerobic, spore-forming bacillus, is widely distributed in nature and is commonly found in soil. The organism is introduced into the human body by a penetrating injury (during gardening, for example). Most cases now occur in intravenous drug users using contaminated needles and syringes.

The spores germinate in anaerobic conditions, producing a powerful exotoxin that is neurotoxic. This process takes 3 to 21 days, depending upon the severity of the wound. The average incubation period is about 10 days. The patient develops painful muscular contractions that initially affect the facial and neck muscles and go on to involve the muscles of the trunk. Involvement of the respiratory muscles leads to compromised breathing. In untreated cases, mortality is high (approximately 60%).

Treatment of a patient with tetanus involves surgical debridement of the wound; the administration of antitoxin, antibiotics and sedative; and intensive care nursing. People who have injured themselves in circumstances where they may have been exposed to tetanus should have the wound cleaned and should be offered vaccine (depending upon their immunisation history) and immunoglobulin. Long-term prevention of tetanus depends upon the childhood immunisation programme.

MUMPS

The mumps virus, a paramyxovirus, is spread by droplets or by direct contact with the saliva of an infected individual. The incubation period is usually about 18 days but may be as short as 12 days or as long as 25 days. The infected child becomes unwell with a headache, sore throat and fever, after which the salivary glands, particularly the parotids, become inflamed. The virus persists in the saliva for several days after the onset of parotitis. Subclinical infection occurs in some children and is important in perpetuating the spread of the virus.

Mumps infection may be complicated by orchitis in post-pubertal males, oophoritis in post-pubertal females, meningitis, encephalitis, and (rarely) pancreatitis. Permanent deafness is a rare consequence of mumps. Routine vaccination of children is the means of controlling mumps.

MENINGOCOCCAL C DISEASE

This is part of the United Kingdom's childhood vaccination programme but is described in the following section on meningitis.

HAEMOPHILUS INFLUENZAE

Haemophilus influenzae is a fastidious, Gram-negative bacillus. Non-capsulated strains of the organism are not invasive and tend to cause secondary infections of the respiratory tract. They are the commonest cause of otitis media in children. Of greater significance, however, are the six capsulated strains, which produce invasive disease.

Haemophilus influenzae type b infection (also known as Hib) used to be the most common bacterial cause of meningitis in children under the age of five years, with a peak incidence at 10 to 11 months of age. A major breakthrough in protecting children against infection by *Haemophilus influenzae* type b occurred with the successful development of a conjugated vaccine that confers high levels of immunity even in very young children. The vaccine was incorporated into the United Kingdom's childhood immunisation programme in October 1992. The incidence of Hib has plummeted since vaccination was introduced (Figure 9.13).

The disease often had an insidious onset with malaise and a high temperature before the characteristic features of meningitis appear: vomiting, headache, neck stiffness and, in infants, a bulging fontanelle. The incubation period is thought to be short (two to four days). The infection is spread by secretions from the respiratory tract, which remain infectious for as long as the organisms are present but are rendered non-infectious 24 to 48 hours after the commencement of antibiotics. Person-to-person spread, giving rise to secondary cases, occurs.

The attack rate was estimated at around 5% prior to the introduction of the vaccine, with children under four years of age being those most at risk. For this reason, antibiotic chemoprophylaxis is recommended for all household contacts of the index case (including adults) when there are other unimmunised under-fours in the family. It should also be considered when two cases occur in children in the same nursery class, but advice on the use of prophylaxis in this specific situation should be sought from the local health protection services.

In addition to meningitis, Hib is also responsible for producing other invasive diseases, such as epiglottitis, pneumonia, cellulitis, septic arthritis and osteomyelitis.

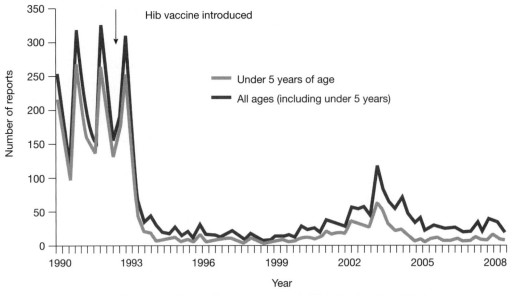

Figure 9.13 Reports of *Haemophilus influenzae* Type b (Hib) in England and Wales

HUMAN PAPILLOMAVIRUS

Cervical cancer is the second most common female cancer worldwide. A total of about 2700 new cases of invasive cervical cancer are diagnosed in the United Kingdom each year, and around 950 women die. Cervical cancer screening has helped to reduce mortality rates over the last 30 years since it was introduced systematically in this country.

Human papillomavirus (HPV) is a double-stranded DNA virus. Although the virus can cause respiratory infections, the more serious concern is its ability to infect the genital and anal tracts. There are more than 100 types of human papillomavirus, and about 40% infect the genital tract. It is the most common viral sexually transmitted infection and affects half of sexually active women at some stage of their lives. Peak incidence is in the teenage years and early twenties (Figure 9.14). The virus can leave someone asymptomatic, but can also cause genital warts, cervical cancer and cancer of the head and neck.

As a result of a full scientific assessment of the benefits and risks, a programme of vaccination against human papillomavirus for 12–13-year-old girls was introduced in 2008.

PNEUMOCOCCUS

Infection with pneumococcus can cause meningitis, septicaemia and pneumonia in babies and children as well as less serious problems, such as ear infections. Children under one year old are particularly susceptible.

A conjugate pneumococcal vaccine was introduced in 2006. Before then, there were around 5000 cases of invasive pneumococcal disease each year in England and Wales, of which 530 occurred in children under two years old. There were 50 deaths of children, the majority from pneumococcal meningitis. Survivors are often left severely disabled.

The conjugate vaccine, now part of the routine childhood immunisation programme, protects against the seven most common strains of *Streptococcus pneumoniae*. By midway through 2008, there had been a major reduction in cases of invasive disease.

OTHER COMMON CHILDHOOD INFECTIONS
CHICKENPOX

Chickenpox is caused by the varicella-zoster virus, which is a member of the herpes virus family. It is a very common infection worldwide, usually causing a mild illness in children. Chickenpox is one of the most highly infectious diseases occurring in humans, spreading rapidly and readily.

It is characterised by the development of fever and a rash that first appears on the trunk. The rash is flat to start with (macular) but swiftly becomes vesicular. The vesicle fluid contains virus particles, although the skin lesions are not as infectious as secretions from the respiratory tract. Transmitted mainly by this means, it is most infectious from a couple of days before the onset of the rash up to about five days after the first crop of vesicles appear. The incubation period is usually 2 to 3 weeks but can be 7 to 26 days.

Usually a mild illness, chickenpox can have a profound effect in immunocompromised individuals, in whom it can be fatal. Occasional deaths in otherwise healthy adults occur because of varicella pneumonia. Neonates are at risk of a severe generalised infection, as are pregnant women. Varicella-zoster immune globulin (VZIG) is indicated in certain circumstances for non-

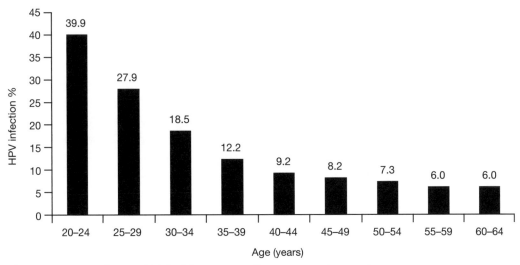

Figure 9.14 Prevalence of high-risk HPV according to age quinquennia
Source: Kitchener HC, Almonte M, Wheeler P, *et al.* HPV testing in routine cervical screening: cross sectional data from the ARTISTIC trial. *Br J Cancer.* 2006; **95**(1): 56–61.

immune pregnant women and for neonates who have been exposed to chickenpox, but it is in short supply and its use is strictly limited – specialist advice must be sought.

Herpes zoster, commonly known as shingles, tends to occur in older adults and is a local manifestation of reactivation of the chickenpox virus. The commonest distribution of the zoster rash is along the skin supplied by the intercostal nerves or over the face in the innervation of the ophthalmic branch of the trigeminal nerve. Severe ophthalmic zoster can permanently damage the cornea. Zoster infection can be treated with antiviral agents (such as acyclovir), which can abort an attack or shorten both the duration of symptoms and the pain associated with herpes zoster infection. Vaccination against chickenpox in children and zoster in older individuals is currently being considered.

HERPES SIMPLEX INFECTION

Although primary infection with herpes virus can occur at any age, it is most common in young children. Most primary infections are subclinical, and it is only when the latent virus is reactivated, forming the typical 'cold sores', that it is apparent that the individual is infected. In young children, however, primary infection can be manifest as a very painful acute ulcerative gingivostomatitis. Whether as a result of primary or recurrent infection, the lesions are highly infectious. The virus is usually spread by direct personal contact such as kissing. Health care workers such as dentists can develop lesions on their hands, the so-called herpetic whitlow, if a patient is excreting virus. The incubation period for herpes virus infection is 2 to 12 days. Halting the spread of infection depends upon avoiding contact with people who have lesions.

In recent years it has been recognised that two forms of herpes virus hominis exist. Type 1 infection leads to the problems described above, while type 2 tends to be sexually transmitted and causes genital herpes, although either virus can cause genital herpes.

CYTOMEGALOVIRUS INFECTION

The importance of this infection, caused by another of the herpes virus group, is in the severe manifestations of congenital infection. It is the commonest cause of congenital infection in developed countries. As many as 5% to 10% of congenitally infected neonates are estimated to develop significant learning disability and permanent blindness.

The infection can be acquired during pregnancy or be a flare-up of a previous infection. In either case it can be transmitted to the baby. Half of pregnant women show evidence of post-cytomegalovirus infection. Amongst the remainder, 1% will acquire the virus during pregnancy.

Cytomegalovirus also causes profound problems in immunocompromised patients, such as transplant recipients, and in individuals infected with HIV. No vaccine is yet available, but some are being trialled.

PARVOVIRUS INFECTION (ERYTHEMA INFECTIOSUM, FIFTH DISEASE, SLAPPED CHEEK SYNDROME)

Infection with human parvovirus B19 is now

probably one of the commonest childhood causes of viral exanthem and is probably mistakenly notified as measles or rubella more often than not. It causes a characteristic erythema on the cheeks (hence slapped cheek syndrome) and a lacy-looking rash on the trunk. The reservoir is human and transmission is predominantly through contact with infected respiratory secretions. The incubation period varies between 4 and 20 days. The infection is usually self-limiting. Although rare, severe complications include transient aplastic crisis. In around 10% of cases of intrauterine infection in the first half of pregnancy, foetal anaemia, hydrops foetalis and foetal death can occur.

INFECTIONS LEADING TO HEPATITIS
HEPATITIS A

Hepatitis A virus is a human picornavirus. Infection is very common in the early years of life in parts of Africa, Asia, Latin America and eastern Europe. In some places, around 95% of children will have been infected by the age of five years. The seroprevalence rates in western Europe are considerably lower, having fallen during the last few decades of the twentieth century; thus an increasing number of adolescents and adults in such countries remain susceptible to hepatitis A infection. Travellers are at greater risk of acquiring infection as they move to areas of higher endemicity.

Many infections with the hepatitis A virus produce no marked symptoms or cause a very mild illness. Other cases have anorexia, abdominal discomfort and pyrexia but no jaundice. Others develop jaundice, which may result in a mild illness lasting

about a week or a severe illness lasting several months. Recovery is slow in the latter instance, but most cases make a complete recovery. Rarely, the disease can involve serious clinical manifestations, including hepatic failure. Hepatitis A is more common in children, but it also affects adults, who usually have a more severe illness. The clinical diagnosis of hepatitis A may be suggested by the history and clinical features, but confirmation depends upon the finding of IgM antibody to hepatitis A virus during the acute phase of the illness.

The incubation period is 15–50 days (usually 28–30 days). The person is most infectious during the latter half of the incubation period and the early stages of the illness. Most people are not infectious after the first week of jaundice. The reservoir is human and some other primates. Transmission is person to person, mainly by the faecal–oral route. Generally the disease occurs when hygiene is poor (for example, in those schools or nurseries where hand washing is not observed and lavatories are kept in a poor state of cleanliness). Transmission can occur between men who have sex with men. Contaminated water and food act as vehicles, and a variety of foods have caused outbreaks – notably shellfish such as mussels, oysters and clams, although these outbreaks are becoming increasingly rare.

Strict isolation of the patient is unnecessary because the stools are virus-free shortly after the jaundice appears. However, it is usual to adopt the standard precautions in handling urine, faeces and blood from the patient. Surveillance of close contacts, new cases and undiagnosed cases should be carried out. It is often difficult to trace the source of an outbreak. The long incubation period and the frequency of mild or asymptomatic illness are reasons for this. There is little to be gained from excluding contacts from school, but it is wise to exclude young people (who are the most susceptible) from food handling for six weeks. A high standard of personal hygiene is especially important when infectious hepatitis is prevalent.

Although human immunoglobulin may give protection for about three months in special circumstances (such as before travelling to endemic areas or as a prophylactic measure after exposure), the protection afforded by immunoglobulin is falling as a consequence of the low incidence of disease (people are not being exposed). Travellers to endemic areas are therefore offered vaccination. The general environmental measures of providing uncontaminated water supply and adequate sewage disposal are important in preventing the spread of infection.

HEPATITIS B

Hepatitis B virus is a hepadna virus. It multiplies within infected liver cells. The disease occurs throughout the world, particularly in Africa, the Far East, South East Asia and parts of Europe. In some individuals, hepatitis B virus persists, resulting in chronic infection. The risks of this are inversely proportional to the age of acquisition, i.e., around 80–90% in neonates but only around 5% in immunocompetent adults.

Chronic carriers of hepatitis B, defined as those with the presence of hepatitis B surface antigen (HBsAg) in the serum for six months or longer, are at increased risk of developing progressive liver disease, including cirrhosis

and hepatocellular carcinoma. In Britain, seroprevalence of HBsAg is low but varies geographically. For example, the prevalence among antenatal women varies between 0.05% in areas such as East Anglia and 1% in some parts of London. In southern Europe, the carrier rate is up to 5% and in the tropics it is up to 10%. In parts of the Far East, some 10–15% of people may have serum that is positive for HBsAg. Although notifications of acute hepatitis B are small in England and Wales, seroprevalence varies within population subgroups such as men who have sex with men and immigrant communities. Most of the carriers in Britain have no previous history of jaundice.

Patients typically present with gradual onset of 'flu-like' symptoms, such as malaise, anorexia, nausea, vomiting, abdominal discomfort and aching of muscles and joints. A rash may occur in this early phase of the illness, but fever is not usually a prominent feature. Clinical jaundice may then ensue or the patient may remain anicteric, the diagnosis being made by liver function and other tests. The fatality rate and likelihood of permanent liver damage with hepatitis B is higher than with hepatitis A infection. In the latter, almost all patients make a full recovery.

Three antigenic components of hepatitis B virus have been identified, each with associated antibodies.

➤ *The surface or capsule antigen (HBsAg)*, also referred to as the Australia antigen, can be detected by various techniques, including radioimmunoassay and electron microscopy; it appears in the late incubation period before the onset of symptoms and remains present in both acute and chronic infection.

➤ *The core antigen (HBcAg)* is not directly detectable in the serum; however, its antibody (anti-HBc) is present during active infection and also persists after recovery and is thus a marker of previous exposure to hepatitis B; the IgM component of anti-HBc predominates during the acute phase and anti-HBc-IgM can be used to detect recent hepatitis B infection.

➤ *The e-antigen (HBeAg)* occurs when there is ongoing active viral replication and is associated with higher infectivity. Chronic carriers with low levels of viral replication are seronegative for HBeAg and seropositive for its associated antibody (anti-HBe) and are less likely to transmit infection.

Other tests, such as hepatitis B DNA or DNA polymerase, are used to assess the infection but tend to be used only in more specialised or research settings.

The incubation period is 45–180 days, with an average of 60–90 days. The individual is infectious as long as hepatitis B surface antigen (HBsAg) is present in the blood. People with chronic hepatitis B infection should not donate blood. The reservoir is human and possibly other primates. Hepatitis B can be transmitted from another case, or more often from a carrier, either parenterally or sexually. Transmission may occur through heterosexual and male to male intercourse, intravenous drug misuse, tattooing, acupuncture, ear piercing as well as medical and dental instrumentation. It is an occupational risk for health care workers and those involved in handling blood products and dialysis equipment. Hepatitis B can be transmitted from infected mothers to their babies at or around the time of birth (perinatal transmission). Blood transfusion is an unlikely method in Britain, as strict screening of donor blood is now carried out.

Isolation of cases is not necessary, but strict precautions are required in the handling and disposal of blood and excreta. Close household and sexual contacts of a case of acute hepatitis B or a chronic carrier of the virus should be screened for hepatitis B markers, and immunisation should be offered to any who are neither immune nor infected. Follow-up of individuals who may have been exposed to hepatitis B infection from a point source, such as a tattooist or to a breakdown in infection control, is indicated. It may be too late for post-exposure prophylaxis to be effective in many cases, but those exposed could become possible sources of infection for their own close contacts.

General preventive measures include adequate precautions as part of the normal routine in all places handling human blood and its products. This includes the correct disposal of used syringes in all settings in which they are used. Specimens must be labelled 'high risk' and sent in special containers. Special risks apply to patients and staff of renal units, where vigilance should be especially high. Many renal units manage HBsAg-positive patients, most often in isolation from other patients and using dedicated machines. While some might feel that infected patients would be better managed at home, patients will need to be admitted to be trained in the use of dialysis; in any case, not all patients would be suitable for home treatment.

Health education is important amongst special and high-risk groups, such as drug takers and men who have sex with men. Adequate sterilisation of instruments should be undertaken, and, wherever possible, disposable needles and instruments should be employed and used once only for each patient. There is a clear need for close supervision of tattooing, body piercing and acupuncture. Patients who are HBsAg-positive should be educated about the mode of spread of the disease and counselled as to behaviour to reduce the risk of transmission.

Perinatal transmission of hepatitis B infection can largely be prevented by the appropriate immunisation, commencing at birth, of infants born to infected mothers. Individuals in groups at increased risk of acquiring infection (for example, injecting drug users, men who have sex with men and bisexual men, close family contacts of a case or carrier and health care personnel) should be immunised. Specific hepatitis B immunoglobulin is available for passive protection and is normally used in combination with hepatitis B vaccine to confer active/passive immunity after exposure (for example, after being pricked by a needle from an infected person) or when immediate protection is required.

HEPATITIS C

Hepatitis C virus (HCV) is a leading cause of chronic liver disease worldwide and is the principal cause of parenterally transmitted non-A non-B hepatitis. It is discussed earlier in the chapter in the section on new and emerging infections.

HEPATITIS D (DELTA HEPATITIS)

Since hepatitis D virus (HDV) requires the presence of hepatitis B for replication, it is always associated with coexisting hepatitis B infection. Hepatitis D infection is therefore either acquired simultaneously with hepatitis B (co-infection) by those susceptible to it, or subsequently by those who are carriers of hepatitis B (super infection). Infection is usually more severe and fatality rates higher than with simple hepatitis B infection. Both natural and vaccine-induced immunity to hepatitis B protect against infection with hepatitis D. Like hepatitis B, the infection is spread by exposure to infected blood or body fluids. The approach to prevention is similar. The incubation period is between two and eight weeks.

HEPATITIS E

Hepatitis E is endemic throughout much of Asia and in some parts of Africa, the Middle East and Central America; cases in the United Kingdom have been most often associated with a history of recent travel to the Indian subcontinent. Hepatitis E shares characteristics with hepatitis A and is spread by the faecal–oral route. Large outbreaks have occurred in some endemic areas in association with faecally contaminated drinking water. It also has been found in pigs (particularly in studies of transmission of the disease in China). The incubation period is 15–64 days and the clinical picture is very similar to hepatitis A. There is no evidence that infection with hepatitis E leads to chronic disease.

INFECTIONS LEADING TO MENINGITIS
MENINGOCOCCAL INFECTIONS

Meningococcus is a Gram-negative diplococcus that is commonly present in the throat and upper respiratory tract but can become pathogenic with severe consequences. *Neisseria meningitidis* forms six serogroups that can cause serious illness: A, B, C, W-135, X and Y.

Meningococcal disease has a worldwide distribution. In Britain *N. meningitidis* is responsible for causing meningitis and septicaemia, which occur both as sporadic cases and in localised outbreaks, particularly in children and young adults. Overcrowded living conditions facilitate its spread. For example, outbreaks occur in boarding schools and military camps where young people are living and sleeping in close proximity. Outbreaks of meningococcus W-135 have been associated with pilgrims returning from the hajj, but the frequency has been reduced by making vaccination a condition of entry into Saudi Arabia.

During the 1980s, a persistent pocket of high incidence of meningococcal infection with fatalities occurred in Stroud, Gloucestershire. The reason for the higher frequency in this area was not elucidated. It gave rise to great public concern, extensive media coverage and the formation of pressure groups that called for more action and research to combat the disease. Between 1100 and 1400 laboratory-confirmed cases of meningococcal disease occur each year in England and Wales. As a result of the meningococcal C vaccination programme, the majority of cases are now group B.

Nasopharyngeal carriage of the organism in asymptomatic individuals can be surprisingly high, with up to 15–20% of individuals being carriers in some age groups. The overall prevalence lies somewhere between 2–4% of the population.

The incubation period ranges from 2 to 10 days, usually 3 to 4 days. The patient is infective for as long as the organism is present in the nasopharynx. Penicillin (the antibiotic of choice in the treatment of meningococcal disease) suppresses the organism but does not eradicate it. This is important, since it means that people who have recovered from meningitis should receive a second antibiotic (usually rifampicin) to eliminate nasopharyngeal carriage of the pathogen.

The reservoir is human. Transmission is by droplet spread following close contact with a carrier of *N. meningitidis*. Only capsulated strains have the capacity to cause invasive disease. Carriage of non-capsulated strains and other commensal *Neisseria* species can help to boost natural immunity. Long-term carriers of pathogenic strains rarely become cases themselves. Their natural defences have learned to cope with the organism.

In cases where meningitis does develop, symptoms are fever, headache, neck stiffness and photophobia. Acute septicaemia, which is rapidly fatal if untreated, is often accompanied by a haemorrhagic rash that does not blanch under pressure (e.g., if a glass is rolled over it). This may be petechial, purpuric or ecchymotic. Other symptoms may occur, such as backache and muscle pains, and other organs (for example, the joints and heart) may be involved. However, septicaemia can occur without typical signs of meningitis; it causes flu-like symptoms, general malaise and can rapidly lead to deterioration and death.

The laboratory diagnosis is made by observing the organism on direct microscopy of cerebrospinal fluid (CSF), by isolating the organism from culture of cerebrspinal fluid or blood or by detecting fragments of the organism's genome in blood or cerebrospinal fluid by non-culture techniques, such as polymerase chain reaction (PCR).

The administration of antibiotics, even before admission to hospital, is vital to reduce mortality from this disease. The organism can be identified by non-culture techniques, so administration of antibiotics should not be delayed in order that it can be grown in culture. Regular health information campaigns are necessary to make the public and parents aware of the symptoms of both meningitis and septicaemia.

Action rests largely with the general practitioner or accident and emergency unit in early treatment. Household contacts and other intimate contacts (for example, kissing contacts) should be traced and offered antibiotic prophylaxis as soon as possible after the diagnosis has been made, preferably within 24 hours. The use of antibiotic chemoprophylaxis is usually limited to people who came into close contact with the infected person in the five days prior to the onset of the illness.

The purpose of antibiotic prophylaxis is to eliminate carriage of meningococcus in the nasopharynx of the close contacts of the case. The fact that a case has occurred usually means that someone in his or her immediate circle is a carrier of the organism. Antibiotic prophylaxis reduces the chance of this carrier causing another case of disease.

The indiscriminate use of antibiotics can do more harm than good. They may eliminate harmless, commensal *Neisseria* from the nasopharynx, which not only boost natural immunity but also prevent pathogenic strains from gaining a foothold. This is especially the case in small children, who tend to be carriers of *Neisseria lactamica*. Clearing carriage of these strains can, paradoxically, leave children open to becoming infected with pathogenic strains. The decision to widen antibiotic prophylaxis beyond close contacts, the only group in which there is compelling evidence of benefit, needs to be taken with care.

Vaccine development is the key to controlling or even eliminating meningococcal disease. The major advance in recent years was the advent of a conjugate vaccine against meningococcus C disease. This was introduced into the childhood vaccination programme in the United Kingdom from 1999 and has brought about a major reduction in the incidence of, and deaths from, meningococcal C disease.

Polysaccharide vaccines to combat A, C, Y and W-135 subtypes have been available for nearly 30 years, but they are not as effective as a conjugate vaccine, providing protection for a relatively short-time (3–5 years). Nor are they effective in very young children. Research to produce conjugate vaccines against these strains is very promising. Developing a vaccine against Meningococcus B is more difficult, but the prospects here are also quite good.

STREPTOCOCCUS PNEUMONIAE (PNEUMOCOCCUS)

Although a less common cause of meningitis than *N. meningitidis* and *H. influenzae* type b, pneumococcal meningitis is important because of its high associated mortality (20–40%). It occurs at all ages but is the commonest bacterial meningitis occurring in the over-50 age group (*see also* sections on 'Infections for which Comprehensive Vaccination Programmes are Available' and 'Respiratory Infections').

OTHER ORGANISMS

In addition to bacterial meningitis, a variety of other organisms cause the disease. These include viruses (for example, mumps, enteroviruses, *Herpes simplex*), mycobacteria (*M. tuberculosis* and *M. bovis*) and, much more rarely, leptospires and fungi (cryptococcal meningitis usually occurs in immunocompromised people, including those with HIV). Listeriosis is a rare but important cause of neonatal meningitis (*see also* the section on food-borne illnesses.)

HEALTH CARE-ASSOCIATED INFECTION

Modern health care has brought untold benefits to millions of patients and their families. Against these benefits, though, must be set the risks. These are extensively described in the section on patient safety in Chapter 4. Prominent within the hierarchy of risks of health care is the risk of infection. This was recognised by Florence Nightingale when she published her *Notes on Nursing* in 1860. Miss Nightingale placed great emphasis on the importance of hygiene, cleanliness and standards of care. She cut death rates from infection in a military hospital in the Crimea.

THE RESURGENCE OF HEALTH CARE-ASSOCIATED INFECTION

By the middle of the twentieth century, infection in hospitals in this country was largely controlled. This was not because it did not occur but because when infection did complicate care, a range of antibiotics was available to treat it quickly and effectively. Complacency set in: fundamentals of hygiene in many hospitals were neglected, leadership in infection control was lacking, training programmes for health care professionals no longer instilled the rigour necessary to prevent infection and pharmaceutical companies did not give priority to research to discover new antibiotics.

As a result, at the end of the first decade of the twenty-first century, the risk of infection in health care settings is a very significant problem and is a matter of major concern for patients, the public, politicians and health care professionals. It is the sort of issue that tests the credibility with the public of those running health services. Challengers often ask why it is that some countries can achieve low levels of infection. They also express incredulity that doctors and nurses do not regularly clean their hands before attending to a patient and that visitors to hospitals see dirty walls and floors.

UNDERLYING CAUSES

There is no single reason for the growth of health care-associated infections. The factors that drive the increase are multiple. They include:

➢ *patient-related factors* – the increase in people with serious illness (e.g., cancer) or treatments (e.g., transplants, cytotoxic drugs) that weaken their immune systems; the mixing of large numbers of patients from different referral sources

➢ *organisational factors* – high bed-occupancy levels; poor staff-patient ratio; increased movement of patients within the hospital

➢ *health care staff factors* – poor hand-hygiene compliance; poor aseptic techniques when carrying out procedures such as insertion of tubes and intravascular lines and cleaning wounds; inadequate skills and training

➢ *environmental factors* – dirty walls, floors and surfaces in clinical areas (although appealing to common sense, the evidence base for this is quite weak); inadequate decontamination and sterilisation of instruments and equipment

➢ *structural factors* – lack of easy access to essential preventive equipment such as hand sanitisers and sinks; low levels of single rooms, isolation cubicles, hand basins and toilets; inadequate waste disposal facilities.

THE SIZE OF THE PROBLEM

Health care-associated infection is a feature of health services in every country of the world to a greater or lesser extent. Two kinds of data are usually presented: firstly, the overall prevalence of infection amongst hospital patients; secondly, the frequency of occurrence of certain specific infections – for example, meticillin-resistant *Staphylococcus aureus* (MRSA) bloodstream infections and *Clostridium difficile*.

Data on health care-associated infection must be collected by surveillance systems, and not all countries have adequate ones in place. In the United Kingdom, the arrangements for surveillance on health care-associated infection consist of mandatory reporting of *S. aureus* bloodstream infection, MRSA bacteraemia, glycopeptide-resistant entero-coccal bacteraemia, *C. difficile* and orthopaedic surgical site infections.

The most common health care-associated infections are urinary tract, respiratory, surgical site and bloodstream. The most common organisms involved are *S. aureus* and *E. coli* (Figure 9.15).

The United Kingdom overall level of health care-associated infection is towards the upper end of the range of other western European countries. International comparisons are not straightforward, because definitions, surveillance systems and laboratories all vary. Studies in developed countries show a range of health care-associated infection prevalence of 5 to 11%, with the United Kingdom at around 8%. The level of MRSA infection is amongst the worst in developed countries (Figure 9.16).

Health care-associated infection represents a heavy burden of disease and cost to the NHS; a total of 5109 deaths involving MRSA and 13 189 involving *C. difficile* were reported in the period 2002–06. Rates of MRSA and *C. difficile* fell during the second half of the 2000s as a result of national policy and local action in the NHS to make reduction of health care-associated infection a priority. Levels were still, however, unacceptably high. The National Audit Office has estimated that there are 300 000 health care-associated infections (5000 deaths) each year, at a cost to the NHS of £1 billion.

HEALTH CARE-ASSOCIATED INFECTION: KEY ORGANISMS

In this section, the key causal organisms are highlighted. There are some areas of overlap with the earlier section on Antimicrobial Resistance.

Meticillin-resistant *Staphylococcus aureus*

Staphylococcus aureus occurs naturally on the skin or in the nasal cavity. It is an important cause of infection, both in the community and in health care settings. The organism has become resistant to many antibiotics, notably meticillin (and other beta-lactam antibiotics), hence the term meticillin-resistant *Staphylococcus aureus* (MRSA). This is described more fully in the section on Antimicrobial Resistance.

MRSA can also be carried harmlessly on the skin of patients. About 3% of the general population carries an MRSA strain (i.e., 10% of all *S. aureus* carriers), but the carriage rate is 6–7% amongst patients screened on admission to hospital. However, it can result in serious infections that are very difficult to treat effectively. These infections prolong hospital stay and can lead to major complications (such as necessitating limb amputation) and death.

MRSA spreads rapidly in hospitals and other health care settings. Colonised patients who are admitted but whose carrier status remains unrecognised can act as a reservoir of infection. The hands of health care workers act as mediators of transmission from one patient to another, and this is the main method of transmission of MRSA (Figure 9.17). Contaminated clinical environments contribute to the likelihood of hand-to-patient transfer of MRSA. Inadequately cleaned equipment is another important factor, as are a lack of proper isolation or cohorting facilities and poor antibiotic prescribing policy and practice (Table 9.13).

Intensive care units of hospitals can be important foci for MRSA spread. They contain many patients who are seriously ill and who have compromised immune systems. Patient care in intensive care units involves multiple contacts between health professionals and patients. Antibiotics are extensively used, which promotes the selection of resistant organisms. The intensive care unit is an important 'hot spot' for other health care infections, not just MRSA.

As with any infection, MRSA infections that show up within 48 hours of hospital admission are usually classified as 'community-acquired' (although many of the patients will have had prior contact with a health care facility). Those occurring later than 48 hours are regarded as 'hospital-acquired'. In recent years, there has been a growth in community-acquired MRSA

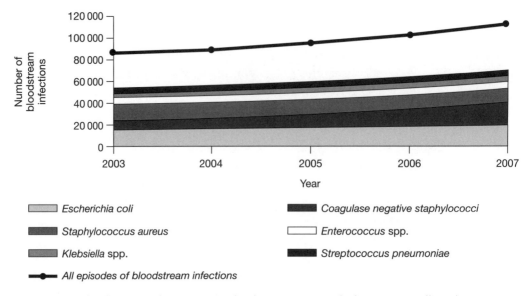

Figure 9.15 Bloodstream infections in England, 2003 to 2007 (voluntary surveillance)
Source: Health Protection Agency. *Surveillance of Healthcare Associated Infections Report: 2008.* London: Health Protection Agency; 2008.

infections. Where there is no prior health care link, they are often different strains to the MRSA that occurs in hospital.

Clostridium Difficile

Clostridium difficile is an anaerobic, spore-forming bacterium that is the commonest cause of diarrhoea acquired by hospital patients. It is present in the gut of a small proportion (about 3%) of healthy people, but the spores are also readily acquired from contaminated surfaces or via the hands of health care workers. They can then grow and produce toxins that cause diarrhoea and colitis when the normal gut flora are disturbed – for example, by the use of antibiotics or by the immune system being suppressed.

C. *difficile* has become an increasing cause of concern in the United Kingdom and other developed countries because of its rising incidence in the early 2000s, but it began to fall towards the end of the decade as it was made a priority for the NHS. It is commoner amongst older patients causing serious and, in some cases, life-threatening infections.

A number of different strains of *C. difficile* occur. Ribotype 001 predominated in the United Kingdom from 1990, but since 2004–05 this country and some other parts of western Europe and North America have been affected by more virulent strains (particularly ribotypes 027 and 106).

C. *difficile* produces spores that can survive in the hospital environment for weeks or months and that are resistant to most non-chlorine-based cleaning agents and disinfectants.

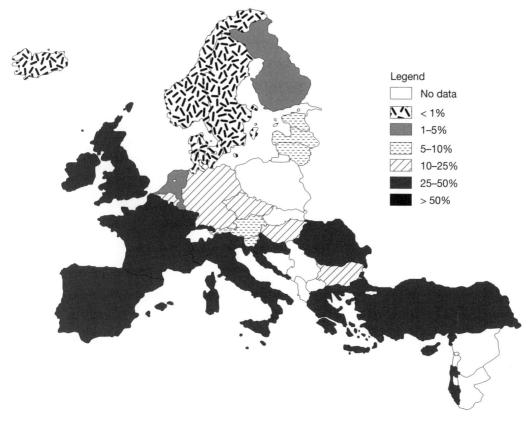

Figure 9.16 Proportion of MRSA isolates in participating countries, 2007
Source: European Antimicrobial Resistance Surveillance System.

Glycopeptide-resistant Enterococci

Glycopeptide-resistant enterococci (GRE) are those that are resistant to glycopeptide antibiotics (e.g., vancomycin, teicoplanin). They usually cause infections in vulnerable patients with multiple underlying conditions and can be responsible for outbreaks of infection. They can cause urinary tract infections, bacteraemia (bloodstream infections) and wound infections. Infections may be difficult to treat because of the limited number of antibiotics effective against these strains (*see also* section on Antimicrobial Resistance).

Prevention is dependent upon prudent antibiotic prescribing, adherence to good hand hygiene, appropriate use of gloves and aprons and good cleaning of the environment. Patients will usually be isolated or cohorted.

Extended-spectrum Beta-lactamases

Extended-spectrum beta-lactamases (ESBLs) are highly multi-drug-resistant Gram-negative organisms first detected in the 1980s. Organisms that display this resistance are *Klebsiellae* and more recently in the United

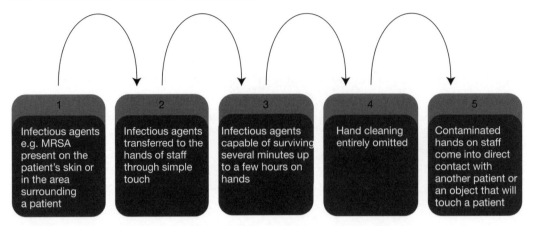

Figure 9.17 Sequential transmission of microbes by hands
Source: World Health Organization, 2006.

Table 9.13 Risk factors associated with MRSA colonisation

- Recent hospitalisation
- Recent (3–6 months) antimicrobial use
- Invasive lines or tube (IV urinary catheters)
- Recent surgery
- Nursing home resident
- Advanced age
- Underlying severe disease
- Exposure to colonised or infected patient
- Morbid obesity
- Orthopaedic implant surgery

Source: Marwick CA, Ziglam HM, Nathwani D. Your patient has a blood culture positive for *Staphylococcus aureus* – what do you do? *J R Coll Physicians Edin.* 2006; **36**: 350–5.

Kingdom, *Escherichia coli*. Most patients will not suffer any harm as a result of colonisation with these organisms, but they can cause urinary tract infection and septicaemia that is difficult to treat (*see also* section on Antimicrobial Resistance).

Those vulnerable to infection are the elderly and neonates, patients with low white blood cells and transplant patients.

Patients with a history of receiving long-term antibiotics are also at risk. Prevention of spread relies on good adherence with hand hygiene, appropriate use of gloves and aprons and high standards of infection control when handling devices. Patients will usually be isolated or cohorted.

Acinetobacter Species

Acinetobacter is a Gram-negative bacterium found widely in the environment, including drinking and surface waters, soil, sewage and various types of food. It lives harmlessly (colonises) on the skin of healthy people, posing very few risks to healthy people. However, some species, particularly *Acinetobacter baumannii*, can cause serious infections – mainly in very ill hospital patients. In these cases, common infections include pneumonia, bacteraemia, wound infections and urinary tract infections. Within the hospital environment, strains of *Acinetobacter* can show resistance to antibiotics and are increasingly difficult to treat. Prevention can be achieved by careful attention to hand hygiene and environmental cleaning and appropriate use of gloves and aprons. Patients will usually be isolated or cohorted

CONTROL OF HEALTH CARE-ASSOCIATED INFECTION

The control of health care-associated infection requires a comprehensive and consistent approach at the level of the health care institution and the health care system as a whole, emphasising:

➤ an organisational culture and leadership and accountability that views health-care-associated infection as a patient safety issue and a priority for action
➤ clear, agreed evidence-based policies and procedures to reduce risk of infection in all care settings
➤ high-quality information to assess the problem, track progress and act as an early warning system
➤ commitment of frontline staff to the highest standards of hand hygiene
➤ competent practitioners supported by robust pre- and post-registration training and education in infection control.

Two high-profile failures in standards of infection control occurred in hospitals in the United Kingdom in the late-2000s. Both involved deaths of patients from *C. difficile*. In both cases, the failure was at the organisational level as well as at the frontline (see Box 9.1). The culture, leadership and working practices had not put patients first.

Infection control policies within institutions are directed at health care workers' hand hygiene, clinical procedures and practices, decontamination of high-risk equipment and design and maintenance of a supportive physical environment and infrastructure. Control of *C. difficile* has some additional special features (Table 9.14).

Hand hygiene improvement is central to ensuring a clean and safe environment for patients and reducing health care-associated infection. Hand-mediated transmission of microbes from one patient to another via health care workers (Figure 9.18) can be interrupted through use of hand sanitisers or hand washing at the sink. During the last 10 years, there has been a growing emphasis on hand hygiene at the point of care, and hand sanitisers (alcohol gels and rubs) have revolutionised hand hygiene improvement methodology, making it possible for health care workers to adhere more easily and effectively to the demands of hand hygiene policies. Hand sanitisers are not a panacea

> ## BOX 9.1 FAILURES IN STANDARDS OF INFECTION CONTROL CAUSING PATIENT DEATHS
>
> In the mid- and late-2000s, the Healthcare Commission investigated three serious outbreaks of *Clostridium difficile* at two hospital NHS trusts in England.
>
> In two outbreaks at Stoke Mandeville Hospital, 334 patients contracted the infection and 33 died. In the outbreak at Maidstone and Tunbridge Wells NHS Trust, 90 patients died.
>
> In both hospitals, the inspectors found poor leadership, a culture that was not orientated to patient safety, failure to act on clinical advice and poor hygiene practice.
>
> — *Source*: Healthcare Commission, 2006 and 2007.

and should not be used on soiled hands or with certain micro-organisms (including *C. difficile*). They act as a safety net for the myriad of microbes that threaten patients in the hospital and have been demonstrated to dramatically increase the likelihood of maximum compliance and to reduce risk.

The Netherlands is commonly cited as the European country that has been successful in keeping MRSA out of its hospitals. It has certainly not had the surge in MRSA seen in the United Kingdom during the 1990s and the early twenty-first century. This is due in part to the so-called 'search and destroy' policy applied in the Netherlands. This involves early identification (including taking nasal swabs) and containment of infection as well as an emphasis on high standards of hand and environmental hygiene. Outbreaks of MRSA can best be controlled if these stringent control measures are employed.

The effectiveness of health care-associated infection control measures is dependent not only on the application of hand hygiene protocols, isolation and cohorting, but also on patient case mix and antibiotic prescribing policies. These factors can differ from one country to another and even within the same country.

Many hospitals have described their infection rates as 'endemic', and strict search-and-destroy strategies were replaced by more flexible approaches. This has been criticised as a key contributor to the unacceptably high levels of this organism. Learning from the best international approaches, including that of the Netherlands, has resulted in an integrated national approach to tackling MRSA, and this appears to be successful. MRSA screening of all elective admissions to NHS hospitals was commenced from 2008.

LEGISLATION

The Health Act 2006 Code of Practice for the Prevention and Control of Health Care Associated Infection requires all health organisations to have management and governance systems in place to prevent and control infection in their institutions and facilities. Compliance with the *Code of Practice* is evaluated by the Care Quality Commission (previously the Healthcare Commission), which can

Table 9.14 Control measures effective against the spread of *C. difficile*

- Isolation or cohorting of infected patients
- Use of gowns and gloves for contact with *C. difficile* patients
- Hand washing with soap and water after contact with patients with *C. difficile* infection
- Rigorous environmental cleaning with chlorine-based products in adequate dosage of rooms occupied by *C. difficile* patients
- Antibiotic stewardship, avoiding broad-spectrum antibiotics, particularly third-generation cephalosporins and fluoroquinolones

issue improvement notices. A revised *Code of Practice* published in 2008 widened the scope, directing, for example, a 'bare below the elbows' policy for health care staff and ensuring adequate isolation facilities and antimicrobial prescribing policy. The *Code of Practice* provides detailed guidance in three main areas:

1 management, organisation and the environment
2 clinical care protocols
3 health care workers.

OCCUPATIONAL AND ENVIRONMENTAL HAZARDS
LEPTOSPIROSIS (WEIL'S DISEASE)

Leptospira is a spirochaetal organism that has two species, *Leptospira biflexa* and *Leptospira interrogans*, with many different serotypes. Two main serotypes cause most cases of disease in Britain – *Leptospira icterohaemorrhagiae* and *Leptospira hardjo*.

The disease is a zoonosis that occurs in all parts of the world. In Britain it was traditionally associated with sewage workers, and it is now seen in farm or abattoir workers or, less commonly, amongst butchers, pest-control workers and veterinary workers.

Contact with water contaminated by animal urine causes the disease. Canoeing and other water sports account for a substantial minority of the cases that occur each year. Imported infections also occur.

The clinical manifestations are sudden onset of pyrexia, headache, severe muscular pain and sometimes vomiting. Occasionally a petechial rash occurs. More severe cases develop jaundice and haemorrhagic complications. This is classical Weil's disease, and up to a fifth of cases can die from it. Spirochaetes can be cultured from patients' blood and sometimes from urine. Antibodies can usually be demonstrated in the serum (a range of tests are available) but not until the end of the first week of illness at the earliest. This means that tests are unhelpful in recognising the disease and initiating treatment in an acutely ill patient. The initial diagnosis should be made on history-taking and physical examination. Early treatment is the most effective, especially in reducing fatalities in severe cases.

The incubation period is usually around 10 days but may extend from 4 to 19 days, and person-to-person transmission is rare. Many animals carry the different serotypes, including rats and other rodents, dogs, cattle, foxes and squirrels. In Britain the main risks are from rats (*Leptospira icterohaemorrhagiae*), dogs and pigs (*Leptospira canicola*) and cattle (largely *Leptospira hardjo*). Cattle become infected through grazing on fields contaminated by the urine of small rodents. In some surveys, over 60% of cattle sera show antibodies to *Leptospira* strains, particularly *L. hardjo*.

Transmission is by direct contact with water, damp soil or vegetation that has been contaminated by the urine of infected animals or, less commonly, transmission occurs directly from the infected urine of animals. The spirochaete enters via broken skin or via mucous membranes, or it may be swallowed.

Health care professionals must exercise caution in handling body excretions, particularly the blood and urine of infected patients. Other people exposed to the primary source must undergo medical surveillance. Protective clothing should be worn by workers in hazardous occupations, and wounds and cuts should be covered. Health education is important. This must be directed both at workers in high-risk occupations and at the general public. The latter should be warned about the dangers of infection through swimming in contaminated water, such as that in disused canals, and through other water sports such as canoeing. The control of the urban rat population is also important. General environmental control measures include extermination of rodents.

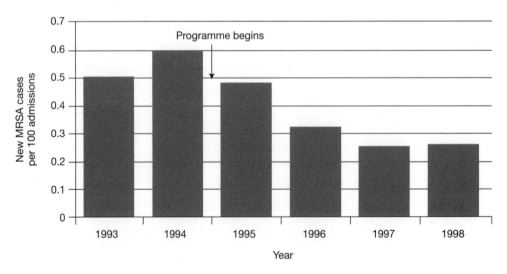

Figure 9.18 New MRSA cases start to decrease after the launch of a hand hygiene programme in Switzerland
Source: Pittet D, Hugonnet S, Harbarth S, *et al.* Effectiveness of a hospital-wide programme to improve compliance with hand hygiene. Infection Control Programme. *Lancet.* 2000; **356**(9238): 1307–12.

TOXOCARA

Toxocara is a nematode (roundworm), and two species cause concern in the British Isles: *Toxocara canis* (the adult form of which occurs in the small intestine of dogs) and *Toxocara cati* (which is found in the cat). Each has a complex but different life cycle. It is the minute larvae (about half a millimetre long) that invade the tissues of many vertebrates and cause symptoms in humans. Human infestation follows the ingestion of infected eggs from dog or cat faeces. The transfer may take place directly from hand to mouth (particularly in children) or possibly on salad vegetables. Surveys have shown that 5–25% of soil samples in gardens, parks and sandpits are contaminated with *Toxocara* eggs. After ingestion the eggs hatch into larvae in the intestine, penetrate the intestinal wall and reach various organs through the bloodstream.

The larvae do not develop into adult worms in humans, but the wandering larvae can invade the lungs, liver, brain and eye. In the various tissues, larvae produce an immune response and become the centre of an inflammatory reaction with subsequent fibrosis and granuloma formation. This gives rise to no symptoms in the great majority of cases, but if the lesion is in a vital organ such as the eye it can lead to disturbance of vision, or if it is in the brain it can result in epilepsy.

It must be remembered that these are rare conditions. There are about 50 cases with ocular involvement reported in Britain each year, mostly children who have been in close contact with dogs. Nevertheless, it is a further reason to ban dogs from beaches, parks and playgrounds. At least 10% of dogs and up to 35% of cats in Britain are infested. Human infection is much more commonly associated with dogs.

BRUCELLOSIS

Brucellosis is caused by *Brucella abortus*, a small, aerobic, Gram-negative coccobacillus that does not produce spores. It induces abortion in cows; the carcasses and the milk both become infected. Other serological types are *Brucella melitensis* (which infects goats and sheep), *Brucella suis* (which infects pigs) and *Brucella canis* (which infects dogs) – none of which are endemic in Britain.

Brucellosis has a worldwide distribution but is more common in Mediterranean areas. By the beginning of the 1990s, following the introduction in Britain in 1971 of a compulsory scheme for eradication of *Brucella* in cattle, the number of laboratory identifications had plummeted. When the disease does occur, it is more often found in rural areas amongst workers (including veterinary surgeons) who are involved with cattle or their untreated milk and also amongst people who drink unpasteurised milk. Some infections are contracted abroad and imported with the traveller.

The illness is not sharply defined. Commonly it produces a so-called undulant fever with febrile periods, followed by intervals with no increase in temperature. The fever often appears in the afternoons. The diagnosis should be considered in any pyrexia of unknown origin, especially in groups with a potential occupational exposure. In about half the cases, the organisms may be isolated in blood cultures taken from the patient in the acute stages of the illness.

Otherwise the diagnosis is often made by serological tests, which are of more value slightly later in the illness.

The incubation period is usually two to four weeks but can often be several months. Person-to-person spread is virtually unknown. There are a number of animal reservoirs of the infection, but in Britain the only animal of importance is the cow. Infection results from direct contact with infected cattle – particularly the products of conception – and from drinking unpasteurised milk from infected cows. The airborne route (inhalation of infected dust) in cattle sheds may occur.

Isolation and surveillance of cases is unnecessary. As human immunisation is not available, health education is important. Farmers should be taught how to avoid infection, and the public should be made aware of the dangers of drinking untreated milk. Outbreaks have usually been traced to an infected herd, if those working with it or drinking its milk become infected.

The general measures of raising herds of cattle that are free from *B. abortus* infection and the pasteurising of milk could entirely eradicate the disease in humans. While the eradication programme in Britain is very well advanced, with most herds free from brucellosis, there are still a small number diagnosed each year. Close cooperation is required between the health and local authorities, together with the veterinary authorities, when cases or outbreaks occur.

LYME DISEASE

Lyme disease was first described in 1975 in Old Lyme, Connecticut, when several children developed acute arthritis. The causal agent, *Borrelia burgdorferi* (a spirochaete), was not identified until 1982. The organism is transmitted by the bite of the *Ixodes ricinus* tick, which lives on wild animals (especially deer). It is not transmissible person-to-person.

Susceptibility to infection is thought to be universal, and the clinical manifestations are divided into two groups. Early symptoms include fever, malaise, headache, lymphadenopathy and a characteristic skin rash called erythema chronicum migrans. Present in about 7% of infected people, the rash develops after about five weeks and spreads slowly during the following months. Late manifestations, which may take years to appear, include arthritis, neurological abnormalities and heart problems.

There have been an increasing number of cases of Lyme disease (Lyme borreliosis) reported in the United Kingdom since surveillance of the disease started in the mid-1980s. Much of the increase has been due to greater awareness, better diagnostic facilities and more complete reporting of cases. The majority (80%) of cases are acquired in the United Kingdom in areas such as Exmoor, the New Forest, the Lake District, the Scottish Highlands and the North Yorkshire Moors. The remaining 20% of confirmed cases are acquired during holidays abroad to other parts of Europe, particularly amongst walkers and mountain-cyclists.

The ticks survive best in moist ground in the summer season and where there are animals such as deer or sheep roaming and grazing. Measures directed at combating this infection include covering exposed areas of skin, particularly legs and ankles, while out walking in the forest. If a tick should bite a person, it should be removed promptly, since transmission of the organism does not seem to occur until the tick has fed for a number of hours.

ORF

This is a common viral disease of sheep and goats, and it is transmitted to humans by occupational exposure. Farmers, shepherds and vets are usually affected by coming into direct contact with lesions on infected animals. The most common presentation is of a single lesion on the hands that develops into a weeping blister. The lesions, which can measure up to 3 cm in diameter, persist for three to six weeks and then disappear. Occurring mainly in rural communities, this self-limiting illness can be confused with anthrax (*see* below) or with malignancy.

ANTHRAX

Anthrax is caused by *Bacillus anthracis*, a large Gram-positive rod that occurs in short chains. The organism grows aerobically and forms heat-resistant spores capable of surviving for many years. It is exceedingly rare in Britain, with only a few cases over a decade. Patients are usually workers dealing with animal products such as carcasses, hides, hairs, wool and bone meal. In late 2008, a man died from inhaled anthrax having made a drum from imported animal skin. Sometimes gardeners using unsterilised bone meal have become infected.

Although now very rare, the relevance of anthrax as a biological-warfare weapon or bioterrorist weapon cannot be overlooked. This was brought home emphatically by the deliberate release of anthrax through packages entering federal buildings in the USA following the 11 September 2001 terrorist attacks on New York City and Washington, DC. The probable perpetrator, a US scientist, committed suicide in the summer of 2008.

The skin is the organ principally affected in this disease. Although respiratory and intestinal forms are uncommon, they may occur and are often fatal. The respiratory form is a particular risk in deliberate releases, where a fine powder can circulate enhanced by air-conditioning systems. In the cutaneous form, a skin lesion develops usually about two to four days after local infection. It becomes vesicular over a period of several days. After rupture of the vesicle, a deep-seated ulcer appears with swollen surrounding skin. It may then become covered by a scab: the characteristic eschar. If left untreated, spread to the bloodstream will lead to a septicaemia that is fatal in as many as 20% of cases.

The diagnosis is usually confirmed by microscopy or isolation of the organism in culture of the skin lesion or blood. The incubation period is between a few hours and seven days. Person-to-person infection has not been reported, but until the patient has received several days of treatment with antibiotics, it is wise to avoid handling the lesion. Lesions should be covered with an occlusive bandage.

Spores, often surviving for many years, are shed from the infected animal. Soil may also contain spores from the remains of dead animals.

Vaccination of workers in conditions where they are exposed to the risk of infection and the education of such workers in personal cleanliness, treatment of minor injuries and the hazards of handling potentially infected material are important control measures for anthrax. Protective clothing, dust reduction and medical supervision of those at risk at work are further preventive steps. Gardeners should take special care when using bone meal known to be unsterilised. General environmental measures include the sterilisation of hair, wool, hides and bone meal – particularly of imported products.

Early diagnosis of affected animals or people and treatment with appropriate antibiotics is essential, as is the rapid identification of outbreaks in animals. The carcasses of animals dying from anthrax should be burned or deeply buried in quicklime, with any contaminated material and equipment sterilised. Primary contacts (those in contact with the original animal source) should have daily medical surveillance for one week. Contacts of human cases do not require such medical surveillance. Close cooperation between health authorities, local authorities and veterinary authorities is necessary when cases or outbreaks occur.

Since 2001 every case (and particularly clusters) must be looked at from the point of view of deliberate release. The police and emergency-planning officials may need to be involved. Decontamination equipment held by the fire services may need to be deployed if a building and its staff are suspected of being targeted.

INFECTIONS RARELY OCCURRING IN THE UNITED KINGDOM AND INFECTIONS ACQUIRED ABROAD

Communicable disease associated with travel is a rapidly changing field, and the account in this section must not be relied upon for the most up-to-date advice for travellers.

MALARIA

Malaria is caused by a protozoan parasite of the *Plasmodium* genus. Four species cause human malaria: two are common (*Plasmodium vivax*, the cause of benign tertian malaria, and *Plasmodium falciparum*, which causes malignant tertian malaria, a non-relapsing and serious disease with a high fatality rate) and two are uncommon (*Plasmodium malariae* and *Plasmodium ovale*).

Malaria is a very common disease in many parts of the tropics and subtropics: the *vivax* form is common in the Indian subcontinent, Central America and Southeast Asia; the *falciparum* form in Africa, South America and Southeast Asia. Cases of malaria reported in the United Kingdom are virtually all imported. They increased steeply during the 1970s then levelled off, but they have increased again since. The pattern has changed: *P. falciparum* has increased markedly, while *P. vivax* has fallen. The imported disease is most common in those who have travelled to see family and friends in West Africa. Most have not taken malaria prophylaxis. Business and holiday travellers are another important group.

Early symptoms can be very non-specific and flu-like. After an initial period of general malaise, pyrexia, shivering and profuse sweating occur in cycles according to the stage of development of the parasite in the human body. These symptoms can vary both in type and severity according to the species of malaria. The diagnosis of malaria should be considered in any patient with a pyrexial illness who has recently been in an endemic area, even if the individual has been taking antimalarial chemoprophylaxis. It is confirmed when the parasite is demonstrated microscopically in blood films.

The incubation period depends on the infecting strain: approximately 7 to 14 days from the infected insect bite for *P. falciparum*; approximately 8 to 14 days for *P. vivax* and *P. ovale*; and 7 to 30 days for *P. malariae*.

The infection is not transmitted within Britain in the usual way (by mosquitoes). The reservoir is human. Transmission is by the bite of an infected female anopheline mosquito. The mosquito bites the person and ingests human blood containing gametocytes (the sexual stages of the parasite). In the mosquito's stomach, these male and female stages join together to form sporozoites. These concentrate in the salivary glands of the mosquito and are injected into the person when the mosquito next feeds. They pass in the bloodstream to the liver, where they develop into merozoites (pre-erythrocytic cycle).

The clinical attack begins when these are released into the bloodstream and invade the red cells, where they can undergo a complete cycle of development (erythrocytic cycle) resulting in further release of merozoites into the bloodstream and a further clinical attack. Some also develop into male and female gametocytes, which can then be taken up by another mosquito. The life cycle in the mosquito spans 8 to 35 days, depending upon the infecting species, the ambient temperature and the pre-erythrocytic cycle in the liver (6 to 9 days for *P. falciparum*, *vivax* and *ovale* and 12 to 16 days for *P. malariae*).

The duration of the erythrocytic cycle varies with the species of parasite: 36–48 hours (*P. falciparum*); 48 hours (*P. vivax* and *P. ovale*); and 74 hours (*P. malariae*). This variation accounts for the different periodicity of clinical attacks in the different forms. A proportion of the merozoites from the pre-erythrocytic cycles continue to develop in the liver (exoerythrocytic cycle): this provides for the source of infection in relapses that may occur several months after a previous attack. Relapses are particularly common with *P. vivax* infections.

Isolation of cases is unnecessary, and surveillance of contacts in Britain is only performed to ensure that fellow travellers have not also contracted the disease. However, it is important that a high index of clinical suspicion is maintained and that malaria is diagnosed and treated early when it does occur. Environmental measures are not required in Britain at the moment.

Travellers going to, or passing through, endemic areas should take appropriate precautions against malaria. This includes prophylactic antimalarial drugs, continued for specific periods after leaving the endemic area. Drug resistance is a problem, and the most up-to-date advice must be given to travellers to particular endemic areas. The World Health Organization issues information annually about areas where drug resistance occurs.

The most important groups for health

education targeting are members of the ethnic minority populations within the United Kingdom, many of whom make relatively frequent trips to their countries of origin and are not always aware of the risks of malaria and the importance of prophylaxis. Business travellers and ordinary holiday-makers should also be included in education programmes. Vigilance is required in ensuring that aircraft do not import the mosquito or expose passengers travelling between non-endemic areas in aircraft that have previously been used on tropical routes. Maintenance of high standards in screening potential blood donors and prevention of cross-infection with blood from infected patients are vital control measures.

In affected areas, the four key elements of prevention are: awareness of risk, prevention of bites by sprays, bed nets, chemoprophylaxis and early diagnosis if prevention fails.

RABIES

The rabies virus is a rhabdovirus. Found in many countries throughout the world, it has an estimated global annual mortality as high as 70 000. The British Isles are at present rabies-free, with only occasional imported cases in animals. Rabies has been detected in wildlife in various parts of western Europe and progressively closer to ports along the English Channel in recent years, although the introduction of oral rabies vaccine into the animal population has led to a reduction in the number of cases overall. Bat rabies occurs in North America and to a lesser extent within the bat population of parts of Europe.

Rabies in people is characterised by an acute encephalitis that is virtually always fatal within a week of first symptoms. The victim is apprehensive, with headache, pyrexia and muscle spasms, which progress to paralysis and death. The fear of water (more accurately of swallowing) has led to the name 'hydrophobia'. The laboratory diagnosis of the disease in the brain of a killed infected laboratory animal confirms the clinical manifestations in the patient.

The incubation period is normally three to eight weeks. It can be as short as nine days or as long as seven years. It depends on the dose of virus and on the nerve supply of the area that is wounded and its proximity to the brain. The virus migrates along peripheral nerves from the site of the bite into the central nervous system. Person-to-person transmission has never been demonstrated, although it is a theoretical risk because human saliva does contain the virus in an infected individual. A rare mode of transmission is via corneal transplant from an infected person who died of the disease, in whom it was not diagnosed.

Dogs and cats are usually infective from between three and 10 days before the onset of clinical illness and remain infectious throughout the course of the illness. A variety of wild animals act as a reservoir, including foxes, wolves, dogs, cats and bats. However, for practical purposes the disease is transferred in the majority of cases by a dog bite (or less often a cat bite). Transmission is by the bite of an infected animal or more rarely by contact between infected animal saliva and the human mucous membrane. The virus cannot penetrate intact skin.

Over many decades, the main strategy for

preventing rabies in the United Kingdom has been strict quarantine regulations coupled with legal penalties to prevent the disease being imported in animals. The United Kingdom has operated a pet travel scheme since the year 2000 that initially related to some European countries but was widened to others such as USA and Canada over time. The scheme applies only to dogs, cats and ferrets travelling between the United Kingdom and certain specified countries. Animals travelling to the United Kingdom from outside the scheme must enter quarantine for six months. Essentially, the scheme involves the pet being vaccinated against rabies, with blood-test confirmation. Each animal must then have a microchip to identify it and a passport and also have been treated against ticks and tapeworms.

Rabies vaccine is recommended for those working with the virus, those who deal with imported animals, licensed bat handlers, those whose work may bring them into contact with rabid animals abroad, and long-stay travellers to rabies endemic areas where access to medical help may be delayed should they be bitten. Health education measures should be employed: travellers to foreign countries should be encouraged to avoid all contact with animals, especially in those countries where rabies is endemic, and people should be warned of the hazards of illegally smuggling animals into this country.

An individual who has been bitten by an animal in which there is a suspicion of rabies or in a foreign country where the disease is endemic should have the wound immediately washed and thoroughly cleansed under medical supervision. Post-exposure treatment with active and passive immunisation (vaccine plus human anti-rabies immunoglobulin) should be considered. The decision whether to proceed with vaccination depends on the likelihood that the animal is infected. If the animal was not captured and rabies is endemic in the particular country, it is prudent to proceed with post-exposure treatment.

In the context of the British patient, all these measures depend on the quality and availability of medical services in the country that is being visited. An increasingly common occurrence as more people travel abroad is a history of animal bite in a returning traveller. Medical care may not have been sought or may not have been available in the country concerned. Personal experience indicates that the public health professional often becomes involved in such a situation. In one example, a party of schoolchildren returning from a school trip abroad contained two members who gave a history of having been bitten by a dog that had exhibited aggressive behaviour towards them. It was only upon return to Britain that parental concern led to the children presenting to the local accident and emergency department some four days after the bite. Through the Department of Health's international links, the animal was located and found to have remained healthy. Post-exposure treatment was not enforced, but it would have been commenced immediately if there was no official record of the incident, if the dog had escaped and could not be traced or if the dog had been killed and diagnosed as suffering from rabies.

Because dog bites are relatively common in the United Kingdom, it is easy to take a casual approach to a dog bite sustained by someone returning from abroad (particularly if they appear fit and well). It is important that such cases are taken seriously. Advice can be obtained from the Health Protection Agency on whether to instigate post-exposure rabies treatment in particular circumstances. There have been some 20 cases in England and Wales since World War II, all imported. Two cases were via bites of animals in Nigeria and the Philippines in 2001. A woman in Northern Ireland died in 2009 having worked in a South African wildlife centre.

If an established case is diagnosed in the United Kingdom, rigid rules of isolation usually apply, although the risk of person-to-person transmission is very slight. Attendant medical and nursing staff and all those potentially exposed to the patient's saliva are offered immunisation. Health care professionals should wear protective gloves and gowns and concurrent and terminal disinfection should be practised. Staff working with imported animals or in quarantine centres must be vaccinated against rabies.

VIRAL HAEMORRHAGIC FEVERS

Some haemorrhagic fevers caused by viruses such as yellow fever have been known from early times. However, since the mid-1950s new haemorrhagic illnesses have been recognised in humans. It is likely that they have been acquired from natural animal hosts. The main public health concern is that the viruses, having been transmitted from their natural host to humans, are then capable of producing person-to-person transmission. This risk is greatly minimised with strict isolation and meticulous medical and nursing procedures. Cases of this group of diseases are very rare in Britain and are almost exclusively imported by travellers from endemic areas.

➤ *Lassa fever* – is caused by a member of the arenavirus family. It was first isolated from an American missionary nurse in the Lassa township in Nigeria during 1969. Since then it has also occurred in Nigeria, Sierra Leone, Liberia and elsewhere in West Africa.

➤ *Marburg disease* – is caused by a virus first described in Marburg in the Federal Republic of Germany in 1967, when 31 cases with seven deaths occurred in Germany and Yugoslavia due to direct contact with the blood, organs and tissues of a batch of African green monkeys originally trapped in Uganda. It is endemic in central and southern Africa.

➤ *Ebola fever* – a very large outbreak of viral haemorrhagic fever with high fatality rates occurred in Southern Sudan and Zaire in 1976, where it still occurs. The causal virus was found to be morphologically identical to the Marburg virus but serologically distinct, and the new strain was named the Ebola virus.

➤ *Hantaan virus* – produces a haemorrhagic fever with renal syndrome and is a major public health problem in China and Korea, where the case fatality rate reaches about 7%. A milder (but also sometimes fatal) disease occurring in Scandinavia and eastern Europe is caused by an antigenic subtype: the Puumala virus.

➤ *Other haemorrhagic fevers* – other infections in this category are endemic in various parts of the world: for example, Dengue Fever (Southeast Asia and the Caribbean), Bolivian haemorrhagic fever (rural areas of Northern Bolivia) and Omsk haemorrhagic fever (parts of Siberia).

A very small number of cases of haemorrhagic fever may be imported into Britain. It should be suspected in patients with unexplained pyrexia who are returning from endemic areas of the world, provided that malaria has been excluded as a diagnosis. Symptoms vary, but often there is an insidious onset with a variety of non-specific symptoms, including general malaise, pyrexia, sore throat and enlarged lymph glands.

Later the patient's condition worsens, with conjunctivitis, chest and abdominal pains, vomiting and occasionally a mild maculopapular rash. Severe bleeding occurs between the fifth and seventh days, most often into the gastrointestinal tract and lung. Other features vary with the haemorrhagic fever concerned. For example, the severe form of Hantaan fever results in kidney symptoms and in some cases in renal failure.

The incubation period varies according to the disease. For example, it is usually 6 to 21 days for Lassa fever, 3 to 9 days for Marburg disease and 2 to 21 days for Ebola disease. The surveillance period for these fevers is usually extended to 21 days as an added precaution.

Where person-to-person transmission occurs, diseases are infectious as long as blood and body secretions contain the virus, which can be several weeks after clinical recovery. The reservoirs vary according to the disease. For Lassa fever, it is a species of wild rodent (*Mastomys natalensis*) in rural West Africa; for Marburg and Ebola disease, the animal reservoir is unknown; and for Haantan fever, the reservoir is field rodents.

Lassa fever is probably acquired through contact with the rodent's urine. Person-to-person spread may occur via the upper respiratory tract in the acute phase but more often is due to contact with infected blood, urine or secretions of the patient.

Although the original outbreak of Marburg disease occurred as a result of contact with African green monkeys, transmission of the disease from an animal to a person has not been demonstrated. Person-to-person spread has usually been due to very close contact with infected individuals. Many outbreaks have been related to hospitals in Africa where unsatisfactory practices have spread the disease amongst patients and staff. In some of these outbreaks, the case fatality rate has been over 50%. Such hospitals acted as amplifiers of the infection, with secondary cases occurring amongst staff and other patients. However, in one outbreak of Ebola fever, the introduction of adequate precautionary measures (care in handling a patient's blood, urine and other secretions) quickly brought the disease under control. In the original outbreak of Marburg fever, a number of secondary cases occurred amongst hospital staff who had been exposed to the patient's blood. In the

United Kingdom, the main risk is to ward and laboratory staff involved in the care of patients with viral haemorrhagic fever.

When a suspected case of viral haemorrhagic fever occurs, an infectious diseases specialist must be contacted to exclude malaria as a diagnosis. Where there are good grounds for suspicion, the consultant in communicable disease control is responsible for arranging the patient's admission to a high-security isolation unit by a special ambulance crew wearing protective clothing and special respirators. The Department of Health and the Health Protection Agency must be informed at the earliest opportunity. Close contacts of the patient, either those in the same household or workmates, are kept under strict daily surveillance for 21 days from the last date of exposure. A daily record is kept of temperature, and if a rise occurs or other signs or symptoms are evident, immediate isolation should be effected and admission to a high security isolation unit considered.

SMALLPOX

Smallpox is caused by the variola virus. Until the 1970s, smallpox was one of the world's major killing infectious diseases and hence has been the subject of an active vaccination programme worldwide. An eradication programme was launched by the World Health Organization in 1967. As a result of this action, the last known natural case of smallpox occurred in Somalia on 26 October 1977. However, in 1978 a medical photographer at Birmingham University contracted the disease as a result of an escape of the virus from a laboratory. She died of smallpox,

but her mother, who was the only other case, survived. Since this accident, rigorous measures have been instituted to reduce the risk of future tragedies of this sort.

Global eradication of the disease was pronounced by the World Health Assembly in 1980. The context has changed significantly since the spectre of bioterrorism presented itself in the early twenty-first century. The remaining supplies of smallpox virus are retained in high-security facilities in Russia and the United States. A number of countries, including the United Kingdom, have stockpiled smallpox vaccine in case the virus should be used in a biological attack.

SEXUALLY TRANSMITTED INFECTIONS

There were substantial increases (30% or more) of certain of the sexually transmitted infections (STIs) amongst teenagers in the mid-to-late 1990s, particularly gonorrhoea and genital chlamydia infection. This was despite the fact that these infections are both easily preventable and easily treatable.

GONORRHOEA

Gonorrhoea is a sexually transmitted disease that is found in all parts of the world. It is caused by a Gram-negative diplococcus, *Neisseria gonorrhoeae*. The initial symptom in men is a urethritis with a purulent discharge. The disease may progress, particularly if treatment is delayed, to cause prostatitis or epididymitis. In women, the shorter female urethra means that symptoms sometimes pass unnoticed. Ascending infection of the female genital tract may cause salpingitis and (in the longer term) infertility. In either sex, joint inflammation or meningitis can occur, though this is rare. The gonococcus may affect the eyes of a baby born to an infected mother, producing ophthalmia neonatorum.

Gonococcal infection is much more common in men who have sex with men than in heterosexual men. They present with anorectal and pharyngeal gonorrhoea (both can also occur in heterosexuals but are much less common) as well as urethral infections.

The diagnosis is usually made clinically and confirmed by stained smears of the infective exudate and, subsequently, culture of the organism. Urethral swabs in heterosexual men and women are the usual clinical investigation. In addition, throat swabs and anorectal swabs (during proctoscopy) are important in men who have sex with men.

In both sexes, the biggest reduction in incidence took place between 1985 and 1988. This was, at least in part, due a massmedia safe-sex campaign designed to reduce the risk of acquiring HIV infection. This rapid decline was, however, short-lived, and an upward trend in the incidence of gonorrhoea has occurred since. Reported gonorrhoea rates are an important marker of unprotected sexual activity, particularly in the high-risk groups. This indicator is even more important given the advent of HIV infection.

GENITAL *CHLAMYDIA TRACHOMATIS* INFECTION

Genital infection with *Chlamydia trachomatis* is the commonest sexually transmitted infection in the United Kingdom. Peak incidence is amongst young men and women aged under 25 years. Although it can cause symptoms similar to gonorrhoea, the discharge is often less obvious and the infection may be overlooked by the individual who gets it. Chlamydia can also be asymptomatic. One of the main risks of the disease is its liability to cause pelvic inflammatory disease in women, with consequent risk of blocked fallopian tubes and infertility.

A national chlamydia screening programme was introduced in the United Kingdom in the mid-2000s and has been gradually rolled out. Screening is provided in a diversity of settings, including contraceptive and abortion clinics, community pharmacies, general practices and youth centres. In England, in the population screened for the first time, the positivity rate was 1 in 10. Further follow-up and treatment is initiated in all positive cases.

TRICHOMONIASIS

The protozoan organism *Trichomonas vaginalis* is mainly an infection in women, though their male partners may be infected. Men remain asymptomatic or have mild symptoms. Women with this infection usually present with a strong-smelling vaginal discharge, soreness of the external genitalia and pain during intercourse (dyspareunia). A vaginal swab examined by microscopy and culture (and if necessary by other more specialised tests) usually confirms the diagnosis. Antimicrobial treatment of both the woman and her partner is necessary to be sure of eradicating the infection.

SYPHILIS

Syphilis, one of the longest-recognised sexually transmitted diseases, is caused by *Treponema pallidum*, a thin spiral organism (spirochaete) that does not stain well and is thus best seen with dark-field illumination microscopy.

It occurs in all parts of the world and is mainly a disease of young adults. In the 1960s and 1970s there was a large increase in the incidence of syphilis, in part due to male-to-male spread of infection. The number of new cases is small in comparison with gonorrhoea cases, but it is more common in seaports and large cities, and there have been a number of recent, well-publicised outbreaks. A fall in the reported incidence of syphilis in men who have sex with men occurred in the late 1980s, believed to be because of fear of AIDS, although heterosexually acquired infection in young adults rose. In the 2000s a number of large outbreaks (in Manchester, for example) amongst gay and bisexual men have presented. This suggests the 'fear factor' of HIV has waned or even that there is active risk-taking.

Syphilis is invariably acquired by sexual contact. The spirochaete does not survive long outside the human body; hence indirect methods of transmission are not usually important. Congenital syphilis arises from prenatal infection via the placenta.

There are three stages of the acquired disease. The primary lesion (chancre) develops as a painless ulcer on the skin or mucous membrane at the site of entry of the spirochaete, usually about three weeks after exposure. Even in untreated cases, the primary lesion disappears and is followed within 6 to 8 weeks by a generalised cutaneous rash heralding secondary syphilis. The tertiary stage develops after 3 to 20 years and can affect various parts of the body, including the bones, liver, cardiovascular system and central nervous system, giving rise to classical tabes dorsalis and general paralysis of the insane. Early treatment with antibiotics has greatly reduced the occurrence of the secondary and tertiary stages. In congenital syphilis, the foetus is frequently aborted or stillborn. If the child survives, handicapping conditions are the usual outcome.

The organism may be seen in specimens under dark-field illumination microscopy or using immunofluorescent techniques. There are also a number of important serological tests that are used to help make the diagnosis.

The patient is infectious during the primary and secondary stages of the disease and may also be intermittently infectious during latent periods. Effective antibiotic treatment makes the patient non-infectious within one or two days.

GENITAL HERPES

Genital herpes is caused by the *Herpes simplex* virus (usually type 2), which is transmitted by sexual intercourse. The type 1 *Herpes simplex* virus is associated with lesions on the mouth and face ('cold sores') but can also cause the genital form of herpes. Genital herpes occurs in male and female heterosexuals and men who have sex with men (in whom it occurs on the penis, in the anorectal area and sometimes in the mouth).

Genital herpes is a relapsing condition. The skin heals and then can break down and ulcerate long after the primary infection.

Symptoms of the primary infection include pain in the genitals and buttocks and sometimes fever, followed by an eruption of vesicles on the skin and mucous membranes of the genital area that gradually break down to produce painful ulcers. Discharge and secondary bacterial infection are common.

Treatment is symptomatic, and antiviral drugs are sometimes effective. The virus becomes latent in the dorsal root ganglia and can then recur at any time, although the number and severity of recurrences varies greatly.

ANAL AND GENITAL WARTS

Warts in the anal and genital areas are caused by viruses, mainly the human papillomavirus (HPV), although another virus also causes a warty-type infection called molluscum contagiosum. Reported cases of anogenital warts have increased in recent years in heterosexuals and gay men. It is likely that this represents a true increase in occurrence, but greater awareness on the part of patients and clinicians has undoubtedly contributed to the increase.

An important association is that between certain types of human papillomavirus and the development of cervical cancer. This topic is discussed in the section on 'Infections for which comprehensive vaccination programmes are available'.

CANDIDIASIS

The yeast *Candida albicans* is a relatively common cause of pruritus, severe vulval discomfort and vaginal discharge. In many cases, the infection is due to spread of the organism from the gastrointestinal tract, where it exists as a commensal, but in some instances it is sexually transmitted. Treatment with antimicrobial pessaries usually resolves the infection.

OTHER DISEASES TRANSMITTED SEXUALLY

A number of other diseases can be transmitted sexually but are not thought of primarily as sexually transmitted diseases. They are discussed elsewhere in the chapter. These include hepatitis B, hepatitis A, scabies and cytomegalovirus.

CONTROL OF SEXUALLY TRANSMITTED DISEASES

In the 1980s and 1990s the whole field of sexually transmitted diseases was transformed from a relatively quiet backwater of clinical and public health practice to one of major international importance by the emergence of the human immunodeficiency virus (HIV), which causes acquired immune deficiency syndrome (AIDS). This subject is covered in the section on new and emerging diseases, but many of the control measures that apply to the control of its spread sexually also apply to other sexually transmitted diseases. Thus HIV-directed health promotion and health education programmes aimed at modifying sexual behaviour and encouraging safer sexual practices, particularly in young people, are equally important to the prevention and control of these other diseases. Well-designed and properly conducted sex education programmes have been demonstrated to bring about a measurable improvement in sexual attitudes and behaviour.

Traditionally, the focus for the prevention and control of sexually transmitted diseases has been the network of genitourinary medicine clinics provided around the country within the National Health Service. Prompt diagnosis and investigation of people presenting is vital, and the tracing of contacts of patients is a key control measure in most diseases. Contact tracing or partner notification (as it is now more commonly called) is a skilled exercise requiring considerable diplomacy, and it is often undertaken by specially trained nurses, health visitors or social workers.

Many of the recent changes in sexually transmitted infection services have been stimulated by experiences of dealing with HIV infection in which it has been important to make sure that risk groups come forward for testing, advice and counselling. The spin-offs for the prevention and control of other sexually transmitted diseases have been important and beneficial.

SOME OTHER PARASITIC DISEASES
ECTOPARASITES
Scabies

Scabies is caused by *Sarcoptes scabiei*, a small mite just visible to the naked eye. The disease occurs in most parts of the world. It appears to fluctuate over a 15-year cycle in Britain. 'The itch', as it was known, has a long history, and it may have been the condition mentioned in the Old Testament for which the treatment advised was bathing in the River Jordan (now known to have a high sulphur content).

Skin lesions caused by burrowing of the mite are most commonly found between the fingers, on the anterior surfaces of the wrist and on the soles of the feet. Symptoms occur when sensitisation develops, with a papular rash that may spread to any part of the body except the face. Itching is intense, especially in bed at night. Scratching may result in secondary infection. The diagnosis is confirmed by extracting the female mite from the burrow and identifying it under the microscope.

The initial infestation passes unnoticed until sensitisation occurs about two months later. In people who have been previously infested, the time is much shorter (one to four weeks). The affected person is infectious until effective treatment is carried out.

The reservoir is human. Scabies in animals (such as dogs) does not transfer to people. Transmission is by close personal contact, such as holding hands or sexual intercourse. It has not been possible to demonstrate transfer by indirect means such as bed linen or clothing. There is no need to isolate the patient after treatment, but contacts should be examined and treated if necessary. It is helpful to treat all family contacts of the patient simultaneously to avoid re-infection. The maintenance of good personal hygiene standards should also be encouraged.

Lice

There are three types of human lice; all are members of the order Anoplura (sucking lice) and are parasites exclusively of mammals. All feed on the blood of the host and parasitise only one species, hence they are strongly host-specific. Moreover, many of the 500 known species of lice are so highly specialised that they only colonise one part of the body of their particular host.

Two genera of lice infest humans, *Phthirus* and *Pediculus*, although only one species of each is involved. When people began to wear clothes, and hair became restricted to the head, axilla and pubic areas, human lice themselves underwent modifications. The crab louse (*Phthirus pubis*) adapted to live on the hair around the human genitalia, while the body louse migrated to clothing, only returning to the host to feed. The head louse became a scalp dweller and specialised to such a degree that its survival depends on being in almost continual contact with its source of food and warmth. There are two varieties of *Pediculus humanus* – *Pediculus humanus humanus* (the body louse) and *Pediculus humanus capitis* (the head louse).

The Body Louse (Pediculus Humanus)

This louse is different from many species of Anoplura in that it lives on the host indirectly (on the clothing), laying its eggs on the seams, near the skin. It visits the body only long enough to obtain meals of human blood. The eggs are laid, attach to the fibres of clothing and, if the temperature is right, hatch within 7 days. The young louse matures in about 7 days and has an average lifespan of 30 days. It is unusual for lice to remain on the body after the clothing has been removed. However, treatment usually consists of an appropriate topical application. A convenient way of delousing clothing is to put it dry into a tumble-drier for five minutes at the maximum temperature, a manoeuvre that kills both lice and eggs.

The Crab Louse or Pubic Louse (Phthirus Pubis)

This parasite has preference for the coarse, widely spaced hair in the pubic area, though occasionally it may be found on legs, beards or eyelashes. The louse tends to feed from the same spot at the base of a hair. It is not easily visible, since it blends in with the skin. The eggs are glued onto the hair and hatched in about eight days. The young louse is mature within a week. Spread is nearly always by sexual contact, and the appropriate current treatment should be chosen by consulting the *British Pharmacopoeia*.

The Head Louse (Pediculus Humanus Capitis)

This louse is strongly host-specific and for all practical purposes is found in only one place: the hair close to the scalp of human beings. The eggs (nits) have been found on the hair of an Egyptian mummy, and there are numerous references to the louse in literature from the time of the Greek classics.

The head louse is about the size of a matchstick head and has a lifespan of 30 days, but few survive in the natural state for so long. The eggs are laid in a glue-like medium that attaches them to a hair shaft, very close to the scalp. Usually they hatch within 7 days into a nymph, which becomes mature within about 10 days. The sole food is human blood. The louse moves quickly but does not readily leave the host. The mode of transmission is almost certainly by the louse walking from one person's head to another when they are in close contact.

Head louse infestation occurs throughout

the world, but it appears to be more common in Western countries. Most infestations are light, and the principal symptoms are itching of the scalp with consequent disturbances of sleep. Secondary infection may occur with scratching, and, since lice can harbour in their intestines bacteria capable of causing impetigo, wounds may become infected in this way.

If someone, particularly a child or young person, presents with an itchy scalp, impetigo or excoriation around the nape of the neck, head infestation must be ruled out. The eggs (nits) are firmly attached to the hair and hence can be distinguished from dandruff. The egg is laid on the hair shaft very close to the scalp and initially is greyish in colour and difficult to see. Later, as the hair grows, the nit becomes pearl white and easily visible. The eggs are frequently located behind the ears, although they may be found anywhere on the head. Eggs found more than a few centimetres from the scalp can be assumed to be dead. The live lice are difficult to see.

The insecticides most appropriate for the treatment of head infestation should be chosen by consulting the current edition of the *British Pharmacopoeia*. The reservoir of infestation is frequently the family, so it is important that the whole family is treated at the same time.

ENDOPARASITES
Enterobiasis (Threadworm Disease)

Threadworm is caused by *Enterobius vermicularis*, a small, whitish, thread-like nematode (roundworm) 5–12 mm long. The disease is found in most parts of the world and is the most common helminth infection affecting people. Up to 15 million people may be infected in the United Kingdom, and more often these are children.

The patient is often symptomless but may notice the threadlike worms on the surface of the stool. The most common symptom is itching around the anus, which may lead to scratching and disturbed sleep. The worm may cause appendicitis or, by migration, vaginitis or salpingitis. These complications are, however, extremely rare, and the majority of patients have very mild symptoms. Diagnosis is made by pressing Sellotape on to perianal skin and then onto a microscope slide. Characteristic eggs are seen under the microscope.

The incubation period is two to six weeks, though it may take longer before symptoms appear, because the number of worms increases with continuous self-reinfections. The patient is infectious for as long as pregnant female worms remain in the gut. An individual worm lives for about two months. The reservoir is human. Similar worms in other animals do not infect people.

The adult worm lives in the caecum and the small and large intestines. The gravid female migrates through the anal orifice and lays small, sticky eggs on the skin of the perianal region. The eggs are then carried by the fingers to the mouth or indirectly to another individual. They are capable of survival for a few days on clothes, bed linen or dust if conditions are cool and moist. However, person-to-person transmission is most common. When swallowed, the eggs hatch out in the small intestine and the cycle recommences.

There is no need to isolate the patient, but the family and other close contacts should be screened. Simultaneous treatment of all infected members of the family is essential to prevent re-infection. In addition, there should be education in personal hygiene, frequency of washing of the perianal region and the need to keep fingernails short and clean. The most important general environmental control measures are frequent washing of personal clothing and bed linen. The hot cycle of the domestic washing machine is sufficient to destroy the eggs. In institutions the eggs may be present in dust, so a general clean-up should accompany treatment of patients.

CONCLUSIONS

Infectious disease surveillance and control remains a central component of public health practice. Despite the decline in the relative importance of infectious disease as a cause of death, it remains a major source of morbidity in the population. Infectious diseases can produce distressing symptoms and complications.

While control of the acute outbreak of illness caused by a micro-organism is vitally important and is the aspect of this field of work that keeps infectious diseases in the public eye, it is only one part of a comprehensive public health approach to control. A detailed understanding of the nature, causes, modes of transmission and clinical features of infectious diseases is also essential to an overall strategy of population control of this group of diseases. So too, as in many other fields of public health, is the availability of accurate information and its proper analysis. There is also a need for clear policies for infectious disease control that

place strong emphasis on prevention and on organisations working in partnership to address the problem.

DEFINITIONS OF TERMS USED FOR INFECTIOUS DISEASES AND PARASITES

Airborne transmission: this is due to the formation of droplet nuclei by evaporation; the particles are small and can be widely dispersed.

Carriers: people who intermittently or continuously harbour infective organisms without suffering the clinical manifestations of the disease. People who excrete the organisms only occasionally are referred to as intermittent carriers. Convalescent carriers are those who remain infective even after recovering from the illness, and the term chronic carrier is applied if this condition persists over months or years. Typhoid carriers may excrete the organism for years, usually because *Salmonella typhi* has infected the gallbladder. Some infections are carried by people who give no history of illness caused by the agent. This healthy carrier state occurs in diphtheria and meningococcal infection.

Commensals: organisms that cause no harm to the host; one or both may gain benefit. If both gain benefit, the state is symbiosis.

Communicable diseases: synonymous with 'infectious diseases' and sometimes referred to as 'contagious diseases' or 'transmissible diseases', communicable diseases are caused by a living organism and transmitted from person to person or from animal or bird to person, either directly or indirectly.

Contact: a person who has the opportunity to acquire infection by virtue of having come into contact with an infected individual or animal or a contaminated environment.

Definitive or primary host: a host in which a parasite reaches maturity or passes through its sexual stage.

Disinfection: the killing of an infectious agent outside the body by direct application of a chemical substance or by physical means such as heat. Concurrent disinfection is the application of disinfective measures to discharges or excreta from the patient as they occur. Terminal disinfection is the use of disinfective measures after the recovery or removal of the patient. It usually applies to rooms and furniture. It is seldom necessary, because thorough cleansing and good ventilation are equally effective.

Disinfestation: the removal or destruction of insects and their ova or larvae associated with an individual and his or her clothing or premises. It also applies to the destruction or removal of rodents.

Droplet transmission: infection caused by a projection of small droplets from the nose or mouth due to sneezing, coughing, talking or exhaling. The range of spread is usually limited to a few feet.

Ectoparasites: parasites that live only on the surface of the host's body and are usually insects.

Endoparasites: parasites that live only inside the host's body; examples are worms and many protozoa.

Endemic: an endemic disease is one that is constantly present in a given geographical area, although it may temporarily increase its incidence to become an epidemic.

Endotoxins: types of toxins (poison) liberated only when the bacterial cell wall is broken; they are important in causing shock.

Epidemic: an increase in the frequency of occurrence of a disease in a population above its baseline level for a specified period of time.

Exotic disease: an infectious condition that is not usually found in Britain but may be imported from overseas.

Exotoxins: toxins produced by bacteria that pass into the tissues of the body. Examples of organisms that produce toxins resulting in illness are diphtheria and tetanus.

Facultative parasites: parasites that are capable of an independent existence outside the host.

Hosts: Animals, birds (also humans) that give support to, and provide a living environment for, an infectious agent. Some parasites pass through their stages of development in different hosts.

Incubation period: the time that elapses between a person becoming infected and the appearance of the first symptoms. Its length is mainly determined by the nature of the infecting organism, but it is also influenced to some extent by the dose of the organism, the route of entry into the body and the susceptibility of the host.

Insect vector: an insect that carries the disease agent either mechanically (on its feet or other parts of its body) or within its body so that the agent is transmitted to the person being infected either by saliva (when the insect bites) or by faeces (deposited on the skin).

Intermediate or secondary host: one in which a parasite is in its larval or asexual stage.

Medical parasitology: although many viruses, bacteria and fungi that cause disease in a strictly biological sense are parasites, it is customary to restrict the term 'medical parasitology' to the branch of medicine that deals with parasites living in or on humans. These parasites are members of the animal kingdom. They fall into three main groups: protozoa (single-cell organisms), helminths (worms) and arthropods (insects).

Nosocomial infection: an infection that occurs in patients or staff and that originated within the hospital or other health setting. Tends to be referred to in day-to-day parlance as 'Health care-associated infection'.

Obligatory parasites: parasites that cannot survive outside the host.

Pandemic: an epidemic of worldwide proportions.

Primary case: the first case that occurs in an outbreak, also referred to as the index case.

Reservoir of infection: any animal, insect, plant or inanimate substance (for example, foodstuff) in which an infectious agent dwells and from which it is capable of being transmitted to a susceptible host.

Sporadic: a term used when cases of infectious diseases are not found to be linked to each other.

Subclinical infection: an infection that gives rise to no reported symptoms or signs in the host.

Vehicle: a contaminated inanimate object (for example, fomites such as toys, blankets, handkerchiefs or soiled linen) or material (for example, food, water, milk, body fluids) allowing an infectious agent to gain entry to a suitable host. The organism might or might not have multiplied on the vehicle.

Zoonoses: Infectious diseases that are transmitted to people from animals. It is estimated that there are some 400 known zoonoses.

REFERENCES

1 Department of Health. *Immunisation Against Infectious Disease: the Green Book*. London: Department of Health; 2008.

2 Murch SH, Andrew A, Casson DH, *et al*. Retraction of an interpretation. *Lancet*. 2004; **363**: 750.

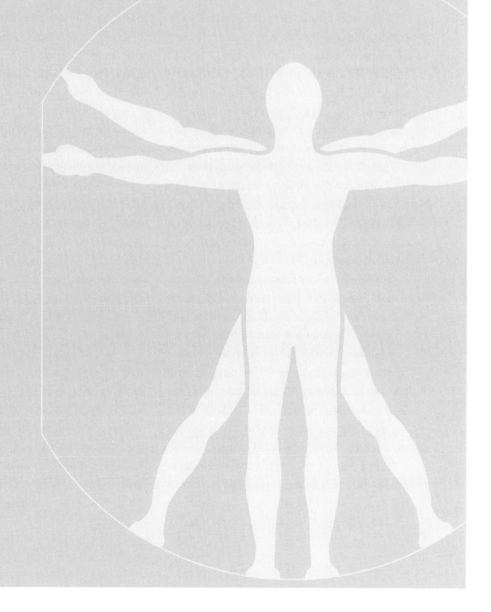

CHAPTER 10
Environment and Health

INTRODUCTION

The links between the environment and human health have long been recognised. In ancient Greece they were recognised because the development of the empire was dependent on the health of the population in the trading centres that it established. In one of the Hippocratic corpus of writings, *Airs, Waters, Places*, the association is made between the conditions affecting inhabitants and the prevailing climate and water quality.

The direct connection between physical conditions and health was a main theory of disease causation until the nineteenth century. The name 'malaria' comes from the medieval Italian for 'bad air' and was also know in English as 'marsh fever' because of its association with swampy ground. The 'miasmatic' theory of disease attributed the origin of serious outbreaks of scourges such as cholera to the airborne carriage of particles of decaying organic matter. It wasn't until the end of the nineteenth century that the germ theory of disease displaced the fear of the miasma.

Some of the conditions for the generation of disease arise from climate and nature independent of the activities of humankind. However, the changes that human activity impose on the natural world play a major role in disease causation. Human activity can prevent disease as well, of course, whether by the draining of malarial swamps or the development of an abundant food supply through conversion of land to agriculture.

The concept of environment encompasses our physical surroundings, either natural or man-made; the air that we breathe; the pollution we create; the quality and availability of our water; the climate and natural life that make up our ecosystem; and the social, economic and political infrastructure that regulates and controls our lives. It is together that these different facets of a complex environment exert their influence on health. This chapter deals with that relationship.

GLOBAL WARMING AND CLIMATE CHANGE

At the very heart of any public health analysis of environment and health in the twenty-first century is global warming. Having been much disputed, often by those with vested interests, there is now a strong consensus that global warming is a fact and also that it is due to the pollution of the environment by humankind. The burning of fossil fuels releases into the atmosphere so-called 'greenhouse gases', which trap heat from the sun in the atmosphere and cause the temperature of the earth's surface to rise (Figure 10.1). The pattern of the earth's weather is changing, and changing rapidly. In particular, the altered pattern of rainfall and increased incidence and severity of adverse weather events pose significant threats.

The change in temperature itself is a major public health problem, with the heatwave in Europe in 2003 contributing to over 35 000 premature deaths. Summer heatwaves are not new, but the warmer baseline means that the heatwave temperature will be higher too. The elderly are particularly vulnerable, and specific community-based plans address the risks in the event of a heatwave.

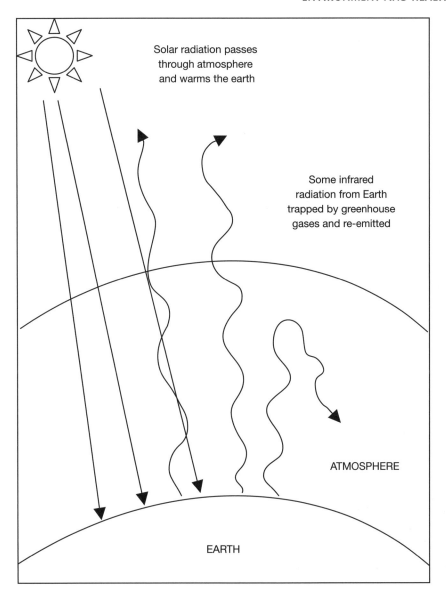

Solar radiation passes
through atmosphere
and warms the earth

Some infrared
radiation from Earth
trapped by greenhouse
gases and re-emitted

ATMOSPHERE

EARTH

Figure 10.1 The effect of greenhouse gases

More important is the global effect that climate change is already having, and this seems certain to intensify in the future. The climate-sensitive global health problems of malnutrition, diarrhoea and malaria will be affected by factors such as changes in water availability and food production and by the altered dynamics of pathogens and vectors. The global health effects of climate change were addressed by the World Health Organization at its 2008 Assembly (Table 10.1).

Table 10.1 Health issues and actions in respect of climate change

Health issues

- Climate change threatens public health security.

- Health impacts will be disproportionately greater in vulnerable populations.

- Mitigating the effects of climate change can have direct and immediate health benefits.

- Adaptation is needed because some degree of climate change is inevitable, even if greenhouse gas emissions were abruptly capped. Failure to respond will be costly in terms of disease, health care expenditure and lost productivity.

Actions

- Raise awareness of the need to ensure public health security by acting on climate change.

- Enhance capacity to deal with public health emergencies.

- Promote health development. National and sub-national health agencies can promote health through assessment of the health implications of decisions taken in other sectors.

- Enhance applied research on health protection from climate change.

- Monitor and evaluate delivery.

- Foster cross-disciplinary partnerships.

Source: Adapted from report from the Secretariat to the World Health Assembly, 2008.

CARBON REDUCTION

In the middle of the nineteenth century, the Irish scientist John Tyndall showed that levels of carbon dioxide (CO_2) have a profound effect on the ability of air to trap infrared radiation. Carbon dioxide traps within the atmosphere the infrared radiation emitted by the Earth's surface. The levels of carbon dioxide in the Earth's atmosphere have varied over hundreds of thousands of years. Today, levels of carbon dioxide in the atmosphere are higher than they have been for over 650 000 years. The atmospheric burden is growing because of carbon releases from the combustion of fossil fuel (oil, coal and gas). Levels of other important greenhouse gases, such as methane, have also been rising.

To take account of all the major green-house gases, a 'carbon dioxide equivalent' figure is used. In 2007 this was deemed to be at the level of about 430 parts per million (ppm). The temperature rise of the atmosphere will continue irrespective of current action because of the lag-time between the levels of carbon and the response of the Earth, particularly the oceans. Urgent action to cut carbon emissions would limit the warming of the Earth to the minimum possible level. The most widely advocated target is to restrict the level to less than 450 ppm.

The United Kingdom government's target is by 2050 to have reduced carbon dioxide emissions by 80% from their 1990 level. Some commentators consider that this level of reduction is insufficient to avoid the worst effects of global warming.

Health services are major users of energy

in their own right. They are also major generators of patient and staff journeys, major consumers of goods and services and major producers of waste. The NHS represents about 10% of gross domestic product and is Europe's largest employer, with 1.3 million employees. The NHS must make the necessary changes in its operation to contribute to the achievement of the targets. The carbon footprint of the NHS in England has been estimated to be 18 million tons of CO_2 (about 3% of total emissions in the country), which makes it the largest public-sector contributor. The different elements of NHS activity show that procurement is a key area for carbon reduction (Figure 10.2).

The public health perspective is not only about avoiding the worst effects of global warming; it is also concerned with identifying the changes required in society to have major beneficial effects on health. For example, a substantial shift to active forms of travel and away from reliance on the internal combustion engine will increase levels of physical activity. Reduction in animal husbandry, a major source of methane emissions, will reduce meat eating and contribute to lower levels of vascular disease and cancer. This interaction between the human race and the planet on which we live has been summed up by the American eco-theologian Thomas Berry.

> Human health is a subsystem of the Earth's health. You cannot have well humans on a sick planet. And that is

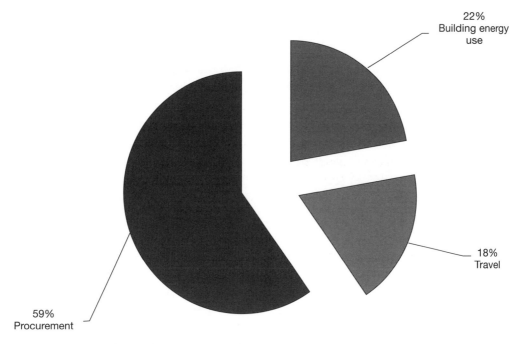

Figure 10.2 Sectoral contribution to NHS carbon emissions, 2004
Source: NHS Sustainable Development Unit. *Saving Carbon, Improving Health: a draft carbon reduction strategy for the NHS in England – a consultation document.* London: Department of Health; 2008.

what we are trying to do, with all our technologies: we are trying to have well humans on a sick planet.

Thomas Berry. The mystique of the earth [Interview]. *Caduceus* magazine. 2003; **59**.

SUSTAINABLE DEVELOPMENT

The interdependence of people and their environment is captured in the concept of sustainable development. In 1992, the United Nations Conference on Environment and Development, also known as the Earth Summit, was held in Rio de Janeiro. It was attended by over 100 heads of government, which made it the largest-ever gathering of world leaders. The action plan, Agenda 21, recommended the formulation of sustainable development strategies by every country.

The standard definition of sustainable development comes from *Our Common Future*, the report of the World Commission on Environment and Development, published in 1987. Sustainable development is development that meets the needs of the present without compromising the ability of future generations to meet their own needs. The United Kingdom Sustainability Development Strategy, *Securing the Future*, which was published in 2005, stated that the goal of sustainable development:

. . . will be pursued in an integrated way through a sustainable, innovative and productive economy that delivers high levels of employment; and a just society that promotes social inclusion, sustainable communities and personal wellbeing. This will be done in ways that protect and enhance the physical and natural environment, and use resources and energy as efficiently as possible.

The strategy is monitored by a national data set of 68 indicators, of which the 20 shown in Table 10.2 are the framework representing the agreed priorities.

HEALTH AND THE BUILT ENVIRONMENT

The connection between housing conditions and health has long been recognised (and is discussed later in this chapter), but many other aspects of the built environment have been neglected. Decisions made by planning authorities and their impact on the health of current and future residents are often not made explicit. The communities in which low-income families live are more likely to contain environmental hazards and less likely to be conducive to physical activity and healthy eating. It is inevitable that such problems will contribute to the burden of ill health and health inequalities suffered by a local population.

Decisions taken at national governmental or local level in many different fields may ultimately have an effect on the health of the population. For example, education has an important bearing on people's health and lifestyle in later life. So a national education policy, while primarily intended to improve an aspect of the education of school-age children, could secondarily have an influence on the health of the population in years

Table 10.2 UK framework indicators for sustainable development

- Greenhouse gas emissions
- Resource use
- Waste arisings
- Bird populations
- Fish stocks sustainability
- River quality
- Ecological impacts of air pollution
- Economic growth
- Active community participation
- Crime
- Employment
- Workless households
- Childhood poverty
- Pensioner poverty
- Educational attainment
- Health inequality
- Mobility
- Social justice
- Environmental equality
- Wellbeing

Source: Department for Environment, Food and Rural Affairs. *Sustainable Development Indicators in Your Pocket 2007.* London: DEFRA; 2007.

to come. Similarly, a local plan to site a new young people's centre alongside a busy dual carriageway, while primarily intended to improve access to leisure facilities, may have the secondary effect of increasing the rate of accidents (young people crossing the road) or asthma attacks from traffic fumes.

The realisation that there may be health consequences to many aspects of public policy and decision-making has led to the development of methodologies to assess them. Health impact assessment (HIA) is a form of appraisal of policy in which full health consequences can be explored. The methodology has been developed from a longer-standing and similar approach used to assess the impact of planned new developments on the environment (environmental impact assessment). The adoption of such an approach to health has been applied to major projects, such as the second runway at Manchester airport.

In the late 1990s, the United Kingdom government decided that major new government policies should be assessed for their impact on health. Local decision-makers must think about what the effects might be on health and in particular how they might reduce inequality. The three key questions used in deciding whether a particular project or policy should be subject to the process are listed in Table 10.4. If at least two of the three questions can be answered in the affirmative, a health impact assessment should be carried out. This development took place as recognition was given to the necessity of carrying out impact assessment on the basis of aspects such as gender, race and disability. The development of integrated impact assessment has been designed to provide a methodology that will cover all areas.

WATER

Water is a resource. Looked at internationally, the provision of safe water to drink, to use in the preparation of food and for sanitation is an aspiration, not a reality. The increased demand for water for domestic use, recreation and leisure, industry and agriculture has meant that water is increasingly seen as a precious resource that cannot be taken for granted. The government issues guidance requiring water companies to agree with the Environment Agency's water resource plan for the long term. Targets to reduce leakage from the water distribution system have also been set for each water company.

The quality of water is also an important public health issue. Micro-organisms, chemicals and pesticides are all potential water pollutants that can affect health. Contamination of the water supply has been a major cause of disease and death in the past and still is in some developing countries. It was the provision of a safe water supply, together with proper disposal of sewage, that constituted one of the triumphs of the public health pioneers in nineteenth-century Britain.

Water is an excellent solvent for most gases and many solids. It also carries other substances in suspension. Surface water is the main source of public supply in Britain. Water flowing over the ground dissolves minerals and can carry suspended matter,

Table 10.3 Seven key elements of the built environment and health

1	Activity-promoting environments: Foster incidental and recreational activity
2	Nutrition-promoting environments: Provide and promote safe, affordable, healthy food
3	Housing: Availability of safe, affordable, available housing
4	Transportation: Safe, reliable, accessible and affordable methods for moving people around
5	Environmental quality: Safe, clean water, soil, air, and building materials
6	Product availability: Availability of safe, health-promoting or unsafe, unhealthy products
7	Aesthetic/ambiance: Well-maintained, appealing, clean environment

Source: Prevention Institute, Oakland, CA.

as well as bacteria, viruses, protozoa, algae and various other plant and animal products. Upland surface water in natural lakes and man-made reservoirs supplies about 35% of drinking water and is relatively free from contamination by human and animal waste. Lowland rivers, which supply about 30% of drinking water, become more polluted as they flow from their source to the sea. In some parts of Britain, it is necessary

Table 10.4 Screening questions for health impact assessment

1 Will your policy have a significant impact on human health by virtue of its effects on the following wider determinants of health?
Income
Crime
Environment
Transport
Housing
Education
Employment
Agriculture
Social cohesion
2 Will there be a significant impact on any of the following lifestyle related variables?
Physical activity
Diet
Smoking, drugs, or alcohol use
Sexual behaviour
Accidents and stress at home or work
Consider risk factors that influence the probability of an individual becoming more or less healthy.
3 Is there likely to be a significant demand on any of the following health and social care services?
Primary care
Community services
Hospital care
Need for medicines
Accident or emergency attendances
Social services
Health protection and preparedness response

Source: Department of Health, London; 2007.

to draw on sources from the lower reaches of rivers, and a full purification treatment may be necessary.

Underground water from deep wells and boreholes requires only minimal treatment, being of good quality and almost free from contamination. This source contributes about one-third of the public water supply. It may be 'hard' water because of the dissolved minerals, but most people find it palatable.

MONITORING THE QUALITY OF WATER

Water for human consumption undergoes regular physical, chemical and bacteriological tests. Physical properties such as taste, colour and smell are high priorities in determining acceptability, although they may have little bearing on whether the water is safe to drink. The responsibility for monitoring drinking water standards rests with the Drinking Water Inspectorate (the Drinking Water Quality Regulator in Scotland), which was established in 1990. There has been a marked improvement in drinking water quality since 1990, although the improvement has been less impressive in Scotland and Northern Ireland.

Chemical analysis to determine the type and importance of various chemicals present in water is well established. The decomposition of organic matter contributes to the presence of nitrogen compounds, either as inorganic ammonia, nitrate and nitrites or in its various organic forms. High concentrations of chlorides suggest contamination by sewage. Calcium and magnesium salts are an indication of the hardness of the water. The absence of dissolved oxygen is strong evidence of heavy pollution. In addition, chemical analysis may reveal the presence of small quantities of potentially dangerous substances, such as lead.

Bacteriological examination has been based mainly on isolating and quantifying faecal-indicator organisms. *Escherichia coli* is an indicator of human or animal faecal pollution, and coliforms are a less-specific indicator. *Cryptosporidium* has been a difficult issue for the water industry to tackle. The disease it causes, cryptosporidiosis, has traditionally shown both spring and autumn peaks. Regulations to combat waterborne *Cryptosporidium* spread appear to have resulted in a reduction in the spring peak but not in the autumn one.

PURIFICATION TREATMENT

The aim of purification is to remove pathogenic bacteria, harmful chemicals, suspended matter and any substance causing colour, odour or undesirable taste. There are a number of methods of water purification, including coagulation filtration, disinfection with chlorine and the use of ozone and activated charcoal. The method most commonly used in Britain is described here. In general, underground water needs less treatment than river water.

Water is first coarse-filtered to remove solid objects and then stored in reservoirs to allow sedimentation. This storage system has the advantage of allowing the supply from the rivers to be cut off if excessive contamination occurs.

The next step in the purification process is filtration, through either slow or rapid filters. Slow sand filters consist of sand resting on layers of graded gravel. The active part is the slime (containing bacteria, protozoa and other organisms) that forms on the surface, trapping fine suspended matter (including bacteria) and consuming and oxidising organic matter. Rapid sand filters are more widely used and are made of coarser sand that allows the water to flow through more quickly. Salts of aluminium or iron are added to the water to form floccules, to help remove suspended matter, colour and organic substances. Some bacteria can pass through, and their destruction depends on the next phase of purification, which is disinfection.

Chlorine is the most widely used disinfectant agent and is automatically delivered, by specialised equipment, at a sufficient concentration so that a residual concentration of 0.5 ppm (parts per million) remains after 30 minutes' contact with the water. Before the water is distributed, the level of chlorine is reduced by sulphur dioxide to 0.1–0.3 ppm; at this residual level, some disinfectant properties remain without causing complaints of chlorine taste or smell.

After purification, water is held in covered service reservoirs and delivered in main pipes sunk deep enough to avoid frosts.

FLUORIDE AND DENTAL HEALTH

The presence of fluoride in drinking water at about 1 ppm has been found to reduce dental decay in the population by some 30–50%. Small amounts of fluoride occur naturally in water that is in contact with the Earth's rocks. In many countries, including parts of Britain, fluoride is also added to the water supply. Higher levels, which sometimes occur naturally, may cause mottling of the dental enamel.

Fluoridation of the public water supply has been controversial, with opponents claiming serious ill effects following the consumption of fluoridated drinking water. However, most authorities have found no evidence to substantiate this claim. Other countries, such as Ireland, have introduced this dental health measure on a national basis.

The geographical distribution of fluoridated water is patchy in Britain, to the disadvantage of many children's dental health. A major obstacle has been the refusal of private water companies to introduce fluoridation; they quote the potential for litigation should evidence of illness causation emerge in the future. This has been dealt with by legislation via the Water Act 2003, which compelled the water companies to fluoridate if requested and set out the approach to consultation to be taken in England.

NITRATE

Agriculture is the main source of nitrate in the water. Nitrogen from the soil and from fertilisers is released into rivers and may seep into underground water. The amount that is leached from agricultural land depends on the farming activities and the climate. Nitrates in deep underground water may therefore be a reflection of agricultural activities in earlier years. Excessive nitrates in the water supply can result in methaemoglobinaemia, a disorder of the oxygen-carrying ability of the bloodstream in young babies.

In parts of Britain the nitrate level in

water sources is higher than the limit set by the European Council directive on drinking water, but these waters are treated before supply by water suppliers using denitrification plants to meet the limit. In order to help overcome this problem, the government has designated nitrate-sensitive areas in which certain agricultural operations are regulated. In addition, farmers may qualify for payments to change their farming operations – such as switching from arable to grassland cultivation.

LEAD

Lead has been recognised as a poison for centuries. Lead in tap water is virtually always derived from the domestic plumbing system, particularly where the water is soft and acidic. Introduction of a European Council directive on drinking water in 1998 reduced the maximum permitted level of lead in drinking water to 10 micrograms per litre by 2013 (with an interim level of 25 micrograms per litre to be met by 2003).

There is evidence that lead can cause intellectual impairment in children, therefore levels of lead in drinking water should be as low as possible. This can be achieved by individuals flushing the pipes before consuming the water and by water undertakings rendering the water more alkaline or adding orthophosphate. Replacement of lead pipes is the most satisfactory solution.

ALUMINIUM

Acidic water sources, such as upland surface waters with substantial peat deposits, may contain relatively high concentrations of naturally occurring aluminium. Aluminium sulphate and other aluminium compounds are also widely used in water treatment to improve the appearance and taste of the drinking water and to aid the efficiency of disinfection. Most aluminium is removed in water treatment. If too much aluminium remains, it causes colour and turbidity problems. The statutory limit is 200 parts per billion (micrograms per litre). Higher concentrations may be allowed when the aluminium is from the water source rather than from water treatment. Research has investigated whether aluminium may be causal in Alzheimer's disease. There is no convincing evidence for this hypothesis thus far.

BATHING WATER

The European Union has set tough standards for bathing water quality. The possible effects on health of bathing in seawater contaminated by sewage or farm-animal manure are a matter of public concern. There are 574 identified bathing waters in the United Kingdom, of which 11 are inland freshwater sites. In England and Wales the water quality is tested 20 times during the bathing season. Campaigning groups such as Surfers Against Sewage have provided additional pressure for improvements in bathing water quality.

WASTE MANAGEMENT AND DISPOSAL

Approximately 330 million tonnes of waste needs disposal in the United Kingdom each year. About a quarter of this is from households and businesses. The bulk comes from sewage works, the construction industry, agriculture and the extractive industries. In England and Wales the Environment Agency operates a permit system for waste disposal, and 163 million tonnes of waste was dealt with in 2006 at facilities operating under the permit system.

Landfill is the commonest means of disposal. Its use is in decline (down 18% between 2001 and 2006), partly due to enormous pressure on landfill capacity. It was estimated in 2006 that there was only seven years of landfill capacity remaining in England and Wales. The problem of capacity is particularly acute in the south of England.

Increasing pressure on landfill sites is a major concern for local authorities and has forced a welcome concentration on waste recycling or, even more desirable, reusing. Landfill sites also produce methane, an important greenhouse gas, but there is increasing interest in harnessing it as an alternative energy source. Greenhouse gas emissions from landfill can be reduced by domestic and municipal composting.

Approximately 10% of waste is incinerated. This proportion remains lower than that of most of Europe but has grown significantly in recent years. Public concern about emissions from incineration plants is frequently expressed during planning consultations. A future trend will be combined heat and power plants that burn waste but use the resulting heat to generate electricity.

The regulatory framework for the disposal of waste has undergone considerable change in response to public concerns about environmental pollution and health. The application of the European Directive on Integrated Pollution Prevention and Control (IPPC) requires operators of new facilities (such as incinerators) to apply for a permit, and the regulator (the Environment Agency in England and Wales) has to engage with statutory consultees (including primary care trusts in England and local health boards in Wales) before reaching a decision. This may involve a health impact assessment.

The European directive takes a 'best available techniques' approach to environmental protection. It also mandates that energy is used efficiently in the process. The Environmental Permitting (England and Wales) Regulations, which came into force in 2008, introduced a simplified system of environmental permits and are designed to achieve the goals of the directive.

SEWAGE TREATMENT

Domestic sewage contains a large number of intestinal organisms and is potentially hazardous to human health. The quantity is roughly equal to the amount of water used. A similar amount of industrial waste, which may contain toxic chemicals, runs into public sewers or directly into rivers, as can agricultural wastewater. From an environmental and public health point of view, therefore, a main concern in the disposal of such waste is to prevent the contamination of the water environment through which drinking water is derived.

Sewage treatment can involve up to three main stages. Primary treatment involves separating the solid from the liquid waste by systems of mechanical grills and settlement channels. This removes large materials such as rags, sanitary products, stones and grit. Sedimentation tanks then typically allow the separation of liquid from solid sewage sludge. Secondary treatment by aerobic action is then applied to the liquid left after sedimentation to turn dissolved organic material into solids, or floc. The solids are removed and the resultant liquid goes on to tertiary treatment, where a variety of approaches are used to disinfect it chemically or biologically (such as with a reedbed) to enable discharge into the sea or watercourse.

There are, however, still places where full treatment does not take place and many where, under some conditions, such as heavy rain, sewage can bypass the treatment system entirely and pollute waterways.

Sewage sludge is a major by-product of the process of sewage treatment, and 1.4 million tonnes is produced every year. The majority is disposed of on farmland, and, following the ending of dumping of sludge at sea in 1998, the next most common disposal method is incineration.

PESTICIDES

The term pesticide encompasses a wide range of substances, such as herbicides, fungicides, insecticides, rodenticides, soil sterilants, wood preservatives and surface biocides. More precise definitions of specific substances and what controls govern their sale, storage and use are contained in United Kingdom and European legislation. Pesticides can enter the human body by inhalation, by ingestion or through the skin. Exposure can be through the environment,

food, water, domestic or garden use and occupation.

An essential step in protecting human health from the risk of pesticides is a formal process of approval that each manufacturer, importer and distributor must go through. Data on the substance must be provided for scrutiny. There is, however, no legal requirement for a farmer, for instance, to tell members of the public what pesticides they are using. Farmers and growers are, however, required by law to take all reasonable precautions to protect human and environmental well-being.

Risk assessment requires the establishment of acceptable daily intakes (ADIs) and maximum residue levels (MRLs) for particular pesticides. The levels of residue both in home-produced and imported food are monitored. In addition, surveys are carried out of residues in humans, wildlife and the environment.

Statutory powers derived from both the United Kingdom and Europe set out the controls that must be applied to protect people, animals and plants from the adverse effect of pesticides, to protect the environment and to make information available to the public.

A number of key bodies assist the government with regulation. The Advisory Committee on Pesticides gives expert advice, undertakes reviews of products and appraises product applications. The Pesticides Safety Directorate is responsible for registering certain categories of agricultural and horticultural pesticide, while the Health and Safety Executive carries out the registration function of non-agricultural pesticides. The Food Standards Agency was established by the government in the year 2000 and has a role in relation to food-related pesticides.

The main interest to public health is the effect of small doses over a long period of time. The health effects of acute exposure and acute poisoning by pesticides are well documented. Illnesses usually follow from either accidental or deliberate ingestion or from skin contamination following careless handling. The symptoms occur shortly afterwards, and there is complete recovery without long-term complications in the majority of cases. The picture for long-term low-dosage exposure is much less clear, and there is a strong feeling that the precautionary principle should apply.

NOISE

Noise is an unwanted sound that causes discomfort to the listener. Sound is a form of energy that is transmitted through the air by rapid cyclic pressure changes. Noise in excess is regarded as a pollutant in the environment. Level, frequency, loudness and time are the four characteristics of sound that are important when assessing noise. Noise may arise from many sources, including sources in the general environment (such as transport traffic or industry), in the neighbourhood (such as domestic noise or human behaviour) or in the workplace.

There is a wide range of literature on the effects of noise on hearing, sleep, communication, work and leisure, as well as on other general physiological and psychological parameters. The evidence is not always convincing, but some studies have found an association between noise and sleep disturbance, poor school performance and hypertension. There is ample evidence of noise causing very high degrees of annoyance to sections of the population.

Workers have a high risk of noise-induced deafness if their environment has noise levels equivalent to a continuous level of 90 dBA or more. However, occupational deafness is the result of fairly lengthy exposure. Permanent deafness may also result from a single, loud explosive sound. Transient deafness (temporary threshold shift) may also be the sequel of exposure to a sudden loud noise or to prolonged intense noise. Employers are required under the Control of Noise at Work Regulations 2005 to take action when noise reaches levels of 80 dBA and to take more stringent action when it reaches 85 dBA.

In England the Environmental Noise (England) Regulations 2006 set out how an approach to environmental noise (also known as ambient noise) is being developed following a European directive. The initial step is noise mapping, and following that action plans are to be developed. Mitigation of road noise can involve interventions such as speed restriction, installation of noise barriers or low-noise road surfacing.

HOUSING

Living accommodation is designed to provide shelter, security, privacy and comfort. Whether it be in the form of a house, a flat, a bed-sitting room, a caravan, a houseboat or a residential institution, all are covered by legislation.

The industrial revolution led to small houses and large tenements crowding the centres of the new towns and cities, in narrow streets with little open space. Those dwellings were poorly ventilated, badly lit and lacking in sanitary facilities, and the practice of burning coal on open fires created a smoke-polluted environment.

The recognition of the association between poor housing and poor health was a main focus of the sanitary reformers of the nineteenth century. In the first half of the twentieth century, with the great improvements in sanitary conditions, emphasis changed to the link between inadequate housing and communicable diseases, particularly tuberculosis. Stress was placed on the need for good ventilation, natural lighting, heating and the eradication of overcrowding. There is general acceptance that these measures contributed to the decline in tuberculosis and other infectious diseases prior to the advent of vaccination and effective therapeutic measures. By the 1950s, the great decline in communicable diseases lessened the emphasis on housing as a factor in ill health.

There has been a paucity of good research into the relationship between housing and health. However, it is now well established that there is a significant association between damp dwellings and respiratory symptoms in children. There is less convincing evidence for this as a cause of an excess of respiratory symptoms in adults or for links between poor housing and other diseases. In studying this problem, it is difficult to eliminate the effect of confounding variables such as social deprivation, which themselves are linked to poor health. However, taken together, evidence shows that the relevance of housing to health is wide-ranging (Table 10.5). The existing evidence points to cold homes being the primary health risk associated directly with the condition of the housing stock, contributing to a proportion of excess winter deaths each year.

Standards for housing are set through local and national legislation and enforced by local authorities. The Housing Health and Safety Rating System (HHSRS) was introduced in England in 2006 and expanded on the previous Housing Fitness Standard by including a wider range of potential hazards to health and well-being. It applies to all residential properties. The most common hazards are fire, falls, cold, lead in water supplies, burns and scalds. Health and social care professionals can inform local authorities of potential hazards that they encounter in the course of their work with vulnerable patients or clients, and the local authority can use its enforcement powers to produce improvement.

The condition of the housing stock in England was ascertained by means of the English House Condition Survey from 2002 until 2008, when it was merged with another housing survey to form the English Housing Survey. The 2006 English House Condition Survey reported that some 8.1 million homes (36.8%) did not meet the 'decent' homes standard. It was in the private rented sector that the level of non-decent homes was highest. Problems associated with cold and falls were the most common.

When allocating social housing, all housing authorities are required by law to give 'reasonable preference' to people with a medical need for settled accommodation or to people currently living in unsanitary, overcrowded or unsatisfactory housing.

Table 10.5 Health manifestations of poor housing

Feature of housing	Example of health effect
Homelessness (including temporary accommodation)	Increased risk of mental illness, alcohol and drug problems, tuberculosis
Quality of housing	
• Damp	
• Cold	
• Lacking amenities	
• Infestation	Asthma, bronchitis, hypothermia, fires, falls, stress, loss of sleep
• Overcrowding	
• Design	
• Noise insulation	
• Air quality	
Urban environment	
• High-rise	
• Access to services	Road traffic accidents, social isolation, violence, stress, poor access to health services
• Transport	
• Recreation	
• Fear of crime	

Source: The Health of Londoners. London: King's Fund Publishing; 1998.

Authorities have different methods of assessing medical priority, but most make decisions on the advice of independent medical experts. The usual system of allocation is a points-based system in which 'housing points' are awarded on the basis of a variety of categories of need.

HOMELESSNESS AND ROUGH SLEEPING

It is estimated by the United Nations that over one billion people are inadequately housed and that approximately 100 million people worldwide are without a place to live. The causes of homelessness can be many and varied; they include conflict and natural disaster, family breakdown and economic failure. Being homeless is about more than simply not having a roof over one's head. The term 'rough sleeping' is often used to describe being at the worst end of the spectrum, where people have to sleep out of doors on a regular basis.

The legal definition of homelessness varies within the United Kingdom but is broadly defined in legislation as having no right to occupy a property as an owner or a tenant or having accommodation not reasonable to continue to occupy. People in temporary accommodation such as a hostel would be classified as homeless although they are not literally out on the streets, as are rough sleepers.

The population of rough sleepers in the United Kingdom can be broadly characterised as being 90% male, 50% alcohol reliant, around 70% misusing drugs and between 30–50% having mental health problems. Between one-quarter and one-third will have been in local authority care as a child or young person. Apart from mental health and addiction problems, rough sleepers are also likely to have a higher incidence of tuberculosis and hepatitis than the general population and to have feet and hands in a poor condition.

Numbers of homeless people and rough sleepers have fallen substantially in recent years. In 2007 the estimated number of rough sleepers on any one night in England was 498; this is a reduction from the 1998 baseline figure of 1850. The public health challenge is to provide rough sleepers and those who are homeless and in temporary accommodation with ready access to health services to protect their physical and mental condition.

ATMOSPHERIC POLLUTION AND AIR QUALITY

In the eighteenth and nineteenth centuries, the industrial revolution brought increasing problems of atmospheric pollution from the chimneys of factories and houses in the new industrial towns. Legislation to control pollution at that time was directed mainly at industry. The zeal of the sanitary reformers more than 150 years ago in achieving safe drinking water and proper disposal of sewage was not matched by an attack on the other environmental evil, air pollution, which had effectively turned the atmosphere over the large towns into a cloud of smoke. Over the years, the public showed little interest. Indeed, a major contributor to air pollution, the domestic open coal fire, was stoutly defended.

A dramatic turning point in attitudes to atmospheric pollution occurred in December 1952. A London 'smog' (the word 'smog' was coined by a public health doctor in the early years of the twentieth century to describe fog filled with smoke) coincided with a steep rise in the number of deaths. Although excess deaths had been noted in other smog episodes, nothing quite as striking had occurred before. More than 4000 excess deaths were estimated to have occurred over the four days of the smog. The matter received wide media coverage, and a curious occurrence made the story even more sensational. A number of prime young cattle at a show in London also succumbed to the effects of pollution.

LEGISLATION

The results of the events in the early 1950s in London led to the first Clean Air Act of 1956 and to subsequent legislation. This set a framework for action and was enhanced by other factors, such as the trend towards the use of gas and electricity for domestic and central heating and the switch in the 1960s to natural gas, which is smoke-free and virtually sulphur-free.

A major feature of the legislation was to create smoke-control areas. In general, it is an offence to emit smoke from a chimney in these areas. They are not 'smokeless zones', because controlled amounts of smoke from specific buildings are permitted (as the result of lighting-up a furnace, for example). The main thrust of the scheme was to reduce smoke from the domestic fire, which had been identified as contributing to 80% of pollution. Householders were provided with grants for conversion to smokeless fuel.

The result was a dramatic improvement. The average visibility on a winter's day in London increased from one to four miles. The concept in the legislation has been adopted by other countries and has been reinforced by air-quality standards in European Commission directives. By 1980 the perceived success of the reduction of atmospheric pollution led to the demise of the very bodies that helped to solve the problem: the Clean Air Council and the Medical Research Council's Air Pollution Unit. Furthermore, much of the monitoring network for air quality was dismantled. The network has expanded again in recent years. The consequence of these measures has been that the high quality research into the effects of atmospheric pollution, which started at the time of the London smog, ceased in the 1980s in Britain and began again only in the early 1990s.

The smog attributed to coal fires has been replaced in recent decades by photochemical smog, which is due to the effect of sunlight on the complex mix of chemicals emitted into the air above modern cities. It is more likely to be present in cities situated in a natural bowl with a large number of motor vehicles and a dry, sunny climate. Los Angeles, Mexico City and Tehran are some of the cities affected. In Beijing special temporary measures were put in place to avoid athletes participating in the 2008 Olympic Games being affected by the smog that frequently hangs over the city.

TYPES OF POLLUTANTS

The 2007 version of the United Kingdom National Air Quality Strategy aims to ensure that polluting emissions and ambient air quality do not harm human health and the environment. It does so by setting standards (taking account of European Commission directives), conducting extensively monitoring and implementing measures. Eight pollutants in particular are targeted in the strategy. These are briefly described in this section.

Sulphur Dioxide

In Britain almost 70% of emissions of sulphur dioxide are from fossil-fuelled power stations, and a substantial proportion also comes from industry. In Northern Ireland the domestic use of coal is a significant factor. Reductions were achieved during the 1980s and early 1990s by reducing emissions arising from electricity generation. Further reductions depend on tight monitoring against standards and a particular focus on replacement of older power stations. The major problem sulphur dioxide causes is constriction of the airways, particularly in those with pre-existing lung disease such as asthma. Sulphur dioxide has effects on human health shortly after exposure, so standards for outdoor levels are set at 15-minute, one-hour and 24-hour limits not to be exceeded a certain number of times per year.

Lead

Lead is a particularly dangerous heavy metal. During the 1980s, concern was expressed that the average blood-lead concentration of the population was high. A major contributor to lead in the atmosphere was the petrol engine. As a result, measures were taken to introduce unleaded petrol, and this was combined with tax incentives. The use of leaded petrol declined rapidly and is now available on a very limited basis. The introduction of unleaded petrol has made possible the use of catalytic converters, which remove a large part of the nitrogen oxides and volatile organic compounds from vehicle exhausts. Catalytic converters have been standard on all cars sold in the United Kingdom since 1993.

Certain industrial processes, smelting in particular, also emit lead into the air. These remain a problem in some areas. The adverse health effects of lead include impaired brain development in children, abnormal synthesis of haemoglobin and effects on certain other organs and systems (including the kidneys and the reproductive system).

Nitrogen Oxides and Ozone

Whereas sulphur dioxide gas is only produced when sulphur is present in the fuel being burned, oxides of nitrogen are formed when any material is burned. The main sources of oxides of nitrogen are power stations, large industrial plants and, in particular, motor vehicles, which contribute 80% of the nitrogen dioxide in urban environments. During the latter part of the 1980s, levels of nitrogen oxides were increasing with growing vehicle emissions, especially in urban centres. This is now being tackled in Europe through vehicle emission standards.

Ozone is formed by the action of sunlight on nitrogen oxides and occurs in increased concentrations when hydrocarbons are present. Levels tend to be highest in southern Britain, and recent research has shown that there are significant effects on health. Because the formation of ozone through the photochemical chain reaction may take place thousands of kilometres from where some of the air pollutants were emitted, the ozone problem needs to be tackled on an international basis.

Nitrogen oxides and sulphur dioxide contribute to the formation of acid rain. The gases that are involved can be carried long distances by the wind and can cross national boundaries to affect neighbouring countries. Consequently, acidic air pollution can have a widespread effect on buildings, fish, wildlife and vegetation.

Particulates

Particulate studies in the United Kingdom, the United States and Europe have shown that particulate air pollution, in particular small particles, is still an important cause of damage to health. They are thought to be causally associated with both respiratory and cardiovascular disease. Particulate matter

(PM) is categorised on the basis of the size of the particulates. For example, PM2.5 consists of particulates less than 2.5 micrometers in diameter. It is believed that smaller particles are the most detrimental to health. Motor vehicles are major sources in urban areas, with particulates being formed from a variety of sources, including engine emissions, brake pads and tyre wear.

Standards defined in term of the mass of particles per volume of air have been introduced. Extensive monitoring of such particle concentrations is now undertaken in the United Kingdom and other developed countries.

Other Pollutants

Emissions of carbon monoxide, which is produced by incomplete combustion of fuel, have increased in the same way and for the same reasons as the oxides of nitrogen. In Britain 85% of carbon monoxide emissions come from car exhausts. The application of European Commission standards should reduce this.

Ammonia, which is mainly derived from agricultural activities, can lead to serious changes in ecosystems and act as a precursor to the formation of particulate matter.

Carcinogenic air pollutants, including benzene, 1,3-butadiene and polycyclic aromatic hydrocarbons, are produced by vehicles and other fuel-burning processes. All three groups of pollutants are carcinogenic, and benzene and 1,3-butadiene have been shown to produce leukaemia. No safe levels can be specified.

In the United Kingdom the National Air Quality Strategy has set standards for these pollutants, and, in addition, European Commission standards are in place. An evaluation of the United Kingdom's performance in reducing air pollution was published in 2005. It concluded that in the period 1990 to 2001 there had been major improvements in air quality, and it drew particular attention to the contribution made by the mandatory fitting of catalytic converters to motor vehicles and also by a shift of electricity production to gas-powered generation. It also concluded that the cost/benefit ratio of these changes was 1:24.

LOCAL AIR QUALITY MANAGEMENT

Local authorities across the United Kingdom have a particular role in monitoring air pollution and acting in order to achieve reductions. The Environment Act 1995 (and the Environment (Northern Ireland) Order 2002) introduced the system of local air quality management, which compelled local authorities to monitor and act in respect of air pollution. Parts of local authority areas that were judged to be particularly polluted had to be designated as air quality management areas (AQMAs), and action plans to reduce pollution were introduced. By 2007 over 200 local authorities in the United Kingdom had designated the whole or parts of their districts in this way. Road-based emissions, nitrogen dioxide and PM10 in particular have been responsible for the majority of those designations.

INDOOR AIR QUALITY

The population spends, on average, 90% of their time indoors, and of that time 70%

is in their own homes. Thus air is breathed primarily in a closed environment, and increasing attention is being paid to this microclimate. Indoor pollution can arise from the activities of individuals (such as cigarette smoking), from combustion of fossil fuels, from the growth of moulds in damp conditions, from materials of which the building is constructed and through emissions from the ground, such as radon, a naturally occurring radioactive gas. The increasingly recognised dangers from radon are discussed in the section on radiation.

Production of carbon monoxide can result from improper installation and maintenance of gas or solid fuel fires where there is an inadequate supply of air. Lethal concentrations are responsible for more than 50 deaths every year in England and Wales. Headaches, tiredness, difficulty in thinking clearly and feeling sick are common symptoms of chronic carbon monoxide poisoning.

Smoking tobacco can give rise to a variety of pollutants in the indoor climate. Children living with people who smoke indoors experience an increased incidence of respiratory illness, and non-smokers in such households experience an increased incidence of lung cancer. It is estimated that several hundred lung cancer deaths a year in Britain can be attributed to passive smoking. In addition, smoking enhances the risk posed by radon, which is estimated to be 10 times greater for the smoker than for the non-smoker. Almost half of the children in the United Kingdom are exposed to tobacco smoke in the home environment. The legislation to introduce smoke-free enclosed public places and working places introduced in different parts of the United Kingdom during 2007 has had a major impact on passive exposure to cigarette smoke.

A wide variety of chemicals are found in modern building materials and household fittings. The presence of organic volatile chemicals in the air in buildings, particularly if new or recently renovated, is associated with sickness in the occupants.

Reports of a higher incidence of symptoms amongst people who work in certain buildings have given rise to the label 'sick building syndrome'. The type of symptoms reported are eye problems, headaches, respiratory tract infections and sore throats. A variety of causes have been suggested, including poor air quality and the design of buildings. Research is continuing but has not yet established a specific link between any of the suggested causative factors and illness. However, improved ventilation seems to be helpful in reducing symptoms.

TRANSPORT

The transport system is responsible for major adverse impacts on health. Road traffic contributes to congestion, accidents, air pollution and noise. Major roads can cause divisions and exclusion in communities, while planning decisions can mean that services, including health services, are sited so that access for some people is difficult and car use is increased for others. The structure of transport systems can also make it difficult to choose healthy forms of transport; for example, fear of accidents and crime means that far fewer children walk or cycle to school than a generation ago. In Britain in 2006, just over half (52%) of trips to school by children aged 5 to 10 were made on foot and 41% were made by car.

While some of these problems can be tackled through 'technical fixes' such as catalytic converters or more fuel-efficient vehicles, it is obvious that in order to maximise benefits to health, transport systems need to be viewed as a whole so that integrated and sustainable improvements can be made (Table 10.6). The concept of 'active travel' recognises the potential contribution of personal movement to the reduction of obesity and is an important area for joint working between public health experts and transport planners.

RADIATION

In this area, concern and attention in environmental and public health has centred primarily on ionising radiation, though reference will be made later to non-ionising radiation, the effects of which are the subject of increasing media scrutiny.

Most elements have stable forms. However, some natural elements such as radium and uranium have no stable form and are said to be *radioactive*, emitting radiation from their nuclei in moving towards a more stable configuration. Radioactive forms of stable elements can be produced artificially – for example, by bombardment with neutrons (widely used in medicine and industry).

Three principal types of radiation are emitted:

1 *alpha particles* – these particles are essentially identical to the helium nucleus, comprising two protons and two neutrons and consequently having a double positive charge and relatively large mass

2 *beta particles* – these are identical to electrons but are emitted from the nucleus after the internal transformation of a neutron into a proton and an electron

3 *gamma rays* – like X-rays, these are electromagnetic radiation and similar to light, but they are of much higher frequency. They may be regarded as quanta (or packets) of photons usually emitted during de-excitation of the nucleus – commonly after emission of a beta particle.

In passing through matter, including tissue, each form of radiation loses energy by ionisation, removing electrons from the orbital shells of atoms or molecules in the matter and leaving behind ions or free radicals as chemically active species.

However, the alpha particle by its nature is densely ionising, depositing more energy per unit track length, having a high linear energy transfer (LET). Consequently, alpha particles have a relatively short range and greater propensity within the body for damaging cells. In contrast to alpha particles, which outside of the body are completely absorbed by a thin sheet of paper or the dead layers of skin, beta and gamma radiation have a lower LET and are more penetrating. Up to 1 cm of aluminium is required to absorb beta radiation and about 4 cm of lead to reduce the gamma ray intensity from, for example, a radium source by a factor of 10. Clearly, beta and gamma radiation can pose a potential risk outside of, as well as inside of, the body.

Table 10.6 Some important elements of healthier policies on transport

- Reducing reliance on motorised transport
- Better coordination and integration of health, environment and transport at national and local level
- Enabling and encouraging forms of transport which support physical activity (e.g., walking and cycling)
- Increasing access to good public transport
- Targeting the reduction of health risks of transport on the most vulnerable (e.g., children, the elderly, the socially excluded)
- Reducing air pollution and noise arising from transport
- Minimising risks arising from transport pollutants and sources of injury

CONCEPTS OF RADIATION DOSE TO INDIVIDUALS AND POPULATIONS

The absorbed dose corresponds to the energy deposited per unit mass. Its unit is the gray (symbol Gy), named after a British scientist, which is equivalent to1 joule per kilogram.

As might be expected, because of its high LET, 1 Gy of alpha radiation in tissue will cause more harm than 1 Gy of beta or gamma radiation. To provide a common measurement of potential harmfulness, the equivalent dose is used which is equal to the absorbed dose multiplied by a factor to take account of the LET for that type of radiation. The unit of equivalent dose is called the sievert (symbol Sv), named after a Swedish scientist. For beta and gamma radiation, the factor is 1, so the absorbed dose and equivalent dose are numerically identical. In the case of alpha particles emitted within the body from inhaled or ingested material, the factor is 20, and an absorbed dose of 1 Gy corresponds to an equivalent dose of 20 Sv.

It is necessary to recognise that the susceptibility of different tissues to the induction of malignancy is not the same. For example, the risk of fatal malignancy per Sv is greater for the lungs than for the thyroid. To take account of these differences and the risk of serious hereditary effects, the equivalent dose is multiplied by a risk-weighting factor for the different tissues, which can then be summed to give the effective dose (commonly abbreviated to 'dose'). A benefit of using the effective dose measure is that the risk to health for non-uniform distribution of equivalent dose in the body can be broadly expressed as a single number. For illustration, as will be seen shortly, the average annual effective dose from natural background radiation to inhabitants of the United Kingdom is 2200 microsieverts.

As the sievert is a relatively large dose of radiation, submultiples are commonly used. The microsievert is one-millionth of a sievert, and the millisievert is one-thousandth of a sievert. The gray and sievert are standard international (SI) units; earlier literature used the previous terminology of the rad (100 rad = 1 gray) for absorbed dose and the rem (100 rem = 1 sievert) for the equivalent dose.

Although radiation doses to individuals are generally of greatest interest, it is sometimes appropriate to have a measure of the total dose from a particular source to groups of people or a whole population. This total dose is expressed as the collective effective dose (commonly abbreviated to 'collective dose'). By analogy with man-hours, the collective dose is expressed in man sieverts (symbol manSv) and is obtained by summing the average effective dose to each group multiplied by the number of people in that group.

As the population of the United Kingdom is about 56 million, the collective dose for the population is the product of this number and the average annual effective dose: that is, about 124 000 manSv. However, it is important to recognise that although the collective dose would be the same for a population half this size and receiving twice the average dose, the personal risk to these individuals would obviously be doubled.

EFFECTS OF IONISING RADIATION ON HEALTH

Soon after the discovery of X-rays by Röntgen in 1895 and of radioactivity by Becquerel in the following year, the harmful effects of radiation were noticed. The effects are dependent on the dose, dose rate and tissues exposed, as summarised in Table 10.7.

Early Effects

Early effects are associated with exposure to high dose and dose rates. At the extreme, an absorbed dose of 5 Gy or more to the whole body delivered almost instantaneously is liable to be fatal because of acute damage to the gastrointestinal, erythropoietic and central nervous systems. Brief exposure of a limited area of the body to a very large dose may be sub-lethal, but some early effects may be generated. Whole-body doses of about 1 to 3 Gy may create the symptoms of acute radiation sickness, including vomiting, diarrhoea and epilation, but with a substantial probability of survival. Exposure of the skin to an almost instantaneous absorbed dose of 5 Gy would probably produce erythema within about a week, and more serious damage would result with higher doses. Such doses to the testes or ovaries would be liable to cause sterility.

With whole-body doses rather less than 1 Gy or larger total doses received more protractedly, no early signs of injury may be apparent but results may be manifested much later as malignancy or hereditary effects in offspring.

Late Effects

The two most important late effects of radiation are the induction of malignant disease and hereditary effects. In studies of groups of people exposed to ionising radiation, such as the Japanese survivors of atomic bombing, a greater incidence of various malignant disease was recorded in those exposed to relatively high doses of radiation some years previously. From these data, risk factors have been derived by the United Nations Scientific Committee on the Effects of Atomic Radiation (UNSCEAR) and the International Commission on Radiological Protection (ICRP) relating the excess of fatal cancers to the radiation dose received. Importantly, it is further assumed that there is no threshold below which fatal cancer

Table 10.7 Principal harmful radiation effects: conditions for occurrence and sources of information

Health consequences	Circumstances of exposure	Sources of information
Early effects		
Death	High dose and dose-rate:	Human data from various sources
Erythema	• to much of the body	
Sterility	• to area of skin	
	• to testes and ovaries	
Late effects		
Various cancers	Any dose or dose-rate	Risk factors for human beings estimated from high doses and dose-rates in human health studies
	Risk depends on dose	
	Appear years later	
Hereditary defects	Any dose or dose-rate	Risk factors for human beings inferred from animal data and the absence of human evidence
	Risk depends on dose	
	Appear in offspring	
Functional damage to organs and tissues	High dose at any rate	Human data from various sources
	Various times to appear	
Learning disability	Dose in the womb	Limited human data
	Appears in the child	

Source: National Radiological Protection Board. *Living with Radiation.* Didcot: NRPB; 1998.

might not be induced by radiation. The number of cancers increase with increasing radiation dose.

Clearly these risk factors are based on relatively high doses received in a short period of time. In the normal course of events, relatively small doses are received over longer periods. It would seem reasonable to expect reduced risks in the latter circumstances, and indeed there is substantial evidence, at least for beta, X and gamma radiation, that the risk is less at low doses and low dose rates. The risk factors, recently revised by ICRP, are expressed as a mathematical probability – for example, 1 in 20 per Sv (or $5' 10-2$ Sv–1) – and incorporate a dose and dose-rate effectiveness factor of 2 to make some allowance for this low dose rate effect.

Similar considerations apply to hereditary effects. However, in human offspring there has been no conclusive evidence for hereditary defects attributable to exposure from natural or artificial radiation. The Japanese data failed to show statistically significant increases in hereditary defects, but these negative findings, representing an upper estimate, were used together with animal data by ICRP to estimate a risk factor for serious hereditary damage in humans.

When all generations subsequent to a radiation exposure are taken into account, the value of the risk factor for severe hereditary effects is about 1 in 100 per Sv (or 1′ 10–2 Sv–1).

To maintain proper perspectives, it is important to recognise corollaries arising from the basic assumption of a proportional relationship between dose and risk, without a threshold. It implies that exposure to any dose of radiation, no matter how small, carries some risk. Consequently, even the smallest additional risks to a population will inevitably lead to a prediction of some associated deaths or hereditary effects, which can be alarming. For example, a very small increase (of 20 microsieverts – about 1% of the average annual dose from natural background radiation) in the average dose to a population would give a calculated additional risk of only one in a million, but for the United Kingdom (population of 56 million) would lead to a prediction of 56 attributable cancer deaths. In other European countries (population 650 million), this would be 650 attributable cancer deaths. It is sometimes necessary to remember that even for a fatal risk of one in 10 000, there is a probability of 99.99% that death will occur from some other cause (Table 10.8).

RADIATION DOSES TO THE GENERAL PUBLIC IN PERSPECTIVE

The principal sources of radiation exposure to the general public include natural background radiation, medical exposures and discharges from the nuclear industry.

Natural background radiation arises from extraterrestrial cosmic rays and through naturally radioactive elements in the earth's crust, notably uranium, thorium and potassium-40. Uranium occurs in soil and rock in concentrations varying from a few parts per million (ppm) to more than 1000 ppm. Uranium-238 is the parent of a long chain of radioactive daughters. The decay products include the alpha-emitting radioactive gas radon (radon-222), some of which escapes to the atmosphere, continuing to decay to radioactive daughters such as polonium-210, which is another natural alpha-emitting element that has a radio toxicity similar to that of plutonium-239. Thorium is similarly distributed in the earth, and radon-220 (called thoron) is akin to radon-222, being a daughter product of thorium-232. Potassium comprises 2.4% by weight of the earth's crust, and naturally radioactive potassium-40 in turn constitutes 120 ppm of the stable element. Consequently, the public is exposed to *external radiation* from cosmic rays and gamma rays from radioactivity in the earth and to *internal radiation* through inhalation of radon and thoron and their daughter products and also through ingestion of foodstuffs and water incorporating natural radioactivity.

The primary source of medical exposures for the public as a whole is through diagnostic X-ray examinations, being much more common than radiotherapy procedures and outweighing the greater individual dose of the latter.

Figure 10.3, published by the former National Radiological Protection Board (NRPB), shows that for the general public, about 85% of the annual radiation dose is attributable to natural sources (primarily radon and its daughter products), about 14%

Table 10.8 Average annual risk of death in the UK from some common causes

Smoking 10 cigarettes a day	5.0×10^{-3}	1 in 200
Heart disease	3.3×10^{-3}	1 in 300
All cancers	2.5×10^{-3}	1 in 400
All causes, 40 years old	1.4×10^{-3}	1 in 700
All radiation (2.6 mSvy^{-1})	1.3×10^{-4}	1 in 7700
Accident in the home	6.9×10^{-5}	1 in 15 000
Accident on the road	5.9×10^{-5}	1 in 17 000
Homicide	1.0×10^{-5}	1 in 100 000
Nuclear discharges (0.14 mSvy^{-1})	7.0×10^{-6}	1 in 140 000
Pregnancy, for mother	6.0×10^{-6}	1 in 170 000

Source: National Radiological Protection Board. *Living with Radiation.* Didcot: NRPB; 1998.

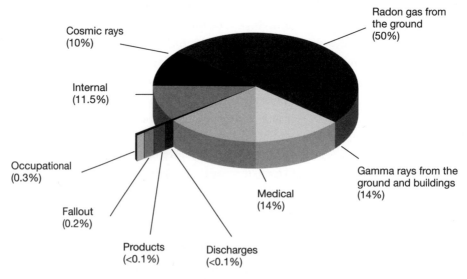

Figure 10.3 Annual radiation doses to the United Kingdom population
Source: National Radiological Protection Board. *Living with Radiation.* Didcot: NRPB; 1998.

is due to medical exposures and less than 0.1% is associated with nuclear discharges. This situation is clearly at variance with public perception. Expressed differently, the average annual dose due to natural background sources is about 2210 units (a unit being one microsievert), the corresponding dose from medical exposures is about 370 units and that from nuclear-waste discharges less than 1 unit, giving a total of some 2581 units.

NON-IONISING RADIATION

Non-ionising radiation is radiation that does not produce ionisation in matter. Non-ionising radiation is broadly of two types: optical (ultraviolet, visible and infrared) and electromagnetic fields (EMF) (microwave, radio frequency and extremely low frequency). Radiations are described in terms of their wavelengths or frequency. For convenience, optical and microwave radiations can be considered as packets of energy (photons) travelling through space. Radio frequency and extremely low-frequency fields can be considered as time-varying electric and magnetic fields moving through space in wave-like patterns. Optical sources of radiation include solar radiation (UV), infrared radiation and lasers. Electromagnetic fields are produced by electrical power-lines and by electrical appliances at home and at work.

Harmful Effects

The harmful effects of non-ionising radiations are of three main types: photochemical, thermal and electrical effects. Photochemical effects result from chemical reactions in the body initiated by the absorption of photons and can be produced by radiations with shortwave lengths, such as solar ultraviolet radiation. However, optical radiation does not penetrate far into human tissue, so the eyes and skin are the organs most at risk.

Examples of adverse photochemical effects are ultraviolet-induced sunburn and snow blindness. There is good evidence that ultraviolet radiation especially can cause non-malignant skin cancer. Cutaneous malignant melanoma is much less common but of considerable public health concern because of its serious nature and its rapid increase during the last few decades. Although direct evidence of a link with ultraviolet radiation is absent, there is epidemiological evidence that short-term intermittent exposure to high levels of solar ultraviolet radiation, especially at an early age, may be a contributory factor in the causation of cutaneous malignant melanoma.

The longer wavelengths in infrared and microwave regions of the non-ionising spectrum do not have enough energy to initiate photochemical reactions but can produce thermal injury resulting from the disruption of the molecular bonds of proteins and enzymes. Intense sources of optical and infrared radiations, such as lasers, can cause thermal burning. The lens of the eye lacks a direct blood supply and is therefore more susceptible to injury from heat. Hence infrared and microwave radiation may increase the risk of cataracts.

At even longer wavelengths (which includes the electric mains), electromagnetic fields can induce electric charge on the surface of the body and electric current within the body, which can occasionally stimulate nerves. Direct contact with electric current will also lead to shock and burns. These immediate effects of human exposure to electromagnetic fields are well understood and restrictions are in place to avoid them.

There has for some time been much speculation about the possible delayed effects of electromagnetic fields on the body – in particular the risk of contracting cancer. Mobile telephones and their base stations have been a particular subject of concern. Epidemiological studies of occupational and population exposures to various electrical and magnetic sources have not so far led to international consensus that there is consistent and persuasive evidence that EMF influence any of the stages of cancer development.

HEALTH RISKS, COMMUNICATION AND PUBLIC UNDERSTANDING

The last decade of the twentieth century saw a major growth in public concern about potential health hazards. This was reflected in widespread media coverage of scientific reports, government actions and human-interest stories that appeared to suggest that a particular environmental or dietary agent carried a risk to human health. In Britain the bovine spongiform encephalopathy (BSE) epidemic in cattle, the use of genetically modified crops and mobile telephones are all examples of issues that became the subject of media attention.

Certain issues where a risk is claimed to exist are more likely to frighten people than others (Table 10.9). While understanding what underlies the public perception of risk is important, the greatest difficulty for public health policy-makers relates to deciding how a risk is assessed, when an intervention to reduce it should be taken and what should be communicated to the public.

The most difficult areas to address are those in which an association is found (or claimed) between a risk factor and an adverse health outcome yet it is not clear whether that association is causal. The question of establishing causality is a constantly recurring theme in this field of public health. Examples of issues that can be portrayed by the media as established 'cause and effect' include a cluster of cases of childhood cancer around an industrial plant, people who take their stories to a tabloid newspaper with a claim that their illness is a result of exposure to a particular environmental hazard and people who believe they are at risk from industrial pollutants. The association may or may not be causal, or the evidence may not be available to prove the case one way or the other. Yet the public will usually expect an immediate response from the scientific community, the government and the public health authorities. There are no easy answers to these questions.

As a first step, a high-quality assessment of the scientific evidence is essential, sometimes coupled with a research investigation. At some point a decision will have to be taken about whether it is appropriate to make an intervention to reduce the risk and what the nature of that intervention should be (for example, legislation, providing public information or advice, altering a manufacturing or production process) (Table 10.10). Although it might be supposed that all the scientific evidence should be to hand before any intervention is contemplated, in practice public concern or media pressure may be so great that early action has to be considered.

This particular aspect of risk – when and how to intervene – became the focus of a great deal of debate in the 1990s in Britain as a result of the BSE crisis. The concept of the 'precautionary principle' has emerged. This has been defined in various ways but essentially is a judgement that must be applied in situations of scientific uncertainty where

Table 10.9 Fright factors

Risks are generally more worrying (and less acceptable) if perceived:
1   To be involuntary (e.g., exposure to pollution) rather than voluntary (e.g., dangerous sports or smoking)
2   As inequitably distributed (some benefit while others suffer the consequences)
3   As inescapable by taking personal precautions
4   To arise from an unfamiliar or novel source
5   To result from man-made, rather than natural sources
6   To cause hidden and irreversible damage; e.g., through onset of illness many years after exposure
7   To pose some particular danger to small children or pregnant women or more generally to future generations
8   To threaten a form of death (or illness/injury) arousing particular dread
9   To damage identifiable rather than anonymous victims
10 To be poorly understood by science
11 As subject to contradictory statements from responsible sources (or, even worse, from the same source)

Source: *Communicating about Risks to Public Health: pointers to good practice.* London: Department of Health; 1997.

Table 10.10 Determining public health policy in relation to a risk

- Assess the risk using the best scientific evidence
- Decide on whether an intervention should be made to reduce the risk
- Choose an appropriate intervention
- Communicate to those exposed to the risk or who perceive there is a risk
- Implement the intervention successfully or (if no intervention is taken) continue to research or monitor

the postulated risk is serious and where action is being contemplated before the results of further research or investigation is to hand. Thus the precautionary principle holds that action to protect the public health should be taken to reduce or control the risk 'in the meantime'.

In the whole area of health and risk, it is essential that there is as much openness and transparency about the issues and the scientific evidence as possible. The guiding principles must be based not only on a rigorous approach to evaluating the risk but also on sharing information with the public (Table 10.11). Without this there will be a breakdown of trust and the value of public health advice will be weakened.

CONCLUSIONS

The importance of the relationship between the quality of the physical environment and people's health has long been recognised. Moreover, in recent years the emergence of consensus about the nature and causation of global warming has heightened the public health engagement in issues to do with the natural and man-made environment. There have been a number of major incidents around the world that have all too dramatically highlighted some of the contemporary threats and hazards both to the well-being of individuals and to the planet itself. The current growth of interest in, and rapidly rising concerns about, wider environmental issues and health are evolving rapidly to the point where the subjects become inextricably linked. One of the important roles of public health will be to engage with environmental issues and campaigns in order to promote this wider view of health, as well as establishing measures to protect populations from the adverse impact of specific environmental hazards.

Table 10.11 Guiding principles

- High quality assessment of science
- Full risk/benefit assessment
- Consistency of approach across risk areas
- Clear framework of interventions
- Approach should have integrity if judged in retrospect
- Protect the vulnerable
- Realistic sharing of uncertainty
- Information should provide insight
- Greater public participation in risk deliberations

Source: *Saving Lives: our healthier nation.* (Cm 4386). London: The Stationery Office; 1999.

Index

Entries in **bold** denote tables, figures or boxes.